The National A
SCIENCES • ENGINE

The Future of Nursing 2020–2030

Charting a Path to Achieve Health Equity

Mary K. Wakefield, David R. Williams, Suzanne Le Menestrel, and Jennifer Lalitha Flaubert, *Editors*

Committee on the Future of Nursing 2020–2030

NATIONAL ACADEMY OF MEDICINE

THE NATIONAL ACADEMIES PRESS
Washington, DC
www.nap.edu

THE NATIONAL ACADEMIES PRESS 500 Fifth Street, NW Washington, DC 20001

This activity was supported by a contract between the National Academy of Sciences and the Robert Wood Johnson Foundation (Grant Number 76081). Any opinions, findings, conclusions, or recommendations expressed in this publication do not necessarily reflect the views of any organization or agency that provided support for the project.

International Standard Book Number-13: 978-0-309-68506-1
International Standard Book Number-10: 0-309-68506-0
Digital Object Identifier: https://doi.org/10.17226/25982
Library of Congress Control Number: 2021938440

Additional copies of this publication are available from the National Academies Press, 500 Fifth Street, NW, Keck 360, Washington, DC 20001; (800) 624-6242 or (202) 334-3313; http://www.nap.edu.

Printed in the United States of America

Suggested citation: National Academies of Sciences, Engineering, and Medicine. 2021. *The future of nursing 2020–2030: Charting a path to achieve health equity.* Washington, DC: The National Academies Press. https://doi.org/10.17226/25982.

The National Academies of

SCIENCES • ENGINEERING • MEDICINE

The **National Academy of Sciences** was established in 1863 by an Act of Congress, signed by President Lincoln, as a private, nongovernmental institution to advise the nation on issues related to science and technology. Members are elected by their peers for outstanding contributions to research. Dr. Marcia McNutt is president.

The **National Academy of Engineering** was established in 1964 under the charter of the National Academy of Sciences to bring the practices of engineering to advising the nation. Members are elected by their peers for extraordinary contributions to engineering. Dr. John L. Anderson is president.

The **National Academy of Medicine** (formerly the Institute of Medicine) was established in 1970 under the charter of the National Academy of Sciences to advise the nation on medical and health issues. Members are elected by their peers for distinguished contributions to medicine and health. Dr. Victor J. Dzau is president.

The three Academies work together as the **National Academies of Sciences, Engineering, and Medicine** to provide independent, objective analysis and advice to the nation and conduct other activities to solve complex problems and inform public policy decisions. The National Academies also encourage education and research, recognize outstanding contributions to knowledge, and increase public understanding in matters of science, engineering, and medicine.

Learn more about the National Academies of Sciences, Engineering, and Medicine at **www.nationalacademies.org**.

The National Academies of
SCIENCES • ENGINEERING • MEDICINE

Consensus Study Reports published by the National Academies of Sciences, Engineering, and Medicine document the evidence-based consensus on the study's statement of task by an authoring committee of experts. Reports typically include findings, conclusions, and recommendations based on information gathered by the committee and the committee's deliberations. Each report has been subjected to a rigorous and independent peer-review process and it represents the position of the National Academies on the statement of task.

Proceedings published by the National Academies of Sciences, Engineering, and Medicine chronicle the presentations and discussions at a workshop, symposium, or other event convened by the National Academies. The statements and opinions contained in proceedings are those of the participants and are not endorsed by other participants, the planning committee, or the National Academies.

For information about other products and activities of the National Academies, please visit www.nationalacademies.org/about/whatwedo.

COMMITTEE ON THE FUTURE OF NURSING 2020–2030

MARY K. WAKEFIELD (*Co-Chair*), Visiting Professor, The University of Texas at Austin

DAVID R. WILLIAMS (*Co-Chair*), Florence and Laura Norman Professor of Public Health and Chair, Department of Social and Behavioral Sciences, T.H. Chan School of Public Health, and Professor, Department of African and African American Studies, Harvard University

MAUREEN BISOGNANO, President Emerita and Senior Fellow, Institute for Healthcare Improvement

JEFFREY BRENNER, Co-Founder and Chief Medical Officer, JunaCare

PETER I. BUERHAUS, Professor of Nursing, College of Nursing, and Director, Center for Interdisciplinary Health Workforce Studies, Montana State University

MARSHALL H. CHIN, Richard Parrillo Family Professor of Healthcare Ethics, Department of Medicine, University of Chicago

REGINA S. CUNNINGHAM, Chief Executive Officer, Hospital of the University of Pennsylvania; Adjunct Professor and Assistant Dean, School of Nursing, University of Pennsylvania

JOSÉ J. ESCARCE, Distinguished Professor of Medicine, David Geffen School of Medicine, and Distinguished Professor of Health Policy and Management, Fielding School of Public Health, University of California, Los Angeles

GREER GLAZER, Schmidlapp Professor of Nursing and Dean, College of Nursing, University of Cincinnati

MARCUS HENDERSON, Charge Nurse, Adolescent Services, Fairmount Behavioral Health System; Lecturer, School of Nursing, University of Pennsylvania

ANGELICA MILLAN, Former Children's Medical Services Nursing Director, County of Los Angeles Department of Public Health

JOHN W. ROWE, Julius B. Richmond Professor of Health Policy and Aging, Mailman School of Public Health, Columbia University

WILLIAM M. SAGE, James R. Dougherty Chair for Faculty Excellence, School of Law, and Professor of Surgery and Perioperative Care, Dell Medical School, The University of Texas at Austin

VICTORIA L. TIASE, Director of Research Science and Informatics Strategy, NewYork-Presbyterian Hospital

WINSTON WONG, Scholar in Residence, University of California, Los Angeles, Kaiser Permanente Center for Health Equity

Study Staff

SUZANNE LE MENESTREL, Study Director (*from June 2020*)
SUSAN B. HASSMILLER, Senior Scholar in Residence and Advisor to the President on Nursing, National Academy of Medicine
JENNIFER LALITHA FLAUBERT, Program Officer
ADRIENNE FORMENTOS, Research Associate
TOCHI OGBU-MBADIUGHA, Senior Program Assistant (*from October 2020*)
CARY HAVER, Study Director (*until June 2020*)
LORI BRENIG, Senior Program Assistant (*until May 2020*)
CAROL SANDOVAL, Senior Program Assistant (*until September 2020*)
ASHLEY DARCY-MAHONEY, National Academy of Medicine Distinguished Nurse Scholar-in-Residence (*August 2020 to August 2021*)
ALLISON SQUIRES, National Academy of Medicine Distinguished Nurse Scholar-in-Residence (*March 2019 to August 2020*)
SHARYL NASS, Senior Board Director, Board on Health Care Services

Reviewers

This Consensus Study Report was reviewed in draft form by individuals chosen for their diverse perspectives and technical expertise. The purpose of this independent review is to provide candid and critical comments that will assist the National Academies of Sciences, Engineering, and Medicine in making each published report as sound as possible and to ensure that it meets the institutional standards for quality, objectivity, evidence, and responsiveness to the study charge. The review comments and draft manuscript remain confidential to protect the integrity of the deliberative process.

We thank the following individuals for their review of this report:

FRANK BAEZ, New York University Langone Health
KENYA V. BEARD, Chamberlain University
PATRICIA FLATLEY BRENNAN, National Library of Medicine
SALLY S. COHEN, New York University
MARY PAT COUIG, The University of New Mexico
FRANCIS J. CROSSON, Kaiser Permanente Bernard J. Tyson School of Medicine
WILLIAM A. DARITY, JR., Duke University
MARGARET FLINTER, Community Health Center, Inc.
BIANCA K. FROGNER, University of Washington
EMILY A. HAOZOUS, The University of New Mexico
BERNADETTE MAZUREK MELNYK, The Ohio State University
TERI A. MURRAY, Saint Louis University
DANIEL J. PESUT, University of Minnesota
KRISTINE QURESHI, University of Hawai'i at Mānoa

ROBERT D. REISCHAUER, The Urban Institute
CAROL A. ROMANO, Uniformed Services University of the Health Sciences
SUSAN E. STONE, Frontier Nursing University and American College of Nurse-Midwives
DANIEL WEBERG, The Ohio State University

Although the reviewers listed above provided many constructive comments and suggestions, they were not asked to endorse the conclusions or recommendations of this report, nor did they see the final draft before its release. The review of this report was overseen by **BOBBIE BERKOWITZ,** Columbia University, and **MAXINE HAYES,** University of Washington. They were responsible for making certain that an independent examination of this report was carried out in accordance with the standards of the National Academies and that all review comments were carefully considered. Responsibility for the final content rests entirely with the authoring committee and the National Academies.

Foreword

The year 2020, the bicentennial of Florence Nightingale's birth, was designated by the World Health Organization (WHO) as the International Year of the Nurse and the Midwife. According to WHO, "Nurses and midwives play a vital role in providing health services. These are the people who devote their lives to caring for mothers and children; giving lifesaving immunizations and health advice; looking after older people and generally meeting everyday essential health needs. They are often, the first and only point of care in their communities."

As president of the National Academy of Medicine (NAM) and as a physician who has worked closely with nurses over the decades, I know the central role of nursing in achieving the high-quality, accessible, and compassionate care that individuals, families, and communities richly deserve. I am proud that we can help commemorate this occasion through the release of our latest report, *The Future of Nursing 2020–2030: Charting a Path to Achieve Health Equity.*

This report is the third in a series on the future of nursing that we at the NAM (formerly known as the Institute of Medicine [IOM]) have been privileged to create with the sponsorship of the Robert Wood Johnson Foundation. The first of these reports, *The Future of Nursing: Leading Change, Advancing Health,* published in 2011, presented a set of bold recommendations to strengthen the capacity, education, and critical role of the nursing workforce. It emboldened nurses to play a central role in improving health care for people, families, and communities around the world. That report, which has served as a blueprint for the nursing profession, is the National Academies' second most downloaded health and medicine report since its release and continues to reach thousands of nurses and other important stakeholders around the world.

The second nursing report, released in 2016, *Assessing Progress on the Institute of Medicine Report* The Future of Nursing, highlighted promising progress made since the 2011 report while noting that much more needed to be done. It outlined three themes central to the future success of the Robert Wood Johnson Foundation/AARP Future of Nursing Campaign for Action (the Campaign):

> the need to build a broader coalition to increase awareness of nurses' ability to play a full role in health professions practice, education, collaboration, and leadership; the need to continue to make promoting diversity in the nursing workforce a priority; and the need for better data with which to assess and drive progress.

Alongside these two reports have been the exemplary and steadfast efforts of the innovative change initiative, the Campaign, in continuing to implement the recommendations from the first report while working to take on the recommendations of the second in a more robust way. Of note, efforts to create a more diverse workforce and to expand ways of working with others in and outside of the health system have served to foreshadow the importance of nurses as key players in achieving health equity in the United States and globally. No one profession or group will achieve the health equity needed in this nation without all health professions, working within and across disciplines, aspiring to advance the culture required. Working across sectors with steadfast vigilance will be a necessary ingredient not only in understanding but also in taking real action to achieve health equity.

With this third report, *The Future of Nursing 2020–2030: Charting a Path to Achieve Health Equity*, the NAM and the Robert Wood Johnson Foundation continue their steadfast collaboration toward promoting a culture of health for all. Both organizations believe that uneven access to conditions needed for good health across the United States has been well documented, as have the poor effects on health that result. The growing visibility of the impacts of systemic racism in almost every aspect of people's lives—policing, health care, the economy, education—is evident. Now more than ever, the nation sees clearly the need for an equitable, just, and fair society—one that promotes racial equity, as well as equity across circumstances, communities, and abilities. The good news is that so many of us are asking, "How can we do better? How can I do better?" In a time marked by COVID-19's unprecedented global health challenges, nurses have stepped up—many times at great personal cost to themselves.

Nurses have seen firsthand this disease's inequitable impact on those they serve. They have also experienced firsthand COVID-19's inequitable impact on the profession. Nurses are more likely to die than are other health care professionals, and nurses of color are far more likely to die. As this report points out with compelling evidence, nurses can play a central role in addressing these inequities across the entire spectrum. The nation cannot achieve true health equity without nurses, which means it must do better for nurses. They must be supported in charting a path for themselves while they work to serve others. This report is intended to do just that.

I am very grateful to the committee for their consensus on the important recommendations in this report—especially the co-chairs, Mary Wakefield and David Williams—and to the National Academies staff, including Suzanne Le Menestrel, Jennifer Flaubert, Adrienne Formentos, and Tochi Ogbu-Mbadiugha, as well as Susan Hassmiller, who served as senior scholar-in-residence and who provided continuity between the first and third reports.

This report calls on many within and around the nursing community to take more definitive action on eliminating systemic racism, whether in schools, institutions, or the profession and its associations. Nurses are powerful in number and in voice and the world needs their actions now more than ever on how individuals, families, and communities might best be served in a more equitable fashion. And in asking nurses to play a central leadership role, I am reminded of the importance of nurse well-being. Nurses have been called on to do so much in this past year throughout the COVID-19 pandemic, and the nation must support them, including giving them all of the necessary tools and equipment to do their job in the best way possible. I am confident that the nursing community and other important stakeholders will use the recommendations in this report and their evidence base to lead the way to a more equitable and healthy society.

Victor J. Dzau, M.D.
President, National Academy of Medicine

Preface

In 2019, the Robert Wood Johnson Foundation (RWJF) sponsored this study to explore the important contributions of nursing to addressing social determinants of health (SDOH) and health equity in the United States. This was to serve as a parallel effort to other National Academy of Medicine reports and initiatives sponsored by RWJF around efforts to create a more robust culture of health in the United States. The work of this committee began in 2019 after years of evidence documenting the relationship between SDOH and health outcomes, as well as broader challenges associated with health and health care equity. By the end of 2020, this report was to be released in a year that was being commemorated by the World Health Organization as the International Year of the Nurse and the Midwife.[1]

Throughout the year, the committee participated in three major town hall meetings; a series of site visits in and around Seattle, Chicago, and Philadelphia; and two other public sessions, recordings and materials from which are available online.[2] We heard time and again how the highly complex health and social needs of people were critical in defining their overall health and well-being, and that of their families and populations at large.

The committee's work continued in 2020 with the goal of launching this report at the end of the year. In March, however, the COVID-19 pandemic hit the

[1] See https://www.who.int/campaigns/annual-theme/year-of-the-nurse-and-the-midwife-2020 (accessed April 13, 2021).

[2] Town hall recordings and materials can be accessed at https://nam.edu/publications/the-future-of-nursing-2020-2030 (accessed April 13, 2021).

United States, and throughout the year it was evident that the challenges outlined in this report were vastly magnified by the most devastating health care event in more than a century. The pandemic, which has since killed nearly 3 million people globally and sickened more than 135 million more,[3] laid bare the depth and breadth of inequity and its impacts on the health and well-being of large swaths of the nation's population, disproportionately impacting people of color, those with low income, and those living in rural areas.

Simultaneously, 2020 taxed the nation's nursing workforce in ways that had never been fully anticipated and planned for. Overcrowded hospitals, countless deaths, and lack of personal protective equipment to secure their safety, in addition to falling sick themselves, pushed nurses to their limits. Many called nurses heroes, but nurses time and again shunned that title and responded by saying they were doing the work they were called to do as nurses, albeit without the equipment, including respirators and personal protective gear, they needed to deliver care safely. Caring for highly infectious patients with dire needs had sweeping adverse impacts on the physical and mental health of scores of thousands of the nation's nurses.

In addition to the crises created by the pandemic and the trauma it caused for society at large and nurses, years of racial injustice culminated in tragic events that also shone a light on inequities for people of color. The tragic deaths of George Floyd, Breonna Taylor, and countless others unleashed decades of pent-up emotion and widespread protests regarding the state of equity in the United States and around the world. These deaths highlighted the reality that serious challenges were being faced, especially by people of color.

This report's release in 2021 comes as the United States and the world have suffered great loss, but also are buoyed by the promise of lessons learned, including witnessing the nursing profession's commitment to health, nursing innovations that improved health care in real time for patients and families impacted by COVID-19, and nurse-driven adaptations in education and practice that will likely drive lasting changes in both. There is now deeper evidence and understanding of the differential impact of generations of inequity associated with racism and bias, socioeconomic status, disabilities, financial poverty, and living in areas with decreased health care access that has fueled compromised health status for many of our fellow Americans. It is against this backdrop that the committee strove to produce a report that would anticipate the needs of the population and the nursing profession for the next decade while advancing a set of recommended actions that can make a meaningful impact on deploying the profession more robustly, so that nurses will be both prepared for disasters in the

[3] The figures as of April 13, 2021, were 135.1 million global cases and more than 2.9 million COVID-related deaths. Nearly 600,000 of these deaths were in the United States. See https://www.who.int/publications/m/item/weekly-epidemiological-update-on-covid-19---13-april-2021 (accessed April 13, 2021).

future and prepared to engage in the complex but essential work of advancing health equity, addressing SDOH, and meeting social needs of individuals and families.

While the 2011 *The Future of Nursing* report was about building the capacity of the nursing workforce, this report clearly answers the question of to what end. Nursing capacity must be brought to bear on the above complex health and social issues and inequities.

By virtue of its history, its focus, and its presence across sectors and populations, the nursing profession is well positioned to bring its expertise to working in partnership with other disciplines and sectors to leverage contemporary opportunities and address deep-seated health and social challenges. And the committee believes that all nurses, at all levels, and no matter the setting in which they work, have a duty and responsibility to work with other health professionals and sectors to address SDOH and help achieve health equity.

As was noted in the preface of the 2011 report, "What nursing brings to the future is a steadfast commitment to patient care, improved safety and quality, and better outcomes."[4] The present report expands that report's focus on outcomes by clearly incorporating and leveraging the profession's own ethics, values, and knowledge assets to address the upstream and midstream work of applying evidence linking health and health care equity to health outcomes for individuals, families, communities, and populations, as well as further building out evidence-based models, health system policies and health-related public policies, and educational approaches. Nurses in particular are well prepared to create, partner in, and lead the complex work of integrating the social and health sectors in support of the health and well-being of individuals, families, and communities. Nurses, working with social services sectors in and across community-based ambulatory care and public health settings to implement health system and point-of-care interventions, can help advance continuous care models that are individual- and population-centered.

In addition to addressing social needs, nurses are called upon to inform and implement policies that will ultimately affect the greatest numbers of people in the most profound ways. For decades, the International Council of Nurses (ICN) has explicitly supported nurses around the world in contributing their expertise to informing health-related public policy. The ICN has also called for policy maker receptivity to nurses' expertise. Nurses recognize that poorly informed public policy, like poor health care and compromised SDOH, can undermine the health of patients, families, and communities. And upstream actions to address SDOH are often rooted in long-standing policies that contribute to inequity in housing, employment, education, and other key precursors to health.

---

[4] IOM (Institute of Medicine). 2011. *The future of nursing: Leading change, advancing health*. Washington, DC: The National Academies Press.

We are grateful to a very committed expert group of committee members who spent countless hours discussing, debating, and then reaching consensus around some very difficult topics. In any consensus-building process, not every individual will agree with every statement in a report such as this, as reflected in a supplemental statement written by one committee member, provided in Appendix E; the response of the rest of the committee to this statement appears in Appendix F. The discussion and ultimate set of recommendations in this report were enhanced by the breadth of expertise brought to bear, expertise that went far beyond the nursing profession. We are also grateful to the talented staff of the National Academies of Sciences, Engineering, and Medicine who worked tirelessly with us to create this report. Finally, we appreciate the foresight of RWJF in valuing the contributions and leadership of nursing in addressing SDOH and health equity and their sponsorship of this report.

Mary K. Wakefield and David R. Williams, *Co-Chairs*
Committee on the Future of Nursing 2020–2030

Dedication

This report is dedicated to the nurses around the world who paid the ultimate price of caring for people during the COVID-19 crisis of 2020–2021. Hundreds lost their lives, and many thousands became sick themselves. And those who escaped the physical symptoms of the illness did not necessarily escape the physical and mental toll of working long hours in grueling circumstances, sometimes without proper personal protective equipment. Their dedication and persistence in the face of adversity saved countless lives. They were also there to ease the suffering of the dying with a hand held, a song sung, or a video call to loved ones.

For them, we look to the future of nursing to help ensure that what happened to the nursing profession this year and those in their care, especially the disadvantaged and people of color, becomes an event of the past.

Acknowledgments

To begin, the committee would like to thank the sponsor of this study. Funds for the committee's work were provided by the Robert Wood Johnson Foundation (RWJF).

Numerous individuals and organizations made important contributions to the study process and this report. The committee wishes to express its gratitude for each of these contributions, although space does not permit identifying all of them here. Appendix A lists the individuals who provided valuable information at the committee's open workshops and its three town halls on the future of nursing. The committee thanks the members of the staff of the National Academies of Sciences, Engineering, and Medicine for their significant contributions to the report: Suzanne Le Menestrel, Susan B. Hassmiller, Jennifer Lalitha Flaubert, Adrienne Formentos, Tochi Ogbu-Mbadiugha, Cary Haver, Lori Brenig, Carol Sandoval, Ashley Darcy-Mahoney, and Allison Squires.

The committee would also like to thank Rona Briere, Allison Boman, Diana Mason, Dalia Sofer, Paul Selker, and Maya Thomas for their writing, editorial, and fact-checking assistance. The committee would like to especially acknowledge Erin Hammers Forstag for her writing and editing contributions. We would like to thank National Academies staff members who provided invaluable support throughout the project: Micah Winograd, senior finance business partner; the late Daniel Bearss and Anne Marie Houppert, research librarians, for assistance with literature searches; and staff that contributed additional writing and research, including Alix Beatty, Bernice Chu, Carolyn Fulco, and Adrienne Stith-Butler. Thank you to Laura DeStefano, Greta Gorman, Andrew Grafton, Talia Lewis, Devona Overton, Esther Pak, and Olivia Ramirez for their communications expertise; Annalee Espinosa Gonzales and Joe Goodman for logistical support in Philadelphia and Seattle; and Sharyl Nass, Tina Seliber, and Lauren Shern for guidance throughout the study process. The committee appreciates the contributions of Molly Ellison and Janet Firshein, who provided strategic communications support for this report through the communications firm Burness. The committee would also like to thank Dave McClinton from African American Graphic Designers for the report cover design and Elena Ovaitt for designing figures and models for the report.

In conjunction with each of its town halls, the committee also visited several clinical and community sites to observe clinics and programs that are nurse-led or where nurses acted as important members of multidisciplinary teams in contributing to health equity and addressing social determinants of health in various settings. The committee greatly appreciates the time and information provided by all of these individuals, especially those who helped to coordinate those visits, including Sue Birch and Azita Emami in Seattle; Kathleen Noonan and Roberta Waite in Camden, New Jersey, and Philadelphia; and Janice Phillips and Sue Swider in Chicago.

The committee also gratefully acknowledges the contributions of the individuals who provided data and research support. Margo Edmunds and Raj Sabharwal of AcademyHealth with a team of research managers, Karen Johnson, Kent Key, Polly Pittman, and Joanne Spetz, who created research products that synthesized, translated, and disseminated information to inform the committee's deliberations. The committee also acknowledges and greatly appreciates the time and effort of David Auerbach and Timothy Bates in analyzing workforce data.

The committee would also like to thank the authors whose commissioned papers added to the evidence base for the study: Amy J. Barton, University of Colorado College of Nursing; Barbara Brandt and Carla J. Dieter, University of Minnesota; and Shanita D. Williams, Health Resources and Services Administration; Jack Needleman, Fielding School of Public Health, University of California, Los Angeles; and Tener Veenema, Johns Hopkins University School of Nursing, with research assistance from Emily Clifford, Johns Hopkins University.

Finally, the committee acknowledges the following individuals who provided additional data, reports, and support to the committee: Michelle Adymec, Mavis Asiedu-Frimpong, Sheila Brown, Laura Buckley, Jess Cordero, Dayna Fondell, Ebony Haley, Lauran Hardan, Mark Humowiecki, Stephanie Jean-Louis, Andrew Katz, Renee Murray, Victor Murray, Jeneen Skinner, Aaron Truchil, and Katie Wood, Camden Coalition of Healthcare Providers; Min An, Kline Galland House; Kate Baber, Downtown Emergency Services Center; Teresita Batayola, Dante Batingan, Rattana Chaokhote, Asqual Getaneh, Sherryl Grey, DoQuyen Huynh, Rachel Koh, Rayburn Lewis, Ian Munar, Jackqui Sinatra, Eric Ric Troyer, and Mayumi Willgerodt, International Community Health Services; Rebecca Bixby, Laniece Coleman, Joan Gray, Mary Katherine Green, Diana Hartley-Kim, Lidyvez Sawyer, and Mary Thornton-Bowmer, Stephen and Sandra Sheller 11th Street Family Health Services, Drexel University; Michelle Cleary, Jesse Dean,

Robin Fleming, Tamarra Henshaw, and Suzanne Swadener, Washington State Health Care Authority; Rebecca Darmoc, Marquis Forman, Mariela Hernandez, and Angelique Richard, Rush University College of Nursing; Candice Douglass, Panome Ratsavong, and Nolan Ryan, University of Washington School of Nursing; Kathy Eaton, Deb Gumbardo, Elizabeth Masse, Erika Miller, Mady Murray, and Debra Ridling, Seattle Children's Hospital; Yolanda Fong, Kitsap Public Health; Theresa Gallagher and Angela Moss, Sue Gin Health Center; Joan Gray, Tarun Kapoor, and Jubril Oyeyemi, Virtua Health System; Jennifer Grenier and Nicole Wynn, The Surplus Project; Patty Hayes and Doreen Hersh, Public Health Seattle & King County; Ayesha Jaco, Westside United and Rush University Medical Center; Jennifer Johnson Joefield, Peninsula Community Health Services; Sally Lemke, Simpson School Based Health Center; Janice Mason, Malcolm X Community College; Brenda Montgomery, Harrison Hospital (CHI Franciscan); Julie Morita, Chicago Department of Public Health; Donna Nickitas, Rutgers School of Nursing–Camden; William Reedy, Thresholds Community Mental Health Center; James Rice, City Colleges of Chicago School of Nursing; Cynda Rushton, Johns Hopkins University School of Nursing; Kelsey Stedman and Jayme Stuntz, Kitsap Connect; and Janet Tomcavage, University of Pennsylvania School of Nursing. We would also like to thank the staff of the Seattle Indian Health Board, Era Living, Ida Culver House, and Salvation Army (Seattle) and everyone at the Port Gamble S'Klallam Health Center.

Contents

ACRONYMS AND ABBREVIATIONS xxix

SUMMARY 1

1 INTRODUCTION 17

2 SOCIAL DETERMINANTS OF HEALTH AND HEALTH EQUITY 31

3 THE NURSING WORKFORCE 59

4 THE ROLE OF NURSES IN IMPROVING HEALTH CARE ACCESS AND QUALITY 99

5 THE ROLE OF NURSES IN IMPROVING HEALTH EQUITY 127

6 PAYING FOR EQUITY IN HEALTH AND HEALTH CARE 147

7 EDUCATING NURSES FOR THE FUTURE 189

8 NURSES IN DISASTER PREPAREDNESS AND PUBLIC HEALTH EMERGENCY RESPONSE 247

9 NURSES LEADING CHANGE 275

10 SUPPORTING THE HEALTH AND PROFESSIONAL WELL-BEING OF NURSES 301

11 THE FUTURE OF NURSING: RECOMMENDATIONS AND RESEARCH PRIORITIES 355

APPENDIXES

A BIOGRAPHICAL SKETCHES OF COMMITTEE MEMBERS AND PROJECT STAFF 377

B DATA COLLECTION AND INFORMATION SOURCES 391

C DATA SOURCES, DEFINITIONS, AND METHODS 405

D GLOSSARY 415

E THE FUTURE OF NURSING 2020–2030: MEETING AMERICA WHERE WE ARE 423

F COMMITTEE RESPONSE TO SUPPLEMENTAL STATEMENT 429

G PROFILES OF NURSING PROGRAMS AND ORGANIZATIONS* 433

* Appendix G is only available online at https://www.nap.edu/catalog/25982.

Boxes, Figures, and Tables

BOXES

S-1 Achieving Health Equity Through Nursing: Desired Outcomes, 2
S-2 The Committee's Recommendations, 13

1-1 Types of Nursing Care Providers, 19
1-2 Statement of Task, 24

2-1 Social Determinants of Health, 33
2-2 Intersectionality, 38

3-1 Internationally Educated Nurses, 65
3-2 COVID-19 and Nurse Staffing in Nursing Homes, 70
3-3 Health Disparities Among American Indians/Alaska Natives, 85
3-4 Agenda for Nursing Health Services Research, 92

4-1 Innovative In-Home Care Programs, 107
4-2 Transitional Care Model, 113
4-3 Culturally and Linguistically Appropriate Services, 115

5-1 Shortcomings of Evaluations of Health Equity Interventions, 130
5-2 Examples of Edge Runner Programs, 138
5-3 Delaware Cancer Consortium, 140

7-1 National League for Nursing's (NLN's) Vision for Integration of the Social Determinants of Health into Nursing Education Curricula, 194
7-2 Domains for Nursing Education, 203
7-3 Competencies for Nursing Education, Depending on Preparation Level, 203
7-4 Discussing Difficult Topics, 205
7-5 Highlights from the Seattle Townhall on Technology and Health Equity and Implications for Nursing Education, 210
7-6 Pine Ridge Family Health Center, 215
7-7 The Community Action Poverty Simulation, 216
7-8 Examples of Supports for Nursing Students, 226

8-1 Pulse Nightclub Shooting, 254
8-2 COVID-19 in Hidalgo County, Texas, 256
8-3 Lessons Learned from Nurses' Role in Evacuation During Hurricane Sandy, 258

10-1 Technological Factors Impacting Nurses' Well-Being, 305
10-2 A Snapshot of the Physical Health of American Nurses, 307
10-3 COVID-19 and Nurses' Health and Well-Being, 309
10-4 Mobile Technology and Mental Health Interventions, 323
10-5 Examples of Nursing Schools' Well-Being Initiatives, 330
10-6 Psychological Personal Protective Equipment (PPE), 332

11-1 Achieving Health Equity Through Nursing: Desired Outcomes, 356

FIGURES

S-1 A framework for understanding the nurse's role in addressing the equity of health and health care, 5

1-1 A framework for understanding the nurse's role in addressing the equity of health and health care, 27

2-1 Conceptual framework of the Commission on the Social Determinants of Health, 35
2-2 Social Determinants of Health and Social Needs Model, 37
2-3 Expected age at death among 40-year-old men and women, by household income percentile, 43

3-1 Number of nursing doctoral graduates by race/ethnicity, 66
3-2 Nurse practitioners by race and ethnicity, 2018, 73
3-3 Scope of practice for nurse practitioners by state, 87

4-1 Licensure staffing patterns (paid and unpaid volunteer) by geography, 110

5-1 Areas of activity that strengthen integration of social care into health care, 129

7-1 Training topics that would have helped registered nurses do their jobs better, by type of work performed and graduation from their nursing program, 2018, 196
7-2 Training topics that would have helped nurse practitioners do their jobs better, by type of work performed and graduation from their nursing education program, 2018, 197

8-1 Disaster nursing timeline, 250

10-1 Systems model of burnout and well-being, 304

TABLES

3-1 Demographic Characteristics of Full-Time Equivalent (FTE) Registered Nurses (RNs), 2000–2018, 63
3-2 Number and Percentage of Nurses with Various Levels of Nursing Education by Race, 2018, 64
3-3 Number of Registered Nurses (RNs) by Employment Setting, Average Annual Earnings, and Age, 2018, 66
3-4 Number of Employed Advanced Practice Registered Nurses (APRNs), 2008 and 2018, 72
3-5 Nurse Practitioner Employment Settings, 2018, 74
3-6 Nurse Practitioner Employment by Clinical Specialty Area, 2018, 76

5-1 Definitions of Areas of Activities That Strengthen Integration of Social Care into Health Care, 129

7-1 Pathways in Nursing Education, 192
7-2 Number of Graduates from Nursing Programs in the United States and Territories, 2019, 193
7-3 Nursing Program Graduates by Degree Type and by Race/Ethnicity, 2019, 218
7-4 Nursing Program Graduates by Degree Type and Gender, 2019, 219
7-5 Diversity and Inclusion in Accreditation Standards, 220

9-1 A Framework for Nurse Leadership, 279

11-1 Research Topics for the Future of Nursing, 2020–2030, 373

C-1 Demographic Characteristics of Full-Time Equivalent (FTE) Registered Nurses, 2001–2018, 406
C-2 Number of Registered Nurses by Employment Settings, Average Annual Earnings, and Age, 2018, 411
C-3 Nurse Practitioner Employment Settings, 2018, 413

Acronyms and Abbreviations

AACN	American Association of Colleges of Nursing
ACA	Patient Protection and Affordable Care Act
ACE	adverse childhood experience
ACEN	Accreditation Commission for Education in Nursing
ACS	American Community Survey
AD	associate's degree
AHA	American Hospital Association
AHRQ	Agency for Healthcare Research and Quality
AMA	American Medical Association
ANA	American Nurses Association
APHA	American Public Health Association
APM	alternative payment model
APRN	advanced practice registered nurse
ASMN	Academy of Medical-Surgical Nurses
BWH	Bureau of Workforce
CAPABLE	Community Aging in Place: Advancing Better Living for Elders
CCNA	Center to Champion Nursing in America
CCNE	Commission on Collegiate Nursing Education
CDC	Centers for Disease Control and Prevention
CMMI	Center for Medicare & Medicaid Innovation
CMS	Center for Medicare & Medicaid Services
CNM	certified nurse midwife
CNS	certified nurse specialist

COVID-19 coronavirus disease 2019
CPT Current Procedural Terminology
CRNA certified registered nurse anesthetist

DNP doctor of nursing practice

EHR electronic health record

FEMA Federal Emergency Management Agency
FNS Frontier Nursing Service
FQHC federally qualified health center

HBR Healthy Baton Rouge
HHS U.S. Department of Health and Human Services
HIV human immunodeficiency virus
HPSA health professional shortage area
HRSA Health Resources and Services Administration

ICD *International Classification of Diseases*
IHI Institute for Healthcare Improvement
IHS Indian Health Service
IOM Institute of Medicine

LVN/LPN licensed vocational nurse/licensed practical nurse

MACPAC Medicaid and CHIP (Children's Health Insurance Plan) Payment and Access Commission
MedPAC Medicare Payment Advisory Commission

NA nursing assistant
NACCHO National Association of County and City Health Officials
NACNEP National Advisory Council on Nurse Education and Practice
NASN National Association of School Nurses
NCLEX-RN National Council Licensure Examination for Registered Nurses
NCSBN National Council of State Boards of Nursing
NFP Nurse-Family Partnership
NIH National Institutes of Health
NINR National Institute of Nursing Research
NLN National League for Nursing
NRC National Research Council
NSSRN National Sample Survey of Registered Nurses

OADN	Organization of Associate Degree Nurses
OECD	Organisation for Economic Co-operation and Development
PACE	Program of All-Inclusive Care for the Elderly
PCMH	patient-centered medical home
PHIN	Public Health Information Network
PHN	public health nurse
PPE	personal protective equipment
RBRVS	resource-based relative value scale
RCT	randomized controlled trial
RHC	rural health clinic
RN	registered nurse
RUC	RVS (relative value scale) Update Committee
RWJF	Robert Wood Johnson Foundation
SAMHSA	Substance Abuse and Mental Health Services Administration
SBHC	school-based health center
SDOH	social determinants of health
SNAP	Supplemental Nutrition Assistance Program
SONSIEL	Society of Nurse Scientists, Innovators, Entrepreneurs and Leaders
VA	U.S. Department of Veterans Affairs
VBP	value-based payment
VHA	Veterans Health Administration
WHO	World Health Organization

Summary[1]

The decade ahead will test the nation's nearly 4 million nurses in new and complex ways. Nurses live and work at the intersection of health, education, and communities. In the decade since the prior *The Future of Nursing* report was issued by the Institute of Medicine, the world has come to understand the critical importance of health to all aspects of life, particularly the relationship among what are termed *social determinants of health* (SDOH), health equity, and health outcomes. In a year that was designated to honor and uplift nursing (the International Year of the Nurse and the Midwife 2020), nurses have been placed in unimaginable circumstances by the COVID-19 pandemic. The decade ahead will demand a stronger, more diversified nursing workforce that is prepared to provide care; promote health and well-being among nurses, individuals, and communities; and address the systemic inequities that have fueled wide and persistent health disparities.

The vision of the Committee on the Future of Nursing 2020–2030, which informs this report, is the achievement of health equity in the United States built on strengthened nursing capacity and expertise. By leveraging these attributes, nursing will help to create and contribute comprehensively to equitable public health and health care systems that are designed to work for everyone. To achieve health equity, the committee also envisions a major role for the nursing profession in engaging in the complex work of aligning public health, health care, social services, and public policies to eliminate health disparities and achieve health equity. Specifically, with implementation of this report's recommendations, the committee envisions 10 outcomes that position the nursing profession to contribute meaningfully to achieving health equity (see Box S-1).

[1] This Summary does not include references. Citations for the discussion presented in the Summary appear in the subsequent report chapters.

BOX S-1
Achieving Health Equity Through Nursing: Desired Outcomes

- Nurses are prepared to act individually, through teams, and across sectors to meet challenges associated with an aging population, access to primary care, mental and behavioral health problems, structural racism, high maternal mortality and morbidity, and elimination of the disproportionate disease burden carried by specific segments of the U.S. population.
- Nurses are fully engaged in addressing the underlying causes of poor health. Individually and in partnership with other disciplines and sectors, nurses act on a wide range of factors that influence how well and long people live, helping to create individual- and community-targeted solutions, including a health in all policies orientation.
- Nurses reflect the people and communities served throughout the nation, helping to ensure that individuals receive culturally competent, equitable health care services.
- Health care systems enable and support nurses to tailor care to meet the specific medical and social needs of diverse patients to optimize their health.
- Nurses' overarching contributions, especially those found beneficial during the COVID-19 pandemic, are quantified, extended, and strengthened, including the removal of institutional and regulatory barriers that have prevented nurses from working to the full extent of their education and training. Practice settings that were historically undercompensated, such as public health and school nursing, are reimbursed for nursing services in a manner comparable to that of other settings.
- Nurses and other leaders in health care and public health create organizational structures and processes that facilitate the profession's expedited acquisition of relevant content expertise to serve flexibly in areas of greatest need in times of public health emergencies and disasters.
- Nurses consistently incorporate a health equity lens learned through revamped academic and continuing education.
- Nurses collaborate across their affiliated organizations to develop and deploy a shared agenda to contribute to substantial, measurable improvement in health equity. National nursing organizations reflect an orientation of diversity, equity, and inclusion within and across their organizations.
- Nurses focus on preventive person-centered care and have an orientation toward innovation, always seeking new opportunities for growth and development. They expand their roles, work in new settings and in new ways, and markedly expand their partnerships connecting health and health care with all individuals and communities.
- Nurses attend to their own self-care and help to ensure that nurse well-being is addressed in educational and employment settings through the implementation of evidence-based strategies.

HEALTH AND HEALTH INEQUITIES

Health inequities, defined as "systematic differences in the opportunities that groups have to achieve optimal health, leading to unfair and avoidable differences in health outcomes," disproportionately impact people of color; the lesbian, gay, bisexual, transgender, and queer (LGBTQ) community; people with disabilities; those with low income; and those living in rural areas. Indeed, growing evidence reveals a clear association between inequities in both health and access to health care and SDOH—the conditions in the environments in which people live, learn, work, play, worship, and age that affect a wide range of health, functioning, and quality-of-life outcomes and risks. SDOH include both the positive and negative aspects of these conditions. Examples of SDOH include education, employment, health systems and services, housing, income and wealth, the physical environment, public safety, the social environment (including structures, institutions, and policies), and transportation. Everyone is affected by SDOH. Some people who have more education or higher incomes will fare better healthwise as they may be able to make more informed choices, have better opportunities to access health care, and have the means to pay for health care. Others, without the benefit of these positive social determinants, are unlikely to fare as well.

A related concept is *social needs*—individual-level, nonmedical, acute resource needs for such things as housing, reliable transportation, and a strong support system at home that are necessary for good health outcomes and health equity. Health equity can be advanced at the individual level by addressing these needs and at the population level by addressing SDOH. Health equity benefits all individuals by promoting such macrostructural benefits as economic growth, a healthier environment, and national security.

For too long, the United States has overinvested in treating illness and underinvested in promoting health and preventing disease. The nation has spent more on medical care than any other high-income country, yet it has seen consistently worse health outcomes than those of its peer countries, including the lowest life expectancy, more chronic health conditions, and the highest rates of infant mortality. At the same time, the COVID-19 pandemic has starkly revealed Americans' unequal access to opportunities to live a healthy life, often resulting from entrenched structural and systemic barriers that include poverty, racism, and discrimination. These two phenomena—suboptimal health outcomes and inequities in health and health care—are not unrelated. If the nation is to achieve better population health, it will have to meet the challenge of mitigating these inequities. Herein lies the greatest contribution of the nursing workforce in the decade ahead.

THE ROLE OF NURSES IN ADVANCING HEALTH EQUITY

A nation cannot fully thrive until everyone—no matter who they are, where they live, or how much money they make—can live the healthiest possible life, and helping people live their healthiest life is and has always been the essential role of nurses. Whether in a school, a hospital, or a community health clinic, they have worked to address the root causes of poor health. The history of nursing is grounded in social justice and community health advocacy. The Code of Ethics for Nurses with Interpretive Statements from the American Nurses Association (ANA), for example, obligates nurses to "integrate principles of social justice into nursing and health policy."[2]

Nurses work in a wide array of settings and practice at a range of professional levels. They often act as the first and most frequent line of contact with people of all backgrounds and experiences seeking care. The nursing workforce also represents the largest of the health care professions—nearly four times the size of the physician workforce. In their various capacities and given their numbers, nurses are uniquely positioned to manage teams and link clinical care, public health, and social services.

STUDY PURPOSE AND APPROACH

Nurses, then, have a critical role to play in achieving the goal of health equity. But to take on the pursuit of that goal, they need robust education, supportive work environments, and autonomy. Accordingly, the Robert Wood Johnson Foundation asked the National Academies of Sciences, Engineering, and Medicine to conduct a study aimed at charting a path forward for the nursing profession to help create a culture of health and reduce disparities in people's ability to achieve their full health potential. To carry out this study, the National Academies convened an ad hoc committee of 15 experts in the fields of nursing leadership, education, practice, and workforce, as well as health policy, economics and health care finance, informatics, population health and health disparities, health care quality and delivery, and health care research and interventions.

To supplement the knowledge and expertise of its members, the committee solicited input from additional experts and interested members of the public at two public sessions held in conjunction with committee meetings. Further input came from several site visits that included town hall meetings. In addition, the committee reviewed the salient peer-reviewed and grey literature not associated with commercial publishers, carried out original data analyses, commissioned papers on topics of particular relevance, and considered public and organizational statements pertinent to this study.

To organize and consolidate this wealth of information, the committee developed the framework depicted in Figure S-1. This framework structures the report's discussion of the key areas for strengthening the nursing profession to meet the challenges of the decade ahead. The heart of this framework is the key areas shown at the top of the figure: the nursing workforce, leadership, nursing

---

[2] See https://www.nursingworld.org/practice-policy/nursing-excellence/ethics/code-of-ethics-for-nurses/coe-view-only (accessed April 13, 2021).

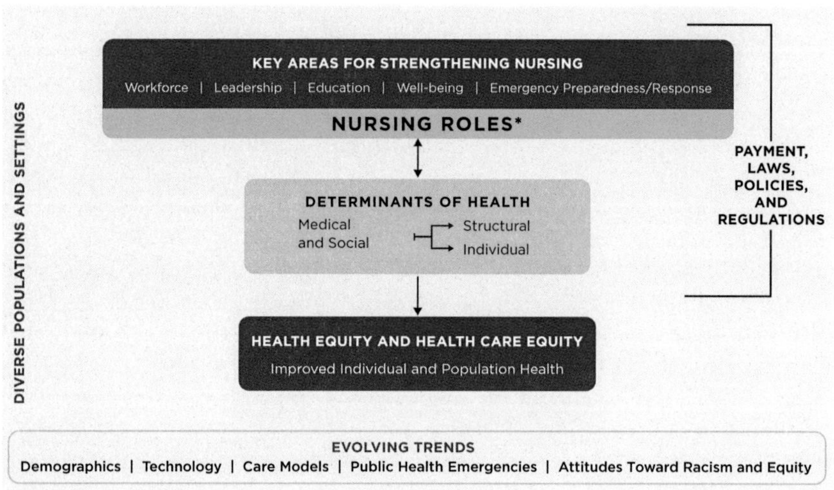

FIGURE S-1 A framework for understanding the nurse's role in addressing the equity of health and health care.

* Examples of nursing roles in acute, community, and public health settings include care coordinator, policy maker, clinician, educator, researcher/scientist, administrator, and informaticist.

education, nurse well-being, and emergency preparedness and response, and the responsibilities of nursing with respect to structural and individual determinants of health. Nurses play multiple roles in acute, community, and public health settings that include, but are not limited to, care team member and leader, primary care provider, patient and family advocate, population health coordinator, educator, public health professional, health systems leader, organizational and public policy maker, researcher and scientist, and informaticist. Through each of these roles, nurses impact the medical and social factors that drive health outcomes and health and health care equity. Nurses can address SDOH through interventions at both the individual level (e.g., referring an individual's family to a food assistance program) and the structural level (e.g., alleviating the problem of food insecurity in the community). Similarly, nurses can address medical determinants of health at both the individual level (e.g., providing patient education and medication management) and the structural level (e.g., implementing a system of team-based multisector care that includes coordination of care across settings and sectors).

ACTING NOW TO IMPROVE THE HEALTH AND WELL-BEING OF THE NATION

The health and well-being of the nation are at an inflection point. In the decade ahead, in addition to growth in the overall size of the U.S. population, other sociodemographic factors and health workforce imbalances will increase the demand for nurses, particularly in areas in which the current registered nurse (RN) and advanced practice registered nurse (APRN) workforce is inadequate to meet the nation's health care needs. For instance, a 2020 report prepared for the American Association of Medical Colleges estimated that by 2033, current physician shortages, seen particularly in the areas of primary care, mental health, and gerontology and in rural areas, could increase—for primary care physicians, ranging between 21,400 and 55,200, and for non–primary care specialty physicians, between 33,700 and 86,700. Salient sociodemographic factors include the aging population, the increasing incidence of mental and behavioral health conditions, increases in lack of access to primary health care, persistently high maternal mortality rates, and worsening physician shortages. For example, the aging of the U.S. population means that over this decade, increasing numbers of people will age into their 70s, 80s, 90s, and beyond. In 2030, 73.1 million people, or 21 percent of the U.S. population, will be older than 65—a population that typically presents with morbidities at higher rates than are seen in younger people.

The strengths of the nursing workforce are many, yet they will be tested by formidable challenges that are already beginning to affect nurses and the health systems and organizations in which they work. These challenges will arise not only from the above changes occurring throughout the broader society but also from changes within the health care system itself and within the nursing and larger health care workforce. Further challenges for nursing will arise from health-related public policies and other factors that affect the scope of practice, size, distribution, diversity, and educational preparation of the nursing workforce. These many challenges include the need to

- increase the number of nurses available to meet the nation's growing health care needs;
- rightsize the clinical specialty distribution of nurses;
- increase the distribution of nurses to where they are needed most;
- ensure a nursing workforce that is diverse and prepared with the knowledge and skills to address SDOH;
- overcome current and future barriers affecting workforce capacity; and
- anticipate long-term impacts of the COVID-19 pandemic on the nursing workforce.

Conclusion 3-1: A substantial increase in the numbers, types, and distribution of members of the nursing workforce and improvements in their knowledge and skills in addressing social determinants of health are essential to filling gaps in care related to sociodemographic and population factors. These factors include the aging population, the increasing incidence of mental and behavioral health conditions, and the increasing lack of access to primary and maternal health care.

Access to comprehensive health services is an essential precursor to equitable, high-quality health care. Nurses can help advance health care equity and improve health outcomes by assisting people in navigating the health care system, providing close monitoring and follow-up across the care continuum, focusing care on the whole person, and providing care that is appropriate and shows cultural humility.[3] In the current system, care is often disjointed. Nurses can provide care management that helps ensure seamless care, serve as advocates for patients and communities, and assist in increasing individuals' trust in and engagement with the health care system.

Lifting Barriers to Expand the Contributions of Nursing

Nurses can address SDOH and help improve health equity by providing care management and team-based care; expanding the capacity of primary care, including maternal and pediatric care, mental health care, and telehealth; and providing care in school, home, work, and public health settings. Yet, their ability to fulfill this potential is limited by state-level regulations restricting nurse practitioners' (NPs') scope of practice. While considerable progress has been made over the past two decades in lifting such regulations, 27 states still do not allow full practice authority for NPs. As of January 2021, 23 states and the District of Columbia allowed full practice authority for NPs, permitting them to prescribe medication, diagnose patients, and provide treatment without the presence of a physician. In 16 states, NPs need a physician's authority to prescribe medication, and in 11 states, they require physician oversight for all practice.

> ***Conclusion 3-2: Eliminating restrictions on the scope of practice of advanced practice registered nurses and registered nurses so they can practice to the full extent of their education and training will increase the types and amount of high-quality health care services that can be provided to those with complex health and social needs and improve both access to care and health equity.***

Designing Better Payment Models

How care is paid for can directly influence access to care. The design of payment systems influences what health care is provided to individuals and communities, where care is provided, and by whom. Positioning health systems to work in partnership with other sectors to meet the complex health and social needs of individuals can help reduce health inequities. However, current payment systems are not designed to pay for services—including those provided by nurses, such as

---

[3] Cultural humility is "defined by flexibility; awareness of bias; a lifelong, learning-oriented approach to working with diversity; and a recognition of the role of power in health care interactions."

supporting team-based care and advancing proven interventions and strategies for reducing health disparities—that address social needs and SDOH. Going forward, payment systems need to be redesigned to recognize the value of those services.

Nurses are essential to whole-person care through their vital roles in coordinating and managing care, helping people navigate the health care system, and providing health education, as well as addressing SDOH and advancing health equity. By supporting team-based care, improved communication, and proven interventions and strategies that can reduce health disparities, payment systems can enable nurses to make these essential contributions to improving care and outcomes for all patients.

Conclusion 6-3: Payment mechanisms need to be designed to support the nursing workforce and nursing education in addressing social needs and social determinants of health in order to improve population health and advance health equity.

New payment models, such as accountable care organizations (ACOs), accountable health communities (AHCs), and value-based payment (VBP), can give health care organizations the flexibility to pursue these goals. Changing the ways in which the nation pays for health care will cause discomfort among some, but will also stimulate those seeking innovative ways of maximizing the population's health. Payment reform represents an opportunity to consider who has access to health care and who does not, what types of services are needed to improve individual and population health, and how the nation's resources can be used most wisely to these ends.

Strengthening Nursing Education

Nursing education needs to be markedly strengthened to prepare nurses to identify and act on the complex social, economic, and environmental factors that influence health and well-being. In particular, their education needs to provide nursing students with substantive, diverse, and sustained community-based experiences, as well as to substantially reorient curricula and reevaluate hiring and admission practices so as to achieve a diverse faculty and student population.

Nursing organizations have developed guidelines for how nursing education should prepare nurses to address health equity issues and SDOH in a meaningful way. The American Association of Colleges of Nursing's (AACN's) *Essentials* provides an outline for the necessary curriculum content and expected competencies for graduates of baccalaureate, master's, and doctor of nursing practice (DNP) programs. Yet, despite this guidance and the numerous calls to incorporate equity, population health, and SDOH into undergraduate and graduate nursing education, these and related concepts are currently not well integrated into nursing curricula.

Conclusion 7-1: A curriculum embedded in coursework and experiential learning that effectively prepares students to promote health equity, reduce health disparities, and improve the health and well-being of the population will build the capacity of the nursing workforce.

Nursing is increasingly practiced in community settings, such as schools and workplaces, as well as through home health care and public health clinics. Other innovative care delivery models are situated in libraries and homeless shelters and implemented through telehealth visits. Nursing students are prepared to practice in hospitals, but do not necessarily receive the same level of training and preparation for community and telehealth settings. Education in the community allows nursing students to learn about the broad range of care environments and to work collaboratively with other professionals who work in these environments, including those from nonhealth sectors.

Conclusion 7-3: Learning experiences that develop nursing students' understanding of health equity, social determinants of health, and population health and prepare them to incorporate that understanding into their professional practice include opportunities to

- ***learn cultural humility and recognize one's own implicit biases;***
- ***gain experience with interprofessional collaboration and multisector partnerships to enable them to address social needs comprehensively and drive structural improvements;***
- ***develop such technical competencies as use of telehealth, digital health tools, and data analytics; and***
- ***gain substantive experience with delivering care in diverse community settings, such as public health departments, schools, libraries, workplaces, and neighborhood clinics.***

Building a diverse nursing workforce is a critical part of preparing nurses to address SDOH and health equity. While the nursing workforce has steadily grown more diverse, nursing schools need to continue and expand their efforts to recruit and support diverse students that reflect the populations they will serve.

Conclusion 7-4: Successfully diversifying the nursing workforce will depend on holistic efforts to support and mentor/sponsor students and faculty from a wide range of backgrounds, including cultivating an inclusive environment; providing economic, social, professional, and academic supports; ensuring access to information on school quality; and minimizing inequities.

Valuing Community Nursing

School and public health nurses play a vital role in advancing health equity. Adequate funding for these nurses is essential if they are to take on that role. School nurses are front-line health care providers, serving as a bridge between the health care and education systems and other sectors. Whether they are hired by school districts, health departments, or hospitals, school nurses focus on the physical and mental health of students in the context of educational environments. They serve as both essential care providers for individuals and links to broader community health issues through the student populations they serve.

School nurses are a particularly critical resource for students experiencing such challenges as food insecurity, homelessness, and living in impoverished circumstances, for whom the school nurse may be the only health care professional they see regularly. Accordingly, access to a school nurse is a health care equity issue for some students, especially in light of the increasing number of students who have complex health needs. School nurses also are well positioned to work with students and families in their neighborhoods and homes to address individual and family social needs, such as access to care, healthy food, and safe and healthy environments/neighborhoods. More school nurses need the practice authority to address in creative ways the complex health and social needs of the populations they serve.

Likewise, the COVID-19 pandemic has highlighted the pivotal role of nurses in improving health care equity. During the pandemic, public health and hospital nurses have had to work synergistically both to help flatten the infection curve and support mitigation strategies (public health nurses) and to care for the sick and critically ill (inpatient and intensive care unit [ICU] nurses). The pandemic also has heightened the need for team-based care, infection control, person-centered care, and other skills that reflect the strengths of community nurses.

Fostering Nurses' Roles as Leaders and Advocates

Creating a future in which opportunities to optimize health are more equitable will require disrupting the deeply entrenched prevailing paradigms of health care, which in turn will require enlightened, diverse, courageous, and competent leadership. Nurses have always been key to the health and well-being of patients and communities, but a new generation of nurse leaders is now needed—one that recognizes the importance of diversity and is able to use and build on the increasing evidence base supporting the link between SDOH and health status. Today's nurses are called on to lead in the development of effective strategies for improving the nation's health with due attention to the needs of the most underserved individuals, neighborhoods, and communities and the crucial importance of advancing health equity. Implementing change to address SDOH and advance health equity will require the contributions of nurses in all roles and all settings; although no one nurse can successfully implement change without the collaboration of others. In addition to collaboration among members of the nursing profession, the creation of enduring change will require the involvement of patients and community members. Rather than a more hierarchal system of leadership, moreover, collaborative leadership assumes that everyone involved has unique contributions to make and that constructive dialogue and joint resources are needed to achieve ongoing goals.

> ***Conclusion 9-1: Nurse leaders at every level and across all settings can strengthen the profession's long-standing focus on social determinants of health and health equity to meet the needs of underserved individuals, neighborhoods, and communities and to prioritize the elimination of health inequities.***

Racism and discrimination are deeply entrenched in U.S. society and its institutions, and the nursing profession is no exception. Nurse leaders can play an important role in acknowledging the history of racism within the profession and in helping to dismantle structural racism and mitigate the effects of discrimination and implicit bias on health. If they are to take on this role, it will be essential to build a more diverse nursing workforce and support nurses of diverse backgrounds in pursuing leadership roles.

> ***Conclusion 9-4: Nurse leaders have a responsibility to address structural racism, cultural racism, and discrimination based on identity (e.g., sexual orientation, gender), place (e.g., rural, urban), and circumstances (e.g., disability, mental health condition) within the nursing profession and to help build structures and systems at the societal level that address these issues to promote health equity.***

Preparing Nurses to Respond to Disasters

The increasing frequency of natural and environmental disasters and public health emergencies, such as the COVID-19 pandemic, reveals in stark detail the critical importance of having a national nursing workforce prepared with the knowledge, skills, and abilities to respond to these events. COVID-19 has revealed deep chasms within an already fragmented U.S. health care system, resulting in significant excess mortality and morbidity, glaring health inequities, and the inability to contain a rapidly escalating pandemic. Most severely—and unfairly—affected are individuals and communities of color, who suffer from the compound disadvantages of racism, poverty, workplace hazards, limited health care access, and preexisting health conditions resulting from the foregoing factors. As other disasters and public health emergencies threaten population health in the decades ahead, articulation of the roles and responsibilities of nurses in disaster response and public health emergency management will be critical to the nation's capacity to plan for and respond to these types of events.

Conclusion 8-2: A bold and expansive effort, executed across multiple platforms, will be needed to fully support nurses in becoming prepared for disaster and public health emergency response. It is essential to convene experts who can develop a national strategic plan articulating the existing deficiencies in this regard and action steps to address them, and, most important, establishing where responsibility will lie for ensuring that those action steps are taken.

Supporting the Health and Well-Being of Nurses

Nurses' health and well-being are affected by the demands of their workplace, and in turn affect the quality and safety of the care they provide. Thus, it is essential to address the systems, structures, and policies that create workplace hazards and stresses that lead to burnout, fatigue, and poor physical and mental health among the nursing workforce. With the emergence of COVID-19, the day-to-day demands of nursing have been both illuminated and exacerbated. Nurses are coping with unrealistic workloads; insufficient resources and protective equipment; risk of infection; stigma directed at health care workers; and the mental, emotional, and moral burdens of caring for patients with a new and unpredictable disease and helping with contact tracing and testing. Moreover, if nurses are to contribute to addressing the many social determinants that influence health, they must first feel healthy, well, and supported themselves. Policy makers, employers of nurses, nursing schools, nurse leaders, and nursing associations all have a role to play to this end.

Conclusion 10-1: All environments in which nurses work affect the health and well-being of the nursing workforce. Ultimately, the health and well-being of nurses influence the quality, safety, and cost of the care they provide, as well as organizations and systems of care. The COVID-19 crisis has highlighted the shortcomings of historical efforts to address nurses' health and well-being.

RECOMMENDATIONS

The committee's recommendations (see Box S-2) call for change at both the individual and system levels, constituting a call for action to the nation's largest health care workforce, including nurses in all settings and at all levels, to listen, engage, deeply examine practices, collect evidence, and act to move the country toward greater health equity for all. The committee's recommendations also are targeted to the actions required of policy makers, educators, health care system leaders, and payers to enable these crucial changes.

BOX S-2
The Committee's Recommendations

Recommendation 1: In 2021, all national nursing organizations should initiate work to develop a shared agenda for addressing social determinants of health and achieving health equity. This agenda should include explicit priorities across nursing practice, education, leadership, and health policy engagement. The Tri-Council for Nursing[a] and the Council of Public Health Nursing Organizations,[b] with their associated member organizations, should work collaboratively and leverage their respective expertise in leading this agenda-setting process. Relevant expertise should be identified and shared across national nursing organizations, including the Federal Nursing Service Council[c] and the National Coalition of Ethnic Minority Nurse Associations. With support from the government, payers, health and health care organizations, and foundations, the implementation of this agenda should include associated timelines and metrics for measuring impact.

Recommendation 2: By 2023, state and federal government agencies, health care and public health organizations, payers, and foundations should initiate substantive actions to enable the nursing workforce to address social determinants of health and health equity more comprehensively, regardless of practice setting.

Recommendation 3: By 2021, nursing education programs, employers, nursing leaders, licensing boards, and nursing organizations should initiate the implementation of structures, systems, and evidence-based interventions to promote nurses' health and well-being, especially as they take on new roles to advance health equity.

Recommendation 4: All organizations, including state and federal entities and employing organizations, should enable nurses to practice to the full extent of their education and training by removing barriers that prevent them from more fully addressing social needs and social determinants of health and improving health care access, quality, and value. These barriers include regulatory and public and private payment limitations; restrictive policies and practices; and other legal, professional, and commercial[d] impediments.

Recommendation 5: Federal, tribal, state, local, and private payers and public health agencies should establish sustainable and flexible payment mechanisms to support nurses in both health care and public health, including school nurses, in addressing social needs, social determinants of health, and health equity.

Recommendation 6: All public and private health care systems should incorporate nursing expertise in designing, generating, analyzing, and applying data to support initiatives focused on social determinants of health and health equity using diverse digital platforms, artificial intelligence, and other innovative technologies.

Recommendation 7: Nursing education programs, including continuing education, and accreditors and the National Council of State Boards of Nursing should

continued

BOX S-2 Continued

ensure that nurses are prepared to address social determinants of health and achieve health equity.

Recommendation 8: To enable nurses to address inequities within communities, federal agencies and other key stakeholders within and outside the nursing profession should strengthen and protect the nursing workforce during the response to such public health emergencies as the COVID-19 pandemic and natural disasters, including those related to climate change.

Recommendation 9: The National Institutes of Health, the Centers for Medicare & Medicaid Services, the Centers for Disease Control and Prevention, the Health Resources and Services Administration, the Agency for Healthcare Research and Quality, the Administration for Children and Families, the Administration for Community Living, and private associations and foundations should convene representatives from nursing, public health, and health care to develop and support a research agenda and evidence base describing the impact of nursing interventions, including multisector collaboration, on social determinants of health, environmental health, health equity, and nurses' health and well-being.

---

[a] The Tri-Council for Nursing includes the following organizations as members: the American Association of Colleges of Nursing, the American Nurses Association, the American Organization for Nursing Leadership, the National Council of State Boards of Nursing, and the National League for Nursing.

[b] The Council of Public Health Nursing Organizations includes the following organizations as members: the Alliance of Nurses for Healthy Environments, the American Nurses Association, the American Public Health Association—Public Health Nursing Section, the Association of Community Health Nursing Educators, the Association of Public Health Nurses, and the Rural Nurse Organization.

[c] The Federal Nursing Service Council is a united federal nursing leadership team representing the U.S. Army, Air Force, Navy, National Guard and Reserves, Public Health Service Commissioned Corps, American Red Cross, U.S. Department of Veterans Affairs, and Uniformed Services University of the Health Sciences Graduate School of Nursing.

[d] The term "commercial" refers to contractual agreements and customary practices that make antiquated or unjustifiable assumptions about nursing.

FINAL THOUGHTS

In conclusion, the nation will never fully thrive until everyone can live the healthiest possible life. Promoting health and well-being has always been nurses' business. Thus, it is essential to harness the vast expertise and untapped potential of nurses at every level and in every setting to build healthy communities for all. As evidenced in this report, nurses are bridge builders and collaborators who engage and connect with people, communities, and organizations to promote health and well-being. But they need ongoing support from the systems that educate, train, employ, and enable them to advance health equity. As of this writing, the COVID-19 pandemic has starkly revealed the challenges nurses face every day.

But this crisis has also given some nurses more autonomy, shifted payment models, and sparked overdue conversations about dismantling racism in health care. Policy makers and system leaders must seize this moment to support, strengthen, and transform the largest segment of the health care workforce so nurses can help chart the nation's course to good health and well-being for all. Over the course of this decade, nurses will face a host of challenges—from addressing the lasting effects of COVID-19 on themselves and their communities to dismantling the racist systems that create and perpetuate inequities. No one is immune from hate and bigotry, but everyone has the capacity for empathy, understanding, and solidarity in a shared hope for a more just and equitable world. The nursing profession is resilient and well positioned to help usher in a new era in which everyone has a chance to live the healthiest possible life.

1

Introduction

It will never be comfortable or easy to advocate for change, but I am a nurse leader because I am comfortable with being uncomfortable.... I am unafraid to use my voice to influence positive change. In doing so, I have taught others how to advocate and inspired others to use their voices as well.

—Andrea Riley, RN, Nebraska 40 Under 40 Leader

Two decades ago, the Institute of Medicine (IOM) published *Crossing the Quality Chasm: A New Health System for the 21st Century* (IOM, 2001). That report delineates six aims for improving health care to reduce the burden of illness, injury, and disability and improve the functioning of the people of the United States. With the explicit purpose of securing these benefits for all people, equity was included as one of the six aims, incorporating a focus on both individuals and the population. In the intervening 20 years, among the six aims, equity in health and health care has been perhaps the least understood, considered, and addressed—until now.

Today, a rapidly growing body of evidence documenting the relationship among social determinants of health (SDOH), inequity in health and health care, and the health status of individuals and populations is generating a widespread call to action. Because of its impact on health status, achieving health equity is urgent. Achieving this goal will require stakeholders, including nurses and the nursing profession, to focus singular attention on closing the chasm between what is known about equity in health and health care and what can be done to achieve it. The 2011 IOM report *The Future of Nursing: Leading Change, Advancing Health* focuses on actions that can build critical capacity in nursing to meet increased demand for care and advance health system improvement. Significant progress has been made in building the capacity called for in that report; however, more remains to be done.

The vision of the Committee on the Future of Nursing 2020–2030, which informs this report, is the achievement of health equity in the United States built on strengthened nursing capacity and expertise. By leveraging these attributes, nursing will help to create and contribute comprehensively to equitable public health and health care systems that are designed to work for everyone. To achieve health equity, the committee also envisions a major role for the nursing profession in engaging in the complex work of aligning public health, health care, social services, and public policies to eliminate health disparities and achieve health equity.

To provide a broad and deep foundation from which to achieve this vision, the committee formulated nine recommendations (see Chapter 11) that touch on virtually every component of the nursing profession. Implementing these recommendations to achieve the committee's vision will require substantive and sustained action by the nursing profession. Nursing will need to consider and reset components of education, leadership, practice, and research, as well as the structures and priorities of vitally important nursing organizations. Nurses will need new knowledge on which to act, and the profession itself will need to reflect the diversity of the populations it serves. Nurses working in all settings will need to be prepared to participate on and lead multidisciplinary teams and multisector partnerships and, through data development, management, and use, identify and respond to challenges that disproportionately affect some segments of the U.S. population, ranging from public health emergencies to community characteristics.

The committee recognizes the significant scope and scale of its recommendations and the associated efforts required to implement them. Mobilizing to take the actions called for in this report will require change, commitment, and perseverance. Nurses will also need courage to engage in difficult conversations about racial inequities, address their own biases and those in the institutions where they work, and then participate actively in calling out and breaking down structural racism. Given the evidence delineating the adverse impacts of inequity on health, operationalizing the recommendations in this report will uphold nursing's social responsibility to improve the health of all people.

The committee also notes, however, that for nursing to make the substantive contributions needed to advance health equity, the profession will require resources, autonomy, and positions of leadership as called for in this report. Across the coming decade, nurses will be key contributors to the substantial progress toward health and health care equity that is needed in the United States. They will do so by taking on expanded roles, working in new settings in innovative ways, and partnering with communities and other sectors. Achieving this vision will require much more rapid, substantive, and widespread efforts than those undertaken to date. If the path set forth in this report and its recommendations are followed, the committee envisions that this decade will usher in a new era of promoting health equity and well-being for all, and the nursing profession will have contributed substantially to making this so.

THE NURSING PROFESSION

Nursing is the nation's largest health profession, numbering close to 4 million nurses in 2018 (HRSA, 2021). There are three categories of nurses, based on education—licensed practical nurses (LPNs)/licensed vocational nurses (LVNs), registered nurses (RNs), and advanced practice registered nurses (APRNs)—practicing in many different specialties and settings (see Box 1-1). More information about the current and future nursing workforce can be found in Chapter 3.

BOX 1-1
Types of Nursing Care Providers

Licensed practical nurses (LPNs)/licensed vocational nurses (LVNs) support the health care team and perform basic tasks, such as taking vital signs; administering medications; changing wound dressings; and ensuring that patients are comfortable and receive nutrition and hydration. LPNs/LVNs complete a 12- to 18-month-long education program at a vocational/technical school or community college, and are required to take a nationally standardized licensing exam in the state where they begin practice (IOM, 2011). In nursing homes, where they predominate, they supervise nurse aides to oversee care. LPNs/LVNs can become registered nurses (RNs) through an associate's degree or a baccalaureate in nursing bridge programs.

Registered nurses (RNs) provide preventive, primary, and acute care in collaboration with other health professionals. Their roles vary enormously by setting but can include such activities as conducting health assessments and taking health histories, looking for signs that health is deteriorating or improving, providing counseling and education to promote health and manage chronic disease, administering medications and other personalized interventions and treatments, and coordinating care. They work across the continuum of care in all health care and public health settings in a variety of interprofessional and multisector teams. RNs are required to take a nationally standardized licensing exam after completing a program at a community college, diploma school, or 4-year college or university. There are more than 50 specialty certifications for RNs, including critical care, home health and hospice, occupational and employee health, oncology, perioperative and operating room, rehabilitation, psychiatric and mental health, and school nursing.

Advanced practice registered nurses (APRNs) hold at least a master's degree in addition to the initial nursing education and licensing required for all RNs, and may continue in clinical practice or prepare for administrative and leadership positions. The responsibilities of an APRN include, but are not limited to, providing primary and preventive health care to the public and prescribing medications and tests when needed. APRNs treat and diagnose illnesses, advise the public on health issues, manage chronic disease, and coordinate care. They work in a variety of interprofessional and multisector teams. There are four categories of APRNs: certified nurse midwife, who provides a "full range of primary health care services to women throughout the lifespan," including gynecologic and obstetric care; clinical nurse specialist, who "integrates care across the continuum [... with a goal of] continuous improvement of patient outcomes and nursing care"; certified registered nurse anesthetist, who provides a "full spectrum of patients' anesthesia care and anesthesia-related care for individuals across the lifespan";

continued

BOX 1-1 Continued

and certified nurse practitioner, who provides a range of specialized services in primary, acute, and specialty health care across settings (APRN Joint Dialogue Group, 2008). Nurse practitioners are "prepared to diagnose and treat patients with undifferentiated symptoms as well as those with established diagnoses" (APRN Joint Dialogue Group, 2008). APRNs engage in continuing education to remain up to date on technological, methodological, pharmacological, and other developments in the field.

STUDY CONTEXT

As of this writing, the world is confronting the pandemic caused by the novel severe acute respiratory syndrome coronavirus 2 (SARS-CoV-2). Daily headlines report the growing numbers of sick and dying around the world. Many nurses are going to work every day, often for extended shifts, to care for patients despite the risk to themselves and their family members. Nurses are on the front lines of this crisis, in many cases without adequate personal protective equipment (PPE) or psychological PPE to promote their mental health and well-being. They are working in emergency rooms, hospitals, schools, and urgent care centers. They are in research labs and at policy-making tables. They are educating the public at the local, state, and national levels. And they are in their communities conducting testing and contact tracing and helping to dispense vaccines.

This crisis has occurred in the context of broader changes in health care in the United States that have important implications for the nursing profession. The nation is still adapting to the passage of the Patient Protection and Affordable Care Act of 2010, but additional policy changes will come in this decade with the recent passage of the American Rescue Plan Act of 2021.[1] Significantly, low- and middle-income individuals and families will receive additional help with their insurance premiums and tax credits and mental health and substance abuse services.

Approaches to health care payment are evolving, with fee-for-service payment increasingly giving way to an emphasis on the use of payment to reward providers for achieving better health outcomes. Attention to the social determinants that influence health and well-being has also increased as researchers have demonstrated the direct effects of such environmental factors as inadequate housing, food insecurity, lack of transportation, lack of or underemployment, social isolation, and unhealthy environments on health, on demands on the health care system, and on health care costs (Adler et al., 2016). Policy makers focusing on these issues are seeking to address not only rising costs but also health inequities

[1] American Rescue Plan Act of 2021, HR 1319, 117th Cong. See https://www.congress.gov/bill/117th-congress/house-bill/1319 (accessed April 10, 2021).

perpetuated by poverty, institutional and systemic racism, and discrimination, and it is important to recognize the key role of nurses in addressing these problems (Pittman, 2019).

A FOCUS ON SOCIAL DETERMINANTS OF HEALTH

The United States has devoted vast resources to medical care to improve the nation's health. Medical care denotes services clinicians provide on a daily basis, such as performing surgeries, checking blood sugar, and titrating blood pressure medications, in settings that include hospitals, surgery centers, and clinics. However, medical care emphasizes disease treatment rather than prevention and rarely addresses SDOH, such as socioeconomic factors and physical environments, that are strong predictors of health outcomes (Hood et al., 2016; Nau et al., 2019). SDOH affect a wide range of outcomes in health, functioning, and quality of life; they affect individuals, communities, and the overall health of the national population; and they have consequences for the economy, national security, business, and future generations (NASEM, 2017). Chapter 2 provides a more detailed overview of SDOH and health equity.

Available evidence suggests that characteristics both of the health care system and of communities and society influence health outcomes and their equity in the United States (IOM, 2013). There are a number of ways to conceptualize the overlapping pursuit of goals for population health, health equity, and better health care. The Centers for Disease Control and Prevention (CDC), for example, describes population health interventions as the harnessing of multiple sectors (e.g., public health, industry, academia, health care, local government) to improve health outcomes (CDC, 2019). And the Institute for Healthcare Improvement has defined the primary objectives for health care improvement as simultaneously improving the patient experience of care, improving the health of populations, and reducing the per capita cost of health care (IHI, n.d.).

Nurses' Accessibility

Nurses have long been advocates for health equity and worked to address the root causes of poor health (Pittman, 2019). Nurses at all levels are present in a wide range of settings outside of traditional health care facilities, working directly in communities to provide care in schools, workplaces, and prisons. They make home visits to families, provide primary care to school-age children, administer vaccines, provide health education, coordinate health care services within and across settings, and educate people on preventive measures for staying healthy (Bodenheimer and Mason, 2016). Nurses routinely work with people who have had adverse life experiences, including not only medical challenges but also social stressors such as trauma, lack of food, or homelessness. They are also key to the provision of long-term, hospice, and palliative care and support for caregivers (Dahlin and Coyne, 2019; Pawlow et al., 2018). Nurse practitioners (NPs) working in primary care are often the only providers caring for low-income or uninsured people, Medicaid beneficiaries, and historically disadvantaged groups in both rural and urban populations (Auerbach et al., 2018; Barnes et al., 2018; Buerhaus, 2018), who cannot always easily access a physician. These interactions give nurses opportunities to get to know and engage meaningfully with people and families on matters related to health and well-being, health care, and the social factors that influence health.

Expansion of Nurses' Responsibilities and Capabilities

Nurses are increasingly developing new kinds of expertise while transitioning to new roles and nurse-led alternative models of care (Pittman, 2019). They are helping to develop new ways of keeping individuals connected to health care services, such as telehealth and home care (Dillon et al., 2018; Glasgow et al., 2018; Machon et al., 2019). And they are increasingly moving into leadership positions in which they are serving as collaborative partners with other health care workers, as well as coordinating with others in non–health care settings and areas of focus (Dyess et al., 2016) to improve overall health.

Even as their capabilities and roles evolve, nurses will face new challenges over the coming decade. By 2030, the nursing profession will look very different than it does today and will need to provide care for a changing America. As the U.S. population changes in diversity, age, and health status, the distribution of people along those spectrums will change, and the roles of nurses will change accordingly. More than 1 million RNs in the baby boom generation, who have amassed a substantial body of knowledge and experience, will retire during this decade. Moreover, as the U.S. population ages, patients will include increasing percentages of older people, many of whom will have multiple comorbid conditions that will increase the complexity and intensity of the nursing care they require. As the population diversifies in race and ethnicity and other factors, nurses will need to be well-versed in providing care that is culturally respectful and appropriate. Nurses also will be called on to address the persistent and in most cases widening disparities in health tied to poverty, structural racism, and discrimination that have been magnified and exacerbated by the COVID-19 pandemic. There is an increasing need as well for mental health care among the general population, stemming from high rates of depression, suicide, anxiety, trauma, and stress due to such challenges as substance abuse, gun violence, and now the lingering effects of the pandemic (Baker et al., 2019). Shifts in care models, where care is delivered, and new technology applications will impact how nurses interface with individuals seeking health care. And nurses will have to expand their roles to supplement a shrinking primary care workforce, provide care to rural populations, help improve maternal health outcomes, and deliver more health and preventive care in community-based settings (Edmonson et al., 2017).

PREVIOUS WORK OF THE NATIONAL ACADEMIES ON THE FUTURE OF NURSING

Before embarking on this study, the National Academies produced two reports on the future of nursing. The first—*The Future of Nursing: Leading Change, Advancing Health* (IOM, 2011)—offered four key messages, embodied in that study committee's recommendations:

- Nurses should practice to the full extent of their education and training.
- Nurses should achieve higher levels of education and training through an improved education system that promotes seamless academic progression.
- Nurses should be full partners, with physicians and other health care professionals, in redesigning health care in the United States.
- Effective workforce planning and policy making require better data collection and information infrastructure.

In support of recommendations offered in *The Future of Nursing*, many organizations worldwide invested in bolstering the nursing workforce over the ensuing decade. The Center to Champion Nursing in America (CCNA) called for the Future of Nursing: Campaign for Action, which was organized to implement solutions to the challenges facing the nursing profession and to build on nurse-based approaches. CCNA, a joint effort of the Robert Wood Johnson Foundation (RWJF), AARP, and the AARP Foundation, is a leading national resource center created to ensure that the nation has the skilled nurses needed to provide care for all Americans, now and in the future. The Future of Nursing: Campaign for Action serves as a focal point for information, public policy research, and analysis at the state, federal, and international levels. The campaign has helped form state action coalitions—groups of nurses and other health care providers, employers, patients, students, and others—in every state to work with health, education, business, and other leaders in promoting better health through nursing to improve health equity and to create communities in which everyone has access to high-quality care. The campaign's focus has been on implementing the recommendations of the 2011 *The Future of Nursing* report, as well as inspiring and specifying strategies for involving nurses in addressing SDOH and health equity.

The second prior National Academies study on the future of nursing is a 2016 assessment of the Campaign for Action's effectiveness in achieving the goals set forth in the 2011 report. The committee that produced the report on that assessment—*Assessing Progress on the Institute of Medicine Report* The Future of Nursing (NASEM, 2016)—noted significant progress in galvanizing nurses at the national and state levels to implement the 2011 report's recommendations. However, the committee strongly encouraged the Campaign for Action to

- engage a broader network of stakeholders to increase awareness of nurses' ability to participate fully in practice, education, collaboration, and leadership among health professionals;
- promote diversity in the nursing workforce; and
- collect better data to assess and drive progress.

STATEMENT OF TASK

With the intent of building on the above two previous reports to engage nursing in efforts to achieve health equity, RWJF developed the Statement of Task for the present study, provided in Box 1-2.

BOX 1-2
Statement of Task

An ad hoc committee under the auspices of the National Academies of Sciences, Engineering, and Medicine will produce a consensus report that will chart a path for the nursing profession to help our nation create a Culture of Health, reduce health disparities, and improve the health and well-being of the U.S. population in the 21st century. The committee will consider newly emerging evidence related to the COVID-19 global pandemic and include recommendations regarding the role of nurses in responding to the crisis created by a pandemic.

The committee will also examine the lessons learned from the Future of Nursing: Campaign for Action as well as the current state of science and technology to inform the assessment of the capacity of the profession to meet the anticipated health and social care demands from 2020 to 2030, with emphasis on multisector teams and partnerships.

In examining current and future challenges, the committee will take into account the dramatically changed context and the rapidly deployed changes in clinical care, nurse education, nursing leadership, and nursing–community partnerships as a result of the pandemic. The committee will consider the following:

- the role of nurses in improving the health of individuals, families, and communities by addressing social determinants of health and providing effective, efficient, equitable, and accessible care for all across the care continuum, as well as identifying the system facilitators and barriers to achieving this goal.
- the current and future deployment of all levels of nurses across the care continuum, including in collaborative practice models, to address the challenges of building a culture of health.
- system facilitators and barriers to achieving a workforce that is diverse, including gender, race, and ethnicity, across all levels of nursing education.
- the role of the nursing profession in assuring that the voice of individuals, families, and communities are incorporated into design and operations of clinical and community health systems.

continued

BOX 1-2 Continued

- the training and competency development skills needed to prepare nurses, including advanced practice nurses, to work outside of acute care settings and to lead efforts to build a culture of health and health equity, and the extent to which current curricula meets these needs.
- the ability of nurses to serve as change agents in creating systems that bridge the delivery of health care and social needs care in the community.
- the research needed to identify or develop effective nursing practices for eliminating gaps and disparities in health care.
- the importance of nurse well-being and resilience in ensuring the delivery of high-quality care and improving community health.
- the role of nurses in response to emergencies that arise due to natural and man-made disasters and the impact on health equity.

In developing its recommendations for the future decade of nursing in the United States, the committee will draw from domestic and global examples of evidence-based models of care that address social determinants of health and help build and sustain a Culture of Health.

STUDY APPROACH

To conduct this study, the National Academies assembled a committee of 15 experts in the fields of nursing leadership, education, practice, and workforce; some members have backgrounds in health policy, economics and health care finance, informatics,[2] population health and health disparities, health care quality and delivery, and health care research and interventions. Biographical sketches of the committee members and study staff are provided in Appendix A.

The committee met eight times, including two meetings during which sessions open to the public were held. In addition, some committee members conducted site visits in Chicago, Philadelphia, and Seattle to better understand the context for the challenges and opportunities facing nurses working in different types of health care settings who are actively addressing social needs and SDOH in their work. The committee also conducted town hall meetings in those same cities to hear from other experts and gather input from interested members of the public.

Further information about the committee's data and information gathering is available in Appendix B. Briefly, in addition to its members' knowledge and expertise, its public sessions, and its town hall meetings, the committee relied on a variety of data and information sources to support its deliberations, including

[2] Nursing informatics is "the specialty that integrates nursing science with multiple information and analytical sciences to identify, define, manage and communicate data, information, knowledge and wisdom in nursing practice" (ANA, 2016).

- staff searches of the published literature, such as a search for evidence-based examples of successful programs that improved health equity in which nurses played essential roles;
- grey[3] literature searches focused on SDOH (including reports and articles from government agencies, universities, foundations, professional associations, and other organizations);
- data and analyses provided by AcademyHealth[4] in response to the committee's requests;
- papers commissioned for this study; and
- public and organizational statements pertaining to the committee's task.

Committee's Interpretation of Its Task

The committee interpreted its Statement of Task (see Box 1-2) as a challenge to map out a path for the nursing profession to help improve all aspects of the U.S. health care system and create a culture of health. As expressed by RWJF, the objective of a culture of health is "to help raise the health of everyone in the U.S." (RWJF, n.d.). The committee interpreted the concept of a culture of health as essentially denoting *health equity,* and therefore considered health equity to be its primary focus as it considered the evolving roles of nurses and the nursing profession in helping to improve population health.

Challenges in Addressing the Task

In its information-gathering process, the committee was challenged by the lack of peer-reviewed, published literature regarding the involvement and/or impact of nurses in new and challenging roles. This paucity of published literature is not surprising, given that the sponsor's charge to the committee was to look to the future. Although some published reports address innovative programs for which there is evidence and that feature nurses in key roles, many such programs are novel and have not yet reported outcomes. In other cases, reports on some programs assumed to rely heavily on nurses do not explicitly describe their roles or responsibilities. To address that challenge, the committee sought reports of potentially scalable, innovative models of care in which nurses have played key roles and for which evidence of improvement in health equity might be avail-

[3] Grey literature is "literature that is produced by and on all levels of government, academia, private industry in both print and electronic formats, and is not associated with commercial publishers" (Farace and Frantzen, 2005).

[4] AcademyHealth supports the production and use of evidence to inform policy and practice. The organization was formed in June 2000, following a merger between the Alpha Center and the Association for Health Services Research, to educate consumers and policy makers about the importance of health services research, secure funding for the field, and provide networking and professional development opportunities.

able. Similarly, new information regarding COVID-19 is continually emerging as knowledge of the novel SARS-CoV-2 is gained. Given all of these challenges, this report relies on the available knowledge base; however, the committee stresses that lessons will continue to be learned and that evidence will continue to build for years after this report has been released.

Study Framework

The committee developed a framework to guide its examination of how nursing can address medical and SDOH to improve the health of individuals and populations and increase equity in health and health care (see Figure 1-1). The framework structures this report's discussion of the key areas for strengthening the nursing profession to meet the challenges of the decade ahead. The heart of this framework is the key areas, specifically the nursing workforce (see Chapter 3), leadership (see Chapter 9), nursing education (see Chapter 7), nurse well-being (see Chapter 10), and emergency preparedness and response (see Chapter 8) and the responsibilities of nursing with respect to structural and individual determinants of health. Nurses play multiple roles in acute, community, and public health settings that include, but are not limited to, care team member and leader, primary care provider, patient and family advocate, population health coordina-

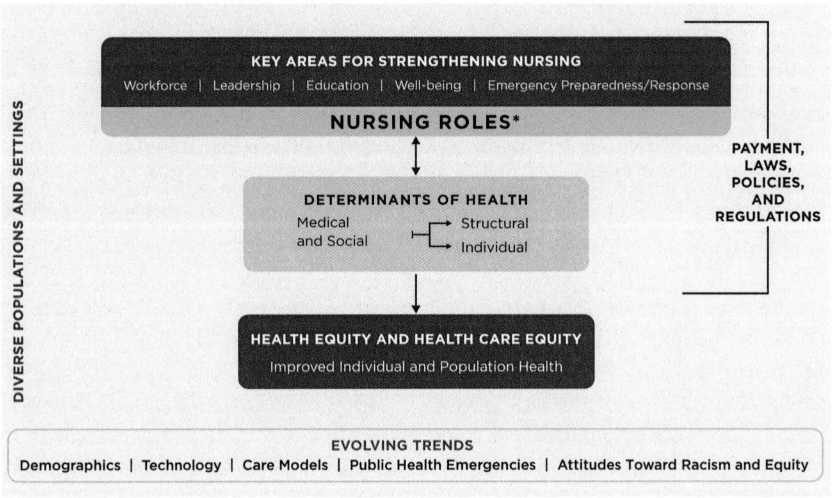

FIGURE 1-1 A framework for understanding the nurse's role in addressing the equity of health and health care.

* Examples of nursing roles in acute, community, and public health settings include care coordinator, policy maker, clinician, advocate, educator, researcher/scientist, administrator, and informaticist.

tor, educator, public health professional, health systems leader, organizational and public policy maker, researcher and scientist, and informaticist. Through each of these roles, they impact the medical and social factors that drive health outcomes and the equity of health and health care. Nurses can address SDOH through interventions at both the individual level (e.g., referring an individual's family to a food assistance program) and the structural level (e.g., alleviating the problem of food insecurity in the community). Similarly, nurses can address medical determinants at both the individual level (e.g., providing patient education and medication management) and the structural level (e.g., implementing a system of team-based multisector care that includes coordination of care across settings and sectors).

Nursing approaches need to be flexible given the complex, multiple, intersecting characteristics of individuals and families and the opportunities and demands of diverse populations and settings, as well as the many evolving trends that affect the nature of their work. Relevant trends include the aging and racial/ethnic diversification of the population, technology advances, evolving models of care, growing recognition of the importance of preparedness for and response to public health emergencies, and increasing awareness of racism and equity issues. Payment methods, laws, organizational policies, and regulations impact the ability of nurses to function successfully in addressing the determinants of health.

ORGANIZATION OF THIS REPORT

Following this introductory chapter, the report continues with Chapter 2, which provides an overview of SDOH and health equity to highlight the challenges nurses are being asked to address—themes that are repeated throughout the report. Chapter 3 explores the workforce needed to prepare the nursing profession of the future. In Chapters 4 and 5, respectively, the committee examines some of the current ways in which nurses are working to improve health care equity and health equity. Chapter 6 describes the financial infrastructure needed to support the nursing profession. Chapter 7 explores the changes in education needed to prepare and engage the nursing profession to address disparities and contribute to achieving equity in health and health care, and Chapter 8 describes the role of nurses in disaster preparedness and public health emergency response. Chapters 9 and 10, respectively, examine nursing leadership, with a focus on ensuring that nurses are leading and engaging across sectors and teams, and the importance of supporting nurses' well-being as they take on new roles and challenges to meet evolving needs. The committee's conclusions are presented in Chapters 2 through 10. Finally, Chapter 11 offers the committee's key messages and perspectives for the future in the form of recommendations and research priorities.

The report's appendixes provide additional information. The biosketches of the committee members and project staff are presented in Appendix A. Additional detail on the committee's information-gathering methods can be found in Appendix B. Appendix C presents a comprehensive overview of the methods used to gather information on the nursing workforce. Appendix D provides a glossary of the terms used throughout the report. Appendix E includes a supplemental statement on the report, followed by Appendix F, presenting the committee's response to that supplemental statement. Appendix G includes illustrative profiles of nursing programs and organizations.

REFERENCES

Adler, N. E., M. M. Glymour, and J. Fielding. 2016. Addressing social determinants of health and health inequalities. *Journal of the American Medical Association* 316(16):1641–1642.

ANA (American Nurses Association). 2016. *Nursing informatics: Scope and standards of practice.* 2nd edition. Silver Spring, MD: American Nurses Association.

APRN (Advanced Practice Registered Nurse) Joint Dialogue Group. 2008. *Consensus model for APRN regulation: Licensure, accreditation, certification & education.* https://www.ncsbn.org/Consensus_Model_for_APRN_Regulation_July_2008.pdf (accessed March 23, 2021).

Auerbach, D. I., D. O. Staiger, and P. I. Buerhaus. 2018. Growing ranks of advanced practice clinicians—Implications for the physician workforce. *New England Journal of Medicine* 378(25):2358–2360.

Baker, M. W., C. Dower, P. B. Winter, M. M. Rutherford, and V. T. Betts. 2019. Improving nurses' behavioral health knowledge and skills with mental health first aid. *Journal for Nurses in Professional Development* 35(4):210–214.

Barnes, H., M. R. Richards, M. D. McHugh, and G. Martsolf. 2018. Rural and nonrural primary care physician practices increasingly rely on nurse practitioners. *Health Affairs* 37(6):908–914.

Bodenheimer, T., and D. Mason. 2016. Registered nurses: Partners in transforming primary care. In *Preparing Registered Nurses for Enhanced Roles in Primary Care.* Conference conducted in Atlanta, GA, sponsored by the Josiah Macy Jr. Foundation. New York: Josiah Macy Jr. Foundation.

Buerhaus, P. 2018. *Nurse practitioners: A solution to America's primary care crisis.* Washington, DC: American Enterprise Institute.

CDC (Centers for Disease Control and Prevention). 2019. *What is population health?* https://www.cdc.gov/pophealthtraining/whatis.html (accessed November 7, 2020).

Dahlin, C., and P. Coyne. 2019. The palliative APRN leader. *Annals of Palliative Medicine* 8(1):S30–S38.

Dillon, J., J. N. Himes, K. Reynolds, and V. Schirm. 2018. An innovative partnership to improve student health: Response to a community health needs assessment. *Journal of Nursing Administration* 48(3):149–153.

Dyess, S. M., B. A. Pratt, L. Chiang-Hanisko, and R. O. Sherman. 2016. Growing nurse leaders: Their perspectives on nursing leadership and today's practice environment. *Online Journal of Issues in Nursing* 21(1).

Edmonson, C., C. McCarthy, S. Trent-Adams, C. McCain, and J. Marshall. 2017. Emerging global health issues: A nurse's role. *Online Journal of Issues in Nursing* 22(1).

Farace, D. J., and J. Frantzen. 2005. *A review of four information professionals—their work and impact on the field of grey literature.* In GL5 Conference Proceedings. http://www.textrelease.com/images/TGJ_V1N3.pdf#page=34 (accessed July 23, 2021).

Glasgow, M. E. S., A. Colbert, J. Vator, and S. Cavanagh. 2018. The nurse–engineer: A new role to improve nurse technology interface and patient care device innovations. *Journal of Nursing Scholarship* 50(6):601–611.

Hood, C. M., K. P. Gennuso, G. R. Swain, and B. B. Catlin. 2016. County health rankings: Relationships between determinant factors and health outcomes. *American Journal of Preventive Medicine* 50(2):129–135.

HRSA (Health Resources and Services Administration). 2021. *Technical report for the national sample survey of registered nurses*. https://bhw.hrsa.gov/data-research/access-data-tools/national-sample-survey-registered-nurses (accessed March 23, 2021).

IHI (Institute for Healthcare Improvement). n.d. *The IHI triple aim*. http://www.ihi.org/Engage/Initiatives/TripleAim/Pages/default.aspx (accessed October 7, 2020).

IOM (Institute of Medicine). 2001. *Crossing the quality chasm: A new health system for the 21st century*. Washington, DC: National Academy Press.

IOM. 2011. *The future of nursing: Leading change, advancing health*. Washington, DC: The National Academies Press.

IOM. 2013. *U.S. health in international perspective: Shorter lives, poorer health*. Washington, DC: The National Academies Press.

Machon, M., D. Cundy, and H. Case. 2019. Innovation in nursing leadership: A skill that can be learned. *Nursing Administration Quarterly* 43(3):267–273.

NASEM (National Academies of Sciences, Engineering, and Medicine). 2016. *Assessing progress on the Institute of Medicine report* The Future of Nursing. Washington, DC: The National Academies Press.

NASEM. 2017. *Communities in action: Pathways to health equity*. Washington, DC: The National Academies Press.

Nau, C., J. L. Adams, D. Roblin, J. Schmittdiel, E. Schroeder, and J. F. Steiner. 2019. Considerations for identifying social needs in health care systems: A commentary on the role of predictive models in supporting a comprehensive social needs strategy. *Medical Care* 57(9):661–666.

Pawlow, P., C. Dahlin, C. L. Doherty, and M. Ersek. 2018. The hospice and palliative care advanced practice registered nurse workforce: Results of a national survey. *Journal of Hospice & Palliative Nursing* 20(4):349–357.

Pittman, P. 2019. Rising to the challenge: Re-embracing the Wald model of nursing. *American Journal of Nursing* 119(7):46–52.

RWJF (Robert Wood Johnson Foundation). n.d. *About RWJF*. https://www.rwjf.org/en/about-rwjf.html (accessed January 13, 2020).

2

Social Determinants of Health and Health Equity

As a nurse, we have the opportunity to heal the heart, mind, soul and body of our patients, their families and ourselves. They may forget your name, but they will never forget how you made them feel.

—Maya Angelou, author, poet, and civil rights activist

The United States spends more money on health care than any other highly industrialized country, yet it has the highest poverty rate, the greatest income inequality, and some of the poorest health outcomes of the developed countries. Although access to health care is important, health is driven by many factors outside of medical care, including the neighborhood where one lives, the kind of job one has, one's economic status, one's level of education, and one's access to such things as healthy foods and reliable transportation. The roots of health inequities are deep and complex. It is critical that today's and tomorrow's nurses understand the extent to which health is shaped by conditions beyond medical care and what it will take to help everyone lead a healthier life. This chapter examines the social determinants of health; how COVID-19 has exacerbated inequities in health among low-income communities and people of color that existed pre-pandemic; and the strategies and tactics that can be used to improve health upstream, midstream, and downstream.

Compared with any other country in the Organisation for Economic Co-operation and Development (OECD), the United States spends more money on health care and still has the highest poverty rate measured by the OECD, the greatest income inequality, and some of the poorest health outcomes among developed countries (Escarce, 2019). For a variety of reasons, low-income individuals, people of color (POC), and residents of rural areas in the United States experience a significantly greater burden of disease and lower life expectancy relative to their higher income, White, and urban counterparts, and this gap has been growing over time (Escarce, 2019). The roots of these inequities are deep and complex, and understanding them can help elucidate how nurses who currently serve a highly diverse population play a pivotal role in addressing social determinants of health (SDOH)—the conditions in the environments in which people live, learn, work, play, worship, and age that affect a wide range of health, functioning, and quality-of-life outcomes and risks—to improve health outcomes and reduce health inequities. To further that understanding, this chapter provides background on SDOH and highlights social factors that disproportionately affect some communities more than others; Chapters 4 and 5, respectively, describe the role of nurses in addressing these inequities in health and health care. This chapter also describes the impact of the COVID-19 pandemic in exacerbating the negative effects of SDOH and health inequities among low-income communities and POC (Garcia et al., 2020; Kantamneni, 2020).

SOCIAL DETERMINANTS OF HEALTH

The growing evidence for inequities in both health and access to health care has brought added scrutiny to SDOH. The term typically refers to "nonmedical factors influencing health, including health-related knowledge, attitudes, beliefs, or behaviors" (such as smoking) (Bharmal et al., 2015, p. 2). Examples of SDOH also include education, employment, health systems and services, housing, income and wealth, the physical environment, public safety, the social environment (including structures, institutions, and policies), and transportation (NASEM, 2019b).

SDOH have consequences for the economy, national security, business, and future generations (NASEM, 2017). Box 2-1 lists SDOH in five areas defined by the U.S. Department of Health and Human Services (HHS)—economic stability, education, social and community context, health and health care, and neighborhood and built environment.

SDOH affect everyone. They include both the positive and negative aspects of the conditions in which people are born, grow, live, work, and age. At their best, SDOH can be protective of good health. Many people, however, exhibit a pattern of social risk factors (the negative aspects of SDOH) that contribute to increased morbidity and mortality (NASEM, 2019a).

A concept related to SDOH is *social needs*—individual-level nonmedical acute resource needs related to SDOH, such as housing, reliable transportation, and a strong support system at home, that must be met for individuals to achieve good health outcomes and for communities to achieve health equity (NASEM, 2019a; Nau et al., 2019). Social needs are a person-centered concept that incor-

BOX 2-1
Social Determinants of Health

Economic Stability
- Employment
- Food Insecurity
- Housing Instability
- Poverty

Education
- Early Childhood Education and Development
- Enrollment in Higher Education
- High School Graduation
- Language and Literacy

Social and Community Context
- Civic Participation
- Discrimination
- Incarceration
- Social Cohesion

Health and Health Care
- Access to Health Care
- Access to Primary Care
- Health Literacy

Neighborhood and Built Environment
- Access to Foods That Support Healthy Eating Patterns
- Crime and Violence
- Environmental Conditions
- Quality of Housing

SOURCE: ODPHP, 2020a.

porates each person's perception of his or her own health-related needs, which therefore vary among individuals (NASEM, 2019a). The nursing community has long focused on the social needs of people and communities, and has worked closely with social workers and community health workers to address individuals' more complex social needs (Foster et al., 2019; Gordon et al., 2020). Nurse-designed models of care, discussed throughout this report, often successfully integrate the social needs of individuals and families, as documented in a recent RAND report (Martsolf et al., 2017).

Improving population health (e.g., through measures that improve life expectancy) means improving health for everyone. However, historically disadvantaged groups trail dramatically behind others by many measures of health. Health equity is achieved by addressing the underlying issues that prevent people from being healthy. At the population level, health equity can be achieved by addressing SDOH, while at the individual level, it can be achieved by addressing social needs. Health equity benefits everyone through, for example, economic growth, a healthier environment, and national security. At both the population and individual levels, work to improve health and health equity will require cross-sector collaborations and, where necessary, enabling policies, regulations, and community interventions.

Conceptual Frameworks for the Social Determinants of Health

Several frameworks have been developed to explain the interactive nature of how social factors can contribute to health. These frameworks help health professionals and others understand and address SDOH to reduce health disparities and improve health equity. Two important frameworks—the conceptual SDOH framework developed by the World Health Organization's (WHO's) Commission on the Social Determinants of Health and the Social Determinants of Health and Social Needs Model of Castrucci and Auerbach (2019)—are described below to show the relationship between health and social factors and strategies for improving health and well-being, providing context for the report's focus on the nurse's role in addressing health and health care equity.

Conceptual Social Determinants of Health Framework of the Commission on the Social Determinants of Health

In 2010, WHO's Commission on the Social Determinants of Health developed a widely used conceptual framework designed to explain the complex relationships between social determinants and health (see Figure 2-1). This framework divides SDOH into two categories: *structural determinants*, defined as SDOH inequities, such as socioeconomic and political context, social class, gender, and ethnicity; and *intermediary determinants*, defined as such SDOH as material circumstances, psychosocial circumstances, and behavioral and biological factors.

The WHO model shows how inequities created by policies and structures (structural determinants) underlie community resources and circumstances (intermediary determinants). In this model, social, economic, and political mechanisms contribute to socioeconomic position, characterized by income, education, occupation, gender, race/ethnicity, and other factors that reflect social hierarchy and status. Social standing is related to an individual's exposures and vulnera-

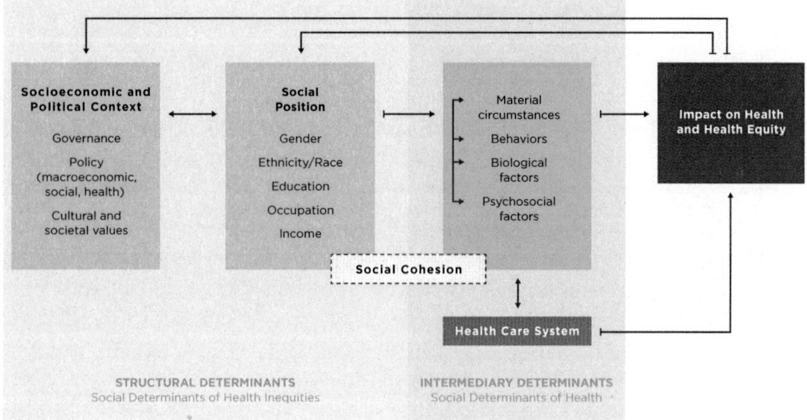

FIGURE 2-1 Conceptual framework of the Commission on the Social Determinants of Health.
SOURCE: Adapted from Solar and Irwin, 2010.

bility to health conditions. Those structural determinants shape the intermediary determinants—material conditions (e.g., living and working conditions, food security), behaviors and biological factors (e.g., alcohol and tobacco consumption, physical activity), and psychosocial factors (e.g., social support, psychosocial stress) that underlie health. All of these factors impact health, and health can also create a feedback loop back to the structural determinants. For example, poor health or lack of education can impact an individual's employment opportunities, which in turn constrains income. Low income reduces access to health care and nutritious food and increases hardship (NEJM Catalyst, 2017; Solar and Irwin, 2010).

The health care system falls in the framework as an intermediary determinant. The impact of the health care system creates another layer of determinants based on differences in access to and quality of care. By improving equitable access to health care and creating multisector solutions to improve health status—such as access to healthy food, transportation, and linkage to other social services as needed—the health care system can address disparities in health (Solar and Irwin, 2010). Furthermore, the health care system provides an opportunity to mediate the indirect consequences of poor health related to deteriorating social status (Solar and Irwin, 2010). Understanding the complex relationship between SDOH and health is essential in order for nurses to address health equity. Accordingly, Chapter 9 highlights the importance of transforming nursing curriculum and continuing education by integrating SDOH to improve health equity.

Social Determinants of Health and Social Needs Model

Throughout this report, the committee uses the Social Determinants of Health and Social Needs Model of Castrucci and Auerbach (2019) to describe the upstream, midstream, and downstream strategies used by nurses to improve individual and population health (see Figure 2-2). *Upstream* factors represent SDOH and affect communities in a broad and inequitable way. Low educational status and opportunity, income disparity, discrimination, and social marginalization are upstream factors that prevent good health outcomes. For example, nurses engage in upstream factors by informing government policies at the local and federal levels. *Midstream* factors represent social needs, or the individual factors that might affect a person's health. These are specific nonmedical acute resource needs that lie on the causal path between SDOH and health inequities (Nau et al., 2019). Midstream factors that might prevent a person from achieving optimal health include homelessness, food insecurity, poor access to education, and trauma. Through midstream efforts, nurses focus on preventing disease and meeting social needs—for example, in federally qualified health centers or through public health departments—by screening for such social risk factors as lack of housing and food access and using these data to inform referrals to government and community resources related to the identified social needs. Activities addressing *downstream* factors include disease treatment and chronic disease management, in which nurses typically engage in settings where health care is delivered, from homes to urgent care clinics to hospitals. Nursing research typically focuses on downstream and midstream factors.

The majority of nurses work in hospitals and clinics; therefore, most work midstream and downstream providing individual-level interventions to patients. Nonetheless, an understanding of the interrelationships among upstream, midstream, and downstream factors and interventions is necessary to fully comprehend and influence the health of individuals and communities. Moreover, all nurses have the opportunity to work upstream through advocacy for policy changes that promote population health. To engage robustly at all three levels, however, nurses need education, training, and support. The following sections review SDOH and social needs at all three levels of this model, along with their health implications.

HEALTH IMPLICATIONS OF SOCIAL FACTORS

This section describes social factors into which people are born, that may change as they age, and that have implications for health outcomes. Additionally, it describes factors in the places where people live, including housing and homelessness, food insecurity, environmental factors, and geography/rurality, that also affect health outcomes. Before proceeding, it is important to note that social determinants intersect, with further implications for health (see Box 2-2).

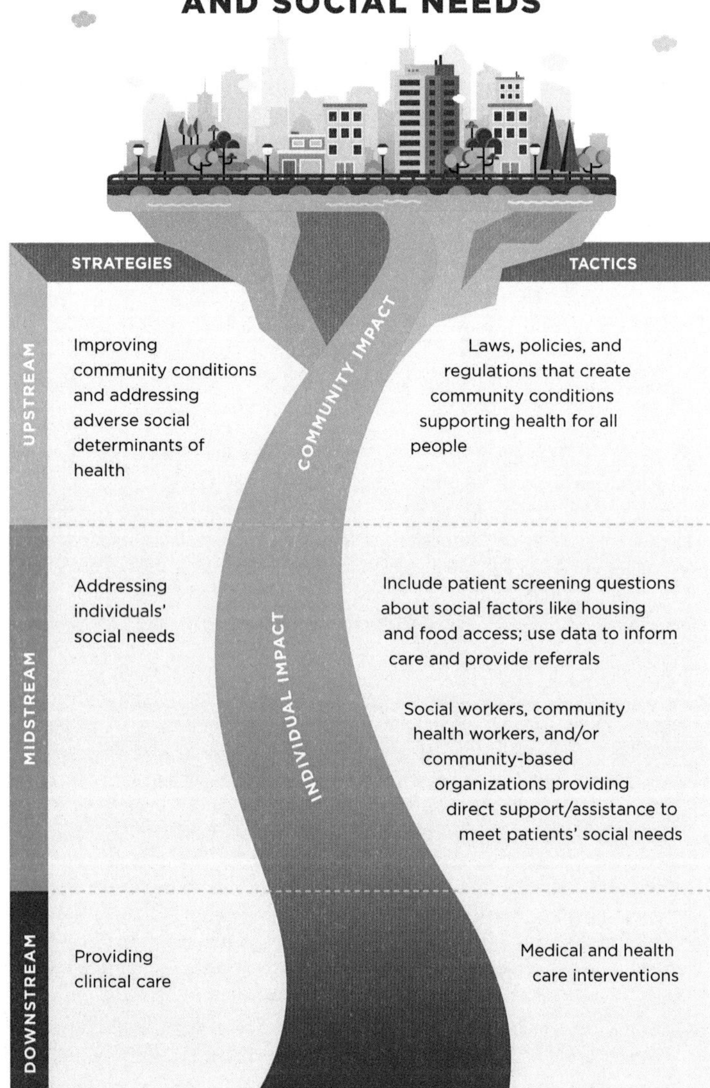

FIGURE 2-2 Social Determinants of Health and Social Needs Model.
SOURCE: Adapted from Castrucci and Auerbach, 2019.

BOX 2-2
Intersectionality

Intersectionality recognizes the complex factors contributing to health inequities by stressing the importance of the intersection of multiple interdependent social determinants that shape the health and well-being of individuals and communities. More specifically, the theoretical framework considers the intersection of these social determinants at the "micro level of individual experience to reflect multiple interlocking systems of privilege and oppression at the macro, social-structural level" (Bowleg, 2012).

In a study examining the intersection of gender, race, and class inequity; HIV-related stigma; and motherhood among African American mothers living with HIV, a majority of data from participant interviews showed that the intersection of social determinants produced an overall negative health response or worked interdependently to negatively influence a participant's health (Caiola et al., 2018). A study participant described her experiences of HIV stigma in being perceived as a sex worker and its significant impact on her psychosocial health. At the individual level, the participant's race and sex intersected with structural-level factors of racism, sexism, and HIV stigma to impact her health and well-being.

In another study, the intersection of race; gender; and socioeconomic status, such as education or income, among American adults either worked to protect against or acted as a risk factor for major depressive episode (MDE) (Assari, 2017). High income protected White women from MDE; education protected African American women; and high income was a risk factor for African American men even after controlling for other socioeconomic indicators. The results of the study show the heterogeneous effects of socioeconomic status across social groups—high income acting as a risk factor for MDE among African American men but protecting White women. The impact of socioeconomic status on a population's life circumstances can be influenced by multiple social determinants that interact to impact health and well-being negatively. Hudson and colleagues (2012) have reported on the diminishing effects of socioeconomic status (characterized by high income and education) in increasing the risk of depression among African American men when racial discrimination is high.

Findings from these studies suggest that the intersection of such social determinants as race, gender, and socioeconomic status is multiplicative rather than additive with respect to health outcomes (Assari, 2017). Although there is a wealth of literature on social determinants of health, less literature is available on the intersection of social determinants and its impact on health outcomes. A full understanding of intersectionality will allow nurses to take a more holistic approach that considers the intersection of multiple interdependent social determinants that impact the health and well-being of individuals and communities.

Race and Racism

Racism, a structural inequity that negatively impacts health and health equity, is "an organized social system in which the dominant racial group, based on an ideology of inferiority, categorizes and ranks people into social groups called 'races' and uses its power to devalue, disempower, and differentially allocate valued societal resources and opportunities to groups defined as inferior" (Williams et al., 2019, p. 106). Williams and colleagues describe three interrelated forms of racism: structural racism, cultural racism, and discrimination.

Structural racism is racism that is embedded in laws, policies, and institutions and provides advantages to the dominant racial group while oppressing, disadvantaging, or neglecting other racial groups (Williams et al., 2019). Structural racism can be seen in residential segregation, the criminal justice system, the public education system, and immigration policy. Williams and colleagues identify structural racism as the most important way in which racism impacts health. A robust body of evidence on the link between residential segregation and poor health, for example, shows that segregation is associated with outcomes that include low birthweight and preterm birth (Mehra et al., 2017) and lower cancer survival rates (Landrine et al., 2017). However, methodological limitations can make structural racism a challenging topic to study. Researchers have developed some novel measures of the phenomenon, including one that combines indicators of political participation, employment and job status, educational attainment, and judicial treatment (Lukachko et al., 2014). In this study, structural racism is defined by state-level racial disparities across those four domains. Using this measure, the researchers found that Blacks living in states with high levels of structural racism were more likely to experience myocardial infarction relative to Blacks living in states with low levels of structural racism (Lukachko et al., 2014). Another group of researchers developed a measure of state-level structural racism that combines indicators of residential segregation, incarceration rates, educational attainment, economic indicators, and employment status. This study found that higher levels of structural racism were associated with a larger disparity between Black and White victims of fatal police shootings (Mesic et al., 2018).

Structural racism has also contributed to the high incarceration rate in the United States, which exceeds the rates of other countries in which POC make up the majority of the population (Acker et al., 2019). Mass incarceration is a public health crisis that disproportionately impacts Black and Hispanic individuals and their families and communities (Brinkley-Rubinstein and Cloud, 2020; Carson, 2020). Individuals who are incarcerated have greater chances of developing chronic health conditions and are exposed to factors, including overcrowding, poor ventilation and sanitation, stress, and solitary confinement, that exacerbate chronic conditions and impact long-term physical and mental health (Acker et al., 2019; Kinner and Young, 2018). Evidence shows that following incarceration, mortality rates increase significantly, and individuals also face limited opportunities in employment, housing, and education (Massoglia and Remster, 2019).

The second form of racism, *cultural racism*, is the "instillation of the ideology of inferiority in the values, language, imagery, symbols, and unstated assumptions of the larger society" (Williams et al., 2019, p. 110). Through cultural racism, people absorb and internalize negative stereotypes and beliefs about race, which can both create and support structural and individual racism and create implicit biases (Williams et al., 2019). Implicit bias can in turn lead to unintentional and unconscious discrimination against others. Important in the context of this study is that implicit bias has been shown to be prevalent in health care (FitzGerald and Hurst, 2017; Hall et al., 2015) and to result in disparate outcomes among individuals of different races. For example, some research suggests that women of color are less likely than their White counterparts to receive an epidural during childbirth because of providers' beliefs about the relationship between race and pain tolerance, as well as poor communication in racially discordant provider–patient relationships (NASEM, 2020). Research has also shown that providers perceive Black individuals as less likely than White individuals to adhere to medical advice, a perception that contributes to poor communication and care (Laws et al., 2014; Van Ryn and Burke, 2000). These experiences of implicit bias, together with a long history of unethical treatment of POC in the health care system, can lead to mistrust and avoidance of the system, thus exacerbating health disparities (Chaturvedi and Gabriel, 2020).

Discrimination is the third—and most researched—form of racism. It occurs when people or institutions treat racial groups differently, with or without intent, and this difference results in inequitable access to opportunities and resources (Williams et al., 2019). Self-reported discrimination, in which the discrimination is perceived by the individual being discriminated against, is often used as an indicator of racism in studies on health care and health outcomes. Self-reported discrimination is believed to impact health by triggering emotional and physiological reactions and by changing an individual's health behaviors (Williams et al., 2019). It has been associated with poor health in multiple areas, including mental health (Paradies et al., 2015), sleep (Slopen et al., 2016), obesity (Bernardo et al., 2017), hypertension (Dolezsar et al., 2014), and cardiovascular disease (Lewis et al., 2014). In addition to the actual experience of discrimination, just the threat of discrimination—and the associated hypervigilance—can negatively impact health. Discrimination can also be experienced through microaggressions, defined as "brief and commonplace daily verbal, behavioral, or environmental indignities, whether intentional or unintentional, that communicate hostile, derogatory, or negative racial slights and insults toward people of color" (Sue et al., 2007, p. 273). Microaggressions have been correlated with outcomes that include poor mental health (Cruz et al., 2019), poor physical health (Nadal et al., 2017), and sleep disturbance (Ong et al., 2017). Moreover, microaggressions that are experienced within the health care setting may undermine the provider–patient relationship and thus the quality of care (Cruz et al., 2019).

The COVID-19 pandemic has brought the issue of racism as a social determinant into sharp focus, illuminating the mechanisms by which it affects health outcomes. COVID-19 has disproportionately affected Black Americans, Hispanic

Americans/Latinos, and American Indians/Alaska Natives (AI/ANs) (Cuellar et al., 2020). Blacks have been more likely to be diagnosed with COVID-19 and more likely to die relative to people of other races. The death rates for COVID-19 among Blacks reported by the Centers for Disease Control and Prevention (CDC) are higher than the rates for non-Hispanic Whites, AI/ANs, Asians, and Hispanics/Latinos (CDC, 2020a). Van Dorn and colleagues (2020) also report disproportionately high rates of COVID-19 deaths among African Americans. As of April 2020, when their article was published, three-quarters of all COVID-19 deaths in Milwaukee, Wisconsin, had occurred among African Americans, who also accounted for all but three COVID-related deaths in St. Louis, Missouri. Still, according to CDC, COVID-19 cases were 3.5 times higher among AI/ANs and 2.8 times higher among Hispanics/Latinos than among non-Hispanic Whites (CDC, 2020b). Van Dorn and colleagues (2020) point out that AI/AN populations have disproportionately high levels of such underlying conditions as heart disease and diabetes that make them more susceptible to the virus, and the Indian Health Service (IHS), which provides health care for the 2.6 million AI/ANs living on tribal reservations, has only 1,257 hospital beds and 36 intensive care units across the United States, so that many people covered by the IHS are hours away from its nearest facility (van Dorn et al., 2020).

Research on the specific mechanisms behind these disparities is ongoing, but there are many potential explanations for the link between race and COVID-19 outcomes. Camara Phyllis Jones, past president of the American Public Health Association, posits that POC are more at risk for four reasons (Wallis, 2020). First, they are more exposed to the risk of infection because they are more likely to live in dense neighborhoods, work in front-line or essential jobs, and be incarcerated or held in immigration facilities (see also van Dorn et al., 2020). This set of risk factors is tied to structural racism, including historical and current residential and educational segregation in the United States. Second, POC are less protected from infection because of cultural norms that devalue their lives and their health. Third, POC are more likely to suffer from underlying conditions that put them at risk of poor outcomes once infected. For example, Black Americans are 60 percent more likely to have diabetes and 40 percent more likely to have hypertension relative to their White counterparts (HHS, 2019, 2020). These conditions, says Jones, are due to the context of their lives—the lack of healthy food choices, more polluted air, and few places to exercise safely. Finally, POC are less likely to have access to quality health care (and thus are more likely to experience unnecessary treatments, inaccurate diagnoses, and medication errors), and more commonly face structural and individual discrimination within the health care system. Yancy (2020) echoes this analysis, noting that social distancing—one of the most effective strategies for reducing transmission of COVID-19—is a privilege that is unavailable to many POC because of where they live and work.

The confluence in 2020 of the COVID-19 pandemic and the Black Lives Matter[1] protests has brought new opportunities for nurses to be involved in dismantling racism. For example, while the American Nurses Association (ANA) issued a position statement in 2018 opposing individual and organizational discrimination (ANA Ethics Advisory Board, 2019), its 2020 resolution took an even stronger stand, calling for an end to systemic racism and health inequities and condemning brutality by law enforcement (ANA, 2020). The executive director of National Nurses United, Bonnie Castillo, stated in June 2020 that "it is racism that is the deadly disease," as reflected in disparities in health, police killings, housing, employment, criminal justice, and other areas (NNU, 2020). Nurses are attending protests to offer aid to injured protestors, despite the threat of tear gas and rubber bullets (Jividen, 2020).

Income and Wealth

Higher income (earnings and other money acquired annually) is associated with a lower likelihood of disease and premature death (Woolf et al., 2015). The relationship of wealth (net worth and assets) to health outcomes shows a similar relationship with disease and premature death. Studies have found longitudinal associations between higher levels of wealth and better health outcomes that include lower mortality, higher life expectancy, slower declines in physical functioning, and decreased risk of smoking and hypertension (Hajat et al., 2010; Kim and Richardson, 2012; Zagorsky and Smith, 2016). Significant health-related differences exist between the income levels of individuals below 100 percent and above 200 percent of the federal poverty level.

With respect to life expectancy, the expected age at death among 40-year-olds is lowest for individuals with the lowest household income and increases as household income rises (Escarce, 2019). Notably, this is a continuous gradient (see Figure 2-3). Between women in the top 1 percent and the bottom 1 percent of income, there is a 10-year difference in life expectancy. This disparity is greater among men, for whom this gap rises to 15 years. These trends have been worsening over time. Since 2000, individuals in all income groups have gained in life expectancy, but the highest earners have had the highest gains, and the gap in life expectancy between the highest and lowest earners is increasing (Escarce, 2019).

Income correlates highly as well with risk factors for chronic disease and mental health conditions. Relative to people with higher family income, for example, people with lower family income have higher rates of heart disease, stroke, diabetes, and hypertension and are more likely to have four or more common chronic conditions (NCHS, 2017). People in families whose income

[1] Black Lives Matter is a global organization whose mission is "to eradicate white supremacy and build local power to intervene in violence inflicted on Black communities by the state and vigilantes" (BLM, n.d.).

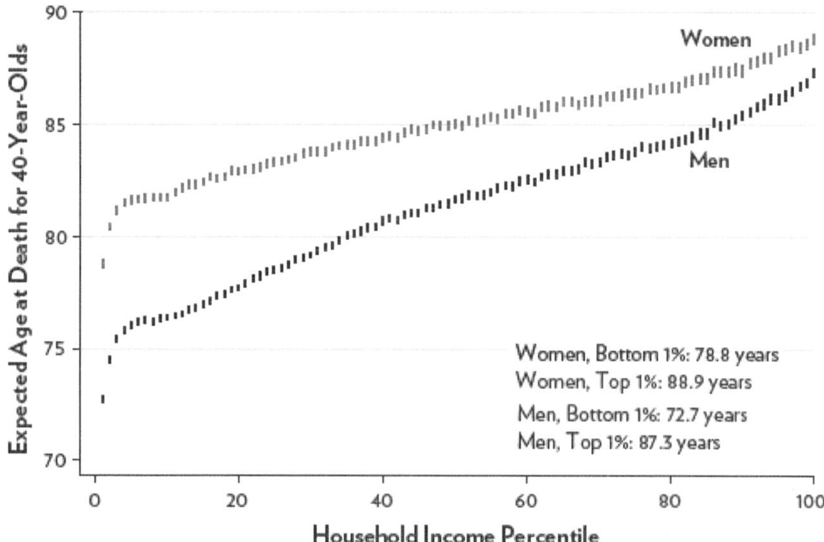

FIGURE 2-3 Expected age at death among 40-year-old men and women, by household income percentile.
SOURCES: Escarce, 2019; reproduced from Chetty et al., 2016.

is below 200 percent of the federal poverty level are more likely than people in families with higher income to be obese and to smoke cigarettes. Adults who live in poverty are also more likely to have self-reported serious psychological distress—6.4 percent of those making less than $35,000 feel sadness and 3.8 percent feel worthlessness, compared with 1.3 percent and 0.6 percent, respectively, of those making $75,000–$99,999 (Weissman et al., 2015; Woolf et al., 2015).

In addition to impacting the safety and quality of neighborhoods and schools, parental income and wealth can affect the resources and support available within families (Chetty and Hendren, 2018). Children in low-income families typically face barriers to educational and social opportunities, which in turn limits their social mobility and good health as adults (Braveman et al., 2018; Killewald et al., 2017; Odgers and Adler, 2018; Owen and Candipan, 2019). As health and socioeconomic disadvantages accumulate over a person's lifetime, this pattern of inequity, exacerbated by structural barriers, can persist across generations, preventing intergenerational social mobility (Braveman et al., 2018; Chetty et al., 2014).

Access to Health Care

Equitable access to health care is needed for "promoting and maintaining health, preventing and managing disease, reducing unnecessary disability and premature death, and achieving health equity" (ODPHP, 2020b). Evidence shows that access to primary care prevents illness and death and is associated with positive health outcomes (Levine et al., 2019; Macinko et al., 2007; Shi, 2012). Access to health care services is therefore an important SDOH, and inequities in multiple factors, such as a lack of health insurance coverage and limited availability of health care providers, limit that access.

Studies have shown that individuals without health insurance are much less likely to receive preventive care and care for major health conditions and chronic diseases (Cole et al., 2018; Seo et al., 2019). In a study of nonelderly adult patients, insured versus uninsured individuals were more likely to obtain necessary medical care, see a recommended specialist, see a mental health professional if advised, receive recommended follow-up care after an abnormal pap test, and get necessary prescription medications (Cole et al., 2018). Lack of insurance is also associated with a lower likelihood of receiving treatments recommended by health care providers and longer appointment wait times (Chou et al., 2018; Fernandez-Lazaro et al., 2019). In one study, two groups posing as new patients discharged from the emergency department requested follow-up appointments. Those who claimed commercial insurance were more likely than the Medicaid-insured group to receive care within 7 days (Chou et al., 2018).

Wide income and racial/ethnic inequities in insurance coverage therefore have a significant effect on access to health care services, thus influencing health equity. In the United States, African American and Hispanic individuals have a higher risk of being uninsured relative to non-Hispanic Whites (Artiga et al., 2020). Census Bureau data indicate that Hispanics face the greatest barriers to health insurance: between 2017 and 2018, the uninsurance rate increased from 16.2 to 17.8 percent for Hispanics, from 9.3 to 9.7 percent for Blacks, from 6.4 to 6.8 percent for Asians, and from 5.2 to 5.4 percent for non-Hispanic Whites (Barnett et al., 2019). American Indians have high uninsured rates; CDC reports that 28.6 percent of these individuals under age 65 are uninsured (HHS, 2018). It is important to note that uninsured people often delay or forgo care because of its cost and are less likely than those with insurance to have a usual source of care or receive preventive care (Amin et al., 2019), which can lead them to experience serious illness or other health problems. Chapter 4 provides information on nursing's role in expanding access to health care.

Access to Education

Lower-income families often live in school districts that are resource-poor, and they lack the resources available to upper-income families for making investments in early childhood enrichment activities. Over time, the gap between the rich and poor with respect to receiving higher education has widened. Children born in 1979–1982 were 18 percent more likely to complete college if their parents were in the highest relative to the lowest income quartile. More recently, this percentage has grown to 69.2 percent (Woolf et al., 2015).

Hahn and Truman (2015) report a strong association between educational attainment and both morbidity and mortality. In the United States, adults with lower educational attainment have higher rates of major circulatory diseases; diabetes; liver diseases; and such psychological symptoms as feelings of sadness, hopelessness, and worthlessness (although those with higher levels of educational attainment experience higher rates of prostate cancer and sinusitis). As for life expectancy, in 2017 a White man in the United States with less than a high school education could expect to live 73.5 years, while his counterpart with a graduate degree could expect to live more than 10 years longer. Likewise, a White woman could expect to live 8 years longer if she had a graduate degree than if she had less than a high school degree (Sasson and Howard, 2019).

Housing Instability and Homelessness

Research shows that people need stable housing to be healthy; people with limited resources and unstable housing are exposed to a number of health risks but often cannot move to better neighborhoods (Woolf et al., 2015). Homelessness also is closely linked to poor physical and mental health. Homeless people experience higher rates of such health problems as HIV, alcohol and drug abuse, mental illness, tuberculosis, and other conditions (Aldridge et al., 2018; Mosites et al., 2020). Providing stable housing coupled with such services as case management has been shown to improve mental health and health status in both children and parents (Bovell-Ammon et al., 2020).

Researchers have identified four pathways by which housing and health are connected (Taylor, 2018):

- *The stability pathway*: As noted above, not having stable housing has negative effects on health. Health problems among youth associated with residential instability include increased risk of teen pregnancy, early drug use, and depression (Taylor, 2018).
- *The quality and safety pathway*: A number of negative environmental factors within homes are correlated with poor health. In-home exposure to lead irreversibly damages the brains and nervous systems of children. Substandard housing conditions, such as water leaks, poor ventilation, poor air quality, dirty carpets, mold, and pest infestation, have been associated with poor health outcomes, most notably asthma (Taylor, 2018).
- *The affordability pathway*: A lack of affordable housing options can affect families' ability to meet other essential expenses and create serious financial strain. Low-income families with difficulty paying rent or utilities are less likely to have a usual source of medical care and more likely to postpone needed treatment (Taylor, 2018).

- *The neighborhood pathway*: Researchers have found that the availability of resources, such as public transportation to one's job, grocery stores with nutritious foods, and safe spaces to exercise, is correlated with better health outcomes (Taylor, 2018).

Food Insecurity

Food-insecure households are those that lack the resources to purchase adequate food to maintain their health. The U.S. Department of Agriculture (USDA) estimates that in 2018, 11.1 percent of U.S. households were food-insecure at some time during the year (USDA, 2020). Residents of low-resource neighborhoods often have limited access to sources of healthy food, such as supermarkets that sell fresh produce and other healthful food options. They are more likely to live in food deserts, characterized by an overconcentration of fast food outlets, corner stores, and liquor stores and a shortage of options for fresh fruits and vegetables and restaurants that offer healthy choices and menu labeling (Woolf et al., 2015).

Gundersen and Ziliak (2015) reviewed the literature on the effect of food insecurity on health in the United States. They found that the majority of research in this area has focused on children, revealing that food insecurity is associated with birth defects, anemia, lower nutrient intakes, cognitive problems, and aggression and anxiety, as well as higher hospitalization rates, poorer general health, asthma, behavioral problems, depression, suicidal ideation, and poor oral health. The authors also found that food insecurity is more common in households headed by an African American or Hispanic person and households with children (Gundersen and Ziliak, 2015). COVID-19 has exacerbated food insecurity; Feeding America estimates that almost 17 million individuals may have experienced food insecurity during the pandemic (Balch, 2020).

Environment and Climate Change

Environmental conditions affect the health of all individuals and communities. Environmental hazards, such as air pollution, harmful agricultural chemicals, and poor water quality, are more likely to exist in low-income communities and those populated by POC, and those communities tend to be more vulnerable to such hazards. Additionally, while natural disasters, such as floods, hurricanes, tornadoes, fires, winter storms, drought, and earthquakes, pose great threats to life and property and strain emergency and health care services wherever they strike, they affect underresourced populations more severely. These populations are more likely to live in geographic areas that are at high risk of natural disasters, such as flood plains, and to live in housing that is less resilient, such as mobile homes. Moreover, low-income residents have less capacity to move when such risks become evident (Boustan et al., 2017). In addition, the impacts of natural disasters depend not only on the magnitude of the event but also on the exposure and vulnerability of the population, which vary with levels of wealth and education; disability and health status; and gender, age, class, and other social and cultural characteristics (IPCC, 2012). These inequities become even more pronounced if populations are displaced or forced to evacuate (Supekar, 2019). Natural disasters have long-term economic impacts on communities as well. Research shows that as damages from natural disasters increase, so, too, does wealth inequity in the long term, especially in relation to race, education, and homeownership (Howell and Elliott, 2018).

Researchers have increasingly found evidence that global climate change is increasing the magnitude and frequency of such severe events, including droughts, wildfires, and damaging storms (McNutt, 2019). Extreme weather (heat, drought), flooding, air and water pollution, allergens, vector- and water-borne diseases (Demain, 2018; IFRC, 2019), fire and its effects on air quality (Fann et al., 2018), and effects on the food supply related to nutrition and migration (NASEM, 2018)—all developments exacerbated by climate change—are already affecting human health around the globe. The changing climate will mean new challenges to health and disproportionate stress on some communities.

Rurality

Geography is associated with barriers to high-quality health care that can impact health outcomes. Rural Americans face numerous health inequities compared with their urban counterparts. More than 46 million Americans, or 15 percent of the U.S. population, live in rural areas (CDC, 2017). Compared with metropolitan areas, rural areas have higher death rates across the five leading causes of death nationally (heart disease, stroke, cancer, unintentional injury, and chronic lower respiratory disease). Among those aged <80 years in 2014, the numbers of potential excess deaths in rural areas for those five leading causes were 25,278 from heart disease, 19,055 from cancer, 12,165 from unintentional injury, 10,676 from chronic lower respiratory disease, and 4,108 from stroke. Death rates for unintentional injuries are 50 percent higher in rural than in metropolitan areas, attributable mainly to motor vehicle crashes and opioid overdoses (Garcia et al., 2017; Moy et al., 2017). Rural relative to urban residents have a higher percentage of several risk factors associated with poorer health. For example, obesity prevalence is significantly higher among rural than urban residents (34.2 percent versus 28.7 percent) (Lundeen et al., 2018).

Inequities within rural areas also exist, particularly at the intersection of geography and race and ethnicity. Based on County Health Rankings data for 2015, rural counties in which the majority of the population was non-Hispanic White had higher median household incomes, lower unemployment rates, fewer households with people younger than 18, and better access to healthy food compared with counties where other racial and ethnic groups made up the majority of the population. Not only did counties with majority Black and majority AI/AN residents have significantly greater potential years of life lost before age 75 relative to counties with predominantly White residents, but also those differences were mediated by sociodemographic characteristics, including household income, unemployment rates, and the number of primary care physicians in the county (Henning-Smith et al., 2019).

Shortages of Health Care Providers

Shortages of health care providers significantly affect access to care in rural areas; as of December 2019, approximately 62.9 percent of primary care health professional shortage areas (HPSAs) were located in rural areas (RHI, 2020). According to the Georgetown University Health Policy Institute, less than 11 percent of U.S. physicians practice in rural areas, while 20 percent of the U.S. population lives in these areas (Georgetown University, n.d.). Adding to this challenge is the closure of more than 160 rural hospitals since 2005 as the result of a number of factors, including decreasing profits, consolidation of the health care system, high rates of uninsured, and waning rural populations to support hospitals (Cecil G. Sheps Center for Health Services Research, 2014a,b). The decline in rural acute care services highlights the increased need for primary care and individual and community-wide education in these areas to help prevent and manage chronic conditions and avoid related health crises that can lead to hospitalization and death (RHI, 2020).

Health Insurance Status

Uninsured rural residents face greater difficulty accessing care compared with their urban counterparts because of the limited supply of rural health care personnel who can provide low-cost or charity health care (Newkirk and Damico, 2014). According to a June 2016 issue brief from HHS, 43.4 percent of uninsured rural residents reported not having a usual source of care (Avery et al., 2016). The brief also states that 26.5 percent of uninsured rural residents had delayed receiving health care in the past year because of cost constraints. The affordability of health insurance is also a barrier for rural residents (Barker et al., 2018).

Transportation and Internet Access

Transportation poses a barrier to accessing appropriate care for all underresourced populations because of the travel time, cost, and time away from work involved. In rural areas, individuals are more likely to have to travel long distances for care, which can be burdensome given the higher rates of rural versus urban poverty. Longer distances can also result in longer wait times for emergency medical services and endanger individuals seeking prompt care for a potentially life-threatening emergency. Moreover, rural areas lack reliable transportation, whereas urban areas often have public transit available as an option for traveling to appointments.

Telehealth can help mitigate the challenges associated with transportation in rural areas; however, adequate broadband access is often limited in these areas. Almost 33 percent of rural individuals lack access to high-speed broadband Internet, defined by the Federal Communications Commission as download speeds of 25 Mbps or higher (FCC, 2015). Without access to broadband Internet, individuals seeking care cannot access video-based telehealth visits. In Michigan, for example, approximately 40 percent of rural residents lack access to high-speed broadband Internet versus just 3 percent of urban residents (FCC, n.d.). Thus, the shift to telehealth during COVID-19 may have exacerbated health disparities for millions of individuals living in rural areas.

THE COVID-19 PANDEMIC AND HEALTH INEQUITIES

The economic impacts of COVID-19 have been wide-reaching in the face of record high unemployment rates (BLS, 2020). The effects of the pandemic on both health and income have been especially severe for low-income individuals and POC. Internationally, rates of job loss have been high among low-income versus high-income people, further impacting their ability to access such essentials as healthy food (Daly et al., 2020; Lopez et al., 2020).

The disproportionate effects of COVID-19 on POC were discussed earlier in the chapter. Undocumented immigrants are another population in the United States that has been particularly vulnerable to the effects of the virus. An estimated 7.1 million undocumented immigrants lack health insurance, and the Patient Protection and Affordable Care Act excludes undocumented immigrants from eligibility for coverage. As a result, many undocumented immigrants lack access to primary care and have relied on emergency departments for years (Page et al., 2020). Although immigrant communities tend to be relatively young and healthy, the prevalence of diabetes, a risk factor for COVID-19, is high (22 percent) among Hispanics (Page et al., 2020). The prevalence of diabetes is also high among AI/ANs—14.7 percent for adults (CDC, 2018). Additionally, as in the African American community, a high proportion of undocumented workers are employed in service industries, such as restaurants and hotels, or in the informal economy, which places them at increased risk of infection.

Another important consideration is the inequity inherent in school closures during the pandemic, which has affected children from underresourced families disproportionately. As with telehealth, access to distance learning is unequal for those who lack access to the Internet or the requisite technologies. Moreover, many underresourced communities rely on subsidized meal programs for adequate nutrition and on school nurses for vaccines and other health care services (Armitage and Nellums, 2020). Schools also may provide safeguarding and supervision, and school closures mean that parents considered essential workers may leave children unsupervised at home or forgo employment to stay at home with them (Armitage and Nellums, 2020). Low-income families have fewer resources to expend on their children's at-home education, meaning that during the pandemic, their children have fallen further behind relative to higher-income classmates who may have easier access to computers and the Internet while they are distance learning.

People in prisons, nursing homes, homeless shelters, and refugee camps constitute other vulnerable populations at higher risk during the pandemic. Many people in certain congregate settings have inadequate access to even basic health care, and many are older and have preexisting conditions, in addition to their close proximity to other people, that have placed them at high risk of infection (Berger et al., 2020). CDC assessed the prevalence of COVID-19 infections in homeless shelters in four U.S. cities during March 27–April 15, 2020, working with local partners to test residents and staff proactively, and found high levels of COVID-19 in both groups. Specifically, they found that 17 percent of residents and 17 percent of staff in Seattle, Washington; 36 percent of residents and 30 percent of staff in Boston, Massachusetts; and 66 percent of residents and 16 percent of staff in San Francisco, California, tested positive for the virus. Clearly, in many congregate care environments both residents and staff have been at high risk for contracting this disease; the latter, many of whom are low-income, are often deemed essential workers.

Emerging morbidity and mortality data further demonstrate that the effects of the pandemic have fallen disproportionately on vulnerable U.S. populations and exacerbate the deeply rooted social, racial, and economic disparities to which these populations are subject. Berger and colleagues (2020) note that underserved communities are distrustful of public health institutions, which have historically mistreated them, and suggest that it is unfair to ask them to act in the public interest by staying home at the expense of supporting themselves and their families. Governments, institutions, and health care facilities all have a role in enacting policies that are respectful and inclusive of vulnerable populations when the nation is faced with a public health emergency such as the COVID-19 pandemic.

In the present context, the global COVID-19 pandemic has exacerbated existing health disparities and health care challenges and long-standing ethical issues that threaten the core values of the nursing profession (Laurencin and McClinton, 2020; see Chapter 3). The roles nurses are playing to address these challenges are described throughout the report. On a positive note, however, the crisis of COVID-19 has brought much-needed attention to these challenges and has accelerated the adoption of tools and approaches for responding to them. For example, while telehealth has long been touted as a way to address issues of access to care, it took COVID-19 for clinicians, payers, and individuals to fully embrace it as a viable—and sometimes even preferred—alternative to in-person care (Shah et al., 2020).

Before the COVID-19 pandemic, the United States was combatting the opioid overdose epidemic, which has led to devastating consequences that include opioid misuse, overdoses, and a rising number of newborns experiencing withdrawal syndrome due to parental opioid use and misuse during pregnancy (NIH, 2021). Data for 2019 show that 70,630 people had died from drug overdose, 1.6 million had experienced an opioid use disorder, and 10.1 million had misused prescription opioids in the past year (HHS, 2021). The opioid epidemic is a public health crisis that impacts both social and economic welfare, and its convergence with the COVID-19 pandemic has exacerbated health disparities and created new health care challenges that need to be addressed.

CONCLUSION

People of lower socioeconomic status, rural populations, and communities of color experience a higher burden of poor health relative to those of higher socioeconomic status, urban populations, and Whites, and the health inequity gap has been growing over time. Such inequities are unnecessary, unjust, and avoidable. The roots of these inequities are shaped by structural determinants, and understanding and acting on those determinants will help nurses play a pivotal role in improving health equity. Improving social conditions upstream and midstream has been found to have positive impacts on health status, and improving those conditions will likely reduce health inequities and improve the health of the U.S. population as a whole. Changes upstream through changes in national policy and midstream at the individual level through integrated social care are needed to connect individuals to social services that include healthy food, affordable housing, and transportation. As an example, although many other developed nations spend less per capita than the United States on medical services, they spend more on social services related to medical care, and their residents lead healthier lives (NASEM, 2019a). Addressing SDOH requires a community-oriented approach that involves aligning health care resources and investments to facilitate collaborations with community and government sectors, and bringing health care assets into broader advocacy activities that augment and strengthen social care resources (NASEM, 2019a).

This report focuses on how the next generation of nurses can contribute to efforts to address SDOH and achieve health equity if provided with appropriate resources, including education, training, and financial support. Later chapters will describe the relatively new efforts of nurses to address SDOH that have been enabled, for example, by new technologies, changes in payment models, and integration of social care.

Conclusion 2-1: Structural racism, cultural racism, and discrimination exist across all sectors, such as housing, education, criminal justice, employment, and health care, impacting the daily lives and health of individuals and communities of color. Nurses have a responsibility to address all of those forms of racism and to advocate for policies and laws that promote equity and the delivery of high-quality care to all individuals.

REFERENCES

Acker, J., P. Braveman, E. Arkin, L. Leviton, J. Parsons, and G. Hobor. 2019. *Mass incarceration threatens health equity in America*. Princeton, NJ: Robert Wood Johnson Foundation.

Aldridge, R. W., A. Story, S. W. Hwang, M. Nordentoft, S. A. Luchenski, G. Hartwell, E. J. Tweed, D. Lewer, S. Vittal Katikireddi, and A. C. Hayward. 2018. Morbidity and mortality in homeless individuals, prisoners, sex workers, and individuals with substance use disorders in high-income countries: A systematic review and meta-analysis. *Lancet* 391(10117):241–250.

Amin, K., G. Claxton, B. Sawyer, and C. Cox. 2019. How does cost affect access to care? *Peterson-KFF Health System Tracker*. https://www.healthsystemtracker.org/chart-collection/cost-affect-access-care/#item-start (accessed November 5, 2020).

ANA (American Nurses Association). 2020. *ANA's membership assembly adopts resolution on racial justice for communities of color*. https://www.nursingworld.org/news/news-releases/2020/ana-calls-for-racial-justice-for-communities-of-color (accessed August 23, 2020).

ANA Ethics Advisory Board. 2019. The nurse's role in addressing discrimination: Protecting and promoting inclusive strategies in practice settings, policy, and advocacy. *Online Journal of Issues in Nursing* 24(3). doi: 10.3912/OJIN.Vol24No03PoSCol01.

Armitage, R., and L. B. Nellums. 2020. Considering inequalities in the school closure response to COVID-19. *Lancet Global Health* 8(5):e644.

Artiga, S., K. Orgera, and A. Damico. 2020. *Changes in health coverage by race and ethnicity since the ACA, 2010-2018*. San Francisco, CA: Kaiser Family Foundation.

Assari, S. 2017. Social determinants of depression: The intersections of race, gender, and socioeconomic status. *Brain Sciences* 7(12).

Avery, K., K. Finegold, and X. Xiao. 2016. Impact of the Affordable Care Act coverage expansion on rural and urban populations. *ASPE Issue Brief*. Washington, DC: U.S. Department of Health and Human Services, Office of the Assistant Secretary for Planning and Evaluation.

Balch, B. 2020. *54 million people in America face food insecurity during the pandemic. It could have dire consequences for their health*. Washington, DC: Association of American Medical Colleges. https://www.aamc.org/news-insights/54-million-people-america-face-food-insecurity-during-pandemic-it-could-have-dire-consequences-their (accessed January 4, 2021).

Barker, A. R., L. Nienstedt, L. M. Kemper, T. D. McBride, and K. J. Mueller. 2018. Health insurance marketplaces: Issuer participation and premium trends in rural places, 2018. *Rural Policy Brief* 2018(3):1–4.

Barnett, M. L., D. Lee, and R. G. Frank. 2019. In rural areas, buprenorphine waiver adoption since 2017 driven by nurse practitioners and physician assistants. *Health Affairs* 38(12):2048–2056.

Berger, Z. D., N. G. Evans, A. L. Phelan, and R. D. Silverman. 2020. COVID-19: Control measures must be equitable and inclusive. *BMJ* 368:m1141.

Bernardo, C. de O., J. L. Bastos, D. A. González-Chica, M. A. Peres, and Y. C. Paradies. 2017. Interpersonal discrimination and markers of adiposity in longitudinal studies: A systematic review. *Obesity Reviews* 18(9):1040–1049. doi: 10.1111/obr.12564.

Bharmal, N., K. P. Derose, M. Felician, and M. M. Weden. 2015. *Understanding the upstream social determinants of health*. Santa Monica, CA: RAND Corporation.

BLM (Black Lives Matter). n.d. *Black Lives Matter: About*. https://blacklivesmatter.com/about (accessed March 4, 2021).

BLS (U.S. Bureau of Labor Statistics). 2020. *Employment situation news release*. https://www.bls.gov/news.release/archives/empsit_01082021.htm (accessed December 14, 2020).

Boustan, L. P., M. E. Kahn, P. W. Rhode, and M. L. Yanguas. 2017. *The effect of natural disasters on economic activity in U.S. counties: A century of data*. Cambridge, MA: National Bureau of Economic Research.

Bovell-Ammon, A., C. Mansilla, A. Poblacion, L. Rateau, T. Heeren, J. T .Cook, T. Zhang, S. de Cuba, and M. T. Sandel. 2020. Housing intervention for medically complex families associated with improved family health: Pilot randomized trial. *Health Affairs (Millwood)* 39(4):613–621.

Bowleg, L. 2012. The problem with the phrase *women and minorities*: Intersectionality—an important theoretical framework for public health. *American Journal of Public Health* 102(7):1267–1273.

Braveman, P., J. Acker, E. Arkin, D. Proctor, A. Gillman, K. A. McGeary, and G. Mallya. 2018. *Wealth matters for health equity*. Princeton, NJ: Robert Wood Johnson Foundation.

Brinkley-Rubinstein, L., and D. H. Cloud. 2020. Mass incarceration as a social-structural driver of health inequities: A supplement to *AJPH*. *American Journal of Public Health* 110(51):S14–S16.

Caiola, C., J. Barroso, and S. L. Docherty. 2018. Black mothers living with HIV picture the social determinants of health. *Journal of the Association of Nurses in AIDS Care* 29(2):204–219.

Carson, E. A. 2020. *Prisoners in 2018*. Washington, DC: U.S. Department of Justice, Office of Justice Programs, Bureau of Justice Statistics.

Castrucci, B., and J. Auerbach. 2019. Meeting individual social needs falls short of addressing social determinants of health. *Health Affairs Blog*. doi: 10.1377/hblog20190115.234942.

CDC (Centers for Disease Control and Prevention). 2017. *Rural health: Death (leading causes)*. https://www.cdc.gov/ruralhealth/cause-of-death.html (accessed November 7, 2020).

CDC. 2018. *Prevalence of diagnosed diabetes*. https://www.cdc.gov/diabetes/data/statistics-report/diagnosed-diabetes.html (accessed March 15, 2021).

CDC. 2020a. *COVID-19 hospitalization and death by race/ethnicity*. https://www.cdc.gov/coronavirus/2019-ncov/covid-data/investigations-discovery/hospitalization-death-by-race-ethnicity.html (accessed August 27, 2020).

CDC. 2020b. *CDC data show disproportionate COVID-19 impact in American Indian/Alaska Native populations*. https://www.cdc.gov/media/releases/2020/p0819-covid-19-impact-american-indian-alaska-native.html (accessed August 27, 2020).

Cecil G. Sheps Center for Health Services Research. 2014a. *Rural hospital closures: More information*. Chapel Hill: University of North Carolina. https://www.shepscenter.unc.edu/programs-projects/rural-health/rural-hospital-closures-archive/rural-hospital-closures (accessed October 14, 2020).

Cecil G. Sheps Center for Health Services Research. 2014b. *176 rural hospital closures: January 2005—present (134 since 2010)*. Chapel Hill, NC: University of North Carolina. https://www.shepscenter.unc.edu/programs-projects/rural-health/rural-hospital-closures (accessed October 23, 2020).

Chaturvedi, R., and R. A. Gabriel. 2020. Coronavirus disease health care delivery impact on African Americans. *Disaster Medicine and Public Health Preparedness* 1–3. doi: 10.1017/dmp.2020.179

Chetty, R., and N. Hendren. 2018. The impacts of neighborhoods on intergenerational mobility I: Childhood exposure effects. *Quarterly Journal of Economics* 133(3):1107–1162.

Chetty, R., N. Hendren, P. Kline, and E. Saez. 2014. Where is the land of opportunity? The geography of intergenerational mobility in the United States. *Quarterly Journal of Economics* 129(4):1553–1623.

Chetty, R., M. Stepner, S. Abraham, S. Lin, B. Scuderi, N. Turner, A. Bergeron, and D. Cutler. 2016. The association between income and life expectancy in the United States, 2001-2014. *Journal of the American Medical Association* 315(16):1750–1766.

Chou, S. C., Y. Deng, J. Smart, V. Parwani, S. L. Bernstein, and A. K. Venkatesh. 2018. Insurance status and access to urgent primary care follow-up after an emergency department visit in 2016. *Annals of Emergency Medicine* 71(4):487–496.

Cole, M. B., A. N. Trivedi, B. Wright, and K. Carey. 2018. Health insurance coverage and access to care for community health center patients: Evidence following the Affordable Care Act. *Journal of General Internal Medicine* 33(9):1444–1446.

Cruz, D., Y. Rodriguez, and C. Mastropaolo. 2019. Perceived microaggressions in health care: A measurement study. *PLoS One* 14(2):e0211620.

Cuellar, N. G., E. Aquino, M. A. Dawson, M. J. Garcia-Dia, E. O. Im, L. M. Jurado, Y. S. Lee, S. Littlejohn, L. Tom-Orme, and D. A. Toney. 2020. Culturally congruent health care of COVID-19 in minorities in the United States: A clinical practice paper from the National Coalition of Ethnic Minority Nurse Associations. *Journal of Transcultural Nursing* 31(5):434–443.

Daly, M. C., S. R. Buckman, and L. M. Seitelman. 2020. The unequal impact of COVID-19: Why education matters. *Federal Reserve Bank of San Francisco Economic Letter* 2020-17.

Demain, J. G. 2018. Climate change and the impact on respiratory and allergic disease: 2018. *Current Allergy and Asthma Reports* 18(4):22.

Dolezsar, C. M., J. J. McGrath, A. J. M. Herzig, and S. B. Miller. 2014. Perceived racial discrimination and hypertension: A comprehensive systematic review. *Health Psychology* 33(1):20–34.

Escarce, J. 2019. *Health inequity in the United States: A primer.* Philadelphia, PA: Penn Leonard Davis Institute of Health Economics.

Fann, N., B. Alman, R. A. Broome, G. G. Morgan, F. H. Johnston, G. Pouliot, and A. G. Rappold. 2018. The health impacts and economic value of wildland fire episodes in the U.S.: 2008–2012. *Science of the Total Environment* 610–611:802–809.

FCC (Federal Communications Commission). 2015. *Data: Broadband.* https://www.fcc.gov/reports-research/maps/connect2health/data.html (accessed September 2, 2020).

FCC. n.d. *Mapping broadband health in America.* https://www.fcc.gov/health/maps (accessed September 2, 2020).

Fernandez-Lazaro, C. I., D. P. Adams, D. Fernandez-Lazaro, J. M. Garcia-González, A. Caballero-Garcia, and J. A. Miron-Canelo. 2019. Medication adherence and barriers among low-income, uninsured patients with multiple chronic conditions. *Research in Social and Administrative Pharmacy* 15(6):744–753.

FitzGerald, C., and S. Hurst. 2017. Implicit bias in healthcare professionals: A systematic review. *BMC Medical Ethics* 18(1):19.

Foster, K., M. Roche, C. Delgado, C. Cuzzillo, J. A. Giandinoto, and T. Furness. 2019. Resilience and mental health nursing: An integrative review of international literature. *International Journal of Mental Health Nursing* 28(1):71–85.

Garcia, M. C., M. Faul, G. Massetti, C. C. Thomas, Y. Hong, U. E. Bauer, and M. F. Iademarco. 2017. Reducing potentially excess deaths from the five leading causes of death in the rural United States. *Morbidity and Mortality Weekly Report* 66(2):1–7.

Garcia, M. A., P. A. Homan, C. García, and T. H. Brown. 2020. The color of COVID-19: Structural racism and the pandemic's disproportionate impact on older racial and ethnic minorities. *Journals of Gerontology, Series B* 76(3):e75–e80.

Georgetown University Health Policy Institute. n.d. *Rural and urban health.* https://hpi.georgetown.edu/rural (accessed September 2, 2020).

Gordon, K., C. Steele Gray, K. N. Dainty, J. DeLacy, P. Ware, and E. Seto. 2020. Exploring an innovative care model and telemonitoring for the management of patients with complex chronic needs: Qualitative description study. *Journal of Medical Internet Research Nursing* 3(1):e15691.

Gundersen, C., and J. P. Ziliak. 2015. Food insecurity and health outcomes. *Health Affairs* 34(11):1830–1839.

Hahn, R. A., and B. I. Truman. 2015. Education improves public health and promotes health equity. *International Journal of Health Services: Planning, Administration, Evaluation* 45(4):657–678.

Hajat, A., J. S. Kaufman, K. M. Rose, A. Siddiqi, and J. C. Thomas. 2010. Do the wealthy have a health advantage? Cardiovascular disease risk factors and wealth. *Social Science & Medicine* 71(11):1935–1942.

Hall, W. J., M. V. Chapman, K. M. Lee, Y. M. Merino, T. W. Thomas, B. K. Payne, E. Eng, S. H. Day, and T. Coyne-Beasley. 2015. Implicit racial/ethnic bias among health care professionals and its influence on health care outcomes: A systematic review. *American Journal of Public Health* 105(12):e60–e76.

Henning-Smith, C., S. Prasad, M. Casey, K. Kozhimannil, and I. Moscovice. 2019. Rural-urban differences in Medicare quality scores persist after adjusting for sociodemographic and environmental characteristics. *Journal of Rural Health* 35(1):58–67.

HHS (U.S. Department of Health and Human Services). 2018. *Crude percent distributions (with standard errors) of type of health insurance coverage for persons under age 65 and for persons aged*

65 and over, by selected characteristics: United States, 2018. Table P-11c. https://ftp.cdc.gov/pub/Health_Statistics/NCHS/NHIS/SHS/2018_SHS_Table_P-11.pdf (accessed March 15, 2021).

HHS. 2019. *Diabetes and African Americans*. https://minorityhealth.hhs.gov/omh/browse.aspx?lvl=4&lvlid=18 (accessed October 20, 2020).

HHS. 2020. *Heart disease and African Americans*. https://minorityhealth.hhs.gov/omh/browse.aspx?lvl=4&lvlid=19 (accessed October 20, 2020).

HHS. 2021. *What is the U.S. opioid epidemic?* https://www.hhs.gov/opioids/about-the-epidemic/index.html (accessed March 6, 2021).

Howell, J., and J. R. Elliott. 2018. Damages done: The longitudinal impacts of natural hazards on wealth inequality in the United States. *Social Problems* 66(3):448–467.

Hudson, D. L., K. M. Bullard, H. W. Neighbors, A. T. Geronimus, J. Yang, and J. S. Jackson. 2012. Are benefits conferred with greater socioeconomic position undermined by racial discrimination among African American men? *Journal of Men's Health* 9(2):127–136.

IFRC (International Federation of Red Cross and Red Crescent Societies). 2019. *Heatwaves: Urgent action needed to tackle climate change's "silent killer."* https://media.ifrc.org/ifrc/press-release/heatwaves-urgent-action-needed-tackle-climate-changes-silent-killer (accessed March 15, 2021).

IPCC (Intergovernmental Panel on Climate Change). 2012. *Managing the risks of extreme events and disasters to advance climate change adaptation: A special report of Working Groups I and II of the Intergovernmental Panel on Climate Change*. Cambridge, UK: Cambridge University Press.

Jividen, S. 2020. *Nurses are going to protests, after work, to help injured people*. Nurse.org. https://nurse.org/articles/nurses-at-protests (accessed November 6, 2020).

Kantamneni, N. 2020. The impact of the COVID-19 pandemic on marginalized populations in the United States: A research agenda. *Journal of Vocational Behavior* 119:103439. doi: 10.1016/j.jvb.2020.103439.

Killewald, A., F. T. Pfeffer, and J. N. Schachner. 2017. Wealth inequality and accumulation. *Annual Review of Sociology* 43:379–404.

Kim, J., and V. Richardson. 2012. The impact of socioeconomic inequalities and lack of health insurance on physical functioning among middle-aged and older adults in the United States. *Health & Social Care in the Community* 20(1):42–51.

Kinner, S. A., and J. T. Young. 2018. Understanding and improving the health of people who experience incarceration: An overview and synthesis. *Epidemiologic Reviews* 40(1):4–11.

Landrine, H., I. Corral, J. G. Lee, J. T. Efird, M. B. Hall, and J. J. Bess. 2017. Residential segregation and racial cancer disparities: A systematic review. *Journal of Racial and Ethnic Health Disparities* 4(6):1195–1205.

Laurencin, C. T., and A. McClinton. 2020. The COVID-19 pandemic: A call to action to identify and address racial and ethnic disparities. *Journal of Racial and Ethnic Health Disparities* 7(3):398–402.

Laws, M. B., Y. Lee, W. H. Rogers, M. C. Beach, S. Saha, P. T. Korthuis, V. Sharp, J. Cohn, R. Moore, and I. B. Wilson. 2014. Provider-patient communication about adherence to anti-retroviral regimens differs by patient race and ethnicity. *AIDS and Behavior* 18(7):1279–1287.

Levine, D. M., B. E. Landon, and J. A. Linder. 2019. Quality and experience of outpatient care in the United States for adults with or without primary care. *JAMA Internal Medicine* 179(3):363–372.

Lewis, T. T., D. R. Williams, M. Tamene, and C. R. Clark. 2014. Self-reported experiences of discrimination and cardiovascular disease. *Current Cardiovascular Risk Reports* 8(1):1–15.

Lopez, M. H., L. Rainie, and A. Budiman. 2020 (May 5). *Financial and health impacts of COVID-19 vary widely by race and ethnicity*. Pew Research Center Factank. https://www.pewresearch.org/fact-tank/2020/05/05/financial-and-health-impacts-of-covid-19-vary-widely-by-race-and-ethnicity (accessed September 2, 2020).

Lukachko, A., M. L. Hatzenbuehler, and K. M. Keyes. 2014. Structural racism and myocardial infarction in the United States. *Social Science and Medicine* 103:42–50.

Lundeen, E. A., S. Park, L. Pan, T. O'Toole, K. Matthews, and H. M. Blanck. 2018. Obesity prevalence among adults living in metropolitan and nonmetropolitan counties—United States, 2016. *Morbidity and Mortality Weekly Report* 67(23):653.

Macinko, J., B. Starfield, and L. Shi. 2007. Quantifying the health benefits of primary care physician supply in the United States. *International Journal of Health Services* 37(1):111–126.

Martsolf, G. R., D. J. Mason, J. Soan, and V. Sullivan. 2017. *Nurse-designed care models: What can they tell us about advancing a culture of health?* Santa Monica, CA: RAND Corporation.

Massoglia, M., and Remster, B. (2019). Linkages between incarceration and health. *Public Health Reports* 134(1 Suppl):8S–14S.

McNutt, M. 2019. Time's up, CO2. *Science* 365(6452):411.

Mehra, R., L. M. Boyd, and J. R. Ickovics. 2017. Racial residential segregation and adverse birth outcomes: A systematic review and meta-analysis. *Social Science & Medicine* 191:237–250.

Mesic, A., L. Franklin, A. Cansever, F. Potter, A. Sharma, A. Knopov, and M. Siegel. 2018. The relationship between structural racism and Black-White disparities in fatal police shootings at the state level. *Journal of the National Medical Association* 110(2):106–116.

Mosites, E., E. M. Parker, K. E. N. Clarke, J. M. Gaeta, T. P. Baggett, E. Imbert, M. Sankaran, A. Scarborough, K. Huster, M. Hanson, E. Gonzales, J. Rauch, L. Page, T. M. McMichael, R. Keating, G. E. Marx, T. Andrews, K. Schmit, S. B. Morris, N. F. Dowling, G. Peacock, and COVID Homelessness Team. 2020. Assessment of SARS-CoV-2 infection prevalence in homeless shelters—Four U.S. Cities, March 27–April 15, 2020. *Morbidity and Mortality Weekly Report* 69(17):521–522.

Moy, E., M. C. Garcia, B. Bastian, L. M. Rossen, D. D. Ingram, M. Faul, G. M. Massetti, C. C. Thomas, Y. Hong, P. W. Yoon, and M. F. Iademarco. 2017. Leading causes of death in nonmetropolitan and metropolitan areas—United States, 1999–2014. *Morbidity and Mortality Weekly Report* 66(1):1–8.

Nadal, K. L., K. E. Griffin, Y. Wong, K. C. Davidoff, and L. S. Davis. 2017. The injurious relationship between racial microaggressions and physical health: Implications for social work. *Journal of Ethnic & Cultural Diversity in Social Work* 26(1–2):6–17.

NASEM (National Academies of Sciences, Engineering, and Medicine). 2017. *Communities in action: Pathways to health equity*. Washington, DC: The National Academies Press.

NASEM. 2018. *Health-care utilization as a proxy in disability determination*. Washington, DC: The National Academies Press.

NASEM. 2019a. *Integrating social care into the delivery of health care: Moving upstream to improve the nation's health*. Washington, DC: The National Academies Press.

NASEM. 2019b. *Vibrant and healthy kids: Aligning science, practice, and policy to advance health equity*. Washington, DC: The National Academies Press.

NASEM. 2020. *Birth settings in America: Outcomes, quality, access, and choice*. Washington, DC: National Academies Press.

Nau, C., J. L. Adams, D. Roblin, J. Schmittdiel, E. Schroeder, and J. F. Steiner. 2019. Considerations for identifying social needs in health care systems: A commentary on the role of predictive models in supporting a comprehensive social needs strategy. *Medical Care* 57(9):661–666.

NCHS (National Center for Health Statistics). 2017. Health, United States. In *Health, United States, 2016: With chartbook on long-term trends in health*. Hyattsville, MD: National Center for Health Statistics.

NEJM (*New England Journal of Medicine*) Catalyst. 2017. *Social determinants of health*. https://catalyst.nejm.org/social-determinants-of-health (accessed November 5, 2019).

Newkirk, V., and A. Damico. 2014. *The Affordable Care Act and insurance coverage in rural areas*. Kaiser Family Foundation. https://www.kff.org/uninsured/issue-brief/the-affordable-care-act-and-insurance-coverage-in-rural-areas (accessed September 2, 2020).

NIH (National Institutes of Health). 2021. *Opioid overdose crisis*. https://www.drugabuse.gov/drug-topics/opioids/opioid-overdose-crisis (accessed March 6, 2021).

NNU (National Nurses United). 2020. *National Nurses United's statement on protests and systemic racism: "Stop blaming underlying health conditions and comorbidities."* https://www.nationalnursesunited.org/press/national-nurses-uniteds-statement-protests-and-systemic-racism (accessed November 6, 2020).

Odgers, C. L., and N. E. Adler. 2018. Challenges for low-income children in an era of increasing income inequality. *Child Development Perspectives* 12(2):128–133.

ODPHP (Office of Disease Prevention and Health Promotion). 2020a. *Social Determinants of Health.* https://www.healthypeople.gov/2020/topics-objectives/topic/social-determinants-of-health (accessed November 9, 2020).

ODPHP. 2020b. *Access to health services.* https://www.healthypeople.gov/2020/topics-objectives/topic/Access-to-Health-Services (accessed November 9, 2020).

Ong, A. D., C. Cerrada, D. R. Williams, and R. A. Lee. 2017. Stigma consciousness, racial microaggressions, and sleep disturbance among Asian Americans. *Asian American Journal of Psychology* 8(1):72–81.

Owens, A., and J. Candipan. 2019. Social and spatial inequalities of educational opportunity: A portrait of schools serving high- and low-income neighbourhoods in U.S. metropolitan areas. *Urban Studies* 56(15):3178–3197.

Page, K. R., M. Venkataramani, C. Beyrer, and S. Polk. 2020. Undocumented U.S. immigrants and COVID-19. *New England Journal of Medicine* 382(21):e62.

Paradies, Y., J. Ben, N. Denson, A. Elias, N. Priest, A. Pieterse, A. Gupta, M. Kelaher, and G. Gee. 2015. Racism as a determinant of health: A systematic review and meta-analysis. *PLoS One* 10(9):e0138511.

RHI (Rural Health Information Hub). 2020. *Healthcare access in rural communities.* https://www.ruralhealthinfo.org/topics/healthcare-access#faqs (accessed April 22, 2021).

Sasson, I., and M. D. Hayward. 2019. Association between educational attainment and causes of death among White and Black U.S. adults, 2010-2017. *Journal of the American Medical Association* 322(8):756–763.

Seo, V., T. P. Baggett, A. N. Thorndike, P. Hull, J. Hsu, J. P. Newhouse, and V. Fung. 2019. Access to care among Medicaid and uninsured patients in community health centers after the Affordable Care Act. *BMC Health Services Research* 19(1):291.

Shah, E. D., S. T. Amann, and J. J. Karlitz. 2020. The time is now: A guide to sustainable telemedicine during COVID-19 and beyond. *American Journal of Gastroenterology* 115(9):1371–1375.

Shi, L. 2012. The impact of primary care: A focused review. *Scientifica* 2012:432892.

Slopen, N., T. T. Lewis, and D. R. Williams. 2016. Discrimination and sleep: A systematic review. *Sleep Medicine* 18:88–95.

Solar, O., and A. Irwin. 2010. *A conceptual framework for action on the social determinants of health: Social determinants of health discussion paper 2.* Geneva, Switzerland: World Health Organization.

Sue, D. W., C. M. Capodilupo, G. C. Torino, J. M. Bucceri, A. M. Holder, K. L. Nadal, and M. Esquilin. 2007. Racial microaggressions in everyday life: Implications for clinical practice. *American Psychologist* 62(4):271–286.

Supekar, S. 2019. Equitable resettlement for climate change-displaced communities in the United States. *UCLA Law Review* 66:1290.

Taylor, L. A. 2018. Housing and health: An overview of the literature. *Health Affairs Health Policy Brief.* doi: 10.1377/HPB20180313.396577.

USDA (U.S. Department of Agriculture). 2020. *Food security and nutrition assistance.* https://www.ers.usda.gov/data-products/ag-and-food-statistics-charting-the-essentials/food-security-and-nutrition-assistance (accessed September 2, 2020).

van Dorn, A., R. E. Cooney, and M. L. Sabin. 2020. COVID-19 exacerbating inequalities in the U.S. *Lancet* 395(10232):1243–1244.

van Ryn, M., and J. Burke. 2000. The effect of patient race and socio-economic status on physicians' perceptions of patients. *Social Science & Medicine* 50(6):813–828.

Wallis, C. 2020 (June 12). Why racism, not race, is a risk factor for dying of COVID-19. *Scientific American: Public Health*. https://www.scientificamerican.com/article/why-racism-not-race-is-a-risk-factor-for-dying-of-COVID-191 (accessed November 6, 2020).

Weissman, J., L. A. Pratt, E. A. Miller, and J. D. Parker. 2015. *Serious psychological distress among adults: United States, 2009–2013*. Hyattsville, MD: National Center for Health Statistics.

Williams, D. R., J. A. Lawrence, and B. A. Davis. 2019. Racism and health: Evidence and needed research. *Annual Review of Public Health* 40:105–125.

Woolf, S. H., L. Aron, L. Dubay, S. M. Simon, E. Zimmerman, and K. X. Luk. 2015. *How are income and wealth linked to health and longevity?* Urban Institute and Virginia Commonwealth University Center on Society and Health.

Yancy, C. W. 2020. COVID-19 and African Americans. *Journal of the American Medical Association* 323(19):1891–1892.

Zagorsky, J. L., and P. K. Smith. 2016. Does asthma impair wealth accumulation or does wealth protect against asthma? *Social Science Quarterly* 97(5):1070–1081.

3

The Nursing Workforce

Health care delivery systems are "held together, glued together, enabled to function ... by the nurses."

—Adapted from Lewis Thomas, physician, essayist, researcher

The nursing workforce will be tested in a variety of ways over the next decade, including responding to an aging population that has more complex and intense medical needs, demand for more primary care capacity, and the need to bridge medical and health care with the social factors that influence people's health and well-being. To build a future workforce that effectively provides the health and health care that society needs will require a substantial increase in the numbers, types, and distribution of the nursing workforce, as well as an education system that better prepares nurses for practicing in community-based settings with diverse populations that face a variety of lived experiences. These improvements will occur more rapidly, more uniformly, and more successfully if programmatic, policy, and funding opportunities can be leveraged by health systems, governments, educators, and payers.

Today in the United States, the health of far too many individuals, families, entire neighborhoods, and communities is compromised by social determinants of health (SDOH), such as food insecurity and poverty, as well as by limited access to health care services. The size, distribution, diversity, and educational preparation of the nursing workforce needed to assist in addressing these health challenges are therefore critically important. Even as the potential for nurses to help improve both SDOH and health outcomes has become clear, however, it has become increasingly apparent that a robust nursing workforce ready to meet these challenges does not yet exist. In fact, some of the data discussed in this chapter highlight the potential for current gaps in the capacity of the nursing workforce to widen over the present decade.

As described in the committee's framework for this study (see Figure 1-1 in Chapter 1), strengthening the nursing workforce is one of the key areas that will enhance nursing's role in addressing SDOH and improving health and health care equity. This chapter focuses on building the nursing workforce needed to respond to SDOH that affect the health care needs of individuals, communities, and society, including the pressing need to reduce health and health care inequities. The chapter begins by placing the nursing workforce in context and summarizing its current state and strengths. Next, it describes key challenges nurses will face over the current decade. Comparison of these challenges against the current state of the nursing workforce illuminates numerous gaps in the workforce that will need to be filled to meet the goal of addressing SDOH and improving health equity. After summarizing research needed to help nurses meet these challenges, the chapter ends with conclusions.

The nursing workforce is composed of actively employed registered nurses (RNs), licensed practical or licensed vocational nurses (LPN/LVNs), and advanced practice registered nurses (APRNs). As described in greater detail at the end of the chapter, the data and methods used to describe the nursing workforce come primarily from the 2008 and 2018 National Sample Survey of Registered Nurses (NSSRN), the U.S. Census Bureau's yearly American Community Survey (ACS) for 2000–2018, and other sources.

THE NURSING WORKFORCE IN CONTEXT

The number of nurses in the United States has grown steadily over the past 100 years. The nursing workforce is the largest among all the health care professions and is nearly four times the size of the physician workforce. RNs practice in a wide variety of care delivery settings, and they provide care to people living in both urban and rural areas and to vulnerable populations, including women, people of color (POC), American Indians/Alaska Natives (AI/ANs), low-income individuals, individuals with disabilities, and people who are enrolled in both Medicare and Medicaid (dual eligible).

The shift in nursing education from hospital-based diploma programs to degrees from colleges and universities has prepared RNs for more highly skilled roles that have expanded their reach and impact, benefiting both nurses and their employers. The emergence and growth of nurse practitioners (NPs) in the mid-1960s, together with other advanced practice nursing roles (certified nurse midwives, nurse anesthetists, and clinical nurse specialists), represent a significant advancement. Nurses also benefit individuals, communities, and society through their efforts as scientists conducting clinical and health services research; as executives and entrepreneurs leading health care organizations; as members of hospital and health system boards; as public health officers and educators; and as members of federal, state, and local governments.

For decades, nurse employment has grown concurrently with increased U.S. spending on acute care, seemingly impervious to either government or market-oriented efforts aimed at constraining the overutilization of costly health care services. With unemployment rates rarely exceeding 1.5 percent, job availability has seldom been a problem for nurses (BLS, 2020; Zhang et al., 2018). Even during economic downturns, RN employment typically has increased, sometimes dramatically. Hospitals added nearly 250,000 nursing full-time equivalents (FTEs) during the Great Recession, for example, including in economically depressed areas of the country (Buerhaus and Auerbach, 2011). Even so, vacancies exist in some areas, including Indian Health Service areas, with uneven distribution across several states, ranging from 10 to 31 percent (GAO, 2018).

RNs and APRNs are among the most highly paid health professionals, making the nursing profession an economic engine for families and communities. In 2018, national RN earnings averaged $76,000, and with an estimated 3.35 million RNs working on an FTE basis in the United States, total RN earnings amounted to roughly $255 billion (not counting nonwage benefits). As a result, the value of the clinical care they deliver typically appears on the cost side rather than the revenue side of earnings statements for provider organizations. When thinking about how nurses can promote health equity, however, one should not lose sight of their contributions to the economic as well as the social and environmental fabric of the places where they live and work.

The COVID-19 pandemic has illuminated the critical importance of nurses, but it also has disrupted long-standing employment patterns and threatened nurses' financial, psychological, and physical resilience. Nurses heroically risked exposure to the coronavirus each day to care for patients and their families, sometimes without adequate personal protective equipment. But the pandemic also exposed nurses' vulnerability to their clinical employers' dependence on reimbursable services, especially elective procedures, to remain in business. With revenue from private health insurers in steep decline, many hospitals and clinics seeking quick reductions in costs have cut back on nursing through furloughs and layoffs (Gooch, 2020). This counterproductive response to the pandemic could cause long-lasting damage to the nursing profession and the health care system. This and other destabilizing effects on the nursing workforce associated with COVID-19 merit close attention.

CURRENT STATE AND STRENGTHS OF THE NURSING WORKFORCE

Although this chapter's main focus is on identifying the challenges and gaps in the nursing workforce that will develop over this decade and describing ways to overcome them, the success of such actions will depend on leveraging the capacity and the many strengths of the current nursing workforce. These strengths represent opportunities to achieve and sustain a workforce of sufficient size, distribution, diversity, and expertise to help achieve equity in health and health care and reverse the trajectory of poor health status seen in communities across the nation.

Registered Nurses

Over the past 20 years, the number of people becoming RNs has increased rapidly, reaching 3.35 million FTEs in 2018 (see Table 3-1). Although the RN workforce continues to be composed largely of White women, the proportion of White RNs decreased from 79.1 percent in 2000 to 69 percent in 2018. The workforce has steadily become more diverse as the proportion of RNs who are Black/African American now approximates that of the nation's population (12 percent), while the proportion of RNs who are Asian (9.1 percent) exceeds that of the population (6 percent). On the other hand, despite doubling since 2001, the proportion of Hispanic RNs in the nursing workforce (7.4 percent) is well below that of the population (18.3 percent). The proportion of men who are RNs had grown to 12.7 percent by 2018.

RNs are increasingly educated at both the undergraduate and graduate levels. It is important to note that the 2011 *The Future of Nursing* report recommends increasing the percentage of nurses with a baccalaureate degree to 80 percent by 2020 (IOM, 2011). The number of employed RNs prepared with at least a bachelor's degree has surpassed the number prepared with an associate's degree. This growth has been driven, in part, by RNs completing RN-to-bachelor of science in nursing (BSN) education programs, which provide additional education needed by RNs with an associate's degree to earn a BSN. The increase in educational attainment has been particularly strong among POC RNs. Table 3-2 shows that nationally, a higher percentage of Black/African American, Hispanic, and particularly Asian RNs relative to White RNs have a BSN.[1] Proportionately, more Black/African American and Asian RNs than White and Hispanic RNs have a master's degree, or a doctor of nursing practice (DNP) or a PhD in nursing. Box 3-1 provides information on the nursing workforce educated in countries outside of the United States.

Analysis of data from the American Association of Colleges of Nursing (AACN) shows that between 2010 and 2017, the number of RNs who obtained a doctoral degree increased rapidly, with those obtaining a DNP far outnumbering those obtaining a PhD (see Figure 3-1). Among White RNs, the number of DNP graduates increased from 982 in 2010 to 4,138 in 2017 (an increase exceeding 3,000 percent), while the number of PhD graduates increased from 363 to 462

[1] It is possible that nurses educated in other countries are more likely to have earned a bachelor's degree, which could partially account for the higher percentage of bachelor's-level education reported by Black/African American and Asian RNs relative to White RNs. When the committee investigated this possibility, it found no supporting evidence with regard to Black/African American nurses but a significant impact for Asian RNs. Additionally, when we examined RNs under age 40, the pattern of results persisted, as a higher proportion of Black/African American (67.3 percent), Asian (76.7 percent), and other (68 percent) RNs compared with White (65 percent) RNs had earned a bachelor's degree in nursing, Hispanics (58 percent) being the exception.

TABLE 3-1 Demographic Characteristics of Full-Time Equivalent (FTE) Registered Nurses (RNs), 2000–2018

		Year			
Characteristics		2000	2004	2008	2018
Total FTE RNs		1,985,944	2,142,353	2,542,703	3,352,461
FTE RNs/ population		7.04	7.32	8.36	10.26
Gender	Men	157,285 (7.9%)	211,891 (9.9%)	244,363 (9.6%)	424,342 (12.7%)
	Women	1,828,709 (92.1%)	1,930,462 (90.1%)	2,298,340 (90.4%)	2,928,119 (87.3%)
Race	White	1,571,136 (79.1%)	1,673,073 (78.1%)	1,906,756 (75.0%)	2,313,002 (69.0%)
	Black/African American	175,669 (8.8%)	191,102 (8.9%)	269,271 (10.6%)	401,755 (12.0%)
	Asian	128,064 (6.4%)	161,598 (7.5%)	211,751 (8.3%)	305,740 (9.1%)
	Other	37,266 (1.9%)	28,027 (1.3%)	37,370 (1.5%)	84,454 (2.5%)
	Hispanic	73,859 (3.7%)	88,553 (4.1%)	117,556 (4.6%)	247,511 (7.4%)
Education	Associate's Degree	703,959 (37.7%)	839,506 (37.4%)	997,671 (38.1%)	910,629 (29.3%)
	Bachelor's Degree	610,735 (32.7%)	778,513 (34.7%)	957,422 (36.6%)	1,411,525 (45.4%)
	Master's Degree/PhD	202,018 (10.8%)	296,245 (13.2%)	361,559 (13.8%)	644,764 (20.7%)
Employment	Hospital	1,307,476 (63%)	1,352,356 (63.1%)	1,606,924 (63.2%)	2,071,034 (61.8%)
	Nonhospital	778,461 (37%)	789,997 (36.9%)	935,779 (36.8%)	1,281,424 (38.2%)
Age	<35	895,759 (23.0%)	486,098 (22.7%)	584,982 (23.0%)	980,779 (29.3%)
	35–49	2,017,925 (51.8%)	968,308 (45.2%)	1,017,328 (40.0%)	1,202,345 (35.9%)
	50+	980,651 (25.2%)	687,947 (32.1%)	940,394 (37.0%)	1,169,337 (34.9%)
	Overall Average	42.68	43.87	44.37	43.69

SOURCE: Calculations of data from the American Community Survey (IPUMS USA, 2020).

TABLE 3-2 Number and Percentage of Nurses with Various Levels of Nursing Education by Race, 2018

Nursing Education	White	Black/ African American	Asian	Hispanic	Other	All
Diploma	118,131 (5.9%)	6,584 (2.9%)	4,794 (2.8%)	13,366 (4.3%)	3,056 (3.6%)	5.3%
Associate's Degree	687,671 (34.6%)	67,163 (29.6%)	26,491 (15.6%)	112,409 (36.2%)	24,429 (29.1%)	33.1%
Bachelor's Degree	968,411 (48.8%)	119,605 (52.07%)	117,425 (69.0%)	155,324 (49.8%)	49,783 (59.2%)	50.8%
Master's Degree	196,362 (9.9%)	28,582 (12.6%)	19,465 (11.4%)	27,701 (8.9%)	6,612 (7.9%)	10.0%
Doctor of Nursing Practice (DNP) or PhD	14,897 (0.8%)	4,841 (2.1%)	1,908 (1.1%)	2,388 (0.8%)	179 (0.2%)	0.9%
Total	1,985,472	226,766	170,083	311,188	84,059	

SOURCE: Calculations of data from the 2018 National Sample Survey of Registered Nurses.

(27 percent). The proportionate growth among POC RNs was even greater. For example, the number of Black/African American RNs who obtained a DNP increased from 139 in 2010 to 826 in 2017 (a nearly 5,000 percent increase), while the number earning a PhD increased from 52 to 107 (105 percent) over this same period. Unfortunately, because RNs who have earned DNPs could not be identified in the 2018 NSSRN public use files, it is impossible to identify the sociodemographic, economic, or employment characteristics of this growing segment of the doctoral-level nursing workforce. It will be important for future NSSRNs to ensure the ability to identify RNs who have obtained a DNP so that the sociodemographic, economic, and practice characteristics of this rapidly growing segment of the nursing workforce can be identified and analyzed, particularly in relation to whether and how DNPs are addressing SDOH.

The average age of the RN workforce has decreased to just under 44 years as the large number of RNs belonging to the baby boom generation (estimated at 1.2 million) have retired and younger RNs have entered the workforce. RNs working in hospitals are younger (42.3) than those working in nonhospital settings (47.0) (see Table 3-1), which suggests that the large numbers of RNs retiring over this decade will likely be among those working in non–acute care settings.

While many policy makers, consumers, and the media often associate RNs with working in hospitals (in fact, hospitals employ almost two-thirds of the RN workforce), what should not be overlooked is that RNs come into contact with individuals in a large number and wide array of settings. Table 3-3 shows more than 30 settings in which some RNs provide direct primary care, while others

BOX 3-1
Internationally Educated Nurses

Internationally educated nurses (IENs) are individuals who have completed nursing education outside of the United States. IENs make up 8–15 percent of the nursing workforce in the United States, with a majority coming from the Philippines (Hohn et al., 2016; HRSA, 2010). To gain employment in the United States, IENs are required to obtain employment-based (EB) visas—EB-2 visas for advanced degree nurses and EB-3 visas for associate's or bachelor's degree nurses. Although employers historically recruited IENs during nursing shortages, this trend has changed since 2000, with greater focus on expanding the domestic nursing workforce (Auerbach et al., 2015). Data from the National Sample Survey of Registered Nurses (NSSRN) show an increase in the proportion of IENs between 2004 and 2008, from 3.5 percent to 5.4 percent (100,791 to 165,539 nurses) (Cho et al., 2011; HRSA, 2010). However, more recent data show decreases in the number of IENs. Data from the Organisation for Economic Co-operation and Development (OECD) demonstrate significant decreases in the annual inflow of IENs, from 24,000 in 2007 to fewer than 6,500 in 2015 (OECD, 2018). The number of first-time internationally educated candidates taking the NCLEX-RN exam decreased between 2007 and 2019, from 33,768 to 15,053 (NCSBN, 2008, 2019). Conversely, the nursing workforce has increased over time in the United States: from 2000 to 2018, the number of RNs increased from 1,985,944 to 3,352,461.

The decreases in IENs can be attributed to factors that include visa retrogression and the economic recession of 2007 to 2009. Visa retrogression occurs "when the number of visa applications within a particular country or category exceeds the number of available visas, causing the cutoff date to move backward in time instead of forward" (Shaffer et al., 2020, p. 30). Retrogression has major impacts on IEN recruitment. For instance, it can delay the waiting period for obtaining a visa, which sometimes exceeds a decade, and there have been times when visas have not been available. During a recession, health care employment typically does not decline since the demand for health care services is constant. Similarly, during the 2007–2009 recession, health care employment grew, with positions being filled mainly by domestic health care workers. The nursing workforce saw less turnover, and there was a decline in IEN recruitment. As the economy recovered, recruitment of IENs slowly increased; however, the numbers of IENs have remained significantly lower than the peak in 2007 (Masselink and Jones, 2014).

supplement the primary care workforce, provide care to rural populations, help improve maternal health outcomes, deliver acute and emergency care, provide health education and preventive care, coordinate patient care, and facilitate continuity of care for patients and families across settings and providers. The table also shows that the average annual earnings of RNs are lowest in settings (e.g., critical access hospitals, nursing homes, inpatient and outpatient mental health facilities, public clinics, public health, school health, and home health) where RNs often interact with people facing multiple social risk factors.

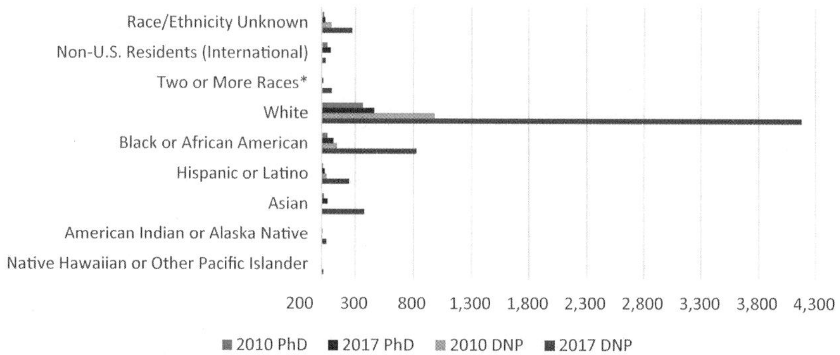

FIGURE 3-1 Number of nursing doctoral graduates by race/ethnicity.
NOTE: DNP = doctor of nursing practice.
* Was not a required reporting categy until 2011.
SOURCE: Data calculated from data from the American Association of Colleges of Nursing.

TABLE 3-3 Number of Registered Nurses (RNs) by Employment Setting, Average Annual Earnings, and Age, 2018

Employment Setting	All RNs	Percentage of All RNs	Average Annual Earnings	RNs Older Than Age 50	Percentage of RNs Older Than Age 50
Hospital (not mental health)					
Critical access hospital	309,822	11.2	$77,122	120,353	38.8
Inpatient unit—not critical access hospital	755,639	27.2	72,668	210,958	27.9
Emergency department—not critical	161,603	5.8	76,577	32,708	20.2
Hospital-sponsored ambulatory care	253,347	9.1	77,826	128,015	50.5
Hospital ancillary unit	54,181	2.0	82,063	23,514	43.4
Hospital nursing home unit	13,288	0.5	72,442	7,564	56.9
Hospital administration	95,543	3.4	110,396	54,103	56.6
Other hospital setting	20,133	0.7	88,454	8,054	40.0
Other hospital setting (consultative)	49,717	1.8	85,924	34,436	69.3
Other Inpatient Setting					
Nursing home unit not in hospital	60,615	2.2	69,479	30,557	50.4
Rehabilitation facility/long-term care	110,554	4.0	74,832	50,160	45.4
Inpatient mental health	55,089	2.0	68,044	24,091	43.7
Correctional facility	13,775	0.5	75,769	5,028	36.5

TABLE 3-3 Continued

Employment Setting	All RNs	Percentage of All RNs	Average Annual Earnings	RNs Older Than Age 50	Percentage of RNs Older Than Age 50
Other inpatient setting	11,938	0.4	70,729	4,414	37.0
Clinic/Ambulatory Setting					
Nursing-managed health center	9,183	0.3	91,244	2,594	28.2
Private medical practice (clinic, physician)	138,291	5.0	72,787	58,379	42.2
Public clinic (rural health center, federally qualified health center [FQHC], Indian Health Service, tribal clinic, etc.)	33,484	1.2	69,983	14,210	42.4
School health service (K–12 or college)	65,015	2.3	57,506	36,718	56.5
Outpatient mental health/substance abuse facility	14,995	0.5	68,288	7,124	47.5
Ambulatory surgery center (freestanding)	8,807	0.3	63,668	3,062	34.8
Other clinical setting	67,182	2.4	71,599	28,773	42.8
Other Types of Settings					
Home health agency/service	175,212	6.3	71,277	96,400	55.0
Occupational health or employee health	11,360	0.4	77,556	8,346	73.5
Public health or community health	41,176	1.5	71,712	16,952	41.2
Government agency other than public/community health or correctional facility	41,229	1.5	81,423	23,777	57.7
Outpatient dialysis center	27,704	1.0	81,032	11,231	40.5
University or college academic department	34,698	1.2	70,857	19,178	55.3
Case management/disease management and insurance company	78,637	2.8	81,324	38,202	48.6
Call center/telenursing center	15,935	0.6	79,754	9,613	60.3
Other type of setting	12,197	0.4	89,431	7,298	59.8
Other type of setting (consultative)	38,130	1.4	92,522	21,366	56.0
All	2,778,476	100.0	76,180	1,137,176	

SOURCE: Calculations based on the 2018 National Sample Survey of Registered Nurses.

Table 3-3 also shows the percentages of RNs in each employment setting who are over the age of 50, many of whom are expected to retire by the end of the decade. Indeed, the number of employment settings in which more than 40 percent of RNs are over age 50 is striking: critical access hospitals (40 percent); outpatient dialysis centers (40.5 percent); public health/community health (41.2 percent); private physician offices (42 percent); public clinics, such as rural health centers, federally qualified health centers (FQHCs), and Indian Health Service facilities (42.4 percent); inpatient mental health facilities (43.7 percent); outpatient mental health/substance units (47.5 percent); case management/disease management (48.6 percent); nursing home units not in hospitals (50 percent); hospital-sponsored ambulatory clinics (50.5 percent); home health agencies (55 percent); school health (56.5 percent); hospital nursing home units (57 percent); call centers (60.3 percent); occupational health (73.5 percent); and other settings (>50 percent). As RNs in these settings retire, they will be replaced by more recently educated nurses who, as discussed below, may not be as prepared for taking care of medically complex patients and addressing SDOH.

Fewer RNs are working in rural areas today than in the past (17 percent in 2005 versus 14.4 percent in 2018). The percentage working in rural hospitals also decreased over these same years (from 16.4 percent to 13.4 percent), as did the percentage of rural RNs working in nonhospital settings (18 percent to 16 percent). Furthermore, the decline in rural practicing RNs occurred more rapidly among younger RNs (under age 40) (from 18.1 percent to 13.7 percent) than among RNs over age 40 (from 16.4 percent to 14.9 percent). If this decrease continues, it will threaten access to care among the nation's rural population. Given the large number of RNs working in critical access hospitals (more than 300,000) and the concern that more rural hospitals will close in the years ahead (Frakt, 2019), the number of RNs and physicians practicing in rural areas could decline further during this decade, complicating policies aimed at increasing access to care for the populations in these areas.

Looking to the future, the size of the FTE RN workforce is projected to grow substantially, from 3.35 million in 2018 to 4.54 million in 2030, enough to replace all the baby boom RNs who will retire over the decade. However, this projected growth will not occur uniformly across the nation because the replacement of the large numbers of retiring RNs by younger nurses will vary by state and by region. Thus, health care delivery organizations in some regions of the country will confront more rapid retirements and slower replacements among their RN workforce relative to other regions, which could in turn result in staffing disruptions. Still, the estimated growth in the RN supply is encouraging and means that large, long-lasting national shortages of RNs are unlikely to be seen during the decade. At the same time, as with all projections, these estimates are based on assumptions that may not hold over the projection period and are subject to unforeseen developments, such as the economic and noneconomic effects of the COVID-19 pandemic.

Licensed Practical/Vocational Nurses

LPN/LVNs (for brevity, referred to here as LPNs) support RNs and APRNs in providing patient care. In 2018, an estimated 701,650 LPNs provided health care to mostly racially and ethnically diverse populations both in the community and in health care organizations. These nurses also add meaningfully to the pipeline for RN and APRN roles and, importantly, allow RNs to concentrate on caring for medically complex patients (NCSBN, 2020). As the U.S. population ages, LPNs are likely to become an important resource for home care, long-term care, and care for individuals with disabilities and otherwise vulnerable groups. As in the case of RNs, the majority of LPNs are White (71.4 percent), but there are proportionately more Black/African American LPNs (18.5 percent) than is the case among RNs (12 percent). Also, as with RNs, the proportion of Hispanic (7.4 percent) and male (7.7 percent) LPNs in 2017 was far below their proportion in the population. Smiley and colleagues (2018) report that newer cohorts of LPNs are younger and more likely to be racially and ethnically diverse (Smiley et al., 2018, p. S46).

As of 2018, more than one-third (38 percent) of LPNs worked in nursing and residential care facilities, considerably more than in hospitals (15 percent), physician offices (13 percent), and home health care facilities (12 percent). Almost one in four LPNs lived in rural areas (166,000). Because nearly one-third of LPNs are over age 55, their impending retirement over the next decade raises concern about a potential shortage of these nurses (Smiley et al., 2018, p. S59). A 2017 Health Resources and Services Administration (HRSA) analysis suggests that, because the demand for LPNs is growing at a slightly faster rate than the supply, a shortfall of roughly 150,000 FTE LPNs is possible by 2030 (HRSA, 2017, p. 13). Such a shortage could mean that home care, long-term care, and care for individuals with disabilities and otherwise vulnerable groups will increasingly have to be provided by the RN workforce.

Box 3-2 provides information on the impacts of COVID-19 on the nursing workforce in nursing homes.

Advanced Practice Registered Nurses

APRNs are nurses who hold a master's degree, post-master's certificate, or practice-focused DNP degree in one of four roles: NP, certified registered nurse anesthetist (CRNA), clinical nurse specialist (CNS), or certified nurse midwife (CNM). As shown in Table 3-4, counting the number of APRNs is complicated because many APRNs are prepared in more than one role (e.g., they could be an NP and also a CNM or a CNS), and because a considerable number are employed in a position that is not what they were prepared for (e.g., an NP might be working as an RN rather than as an NP, or a CNM working as an NP). For consistency, this section focuses on APRNs who are employed in nursing and are working in the role for which they were prepared. Also, because of the larger numbers of APRNs practicing in the NP role relative to other advanced practice roles, this section focuses largely on NPs.

BOX 3-2
COVID-19 and Nurse Staffing in Nursing Homes

As of 2020, there were 15,417 long-term care facilities in the United States (CMS, 2020), and in 2017, these facilities housed just over 1.3 million people (Chidambaram, 2020). As of the end of May 2020, there were 95,515 cumulative confirmed cases of COVID-19 among nursing home residents in the United States and 30.2 deaths per 1,000 residents. Almost one-third (31,782) of the 103,700 people who died from COVID-19 in the United States through the end of May were residents of nursing homes (CMS, 2020). As of the end of July 2020, more than 60,000 deaths had occurred in nursing homes and long-term care facilities in the United Sates, and close to 800 staff had died (McGarry et al., 2020).

A 2019 study (Geng et al., 2019) assessed nursing home staffing prior to the spread of COVID-19 using various data available from the Centers for Medicare & Medicaid Services (CMS). Among the study's findings were the following:

- Seventy-five percent of nursing homes were almost never in compliance with what CMS expected their registered nurse (RN) staffing levels to be, based on residents' acuity.
- Across staffing categories (RN, licensed practical nurse [LPN], and nurse aide), staffing levels, especially for RNs, were stable during weekdays but dropped on weekends. On average, weekend RN staffing in terms of time spent per resident was 17 minutes (42 percent) less than weekday staffing, LPN staffing 9 minutes (17 percent) less, and nurse aide staffing 12 minutes (9 percent) less.

Larger facilities, on average, had a larger decrease in staffing time per resident during weekends. Decreases were smaller among facilities with higher five-star overall ratings and with lower shares of Medicaid residents.

A 2020 study (McGarry et al., 2020) examined access to personal protective equipment (PPE), staffing, and facility characteristics associated with shortages of PPE and staffing from May through the end of July 2020. Findings included the following:

- One in five nursing homes reported facing a severe shortage of PPE or staff shortage in early July 2020. Rates of both PPE shortages and staff did not meaningfully improve from May to July 2020.
- PPE shortages were magnified in nursing homes with COVID-19 cases among staff or residents and those with low quality scores.
- Staff shortages were greater in facilities with COVID-19 cases, particularly among those serving a high proportion of disadvantaged patients on Medicaid and those with lower quality scores, including pre-pandemic staffing score.
- Most prominent staff shortages were for nurses and nursing aides as opposed to other providers or staff.

As shown in the table below, by a wide margin, the numbers of LPNs, home and personal care aides, nursing assistants, and other support staff working in skilled nursing facilities (SNFs) far exceeded the numbers of professionals over the 5-year period 2014–2018. There are also large proportions of Black/African American LPNs, personal care aides, and nursing assistants staffing SNFs in the United States. Nursing homes are ill prepared to manage infectious disease epidemics such as COVID-19. The burden of care falls disproportionately on the nursing staff, which too often is inadequate in numbers and insufficiently trained and protected to deal with such situations. Indeed, a recent study (Figueroa et al., 2020) of 4,254 nursing homes across eight states found that those that were high-performing with respect to nurse staffing had fewer COVID-19 cases relative to their low-performing counterparts. These findings suggest that poorly resourced nursing homes with nurse staffing shortages may be more susceptible to the spread of COVID-19 (Figueroa et al., 2020).

Employment in Skilled Nursing Facilities, 2014–2018

Occupation	White	Black or African American	Asian	Hispanic	Other	Total
Social Worker	72.9%	13.3%	3.0%	9.0%	1.9%	22,905
Occupational Therapist	77.1%	6.1%	10.9%	5.1%	0.8%	12,547
Physical Therapist	65.7%	5.8%	21.5%	5.4%	1.5%	15,911
Registered Nurse	63.8%	18.7%	9.5%	5.6%	2.4%	237,230
Licensed Vocational Nurse	54.8%	29.1%	5.5%	8.0%	2.6%	219,974
Home Health Aide	44.5%	37.2%	3.7%	11.7%	2.8%	115,582
Personal Care Aide	42.5%	30.3%	7.9%	15.7%	3.5%	71,914
Nursing Assistant	44.8%	36.8%	4.3%	10.7%	3.4%	470,183
Other Health Care Support Aides/ Assistants*	60.8%	19.9%	6.0%	10.8%	2.5%	37,726

* Includes occupational and physical therapy aides, orderlies, psychiatric aides, and medical assistants.

NOTE: Data should be interpreted as 5-year averages over the 2014–2018 period.

SOURCE: Calculations based on the American Community Survey 2014–2018, 5-Year Public Use Micro Sample file.

Size and Sociodemographic Characteristics

The total number of APRNs increased considerably in the 10-year period between the last two NSSRNs (2008 to 2018), reaching nearly 375,000 in 2018 (see Table 3-4), although APRN shortages remain in Indian Health Service areas—with vacancy rates ranging between 12 and 47 percent for NPs (GAO, 2018). By a wide margin, NPs outnumber any other APRN role, and their numbers grew more rapidly relative to other APRN roles, nearly doubling over this period. The number of APRNs working in the role of a CNS also increased. Although the total number of RNs prepared as a CRNA-only decreased, the number of CRNAs who were also prepared in another APRN role increased substantially. With regard to CNMs, difficulties associated with question wording in the 2008 and

TABLE 3-4 Number of Employed Advanced Practice Registered Nurses (APRNs), 2008 and 2018

	2008	2018
All APRN-Prepared Registered Nurses (RNs) Employed in Nursing		
Prepared in a single APRN role	205,074	347,861
Prepared in more than one APRN role	18,015	2,968
Total	223,089	373,829
Share of all APRNs prepared in more than one role	8%	7%
Nurse Practitioner (NP)–Prepared RNs Employed in Nursing		
Prepared in the role of an NP only	125,264	258,241
Prepared as an NP and also in another APRN role	17,527	24,395
Total	142,791	282,636
Share of all NP-prepared APRNs also prepared in another APRN role	12%	9%
Clinical Nurse Specialist (CNS)–Prepared RNs Employed in Nursing		
Prepared in the role of a CNS only	34,987	55,111
Prepared as a CNS and also in another APRN role	14,806	15,626
Total	49,793	70,737
Share of all CNS-prepared APRNs also prepared in another APRN role	30%	22%
Certified Registered Nurse Anesthetist (CRNA)–Prepared RNs Employed in Nursing		
Prepared as a CRNA only	31,156	29,869
Prepared as a CRNA and also in another APRN role	871	7,542
Total	32,027	37,411
Share of all CRNA-prepared APRNs also prepared in another APRN role	3%	20%

SOURCE: Calculations based on the 2008 and 2018 National Sample Survey of Registered Nurses.

2018 NSSRNs, combined with small numbers of CNMs sampled in each survey, make estimating the numbers of CNMs problematic. Instead, using data from the American Midwifery Certification Board (AMCB), the number of AMCB-certified nurse midwives in the United States increased from an estimated 11,262 in 2014 to 12,276 in 2018 (AMCB, 2019).

The racial/ethnic composition of NPs has become more diverse (see Figure 3-2), though it lags behind the gains of the basic RN workforce. The proportion of Hispanic NPs increased the most between 2008 and 2018, from 3.8 percent of all NPs to 9.2 percent (an increase of 12,900). The number of Black/African American NPs also increased over this period, from just under 8,000 to nearly 13,000, while the numbers of Asian and other POC NPs increased more slowly.

Similar to the basic RN workforce, NPs and CNSs have remained overwhelmingly women (in 2018, 90.3 percent and 96.7 percent, respectively). The number of male NPs increased slowly between 2008 and 2018, accounting for about 10 percent of NPs in the latter year. In contrast, the proportion of male CRNAs exceeded 40 percent in 2008 but had decreased to 32.7 percent by 2018. CNMs are predominantly female (99 percent) and White (87 percent), with only 6 percent Black or African American (AMCB, 2019).

Employment Settings and Clinical Specialties

Table 3-5 shows that NPs provide access to care for millions of Americans in a wide variety of settings. In 2018, more than 100,000 NPs (52 percent of all NPs) worked in different types of clinics or ambulatory settings (including nurse-managed health centers; private medical practices; school health services;

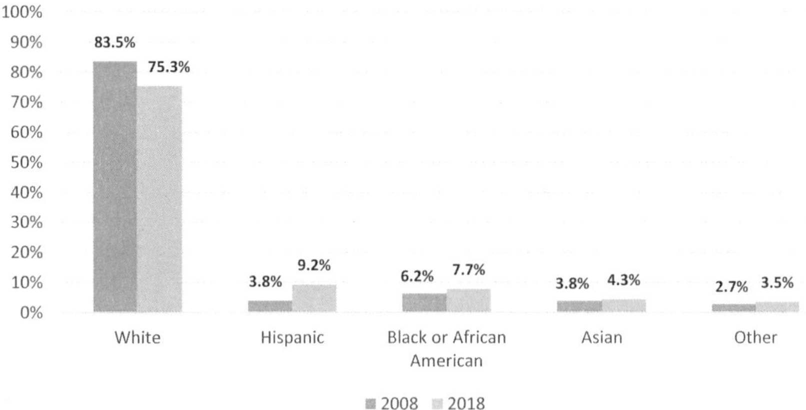

FIGURE 3-2 Nurse practitioners by race and ethnicity, 2018.
SOURCE: Calculations based on data from the 2018 National Sample Survey of Registered Nurses.

TABLE 3-5 Nurse Practitioner Employment Settings, 2018

Employment Setting	Number	Percentage	Median Full-Time Equivalent (FTE) Annual Earnings
Clinic or Ambulatory Care Settings			
Nurse-managed health center	1,736	0.9	$99,000
Private medical practice (e.g., clinic, physician office)	63,155	32.6	100,000
Public clinic (e.g., rural health center, federally qualified health center [FQHC], Indian Health Service [IHS])	16,309	8.4	97,000
School health service (K–12 or college)	4,060	2.1	90,000
Outpatient mental health/substance abuse facility	5,528	2.9	110,000
Other clinic/outpatient/ambulatory care setting	9,742	5.0	106,000
Total	100,529	51.9	
Other Settings			
Home health agency/service	4,118	2.1	$105,000
Occupational health/employee health service	1,459	0.8	106,000
Public health/community health agency	995	0.5	100,000
Government agency, other than public/community health or correctional facility	3,558	1.8	110,000
University or college academic department	2,021	1.0	91,000
Case mgmt./disease mgmt. in insurance company	970	0.5	114,000
Other setting (outpatient dialysis center, call center)	1,064	0.5	100,000
Total	14,185	7.3	105,000
Hospitals			
Critical access hospital (CAH)	7,971	4.1	$112,000
Inpatient unit, non-CAH	28,855	14.9	110,000
Hospital-sponsored ambulatory care	21,464	11.1	109,000
Emergency department, non-CAH	6,077	3.1	120,000
Other hospital-based setting	3,758	1.9	105,000
Total	68,125	35.2	112,000
Other Inpatient Settings			
Nursing home, nonhospital	2,687	1.4	$105,000
Rehabilitation facility/long-term care	3,705	1.9	105,000
Inpatient mental health/substance abuse	2,502	1.3	111,000
Correctional facility	1,567	0.8	108,000
Other inpatient setting	288	0.1	103,000
Total	10,749	5.6	

SOURCE: Calculations from data in the 2018 National Sample Survey of Registered Nurses.

outpatient mental health/substance abuse facilities; and public clinics, including rural health centers, FQHCs, and Indian Health Service facilities). Another 14,000 (7.3 percent of all NPs) worked in various other settings, such as home health agencies, occupational health/employee health services, and universities or colleges. Roughly 68,000 (35 percent of all NPs) worked in hospitals, ranging from critical access hospitals to inpatient units, hospital ambulatory clinics, and emergency departments. Nearly 11,000 (5.6 percent of all NPs) worked in other inpatient settings, including nursing homes, rehabilitation and long-term care facilities, and correctional facilities. With regard to annual earnings, NPs' median earnings varied considerably by setting, ranging from a low of $90,000 for those employed in school health settings to $120,000 for those working in emergency departments in non–critical access hospitals.

In 2018, a little more than half of NPs (54.7 percent or nearly 106,000) were certified as a family NP. The next largest group were NPs certified in the care of adults (33,620) and in pediatrics (21,622). The numbers of NPs certified in gerontology and psychiatric and mental health care grew the least between 2008 and 2018—9.7 percent and 5.3 percent, respectively, and in 2018 numbered only 15,921 and 10,174, respectively.

Within the different settings in which they work, NPs provide a vast array of clinical specialty care. Of the nearly two dozen clinical specialties shown in Table 3-6, NPs were most likely to provide primary and ambulatory care (39.2 percent), followed by general medical surgical care (9.1 percent), psychiatric or mental health care (6.4 percent), critical care (5.9 percent), and gynecology and women's health care (4.3 percent). The remaining 35 percent of NPs provided care in 17 other specialties, ranging from oncology (3.9 percent) to infections/communicable diseases (0.8 percent).

Care for People of Color and People with Limited English Proficiency

Analysis of the 2018 NSSRN shows that a majority (70.6 percent) of NPs who reported managing a panel of patients as a primary provider said at least 25 percent of their patient panel consisted of "racial/ethnic minority groups"; one in five indicated that this was the case for 75 percent or more of their panel. Slightly more than one-quarter of NPs (25.9 percent) also reported that 25 percent or more of their patient panel had limited proficiency in English. Additionally, the vast majority of NPs indicated that to a "great or somewhat extent" (versus "very little" or "not at all"), they participated in team-based care (85.8 percent), and felt confident in their ability to practice effectively in interprofessional teams (96.1 percent) and to use health information technology effectively in their practice to manage their patient population (81.1 percent). Most NPs had observed their organization emphasizing team-based care (84 percent) and evidence-based care (97 percent); only 60 percent reported observing their organization emphasizing discharge planning to a great extent or

TABLE 3-6 Nurse Practitioner Employment by Clinical Specialty Area, 2018

Clinical Specialty	Number	Percentage
Primary Care	47,176	24.4
Ambulatory Care (including primary care outpatient setting, except surgical)	28,787	14.9
General Medical Surgical	17,564	9.1
Psychiatric or Mental Health (substance abuse and counseling)	12,460	6.4
Critical Care	11,462	5.9
Gynecology	8,289	4.3
Oncology	7,556	3.9
Chronic Care	7,538	3.9
Dermatology	7,337	3.8
Cardiac or Cardiovascular Care	5,224	2.7
Neurology	4,373	2.3
Home Health/Hospice	3,809	2.0
Obstetrics	3,406	1.8
Orthopedics	2,854	1.5
Gastrointestinal	2,633	1.4
Pulmonary/Respiratory	2,347	1.2
Occupational Health	2,248	1.2
Other Specialty (neonatology)	2,048	1.1
Renal/Dialysis	1,508	0.8
Infectious/Communicable Disease	1,467	0.8
Labor and Delivery	1,019	0.5
Other Specialty (including school health service, gerontology, and radiology)	12,482	6.4
Total	193,587	

SOURCE: Calculations based on data from the 2018 National Sample Survey of Registered Nurses.

somewhat. Refer to Chapter 7 for more detailed information on interprofessional education and training.

Growth in the Size of the Nurse Practitioner Workforce

The NP workforce is growing rapidly. Using data from the 2001–2016 American Community Survey (ACS), Auerbach and colleagues (2018) project that the number of FTE NPs will more than double from 157,025 in 2016 to 396,546 in 2030 (increasing 6.8 percent annually). As discussed later, the contributions of the growing NP workforce will be useful to overcome projections of primary care and specialty physician shortages over the decade.

CHALLENGES FOR THE NURSING WORKFORCE THROUGH THE CURRENT DECADE

Looking out over this decade, the nursing workforce is growing and providing many different types of care in a variety of settings, giving them opportunities to understand and interact with people who face substantial social risk factors. The strengths of the nursing workforce are many, yet they will be tested by formidable challenges that are already beginning to affect nurses and the health care systems and organizations in which they work. These challenges will arise from changes occurring throughout the broader society that are increasing the number of people who need health care; from within the nursing and larger health care workforce; and from health-related public policies and other factors that affect the size, distribution, diversity, and educational preparation of nurses. These challenges include the need to

- increase the number of nurses available to meet the nation's growing health care needs;
- rightsize the clinical specialty distribution of nurses;
- increase the distribution of nurses to where they are needed most;
- ensure a nursing workforce that is diverse and prepared with the knowledge and skills to address SDOH;
- overcome current and future barriers affecting workforce capacity; and
- anticipate long-term impacts of the COVID-19 pandemic on the nursing workforce.

These challenges will unfold simultaneously over the decade, and will expose shortcomings throughout the nursing workforce, widening current gaps that should be filled if nurses are to fully leverage their expertise in helping to address SDOH for individuals, communities, and society.

Increasing the Number of Nurses Available to Meet the Nation's Growing Health Care Needs

In addition to growth in the overall size of the U.S. population, other factors and health workforce imbalances will increase the demand for nurses, particularly in areas where the RN and APRN workforce are already undersized. Salient sociodemographic factors include the aging population, increases in mental and behavioral health conditions, increases in lack of access to primary health care, persistently high maternal mortality rates, and worsening physician shortages.

The Aging Population

The aging of the U.S. population means that over this decade, increasing numbers of people will age into their 70s, 80s, 90s, and beyond. In 2030, 73.1 million people or 21 percent of the U.S. population, including all baby boomers, will be older than 65 (Vespa et al., 2020). The prevalence of multiple comorbid chronic conditions (e.g., diabetes, heart disease, obesity, cancer, disabilities, mental illness, Alzheimer's disease, dementia) is high among older people and greatly increases the complexity of their care (Figueroa et al., 2019). Increases can also be expected in the number of frail older adults—those who need assistance with multiple activities of daily living, are weak and losing body mass, have multiple chronic or complex illnesses, and have an increased risk of dying within the next 2–3 years (Collard et al., 2012; Fried et al., 2001). The old-age dependency ratio (the number of people aged 65 and over per 100 people aged 20–64) in the United States will increase from 21 in 2010 to more than 35 by the end of the decade (Vespa et al., 2020). The nation's aging population will pose extraordinary challenges for society at large and for health care delivery organizations, nurses, social workers, and families.

There are wide disparities in the economic and physical welfare of older adults by gender, racial/ethnic group, and geographic location. Older women are more likely than men to live alone and are twice as likely to be poor. At age 50, Black men and women still have lower life expectancies relative to their White counterparts. Among adults aged 65 and older, POC individuals are much more likely than Whites to rely solely on Social Security for their family income. In addition to the increased risk of age-associated mental health problems and cognitive degenerative diseases, older adults living in rural areas are more likely than their counterparts living in urban areas to be poor; to experience social isolation; and to have significantly less access to fewer health and social resources, including mental health services (Administration on Aging, 2013). It is essential for policy makers and others to pay attention to these gender and racial/ethnic gaps and geographic trends, which could undermine progress in advancing the well-being of older Americans in the present decade.

As the nation's health care and social support systems come to terms with caring for increasing numbers of older people, increases will be seen not only in the demand for nurses but also in the intensity and types of nursing care required to care for these older adults, extending across inpatient, community-based, and home settings. The gap in the ability of nurses to respond to these needs is already deep and worrisome; according to the 2018 NSSRN, relatively few RNs work in a long-term care facility (60,000) or provide home care (91,000). Similarly, relatively few NPs work in nursing homes (in 2018, 2,700 or 1.4 percent of all employed NPs) or provide home health care services (4,100 NPs or 2.1 percent).

Increases in Mental and Behavioral Health Conditions

Prior to the COVID-19 pandemic, sharp increases in suicide, substance abuse, the opioid crisis, gun violence, and severe depression among younger people were placing growing demands on the mental and behavioral health care workforce, including nurses. Yet, the rising demand for mental and behavioral health services, let alone treatment for the 44 million American adults who are estimated to have a diagnosable mental health condition, is occurring in the face of a shortage of behavioral health professionals that the HRSA (2016) projects could worsen to a shortfall of as many as 250,000 workers by 2025.

Despite current and projected shortages of mental and behavioral health workers, the regulatory policies of many states limit the capacity of existing NPs who provide psychiatric and mental health care. For example, a study by Alexander and Schnell (2019) assessing independent practice authority for NPs between 1990 and 2014 showed that broadening prescriptive authority was associated with improvements in self-reported mental health and decreases in mental health–related mortality, including suicides. These improvements were concentrated in areas underserved by psychiatrists and among populations traditionally underserved by mental health providers. According to the authors, "results demonstrate that extending prescriptive authority to NPs can help mitigate physician shortages and extend care to disadvantaged populations" (Alexander and Schnell, 2019, p. ii).

Similarly, Barnett and colleagues (2019) examined the issuing to NPs and physician assistants of federal waivers for prescribing buprenorphine following passage of the 2017 Comprehensive Addiction and Recovery Act. The waiver expansions were intended to increase patients' access to opioid use treatment, which is particularly important in rural areas underserved by physicians. The study found that between 2016 and 2019, the number of waivered clinicians per 100,000 population in rural areas increased by 111 percent, with NPs and physician assistants accounting for more than half of this increase. Furthermore, rural counties in states that granted full scope-of-practice authority to NPs saw significantly faster growth in NPs' buprenorphine treatment capacity compared with states with restrictive scope-of-practice regulations. "By March 2019 this pattern of growth had led to rural counties in states with full scope of practice having twice as many waivered NPs per 100,000 population, compared to those in states with restricted scope of practice (5.2 versus 2.5)" (Barnett et al., 2019, pp. 2051–2052).

The COVID-19 pandemic has added new stresses for many people, particularly those living in or near places with large outbreaks of the virus, increasing the need for mental and behavioral health treatment. As nurses continue to care for people with COVID-19, many will experience added stress; feelings of inadequacy, guilt, compassion fatigue, and physical exhaustion; and uncertainty over their employment. Some of these nurses may leave the profession, many will need help, and too many will suffer alone (Lai et al., 2020).

Increasing demand for mental and behavioral health care in the face of the decreasing capacity of mental and behavioral health care professionals implies that the nursing workforce will be relied upon to help address gaps in this care (Henderson, 2020). In addition to the capacity-reducing effect of regulations, however, the nursing workforce is unlikely to fill these gaps over the current decade because such a small percentage of RNs (3.5 percent or 78,300) provide care in psychiatric, mental health, or substance abuse settings. Similarly, small numbers of NPs work in inpatient (2,500 NPs in 2018) and outpatient (5,500) mental health/substance abuse settings.

Increases in Lack of Access to Primary Health Care

On the eve of the Patient Protection and Affordable Care Act's (ACA's) 2014 health insurance expansions, nearly 60 million people had inadequate access to primary care in the United States (Graves et al., 2016), and HRSA reported 5,900 health professional shortage areas (HPSAs). While the ACA eventually expanded insurance coverage to an estimated 20 million individuals, not all of those who gained coverage had adequate access to health care. Unfortunately, the size of the population with inadequate access to health care is rising: in March 2020, HRSA reported that the number of HPSAs nationwide had increased to 7,059, affecting 80.6 million people.

The persistent lack of access to primary health care has led to recommendations to increase the number of nurses practicing in primary care and community-based settings (Bodenheimer and Bauer, 2016). A 2016 report of the Josiah Macy Jr. Foundation, *Registered Nurses: Partners in Transforming Primary Care* (Bodenheimer and Mason, 2016), emphasizes the need to overcome the limited ways in which many primary care practices currently use RNs (e.g., telephoning prescriptions to pharmacies, performing administrative duties). Instead, the report urges primary care practices to expand the role of RNs in providing primary care services and allow them to practice to the full extent of their education and training (e.g., by managing stable patient panels with controlled diabetes, hypertension, and other conditions). As discussed in Chapter 7, nursing education programs have historically emphasized preparing students for inpatient acute care and medical and surgical nursing. Consequently, too few nurses today are adequately prepared to practice in non–acute care settings. To address the growing need for primary care providers, educators will have to increase coursework and student clinical experiences in primary care settings, which in turn could lead to more graduates choosing careers in primary care and ambulatory and community-based settings.

Fortunately, more than 160,000 NPs certified in either family health, adult health, or pediatrics provide primary care. And a large and growing body of evidence shows that primary care NPs are more likely than their physician counterparts to practice in rural areas—areas characterized by more uninsured individuals and chronic physician shortages—and to provide care to vulnerable populations that are impacted by SDOH (Barnes et al., 2018; Buerhaus, 2018; Buerhaus et al., 2015; DesRoches et al., 2017; Xue et al., 2019). Yet, despite the growing shortage of physicians practicing primary care and growing calls from public- and private-sector organizations to expand the roles and uses of NPs, many states, hospitals, and health systems continue to restrict NPs' scope of practice. These restrictions limit access to the high-quality primary care needed by millions of Americans.

Persistently High Maternal Mortality Rates

In addition to filling gaps in the delivery of mental and behavioral and primary care, momentum is growing to address the increasing rates of maternal morbidity and mortality that are disproportionately affecting Black/African American and AI/AN women (Leonard et al., 2019; Petersen et al., 2019). As discussed in Chapter 4, these inequities can be reduced by using RNs and expanding the number of CNMs and nurses prepared to provide women's health care to help improve the health status of and health care provided to pregnant women. Although perinatal RNs currently serving this population are concentrated in acute care hospitals, they could become a community resource in antenatal and postpartum maternity care. This use of RNs could be particularly effective if informed by established, evidence-based public health home visiting models.

Crucial gaps in the APRN workforce need to be filled to improve maternal health. At a time when CNMs are needed more than ever, their numbers are growing slowly. There were 3.745 million U.S. births in 2019 (Hamilton et al., 2020). Acute care hospitals are the site of 98 percent of U.S. births (MacDorman and Declercq, 2019), and only about 2,900 hospitals provide maternity care (AHA, 2018). If the supply of CNMs, NPs, and CNSs who specialize in perinatal care/women's health is not expanded (let alone maintained), millions of women will continue to be excluded from critical APRN services at a time when maternal care is increasingly complex, and improving the quality, safety, and equity of maternal care is paramount. Additionally, evidence of disparate care provided by White clinicians to Blacks, AI/ANs, and other POC (Altman et al., 2019; Davis, 2019; Johnson et al., 2019; McLemore et al., 2018; Serbin and Donnelly, 2016; Vedam et al., 2019; Williams et al., 2020) highlights the crucial need to strengthen efforts to increase the racial and ethnic diversity of the nursing workforce providing care for pregnant women. Finally, a recent study by McMichael (2020) examined all births in the United States between 1998 and 2015 (n = 69 million) and found "consistent evidence that allowing APRNs and PAs [physician assistants] to practice with more autonomy reduces the use of medically intensive procedures" (p. 880), specifically caesarean section rates, which place both mothers and infants at risk. This study adds new evidence of how restrictive scope-of-practice regulations (discussed further below) negatively affect maternal and child well-being.

Worsening Physician Shortages

A 2020 report prepared for the American Association of Medical Colleges estimates that by 2033, current physician shortages could increase, ranging between 21,400 and 55,200 for primary care physicians, and between 33,700 and 86,700 for non–primary care specialty physicians (AAMC, 2020). These projections, made prior to the COVID-19 pandemic, took into account decreasing hours worked by physicians, accelerating retirements, and increasing demands for medical care among aging baby boomers. Separately, HRSA projected a shortage of 24,000 primary care physicians by 2025, due mainly to population aging and overall population growth exceeding the growth in physician supply (HRSA, 2016). Current and projected shortages of primary care and specialty care physicians over the next 10 years mean that both RNs and APRNs will increasingly be called upon to fill gaps in individuals' access to care.

Rightsizing the Clinical Specialty Distribution of Nurses

As described above, the health and social ramifications associated with the nation's aging population, growth in mental and behavioral health conditions, inadequate access to primary care, and unacceptably high maternal mortality rates will increasingly fall on the nursing workforce. Not only are there too few nurses and APRNs working in the settings where these populations receive care, but also the number of nurses specializing in these clinical areas needs to increase.

Despite the availability of many fellowship programs and the high career satisfaction reported by clinicians in geriatrics, the number of physicians entering the specialty has consistently been far below the need. Currently, there are 6,671 board-certified geriatricians in the United States—1 for every 7,242 older Americans (Fried and Rowe, 2020). According to the 2018 NSSRN, fewer than 1 percent of RNs (0.4 percent) cited gerontology as the type of specialty care they provide in their primary employment position, and only 8.2 percent of NPs (just under 16,000) were certified in gerontology. With regard to mental and behavioral health, despite current and projected shortages of psychiatrists, only 4 percent of RNs (91,750) spent most of their time providing patient care, including substance abuse treatment and counseling, in psychiatric or mental health care settings, and just 5.3 percent of NPs (10,173) were certified in psychiatric or mental health care. It is not enough merely to increase the number of RNs and APRNs during the decade ahead; rather, there is an urgent need to increase the numbers of nurses in gerontology, mental and behavioral health care, primary care, and maternal health.

Increasing the Distribution of Nurses to Where They Are Needed Most

A third major challenge facing the nursing workforce over this decade is to address the large portions of the U.S. population that are unable to access affordable health care because of geography, insurance status, and other circumstances. In 2018, HRSA reported that 66 percent of HPSAs for primary care and 62 percent of those for mental health care were located in rural or partially rural areas. Because of a lack of education or transportation and competing needs, such as housing and food, individuals and families living in rural areas too often are unable to manage their health and chronic conditions. NPs and the expertise they possess have in many cases markedly expanded access to care in rural and other underserved locations, making them an important resource to help meet individual and community health care needs. As noted earlier, however, too often reimbursement policies and limitations on NPs' scope of practice impede their effective deployment to help address these challenges. Indeed, as discussed below, state-level restrictions on the practice authority of NPs are associated with decreased access to primary care.

Beyond current and growing physician shortages discussed above, particularly in the areas of primary care, mental health, and gerontology, the physician workforce has historically been unevenly distributed. Unfortunately, this trend is expected to worsen during this decade, with the number of physicians per 10,000 population in rural areas projected to decrease by 23 percent between 2017 and 2030 (from 12.2 to 9.4 physicians per 10,000 population) (Skinner et al., 2019). Over the same years, by contrast, the number of physicians per capita practicing in metropolitan areas will remain roughly constant at 31 per 10,000 population. The major reason for the forecast decline in rural physicians is the large number expected to retire over the decade and the need to be replaced by smaller cohorts of younger physicians. As a result, current large disparities in physician supply between rural and nonrural areas will grow over the decade, with resultant gaps in unmet needs for care falling increasingly on the nursing workforce.

As noted earlier, however, fewer RNs are working in rural areas and in rural hospitals today than in the past, a decrease occurring most rapidly among younger RNs. If this trend continues, it will threaten access to care among the nation's rural populations at a time when nurses will be counted on to fill gaps in their care. Moreover, given the large number of RNs working in critical access/rural hospitals (more than 300,000) and the number of such hospitals that could close in the years ahead, the number of nurses practicing in rural areas could decline even more during the decade, further complicating policies aimed at increasing access to care for rural populations.

With respect to the NP workforce, studies show that NPs providing primary care are more likely to practice in rural areas than are physicians, and states that do not versus those that do restrict NPs' scope of practice have a much larger supply of NPs per capita (Barnes et al., 2018; Graves et al., 2016; Xue et al.,

2019). For nurses to respond successfully to rural access problems associated with growing physician shortages and falling numbers of rural physicians projected over the next 10 years, restrictive scope-of-practice provisions will need to be removed and the trend of fewer RNs working in rural areas to be reversed.

Ensuring a Nursing Workforce That Is Diverse and Prepared with the Knowledge and Skills to Address Social Determinants of Health

A fourth challenge facing the nursing workforce over the current decade is to ensure that nurses reflect the people and communities with whom they interact. In addition, nurses need to be prepared to address SDOH that negatively affect health and well-being.

Ensuring a Diverse Workforce

Over the next decade (and beyond), the U.S. population is expected to become more racially and ethnically diverse. Based on data reported by the U.S. Census Bureau, while the number of White individuals will increase by roughly 4 percent, the numbers of all other races will grow much more rapidly: Blacks/African Americans and AI/ANs both by 10 percent, Hispanics by 20 percent, and Asians by 22 percent (Vespa et al., 2020). The fastest growth will be seen among people of two or more races. Box 3-3 provides information on the health disparities that the AI/AN population face and the critical need for nurses to provide culturally competent care. Of note, data on the AI/AN population are limited. More accurate and timely collection of data on AI/AN populations living in and outside tribal lands in the United States is needed to help in determining the allocation of essential resources and services to improve health equity for these populations.

On the other hand, increases in the racial diversity of the APRN workforce have not kept pace with those in the basic RN workforce. Today, most APRNs are White and female (with the exception of CRNAs, who are 30 percent male); the proportion of men who are APRNs (with the exception of CRNAs) is lower than the proportion of men in the basic RN workforce. While higher proportions of POC individuals (with the exception of Hispanics) are obtaining a master's or PhD degree, and especially a DNP degree, APRNs have a long way to go to match RNs in achieving a more diverse workforce. At the same time, it is important to keep in mind that although three-quarters of NPs are White, a strong majority provide care to people who are poor, lack insurance, are female, and are POC with complex health and social needs, and are more likely to practice in rural areas. Despite these attributes, however, the APRN workforce will need to rapidly become more diverse over the decade or it will fall further behind in reflecting the racial make-up of many of the people it serves. Chapters 7 and 9 on leadership and education, respectively, provide further information on the need for diversity in nursing.

BOX 3-3
Health Disparities Among American Indians/Alaska Natives

The American Indian/Alaska Native (AI/AN) population has faced significant health inequities that have contributed to poorer health outcomes compared with non-AI/AN populations. According to the Indian Health Service (IHS), life expectancy for AI/AN people is 5.5 years less than life expectancy for all races in the United States (73 versus 78.5 years) (GAO, 2018; IHS, 2019). In addition, AI/AN populations have higher rates of mortality associated with preventable conditions, including chronic liver disease and cirrhosis, diabetes mellitus, unintentional injuries, assault/homicide, intentional self-harm/suicide, and chronic lower respiratory diseases (IHS, 2019; Leavitt et al., 2018). Specifically, AI/ANs have high rates of obesity and diabetes. In 2018, 48.1 percent of AI/AN people were obese compared with 31 percent of White people. Diabetes is the fourth leading cause of death for AI/ANs. The prevalence of diabetes among AI/ANs is almost double the percentage for Whites (15.1 versus 7.4 percent) (Carron, 2020). Historical trauma has had lasting effects on physical, mental, social, and environmental determinants of health for AI/AN populations (Smallwood et al., 2020).

The significant health inequities that AI/ANs experience underscore the critical need for an adequate supply of nurses to address these disparities and provide culturally competent care. There are sizable provider shortages in areas serving AI/ANs, which negatively affect their access to and quality of care (GAO, 2018). In 2017, 27 percent of positions for nurses were vacant across eight areas (Albuquerque, Bemidji, Billings, Great Plains, Navajo, Oklahoma City, Phoenix, and Portland) in which IHS provides substantial direct health care to AI/ANs (GAO, 2018). For nurse practitioners (NPs), there was a 32 percent vacancy rate, ranging from 12 percent in Oklahoma City to 47 percent in Albuquerque (GAO, 2018). IHS has reported considerable difficulty in filling provider vacancies because of the rural location, geographic isolation, and insufficient housing that characterize AI/ANs. It is also especially difficult to recruit and retain providers for health care facilities on tribal lands. To increase the number of nurses who can provide culturally competent care to AI/AN populations, it will be important to educate nurses on culturally appropriate care specific to AI/ANs and employ strategies for recruiting and retaining these nurses that include financial incentives, professional development opportunities, and access to housing (Carron, 2020).

As recommended in the 2016 report *Assessing Progress on the Institute of Medicine Report* The Future of Nursing, recruitment and retention of a diverse nursing workforce is a priority (NASEM, 2016). As the nation's population becomes more diverse, it will be important to sustain efforts to diversify the racial, ethnic, and gender composition of the nursing workforce—particularly with respect to increasing the number of Hispanics and their educational attainment. Educators can target efforts to ensure more diverse graduates and better-prepared nurses to match population and community needs by understanding the racial and ethnic characteristics of their communities, expected future trends in racial and ethnic diversity, and opportunities to capitalize on nurses' ability to provide culturally and racially concordant care.

Overcoming Deficits in the Knowledge and Skills Needed to Address Social Determinants of Health

Nurses often treat people with multiple comorbid conditions who live in environments that exacerbate social risk factors that negatively affect their health. Yet, as described earlier, many RNs and NPs perceive gaps in their preparation in areas that would help them do their jobs better—mental and behavioral health, SDOH, population health, working in underserved communities, and care for people with complex medical/social needs. Nurses working in schools, public and community health agencies, emergency rooms and urgent care settings, and long-term care settings were most likely to identify these gaps. Furthermore, both RNs and NPs who had graduated since 2010 were more likely to indicate that they would benefit from training in these areas. If RNs and NPs in both the current and future workforce are to be relied on to address social risk factors and respond effectively to the needs of complex individuals, it is critical for them to receive education and training in these areas.

Overcoming Current and Future Barriers Affecting Workforce Capacity

A fifth major challenge facing the nursing workforce over the current decade involves overcoming regulatory restrictions placed on nurses' scope of practice and avoiding disruptions in care associated with the retirement of large numbers of baby boom RNs. Such restrictions limit access to care generally and to the high-quality care offered by APRNs. Those supporting these restrictions maintain that nonphysician providers are less likely to provide high-quality care because they are required to receive less training and clinical experience. However, evidence does not show that scope-of-practice restrictions improve quality of care (Perloff et al., 2019; Yang et al., 2020). Rather, these regulations restrict competition and can contribute to higher health care costs (Adams and Markowitz, 2018; Perloff et al., 2019).

Scope-of-Practice Restrictions That Reduce the Productive Capacity of Registered Nurses and Nurse Practitioners

Frogner and colleagues (2020) write:

> Ongoing payment reforms are pressing health systems to reorganize the delivery of care to achieve greater value, improve access, integrate patient care across settings, provide population health, and address social determinants of health. Many organizations are experimenting with new ways to unleash the potential of

> their workforce by using telehealth, various forms of digital technology and developing team- and community-based delivery models. Such approaches require flexibility to reconfigure provider roles yet states and health care organizations often place restrictions on health professionals' scope of practice (SoP) that limit their flexibility. These restrictions are inefficient, increase costs, and decrease access to care. (p. 591)

While considerable progress has been made over the past two decades in lifting state-level regulations restricting NPs' scope of practice, however, 27 states still do not allow full practice authority for NPs (AANP, 2020). As of January 2021, 23 states and the District of Columbia allow full practice authority for NPs (see Figure 3-3), allowing them to prescribe medication, diagnose patients, and provide treatment without the presence of a physician. Conversely, 16 states restrict NPs' ability to prescribe medication, requiring a physician's authorization, while 11 states require physician oversight for all NP practice (AANP, 2020). Some states have stipulations on the kinds of medications NPs can prescribe. In Arkansas, Georgia, Louisiana, Missouri, Oklahoma, South Carolina, Texas, and West Virginia, for example, NPs are prohibited from prescribing any Schedule II medications (AMA, 2017). CNMs are likewise restricted by scope-of-practice laws: they can practice independently in 27 states and the District of Columbia; a collaborative agreement with a physician is required in 19 states; and the 4 remaining states allow them to practice independently, but without the ability to prescribe medications (Georgetown University, 2019).

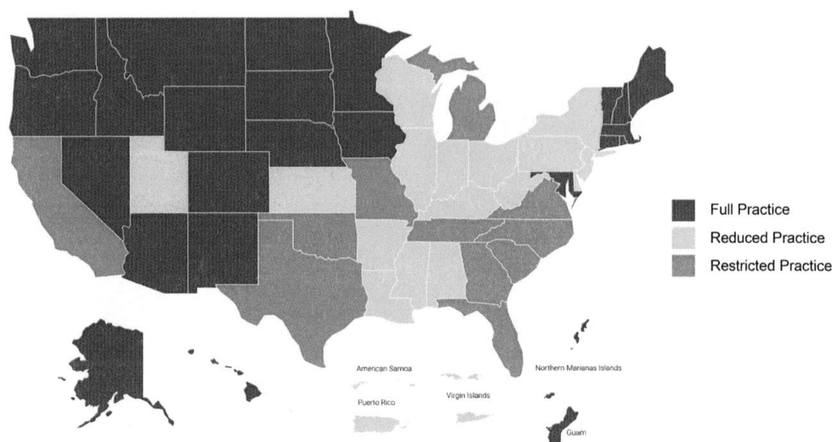

FIGURE 3-3 Scope of practice for nurse practitioners by state.
SOURCE: AANP, 2020.

Not permitting NPs and CNMs to practice to the full extent of their license and education decreases the types and amounts of health care services that can be provided for people who need care. As noted earlier, this artificially imposed reduction in NP and CNM capacity has significant implications for addressing the disparities in access to health care between rural and urban areas. According to the above-cited study by Graves and colleagues (2016), state-level scope-of-practice restrictions on NPs were associated with up to 40 percent fewer primary care NPs per capita in restrictive versus full-practice states, and people living in states allowing for the full practice authority of NPs had significantly greater access to primary care (63 percent) relative to those living in states that reduced (47 percent) or restricted (34 percent) NPs' scope of practice.

The harmful consequences of restricting NPs' scope of practice become starker in light of the findings of a 2018 UnitedHealth report on primary care and NP scope-of-practice laws. According to that report, if all states were to allow NPs to practice to the full extent of their graduate education, advanced clinical training, and national certification, the number of U.S. residents living in a county with a primary care shortage would decline from 44 million to fewer than 13 million (a 70 percent reduction). Furthermore, the number of rural residents living in a county with a primary care shortage would decline from 23 million to 8 million (a 65 percent reduction).

A 2020 study (Xu et al., 2021) examined the geographic locations of dual eligibles and primary care providers and found that one-third (n = 271) of the 791 counties with the highest density of dual eligibles in the United States were designated as HPSAs. These counties were more likely to be rural, located in the Southeast region of the country, and encumbered by high poverty rates and a heavy burden of chronic conditions. The investigators found that in nearly half (n = 128) of the 271 counties with both a high-density dual eligible population and a primary care physician shortage, the density of primary care NPs (PCNPs) was the highest, meaning that the distribution of PCNPs was within the highest quartile of the overall supply of PCNPs in the country. The study found that Southeastern states "impose the most restrictive scope of practice regulations that limit the capacity of NPs. Such restrictions may also increase NPs' reluctance to locate in these states. Thus, a first step to expand access to care is to lessen the state-imposed restrictions on scope of practice for the NPs" (Xu et al., 2021).

The damaging effects of scope-of-practice restrictions on access to care were recently acknowledged during the COVID-19 pandemic when several states (Florida, Kentucky, Louisiana, New Jersey, New York, Tennessee, West Virginia, and Wisconsin) and the Centers for Medicare & Medicaid Services eased supervision and other restrictions placed on NPs to increase the capacity of the health care workforce. It is uncertain whether these restrictions will be reinstated after the pandemic subsides (Yuanhong et al., 2020). Clearly, however, if government leaders concluded that removing restrictions on NPs was beneficial in expanding the public's access to care during the pandemic, it would be counterproductive to reimpose those restrictions once the pandemic eases, thereby decreasing access to care.

Until all APRNs are permitted to practice to the full extent of their education and training, significant and preventable gaps in access to care will continue. Millions of people who need health care will be unable to obtain needed care as readily as others who happen to live in states where NPs' scope of practice is not restricted. For many people, delays in obtaining care lead to worsening of symptoms and disease progression, and to greater costs when care is ultimately provided. Allowing APRNs to practice to the full extent of their education and training as recommended in the 2011 *The Future of Nursing* report would help remediate inequities in access to health care and enable more people to enjoy the benefits of care provided by NPs and other APRNs.

Disruptions in Care Delivery Associated with the Retirement of Baby Boom Registered Nurses

An estimated 600,000 baby boom RNs have not yet retired and are expected to leave the workforce by 2030. The exit from the workforce by so many experienced RNs (about 70,000 per year) means that health care delivery organizations that depend on RNs will face a significant loss of nursing knowledge, clinical expertise, leadership, and institutional history. The number of experience-years lost from the nursing workforce is estimated to exceed 2 million each year in the current decade (Buerhaus et al., 2017). As shown earlier in Table 3-3, in 2018 more than one-third and in many cases more than half of RNs working in noninpatient settings, including many settings where nurses are vital in ensuring access to care for minority and other vulnerable populations, were over age 50. The loss of nursing knowledge, clinical expertise, leadership, and institutional history associated with the retirement of baby boom RNs is likely to increase gaps in nurses' ability to provide needed care to vulnerable populations, who often have complex clinical conditions. It is crucial for nurses who enter the workforce during this decade to be well prepared for their role in addressing SDOH and reducing health inequities.

Anticipating Long-Term Impacts of the COVID-19 Pandemic on the Nursing Workforce

A final challenge concerns the pandemic's economic and noneconomic impacts on the nursing workforce over the immediate (next few years) and longer-term future. The impacts are difficult to predict because of uncertainties about the length and severity of the pandemic; its effects on health care systems and other health care professions; and whether it leads to a deep or shallow economic recession, how long the recession lasts, and the speed with which the economy recovers.

During the first half of 2020, health care systems reoriented their operations to manage a substantial influx of COVID-19-related testing, hospitalizations, and use of postacute care. Stay-at-home orders and social distancing then led to a massive reduction in hospital admissions, surgeries, tests, diagnostic procedures, and elective procedures. As revenues fell, hospitals took actions to decrease their costs, including furloughing nurses. Many physician offices and clinics similarly reduced their staffing. The magnitude of these short-run cost-cutting actions has varied by region and type of employer and may result in disparities in impacts by providers' race, ethnicity, gender, and age. In the longer run, the pandemic may lead to fundamental shifts in the demand for and supply of nurses. On the demand side, there may be a substantial restructuring of care delivery (e.g., toward telehealth or permanent staffing reductions in hospitals) that affects the nursing workforce. On the supply side, the pandemic may either increase or decrease entry into nursing and accelerate or slow retirement from nursing among the older members of the nursing workforce.

RESEARCH NEEDS TO HELP NURSES MANAGE THESE CHALLENGES

This chapter has provided information about the state of the nursing workforce, its strengths, and the many formidable challenges nurses will face in the coming years. Throughout this report, many ideas are provided for how nurses can address SDOH. What will be useful is to conduct research on how well nurses are implementing these ideas and evaluate whether the desired results are being achieved. For example, nurses are urged to become more active in community-based settings, and nurse educators are urged to modify their curriculum to expand the diversity of the workforce and better prepare nurses for practicing effectively in such settings. Over the decade, then, it will be important to assess whether and how effectively educators and nurses have responded to the ideas put forth in this report and determine whether and how their efforts have impacted SDOH that negatively affect health.

Research is also needed in many other areas to generate information and evidence on what is working and fill gaps in knowledge. Box 3-4 provides questions that can be addressed through a robust research agenda. These questions were generated by experts in nursing health services research and represent their views on the most important and feasible research questions that need to be investigated to increase nurses' ability to

- improve access to mental and behavioral health care and assess the effectiveness of interventions and services;
- improve access to primary health care and the effectiveness of primary care delivery systems;

- improve maternal health outcomes and the delivery of maternal health care;
- improve the care provided to the nation's aging population, particularly frail adults; and
- control health care spending, reduce costs, and increase the value of nurses' contributions to improving health and health care delivery.

As can be seen, these questions mirror many of the concerns about the gaps in the nursing workforce and their implications for SDOH that have been discussed throughout this chapter.

CONCLUSIONS

The many strengths of the nursing workforce—its large and growing numbers of increasingly educated nurses; provision of basic and advanced specialty care in numerous types of acute care and community-based settings; delivery of public health, school health, and home health services; and compassion in caring for vulnerable populations in rural and undeserved locations, as well as the public's positive perceptions of and trust in nurses, will be tested by a variety of challenges that will develop over this decade. These challenges will widen gaps in the size, distribution, diversity, and expertise of the full spectrum of the nursing workforce, gaps that will need to be addressed to help achieve health equity and reverse the trajectory of poor health status too often found in communities across the nation.

Among these challenges is the growing population of older people, many of whom, particularly frail older adults, have multiple comorbid conditions that increase the complexity and intensity of the nursing care they require. Nurses at all levels will also be challenged to help expand the capacity of the primary care workforce, provide care to rural populations, improve maternal health outcomes, and deliver more health and preventive care in community-based settings. And nurses will be called on to provide mental and behavioral health care to treat growing numbers of Americans with mental health conditions and help stem increases in substance abuse, suicide, and gun violence. Projected shortages of physicians in both primary care and non–primary care specialties, combined with projections of decreasing numbers of physicians practicing in rural areas, will increase the demand for RNs and APRNs. Yet, scope-of-practice restrictions that persist in many states and within many health care organizations will reduce the capacity of the nursing workforce when and where it is most needed. Meanwhile, various health care reforms expected to evolve over the decade will require a well-prepared and engaged nursing workforce if they are to succeed.

All of these challenges will be faced by a nursing workforce that will be expanding unevenly across the nation and whose composition and capabilities will be changing as the most experienced nurses in the nation's history retire,

BOX 3-4
Agenda for Nursing Health Services Research

In July 2019, a meeting of 38 individuals was convened in Bozeman, Montana, to develop a nursing health services research (NHSR) agenda for the 2020s. Experts in the fields of health services and social sciences research, survey and outcomes research, informatics, health workforce research, economics and policy, as well as physicians, and leaders in nursing education and public health, focused on identifying the key research questions that, if acted upon over the next decade, would generate evidence needed to help nurses meet the challenges of the current decade:

1. Improve Access to Behavioral Health and the Effectiveness of Interventions and Services
   - What are the emerging roles and functions of RNs and APRNs providing behavioral and mental health as health care delivery becomes increasingly value-based?
   - What are the behavioral health competencies needed for all nurses, RNs and APRNs?
   - What are the specific roles and functions of RNs and APRNs providing behavioral healthcare generally, and how do they vary by severity of behavioral health issues?
   - How is team-based care affecting the delivery of behavioral health care, and what is the role of the nurse? What is the optimal configuration of teams to provide effective behavioral health care, and what role(s) do nurses play in such teams?
   - How are hospitals and healthcare systems using nurses to address SDOH that negatively affect health and well-being? What is the role of nurses in addressing these SDOH?
2. Improve Access to Primary Care and Improve the Effectiveness of Primary Care Delivery Systems
   - How do we measure the value of primary care provided by nurses and measure their productivity in achieving desired primary care outcomes?
   - How do APRN scope of practice (SOP) restrictions imposed by organizations and health systems impact access to care and effectiveness of primary care delivery systems?
   - What are models of high-performing team-based primary care and how do RNs and APRNs contribute?
   - How can nurse practitioners (NPs) transition into primary care practice be improved?
   - What are the innovations in training RNs for careers in primary care? How can effective innovations be replicated?
3. Improve Maternal Health Outcomes and the Delivery of Maternal Health Care
   - What is the current and future capacity of the nursing workforce to provide the full spectrum of women's health care along the reproductive life course (not just in the perinatal period)?

- What are the maternal health outcomes that are directly and indirectly influenced by nurses and nursing practice?
- How can evidence-based practices in maternal care be implemented consistently across care delivery settings?
- Why are maternal mortality rates increasing overall in the US, and what accounts for the severe disparities in mortality rates between racial and ethnic groups?
- What are the patterns and drivers of postpartum complications and deaths, and what can nurses do to address them?
- What are the effects of hospital and obstetric unit closures on the delivery of maternal care and on the nursing workforce skilled in delivering this care?

4. Improve Care of the Nation's Aging Population, Including Frail Adults
   - What are the roles and composition of teams caring for older people and frail adults? How do nurses contribute to team-based care serving this population?
   - What are the knowledge and skills needed by nurses to work effectively with informal and unregulated care givers?
   - How do other countries care for their aging populations? What can be learned from other countries in how they use nurses to provide care for older adults? What is the SOP of nurses caring for older and frail adults in other countries?
   - How well educated and skilled are nurses in providing long-term care, home-based care, and care coordination? What can be done to prepare more nurses to work in non-acute settings?
   - How can collaboration be improved between nurses and public health and community partners to address SDOH?

5. Help Control Healthcare Spending, Reduce Costs, and Increase the Value of Nurses' Contribution to Health and Health Care Delivery
   - What are the drivers of variation in the productivity of individual nurses and can studying individual variation identify ways to improve nurse's contribution to value of services provided to patients and consumers?
   - What are examples of successful nurse-led innovations that improve the value of health care? What are the outcomes of such innovations? What are the elements of successful innovation models?
   - What are the contributions of nurses under a shared/alternative savings model of care delivery?
   - What impact do nurses have on addressing the SDOH that negatively affect health and well-being?
   - How are nurses contributing to or helping eliminate waste in the health care system? What are the financial, resource, ethical, and environmental dimensions of waste reduction? What forms of waste are of concern to nurses and how can systems empower nurses to reduce waste?

SOURCE: Excerpted from Cohen et al., 2020.

leading to fewer RNs practicing in rural areas and many nurses being ill prepared to practice in non–acute care settings. Furthermore, the number of nurses in the specialties that are most needed to serve all Americans and achieve improved population health are woefully lacking. While each of these challenges is uniquely consequential, it is important to recognize that the nursing workforce in the United States will confront all of these challenges simultaneously. And not to be forgotten are the unknown effects of the COVID-19 pandemic on the near- and longer-term supply of and demand for nurses.

The many gaps in the capacity of the current nursing workforce will need to be overcome if the nation is to build a future workforce that can provide the health care it needs. Such a workforce would address social risk factors that negatively affect individual and overall population health and help ensure that all people can attain their highest level of well-being. Currently, there are insufficient numbers of nurses providing enough of the right types of care to the people who need health care the most, particularly in underserved locations. To overcome these deficits, substantial increases in the numbers, types, and distribution of the nursing workforce, as well as improvements in the knowledge and skills needed to address SDOH, will be needed. These improvements will occur more rapidly, more uniformly, and more successfully if programmatic, policy, and funding opportunities can be leveraged by health systems, government, educators, and payers, as well as stakeholders outside of the health care sector.

Conclusion 3-1: A substantial increase in the numbers, types, and distribution of members of the nursing workforce and improvements in their knowledge and skills in addressing social determinants of health are essential to filling gaps in care related to sociodemographic and population factors. These factors include the aging population, the increasing incidence of mental and behavioral health conditions, and the increasing lack of access to primary and maternal health care.

Conclusion 3-2: Eliminating restrictions on the scope of practice of advanced practice registered nurses and registered nurses so they can practice to the full extent of their education and training will increase the types and amount of high-quality health care services that can be provided to those with complex health and social needs and improve both access to care and health equity.

Conclusion 3-3: As the nation's population becomes more diverse, sustaining efforts to diversify the racial, ethnic, and gender composition of the nursing workforce will be important.

REFERENCES

AAMC (Association of American Medical Colleges). 2020. *New AAMC Report Confirms Growing Physician Shortage*. https://www.aamc.org/news-insights/press-releases/new-aamc-report-confirms-growing-physician-shortage (accessed January 10, 2021).

AANP (American Association of Nurse Practitioners). 2020. *State practice environment*. https://www.aanp.org/advocacy/state/state-practice-environment (accessed June 13, 2020).

Adams, E. K., and S. Markowitz. 2018. Improving efficiency in the health-care system: Removing anticompetitive barriers for advanced practice registered nurses and physician assistants. *Policy Proposal* 8:9–13.

Administration on Aging. 2013. *Issue Brief No. 11: Reaching diverse older adult population and engaging them in prevention services and early intervention*. Washington, DC: Administration on Aging.

AHA (American Hospital Association). 2018. *AHA hospital statistics, 2018 edition*. https://www.aha.org/statistics/2016-12-27-aha-hospital-statistics-2018-edition (accessed June 15, 2020).

Alexander, D., and M. Schnell. 2019. Just what the nurse practitioner ordered: Independent prescriptive authority and population mental health. *Journal of Health Economics* 66:145–162.

Altman, M. R., T. Oseguera, M. R. McLemore, I. Kantrowitz-Gordon, L. S. Franck, and A. Lyndon. 2019. Information and power: Women of color's experiences interacting with health care providers in pregnancy and birth. *Social Science and Medicine* 238:112491.

AMA (American Medical Association). 2017. *State law chart: Nurse practitioner prescriptive authority*. https://www.ama-assn.org/sites/ama-assn.org/files/corp/media-browser/specialty%20group/arc/ama-chart-np-prescriptive-authority.pdf (accessed September 3, 2020).

AMCB (American Midwifery Certifications Board). 2019. *American Midwifery Certification Board 2019 demographic report*. https://www.amcbmidwife.org/docs/default-source/reports/demographic-report-2019.pdf?sfvrsn=23f30668_2 (accessed February 24, 2021).

Auerbach, D. I., P. I. Buerhaus, and D. O. Staiger. 2015. Will the RN workforce weather the retirement of the baby boomers? *Medical Care* 53(10):850–856.

Auerbach, D., D. Staiger, and P. Buerhaus. 2018. Growing ranks of advanced practice clinicians—Implications for the physician workforce. *New England Journal of Medicine* 378(25):2358–2360.

Barnes, H., M. R. Richards, M. D. McHugh, and G. Martsolf. 2018. Rural and non-rural primary care physician practices increasingly rely on nurse practitioners. *Health Affairs* 37(6):908–914.

Barnett, M. L., D. Lee, and R. G. Frank. 2019. In rural areas, buprenorphine waiver adoption since 2017 driven by nurse practitioners and physician assistants. *Health Affairs* 38(12):2048–2056.

BLS (U.S. Bureau of Labor Statistics). 2020. *Occupational outlook handbook: Registered nurses*. https://www.bls.gov/ooh/healthcare/registered-nurses.htm (accessed December 8, 2020).

Bodenheimer, T., and L. Bauer. 2016. Rethinking the primary care workforce—An expanded role for nurses. *New England Journal of Medicine* 375:1015–1017.

Bodenheimer, T., and D. Mason. 2016. Registered nurses: Partners in transforming primary care. In *Preparing registered nurses for enhanced roles in primary care*. Conference conducted in Atlanta, GA, sponsored by the Josiah Macy Jr. Foundation. New York: Josiah Macy Jr. Foundation.

Buerhaus, P. 2018. *Nurse practitioners: A solution to America's primary care crisis*. Washington, DC: American Enterprise Institute.

Buerhaus, P. I., and D. I. Auerbach. 2011. The recession's effect on hospital registered nurse employment growth. *Nursing Economics* 29(4):163–168.

Buerhaus, P. I., C. M. DesRoches, R. Dittus, and K. Donelan. 2015. Practice characteristics of primary care nurse practitioners and physicians. *Nursing Outlook* 63(2):144–153.

Buerhaus, P. I., L. E. Skinner, D. I. Auerbach, and D. O. Staiger. 2017. Four challenges facing the nursing workforce in the United States. *Journal of Nursing Regulation* 8(2):40–46.

Carron, R. 2020. Health disparities in American Indians/Alaska Natives: Implications for nurse practitioners. *Nurse Practitioner* 45(6):26–32.

Chidambaram, P. 2020. *Data note: How might Coronavirus affect residents in nursing homes?* Kaiser Family Foundation. https://www.kff.org/coronavirus-covid-19/issue-brief/data-note-how-might-coronavirus-affect-residents-in-nursing-facilities (accessed March 23, 2021).

Cho, S-H., L. E. Masselink, C. B. Jones, and B. A. Mark. 2011. Internationally educated nurse hiring: Geographic distribution, community, and hospital characteristics. *Nursing Economics* 29(6):308.

CMS (Centers for Medicare & Medicaid Services). 2020. *Long term care facility reporting on COVID-19*. https://www.cms.gov/files/document/covid-nursing-home-reporting-numbers-5-31-20.pdf (accessed April 26, 2021).

Cohen, C. C., H. Barnes, P. I. Buerhaus, G. R. Martsolf, S. P. Clarke, K. Donelan, and H. L. Tubbs-Cooley. 2020. Top priorities for the next decade of nursing health services research. *Nursing Outlook*. doi: 10.1016/j.outlook.2020.12.004.

Collard, R., H. Boter, R. Schoevers, and R. Oude Voshaar. 2012. Prevalence of frailty in community-dwelling older persons: A systematic review. *Journal of American Geriatric Society* 60(8):1487–1492.

Davis, D. A. 2019. Obstetric racism: The racial politics of pregnancy, labor, and birthing. *Medical Anthropology* 38(7):560–573.

DesRoches, C. M., S. Clarke, J. Perloff, M. O'Reilly-Jacob, and P. Buerhaus. 2017. The quality of primary care provided by nurse practitioners to vulnerable Medicare beneficiaries. *Nursing Outlook* 65(6):679–688.

Figueroa, J. F., L. G. Burke, J. Zheng, E. Orav, and A. K. Jha. 2019. Trends in hospitalization vs observation stay for ambulatory care–sensitive conditions. *JAMA Internal Medicine* 179(12):1714–1716.

Figueroa, J., R. Wadhera, and I. Papanicolas. 2020. Association of nursing home ratings on health inspections, quality of care, and nurse staffing with COVID-19 cases. *Journal of the American Medical Association* 324(11):1103–1105.

Frakt, A. B. 2019. The rural hospital problem. *Journal of the American Medical Association* 321(23):2271–2272.

Fried, L. P., and J. W. Rowe. 2020. Health in aging—Past, present, and future. *New England Journal of Medicine* 383(14):1293–1296.

Fried, L. P., C. M. Tangen, J. Walston, A. B. Newman, C. Hirsch, J. Gottdiener, and M. A. McBurnie. 2001. Frailty in older adults: Evidence for a phenotype. *Journals of Gerontology Series A: Biological Sciences and Medical Sciences* 56(3):M146–M157.

Frogner, B. K., E. P. Fraher, J. Spetz, P. Pittman, J. Moore, A. J. Beck, and P. Buerhaus. 2020. Modernizing scope-of-practice regulations—Time to prioritize patients. *New England Journal of Medicine* 382(7):591–593.

GAO (U.S. Government Accountability Office). 2018. *Indian Health Service: Agency faces ongoing challenges filling provider vacancies*. Washington, DC: U.S. Government Accountability Office.

Geng, F., D. G. Stevenson, and D. C. Grabowski. 2019. Daily nursing home staffing levels highly variable, often below CMS expectations. *Health Affairs* 38(7):1095–1100.

Georgetown University. 2019. *How does the role of nurse-midwives change from state to state?* https://online.nursing.georgetown.edu/blog/scope-of-practice-for-midwives/#practice%20 environment (accessed December 17, 2020).

Gooch, K. 2020 (June 5). Record number of healthcare workers laid off, furloughed during pandemic. *Becker's Hospital Review*. https://www.beckershospitalreview.com/workforce/record-number-of-healthcare-workers-laid-off-furloughed-during-pandemic.html (accessed December 8, 2020).

Graves, J. A., P. Mishra, R. S. Dittus, R. Parikh, J. Perloff, and P. Buerhaus. 2016. Role of geography and nurse practitioner scope-of-practice in efforts to expand primary care system capacity. *Medical Care* 54(1):81–89.

Hamilton, B. E., J. A. Martin, M. J. Osterman, and L. M. Rossen. 2020. *Births: Provisional data for 2018*. NVSS Vital Statistics Rapid Release, Report No. 007. Hyattsville, MD: National Center for Health Statistics, Centers for Disease Control and Prevention.

Henderson, M. 2020. Legislative: COVID-19 and mental health: The inevitable impact. *Online Journal of Issues in Nursing* 25(3).

Hohn, M. D., J. Witte, J. Lowry, and J. Fernández-Peña. 2016. *Immigrants in health care: Keeping Americans healthy through care and innovation*. Washington, DC: Immigrant Learning Center.

HRSA (Health Resources and Services Administration). 2010. *The registered nurse population: Initial findings from the 2008 National Sample Survey of Registered Nurses*. Rockville, MD: Health Resources and Services Administration.

HRSA. 2016. *National projections of supply and demand for selected behavioral health practitioners: 2013–2025*. Rockville, MD: Health Resources and Services Administration.

HRSA. 2017. *National and regional supply and demand projections of the nursing workforce: 2014–2030*. Rockville, MD: Health Resources and Services Administration.

IHS (Indian Health Service). 2019. *Disparities*. https://www.ihs.gov/newsroom/factsheets/disparities (accessed November 9, 2020).

IOM (Institute of Medicine). 2011. *The future of nursing: Leading change, advancing health*. Washington, DC: The National Academies Press.

IPUMS (Integrated Public Use Microdata Series) USA. *Select samples*. https://usa.ipums.org/usa-action/samples (accessed December 8, 2020).

Johnson, J. D., I. V. Asiodu, C. P. McKenzie, C. Tucker, K. P. Tully, K. Bryant, and A. M. Stuebe. 2019. Racial and ethnic inequities in postpartum pain evaluation and management. *Obstetrics & Gynecology* 134(6):1155–1162.

Lai, J., S. Ma, Y. Wang, Z. Cai, J. Hu, N. Wei, and H. Tan. 2020. Factors associated with mental health outcomes among health care workers exposed to coronavirus disease. *JAMA Network Open* 3(3):e203976.

Leavitt, R. A., A. Ertl, K. Sheats, E. Petrosky, A. Ivey-Stephenson, and K. A. Fowler. 2018. Suicides among American Indian/Alaska Natives—National violent death reporting system, 18 states, 2003–2014. *Morbidity and Mortality Weekly Report* 67(8):237.

Leonard, S. A., E. K. Main, K. A. Scott, J. Profit, and S. L. Carmichael. 2019. Racial and ethnic disparities in severe maternal morbidity prevalence and trends. *Annals of Epidemiology* 33:30–36.

MacDorman, M. F., and E. Declercq. 2019. Trends and state variations in out-of-hospital births in the United States, 2004–2017. *Birth* 46(2):279–288.

Masselink, L. E., and C. B. Jones. 2014. Immigration policy and internationally educated nurses in the United States: A brief history. *Nursing Outlook* 62(1):39–45.

McGarry, B. E., D. C. Grabowski, and M. L. Barnett. 2020. Severe staffing and personal protective equipment shortages faced by nursing homes during the COVID-19 pandemic. *Health Affairs* 39(10). doi: 10.1377/hlthaff.2020.01269.

McLemore, M. R., M. R. Altman, N. Cooper, S. Williams, L. Rand, and L. Franck. 2018. Health care experiences of pregnant, birthing and postnatal women of color at risk for preterm birth. *Social Science & Medicine* 201:127–135.

McMichael, B. 2020. Healthcare licensing and liability. *Indiana Law Journal* 95(3):821–882.

NASEM (National Academies of Sciences, Engineering, and Medicine). 2016. *Assessing progress on the Institute of Medicine report* The Future of Nursing. Washington, DC: The National Academies Press.

NCSBN (National Council of State Boards of Nursing). 2008. *Number of candidates taking NCLEX examination and percent passing, by type of candidate*. https://www.ncsbn.org/Table_of_Pass_Rates_2007.pdf (accessed November 9, 2020).

NCSBN. 2019. *Number of candidates taking NCLEX examination and percent passing, by type of candidate*. https://www.ncsbn.org/table_of_pass_rates_2019.pdf (accessed November 9, 2020).

NCSBN. 2020. *NCSBN's environmental scan: A portrait of nursing and healthcare in 2020 and beyond*. https://www.ncsbn.org/2020_JNREnvScan.pdf (accessed on June 4, 2021).

OECD (Organisation for Economic Co-operation and Development). 2018. *Health workforce migration: Migration of nurses*. Dataset. https://stats.oecd.org/Index.aspx?DataSetCode=HEALTH_WFMI (accessed March 23, 2021).

Perloff, J., S. Clarke, C. M. DesRoches, M. O'Reilly-Jacob, and P. Buerhaus. 2019. Association of state-level restrictions in nurse practitioner scope of practice with the quality of primary care provided to Medicare beneficiaries. *Medical Care Research and Review* 76(5):597–626.

Petersen, E. E., N. L. Davis, D. Goodman, S. Cox, N. Mayes, E. Johnston, and W. Barfield. 2019. Vital signs: Pregnancy-related deaths, United States, 2011–2015, and strategies for prevention, 13 states, 2013–2017. *Morbidity and Mortality Weekly Report* 68(18):423–429.

Serbin, J., and E. Donnelly. 2016. The impact of racism and midwifery's lack of racial diversity: A literature review. *Journal of Midwifery & Women's Health* 61(6):694–706.

Shaffer, F. A., M. A. Bakhshi, N. Farrell, and T. D. Álvarez. 2020. CE: Original research: The recruitment experience of foreign-educated health professionals to the United States. *American Journal of Nursing* 120(1):28–38.

Skinner, L., D. O. Staiger, D. I. Auerbach, and P. Buerhaus. 2019. Implications of an aging rural physician workforce. *New England Journal of Medicine* 381(4):299–301.

Smallwood, R., C. Woods, T. Power, and K. Usher. 2020. Understanding the impact of historical trauma due to colonization on the health and well-being of indigenous young peoples: A systematic scoping review. *Journal of Transcultural Nursing* 32(1):59–68. doi: 1043659620935955.

Smiley, R. A., P. Lauer, C. Bienemy, J. G. Berg, E. Shireman, K. A. Reneau, and M. Alexander. 2018. The 2017 national nursing workforce survey. *Journal of Nursing Regulation* 9(3):S1–S88.

Vedam, S., K. Stoll, T. K. Taiwo, N. Rubashkin, M. Cheyney, N. Strauss, and L. Schummers. 2019. The Giving Voice to Mothers study: Inequity and mistreatment during pregnancy and childbirth in the United States. *Reproductive Health* 16(1):77.

Vespa, J., L. Medina, and D. M. Armstrong. 2020. *Demographic Turning Points for the United States: Population Projections for 2020 to 2060*. Current Population Reports, P25-1144. Washington, DC: U.S. Census Bureau.

Williams, J. C., N. Anderson, M. Mathis, E. Samford III, J. Eugene, and J. Isom. 2020. Colorblind algorithms: Racism in the era of COVID-19. *Journal of the National Medical Association* 112(5):550–552. doi: 10.1016/j.jnma.2020.05.010.

Xu, W., S. Retchin, and P. Buerhaus. 2021. Dual eligibles and inadequate access to primary care providers. *American Journal of Managed Care* 27(5).

Xue, Y., J. A. Smith, and J. Spetz. 2019. Primary care nurse practitioners and physicians in low-income and rural areas, 2010–2016. *Journal of the American Medical Association* 321(1):102–105.

Yang, B. K., M. E. Johantgen, A. M. Trinkoff, S. R. Idzik, J. Wince, and C. Tomlinson. 2020. State nurse practitioner practice regulations and US health care delivery outcomes: A systematic review. *Medical Care Research and Review*. doi: 1077558719901216.

Yuanhong, A., S. Skillman, and B. Frogner. 2020. Is it fair? How to approach professional scope-of-practice policy after the COVID-19 pandemic. *Health Affairs Blog*. doi: 10.1377/hblog20200624.983306.

Zhang, X., D. Tai, H. Pforsich, and V. W. Lin. 2018. United States registered nurse workforce report card and shortage forecast: A revisit. *American Journal of Medical Quality* 33(3):229–236.

4

The Role of Nurses in Improving Health Care Access and Quality

Of all the forms of inequality, injustice in health care is the most shocking and inhumane.

—Dr. Martin Luther King, civil rights activist

Nurses can be key contributors to making substantial progress toward health care equity in the United States in the decade ahead by taking on expanded roles, working in new settings in innovative ways, and partnering with communities and other sectors. But the potential for nurses to help people and communities live healthier lives can be realized only if the barriers to their working to the full extent of their education and training are removed. To this end, it will be necessary to revise scope-of-practice laws, public health and health system policies, state laws regarding the use of standing orders, and reimbursement rules for Medicare and other payers. Major shifts occurring both within society at large and within health care will transform the environment in which the next generation of nurses will practice and lead. If health care equity is to be fully achieved, nursing schools will need to focus on ensuring that all nurses, regardless of their practice setting, can address the social factors that influence health and provide care that meets people where they are.

Health care equity focuses on ensuring that everyone has access to high-quality health care. As shown in the Social Determinants of Health and Social Needs Model of Castrucci and Auerbach (2019) (see Chapter 2), health care is a downstream determinant of health, but disparities in health care access and quality can widen and exacerbate disparities produced by upstream and midstream determinants of health outcomes.

According to Healthy People 2020, access to quality health care encompasses the ability to gain entry into the health care system through health insurance, geographic availability, and access to a health care provider. Health care quality has been defined as "the degree to which health care services for individuals and populations increase the likelihood of desired outcomes and are consistent with current professional knowledge" (IOM, 1990, p. 4). The Agency for Healthcare Research and Quality (AHRQ) defines quality health care "as doing the right thing for the right patient, at the right time, in the right way to achieve the best possible results" (Sofaer and Hibbard, 2010). Nurses deliver high-quality care by providing care that is safe, effective, person-centered, timely, efficient, and equitable (IOM, 2001).

As noted, frameworks for social determinants of health (SDOH) place the health care system downstream, often operating in response to illness, rather than upstream, impacting the underlying causes of health outcomes (Castrucci and Auerbach, 2019). Therefore, health care itself does not address most of the upstream factors, or root causes of illness, that affect health equity; such upstream social factors as economic and housing instability, discrimination and other forms of racism, educational disparities, and inadequate nutrition can affect an individual's health before the health care system is ever involved (Castrucci and Auerbach, 2019). Health equity is discussed in detail in Chapter 5. Some estimates indicate that a small portion of health outcomes is related to health care, while equity in health care is an important contributing factor to health equity (Hood et al., 2016; Remington et al., 2015).

Major shifts occurring both within society at large and within health care will transform the environment in which the next generation of nurses will practice and lead. These shifts encompass changing demographics, including declining physical and mental health; increased attention to racism and equity issues; the development and adoption of new technologies; and changing patterns of health care delivery. The widespread movement for racial justice, along with the stark racial disparities in the impacts of COVID-19, has reinforced the nursing profession's ethical mandate to advocate for racial justice and to help combat the inequities embedded in the current health care system. The commitment to social justice is reflected in provision 9 of the Code of Ethics of the American Nurses Association (ANA, 2015), and its priority has been elevated by the increased demand for social justice within communities and society at large.

Changing health outcomes will require action at all levels—upstream, midstream, and downstream—and nurses have a major role at all levels in reducing gaps in clinical outcomes and improving health care equity. Nurses can strengthen their commitment to diversity, equity, and inclusion by leading large-scale efforts to dismantle systemic contributors to inequality and create new norms and competencies within health care. In that process, nurses will need to meet the complex ethical challenges that will arise as health care reorients to respond to the rapidly changing landscape (ANA, 2020; Beard and Julion, 2016; Koschmann et al., 2020; Villarruel and Broome, 2020). To ensure nursing's robust engagement with these major shifts in health care and society, investments in the well-being of nurses will be essential (ANA, 2015) (see Chapter 10).

This chapter examines ways in which nurses today work to improve health care equity, as well as their potential future roles and responsibilities in improving equity through efforts to expand access to and improve the quality of health care. Existing exemplars are also described, as well as implications of COVID-19 for health care access and quality.

NURSES' ROLES IN EXPANDING ACCESS TO QUALITY HEALTH CARE

The United States spends more than $3.5 trillion per year on health care, 25 percent more per capita than the next highest-spending country, and underperforms on nearly every metric (Emanuel et al., 2020). Life expectancy, infant mortality, and maternal mortality are all worse in the United States than in most developed countries. In the United States, moreover, disparities in health care access and health outcomes are seen across racial lines; however, being able to use social and financial capital to buy the best health care is not necessarily associated with the world's best health outcomes. Even among White U.S. citizens and those of higher socioeconomic status (SES), U.S. health indicators still lag behind those in many other countries (Emanuel, 2020). The U.S. population will not fully thrive unless all individuals can live their healthiest lives, regardless of their income, their race or ethnicity, or where they live. As discussed in Chapter 2, however, race and ethnicity, income, gender, and geographic location all play substantial roles in a person's ability to access high-quality, equitable, and affordable health care. A variety of professionals from within and outside of health care settings participate in efforts to ensure equitable access to care. But the role of nurses in these efforts is key, given their interactions with individuals and families in providing and coordinating person-centered care for preventive, acute, and chronic health needs within health settings, collaborating with social services to meet the social needs of individuals, and engaging in broader population and community health through roles in public health and community-based settings.

Both in the United States and globally, the rapid growth in the number of older people in the population will likely lead to increased demand for services and programs to meet their health and social care needs (Donelan et al., 2019; Spetz et al., 2015), including care for chronic conditions, which account for approximately 75 percent of all primary care visits (Zamosky, 2013). The aging population will also bring change in the kinds of care the patient population will need. Older people tend to require more expensive care, and to need increasing support in managing multiple conditions and retaining strength and resilience as they age (Pohl et al., 2018). These realities underscore the importance of designing, testing, and adopting chronic care models, in which teams are essential to managing chronic disease, and registered nurses (RNs) play a key role as chronic disease care managers (Bodenheimer and Mason, 2016). Studies of exemplary primary care practices (Bodenheimer et al., 2015; Smolowitz et al., 2015) define key domains of RN practice in primary care, including preventive care, chronic illness management, practice operations, care management, and transition care.

Since the passage of the Patient Protection and Affordable Care Act, substantial changes have occurred in the organization and delivery of primary care, emphasizing greater team involvement in care and expansion of the roles of each team member, including RNs (Flinter et al., 2017). Including RNs as team members can increase access to care, improve care quality and coordination for chronic conditions, and reduce burnout among primary care practitioners by expanding primary care capacity (Fraher et al., 2015; Ghorob and Bodenheimer, 2012; Lamb et al., 2015).

In primary care, RNs can assume

> at least four responsibilities: 1) Engaging patients with chronic conditions in behavior change and adjusting medications according to practitioner-written protocols; 2) Leading teams to improve the care and reduce the costs of high-need, high-cost patients; 3) Coordinating the care of chronically ill patients between the primary care home and the surrounding healthcare neighborhood; and 4) Promoting population health, including working with communities to create healthier spaces for people to live, work, learn, and play. (Bodenheimer and Mason, 2016, pp. 11–12)

Findings from a 2013 study of The Primary Care Team: Learning from Effective Ambulatory Practices (LEAP) suggest that a large majority of LEAP primary care practices, regardless of practice type or corporate structure, use RNs as a key part of their care team model (Ladden et al., 2013). This contrasts with a study of 496 practices in the Centers for Medicare & Medicaid Services (CMS) Comprehensive Primary Care initiative (Peikes et al., 2014) that found that only 36 percent of practices had RNs on staff, compared with 77 percent of LEAP sites (Flinter et al., 2017).

The health needs of individuals exist across a spectrum, ranging from healthy people, for whom health promotion and disease prevention efforts are most appropriate, to people who have limited functional capacity as a result of disabilities, severe or multiple chronic conditions, or unmet social needs or are nearing the end of life. Access to quality health care services is an important SDOH, and equitable access to care is needed for “promoting and maintaining health, preventing and managing disease, reducing unnecessary disability and premature death, and achieving health equity” (ODPHP, 2020). Likewise, “strengthening the core of primary care service delivery is key to achieving the Triple Aim of improved patient care experiences, better population health outcomes, and lower health care costs" (Bodenheimer and Mason, 2016, p. 23). The 2011 *The Future of Nursing* report echoes these themes:

> while changes in the healthcare system will have profound effects on all providers, this will be undoubtedly true for nurses. Traditional nursing competencies, such as care management and coordination, patient education, public health intervention, and transitional care, are likely to dominate in a reformed healthcare system as it inevitably moves toward an emphasis on prevention and management rather than acute [hospital] care. (IOM, 2011, p. 24)

Given the increased evidence supporting the focus on addressing social needs and SDOH to improve health outcomes, these competencies are even more important a decade later. While progress has been made, there is still work to be done, and leveraging and expanding the roles and responsibilities of nurses can help improve access to care (Campaign for Action, n.d.).

For people who have difficulty accessing health care because of distance, lack of providers, lack of insurance, or other reasons, nurses are a lifeline to care that meets them where they are. Nurses work in areas that are underserved by other health care providers and serve the uninsured and underinsured. They often engage with and provide care to people in their homes, they work in a variety of clinics, they use telehealth to connect with people, and they establish partnerships and create relationships in schools and communities. In addition to expanding the capacity of primary care, nurses serve in vital roles during natural disasters and public health emergencies, helping to meet the surge in the need for care (see Chapter 8). Yet, the potential for nurses to advance health equity through expanded access to care is limited by state and federal laws and regulations that restrict nurses' ability to provide care to the full extent of their education and training (see Chapter 3). Ways in which nurses can fulfill this potential to increase access to care for populations with complex health and social needs are discussed below.

INCREASING ACCESS FOR POPULATIONS WITH COMPLEX HEALTH AND SOCIAL NEEDS

Many individuals cannot access health care because of lack of insurance, inability to pay, and lack of clinics or providers in their geographic area. To bridge this gap, access to care is expanded through a variety of settings where nurses work, including federally qualified health centers (FQHCs), retail clinics, home health and home visiting, telehealth, school nursing, and school-based health centers, as well as nurse-managed health centers. Across all of these settings, nurses are present and facilitate access to health services for individuals and families, often serving as a bridge to social services as well.

Federally Qualified Health Centers

Through FQHCs—outpatient facilities located in a federally designated medically underserved area or serving a medically underserved population—nurses expand access to services for individuals regardless of ability to pay by helping to provide comprehensive primary health care services, referrals, and services that facilitate access to care. The role of advanced practice registered nurses (APRNs) in FQHCs has grown over time (NACHC, 2019). The emerging role of RNs in FQHCs is seen in increased interactions with patients, involvement in care management, and autonomy in the delivery of care. Nurses also work to address key social factors in partnership with care coordinators, health coaches, and social workers to improve health outcomes (Flinter et al., 2017).

Retail Clinics

Health care delivery in the United States has been undergoing transformation, and these changes provide new opportunities for more patients and greater access to nurses as new policies are implemented, new payment models take hold, resources are focused on SDOH, and consumerism shapes care choices. One change in particular since the prior *The Future of Nursing* report (IOM, 2011) has been and will continue to be impactful for nursing: the emergence of nontraditional health care entities, such as retail clinics. The evolution and rapid growth of these established retail clinics provide increased accessibility of basic care, health screenings, vaccines, and other services for some populations (Gaur et al., 2019). The number of such is growing rapidly, from around 1,800 in 2015 to 2,700 operating in 44 states and the District of Columbia by 2018.

Retail clinics provide more accessible primary care for some populations. In 2016, 58 percent of retail clinic visits represented new utilization instead of substitution for more costly primary care or emergency department visits (Bachrach and Frohlich, 2016). Many individuals and families use retail clinics for their convenience, which includes long hours of operation, accessible location, and walk-in policies, as well as low-cost visits. These attributes are important for those with lower income or without insurance who may not have a regular source of care or be able to access a primary care provider (Bachrach and Frohlich, 2016). However, research shows retail clinics are typically placed in higher-income, urban, and suburban settings with higher concentrations of White and fewer Black and Hispanic residents (RAND Corporation, 2016). The RAND Corporation (2016) study found that while 21 percent of the U.S. population lived in medically underserved areas, only 12.5 percent of retail clinics were located in these areas. RAND concluded that "overall, retail clinics are not improving access to care for the medically underserved." Thus, while these new models of care have the potential to advance health care equity and population-level health, the available data do not indicate that this potential has been realized (RAND

Corporation, 2016). The equity impact of these retail clincs depends in large part on who utilizes the services, and whether the utilization patterns are similar to or different from those of traditional health care.

Retail clinics are staffed largely by nurse practitioners (NPs) (Carthon et al., 2017). These clinics in pharmacies and grocery stores often have been constrained by restrictive scope-of-practice laws. In 2016, a study by the University of Pennsylvania School of Nursing's Center for Health Outcomes and Policy Research investigated scope-of-practice regulatory environments and retail-based clinic growth. Looking at three states with varying levels of scope-of-practice restrictions, the study found an association between relaxation of practice regulations and retail clinic growth. Evidence suggests that optimization of innovative health care sites such as retail clinics will require moving toward the adoption of policies that standardize the scope of practice for NPs, the providers who largely staff retail clinics (Carthon et al., 2017).

Home Health and Home Visiting

Visiting people in their homes can advance equitable access to quality health care. Home health care has increased access to care for many Americans, from older individuals to medically fragile children. Yao and colleagues (2021) recently explored trends in the U.S. workforce providing home-based medical care and found that less than 1 percent of physicians participating in traditional Medicare provide more than 50 home visits each year (a rate unchanged between 2012 and 2016). By contrast, the number of NPs providing home visits nearly doubled during that same period. Home health nurses address a fragmented system by coordinating care for patients transitioning from a tertiary care facility to ongoing health care within their own homes. Since the onset of the COVID-19 pandemic, these nurses have increasingly provided families with respite for caregivers and offered mental health services in many forms, but certainly in decreasing social isolation for elderly people. Delivering care at home has offered a window for physicians and NPs to see where patients live, to engage in telehealth video calls with family members present, and to see the features of neighborhoods that impact health (e.g., sidewalks, playgrounds, stairs).

With the expansion in the home health care industry driven by an aging population, home visiting nurses are essential to providing care and enhancing health care equity (Walker, 2019). Prior to 2020, Medicare rules allowed only physicians to order home health services for Medicare beneficiaries. However, the Coronavirus Aid, Relief, and Economic Security (CARES) Act permanently authorizes physician assistants and NPs to order home health care services for Medicare patients. In addition, CMS has instituted new policies outlining comprehensive temporary measures for increasing the capacity of the U.S. health care system to provide care to patients outside a traditional hospital setting amid the rising number of COVID-19-related hospitalizations nationwide. These measures include both the Hospital Without Walls and Acute Hospital Care At Home programs, both initiated during the pandemic. Under previous federal requirements, hospitals had to provide services within their own buildings, raising concerns about capacity for treating COVID-19 patients, especially those requiring ventilator and intensive care. Under CMS's temporary new rules, hospitals can transfer patients to outside facilities, such as ambulatory surgery centers, inpatient rehabilitation hospitals, hotels, and dormitories, while still receiving hospital payments under Medicare. Provision for at-home care, which is often preferred by patients, is especially important during a crisis such as the pandemic, when hospital care means family and/or caregivers cannot be present. Moreover, some research has shown home care to be less costly and to result in fewer readmissions relative to hospital care (Levine et al., 2020). These programs also will create new demand for nurses to work in the community and are the types of adaptations that occurred as a result of the COVID-19 pandemic that should remain permanent to expand high-quality access to care.

The locus of care delivery will continue to follow personal preferences of individuals and families. To improve health care access, nurses will need to be intentional about meeting patients where they are in the most literal sense, and to serve as advocates with and within public health, retail clinics, and health systems to ensure that patients can access the care they need in their homes and neighborhoods. Box 4-1 describes several innovative nurse-led, in-home care programs.

In addition to home health, nurse home visiting programs often include such services as health check-ups, screenings, referrals, and guidance in navigating other programs and services in the community (Child and Family Research Partnership, 2015). Growing evidence suggests that home visits by nurses during pregnancy and in the first years of a child's life can improve the health and well-being of both child and family, including by promoting maternal and child health, prevention of child abuse and neglect, positive parenting, child development, and school readiness. This positive impact has been found to continue into adolescence and early adulthood (NASEM, 2019).

Telehealth

The proliferation of mobile devices and applications offers an opportunity for nurses to use telehealth more broadly to connect with individuals. Telehealth, including video visits, email, and distance education, serves as a tool to connect with people on an ongoing basis without their having to leave their homes, workplaces, or other settings, and allows for long-distance patient and clinician contact for purposes of clinical interventions, health promotion, education, assessment, and monitoring. The use of telehealth is especially helpful for those who have difficulty traveling to obtain care and those who reside in rural or remote areas. Vulnerable populations with multiple chronic illnesses, poor health literacy, and lack of supportive resources may benefit the most from telehealth use. However, use of telehealth or virtual health tools is limited by access to reliable Internet

BOX 4-1
Innovative In-Home Care Programs

The aging population's health and social needs will call for more programs that meet those needs in elderly people's homes and communities. Examples of such programs are described below.

CAPABLE: The Community Aging in Place—Advancing Better Living for Elders (CAPABLE) program targets low-income seniors and provides comprehensive services to improve daily function, improve quality of life, and reduce mortality risk. It is a multidisciplinary, nurse-led home visiting intervention with the goal of helping older adults age in place. CAPABLE has been studied in randomized controlled trials (RCTs) funded by Medicaid and Medicare in 13 cities and 8 states. It has successfully reduced hospital and nursing home admissions, reduced incorrect medication dosing, and improved nutrition and diet. It has yielded reported savings of more than $10,000 per member per year for Medicare (Szanton et al., 2019).

House Calls: This United HealthCare program provides Medicare Advantage recipients with nurse home visits. The nurse visits are meant to identify care opportunities that may not be readily apparent in primary care provider office visits, and then to coordinate care to ensure that those needs are addressed. The program was found to yield a 14 percent decrease in member hospital admissions, a 90 percent decrease in the risk for long-term care stays, a 6 percent reduction in emergency department visits, and a 2–6 percent increase in primary care provider office visits (United HealthCare, 2018).

Nurse-Family Partnership: The Home Visiting Evidence of Effectiveness project, established by the Administration for Children and Families (ACF) in the U.S. Department of Health and Human Services, identified 20 home visiting models as meeting criteria for effectiveness that warranted recommending them for state-based home visitation programs (OPRE, 2020). Based on the available high- or moderate-quality studies identified, the review showed that most of these programs have multiple favorable effects with sustained impact, with Healthy Families America and the Nurse-Family Partnership (NFP) showing favorable impact across the greatest breadth of outcomes

The NFP, a program of intensive pre- and postnatal home visitation by registered nurses targeting low-income mothers and their first children, has been evaluated in six RCTs and several more limited analyses of operational programs.The program has demonstrated multiple positive outcomes. It was found to have reduced both emergency department visits for children (Michaleopoulos et al., 2019) and domestic violence reports (Eckenrode et al., 2017). Mothers receiving visits from nurse home visitors had fewer health care encounters for injuries and higher ratings on the home environment and parents' reports of caregiving (Kitzman et al., 1997; Olds et al., 2019). Estimates indicate that by 2031, NFP program enrollments in 1996–2013 will have prevented an estimated 500 infant deaths, 10,000 preterm births, 13,000 dangerous closely spaced second births, 4,700 abortions, 42,000 child maltreatment incidents, 36,000 intimate partner violence incidents, 90,000 violent crimes by youth, 594,000 property and public order crimes (e.g., vandalism, loitering) by youth, 36,000 youth arrests, and 41,000 person-years of youth substance abuse (Miller, 2015).

connections and the availability of the necessary hardware, including smartphones, computers, or webcams. A recent report in the *Journal of the American Medical Association* looks at 41 FQHCs serving 1.7 million patients. Prior to the COVID-19 pandemic, there was minimal telehealth use at these facilities. During March 2020, FQHCs rapidly substituted in-person visits with telephone and video visits. For primary care, however, 48.5 percent of telehealth visits occured by telephone and 3.4 percent by video. In addition, CMS estimated that 30 percent of telehealth visits were audio-only during the pandemic. These numbers indicate that telehealth appointments for lower-income Americans were in large part audio-only, raising questions about the quality of care (Uscher-Pines et al., 2021).

There have been examples of telehealth activities that have demonstrated great success. The Mississippi Diabetes Telehealth Network, for example, implemented a program that uses telehealth in the home as a viable way to bring a care team to patients to assist them as they manage their illnesses. NPs provide daily health sessions and remote monitoring for individuals with diabetes (Davis et al., 2020; Henderson et al., 2014). A prospective, longitudinal cohort study design evaluated the relationship between using telehealth for chronic care management and diabetes outcomes over a 12-month period, finding a significant difference in HbA1c values from baseline to 3-, 6-, 9-, and 12-month values (Davis et al., 2020). In another example, Mercy Hospital, a virtual care center, delivers telehealth services to rural communities in Arkansas, Kansas, Missouri, and Oklahoma. One of its many services is Nurse on Call, which provides timely clinical advice and is available around the clock. In still another example, Banner Health's skilled nursing model delivers home care combined with telehealth services to people at home instead of their having to move to a nursing home facility (Roth, 2018).

School Nursing

School nurses are front-line health care providers, serving as a bridge between the health care and education systems. Hired by school districts, health departments, or hospitals, school nurses attend to the physical and mental health of students in school. As public health sentinels, they engage school communities, parents, and health care providers to promote wellness and improve health outcomes for children. School nurses are essential to expanding access to quality health care for students, especially in light of the increasing number of students with complex health and social needs. Access to school nurses helps increase health care equity for students. For many children living in or near poverty, the school nurse may be the only health care professional they regularly access.

School nurses treat and help students manage chronic health conditions and disabilities; address injuries and urgent care needs; provide preventive and screening services, health education, immunizations, and psychosocial support; conduct behavioral assessments; and collaborate with health care providers, school staff, and the community to facilitate the holistic care each child needs (Council on School Health, 2008; Holmes et al., 2016; HRSA, 2017; Lineberry and Ickes, 2015; Maughan, 2018). By helping students get and stay healthy, school health programs can contribute to closing the achievement gap (Basch, 2011; Maughan, 2018). According to Johnson (2017),

> Healthy children learn better; educated children grow to raise healthier families advancing a stronger, more productive nation for generations to come. School nurses work to assure that children have access to educational opportunities regardless of their state of health. (p. 1)

Meeting the mental health needs of children can be particularly challenging. Researchers estimate that about a quarter of all school-age children and adolescents struggle with mental health issues, such as anxiety and depression. Approximately 30 percent of student health visits to the school nurse are for mental health concerns, often disguised by complaints of headaches and stomachaches (Foster et al., 2005). School nurses have experience with screening students at risk for a variety of such concerns and can assist students in addressing them (NASN, 2020a). However, most youth—nearly 80 percent—who need mental health services will not receive them (Kataoka et al., 2005); schools are not always equipped to deal with students' emotional needs, and parents often lack the awareness or resources to get help for their children. Additionally, a recent study found disparities in access to mental health treatment for students along racial and ethnic lines (Lipson et al., 2018), and structural racism undergirds many risk factors for mental illness (see Chapter 2). The COVID-19 pandemic has revealed—and exacerbated—inequities among children of different incomes and races/ethnicities. School closures and social isolation have affected all students, but especially those living in poverty. In addition to the damage to student learning, the loss of access to mental health services that were offered by schools has resulted in the emergence of a mental health crisis (Leeb et al., 2020; Patrick et al., 2020; Singh et al., 2020).

Schools are increasingly being recognized not just as core educational institutions but also as community-based assets that can be a central component of building healthy and vibrant communities (NASEM, 2017). Accordingly, schools and, by extension, school nurses are being incorporated into strategies for improving health care access, serving as hubs of health promotion and providers of population-based care (Maughan, 2018). Yet, while there have been calls for every school to have access to a nurse (Council on School Health, 2016; NASN, 2020b), only 39.9 percent of schools employed a full-time nurse in 2017. The remainder of schools (39.3 percent) employed a part-time nurse or did not employ a nurse at all (25.2 percent) (Willgerodt, 2018). The availability and staffing levels of school nurses vary greatly by geography (Willgerodt, 2018) (see Figure 4-1).

To address the lack of health care resources in rural school settings, telehealth programs have been implemented with success (RHI, 2019). An example is

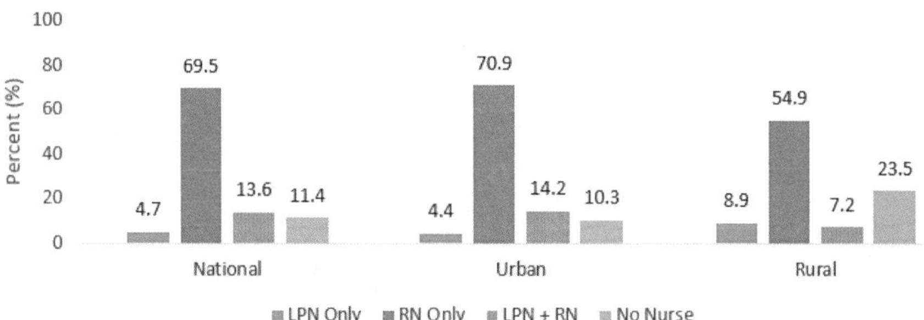

FIGURE 4-1 Licensure staffing patterns (paid and unpaid volunteer) by geography.
SOURCE: Data from Willgerodt, 2018.

Health-e-Schools, in which onsite school nurses connect sick students with health care providers. The program employs a full-time, off-site family NP who uses telehealth to evaluate and diagnose patients with such health issues as earaches, sore throats, colds, and rashes, as well as to provide sports physicals, medication, chronic disease management, and behavioral health care. It began as a telehealth program implemented by only 3 schools in 2011 and has since expanded to more than 80 schools serving more than 25,000 students. Health-e-Schools has helped increase classroom attendance and decrease the amount of time parents or guardians must take off from work to bring their children to appointments. This model relies heavily on the school nurses employed within each school district to serve as primary telehealth providers, thus requiring that funding be allocated to provide a school nurse in each school.

School-Based Health Centers

School-based health centers (SBHCs) also make care accessible to students in the school setting. In 2017, 2,584 SBHCs were operating in the United States (Love et al., 2019). SBHCs often operate as a partnership between the school and a community health organization, such as a community health center, hospital, or local health department; more than half are supported by or are an extension of FQHCs (SBHA, n.d.). SBHC services include primary care, mental health care, social services, dentistry, and health education, but vary based on community needs and resources as determined through collaborations among the community, the school district, and health care providers (CPSTF, 2015; HRSA, 2017). Services are provided by interprofessional teams of health care professionals that include nurses, mental health care providers, physicians, nutritionists, and others. As of 2017, NPs provided primary care services onsite and through telehealth services at 85 percent of SBHCs (Love et al., 2019; SBHA, 2018).

One example of an SBHC is the nurse-run Vine School Health Center (VSHC) located at the Vine Middle Magnet School in Knoxville, Tennessee, a

Title I school where 100 percent of the students qualify for free lunch. VSHC provides onsite and telehealth services to anyone up to 21 years of age who lives in the county. It also serves 10 other Title I schools through direct health care or telehealth services. The clinic is a partnership between the University of Tennessee College of Nursing and Knox County Schools and is staffed by nurses, nursing students, social workers, and special education professionals. Staff assist families with social needs, including food, housing, clothing, linkages to health insurance, and financial support for rent and utilities (AAN, 2015; Pittman, 2019). Services rendered during the 2016–2017 school year included 1,110 early and periodic screening, diagnostic and treatment (EPSDT) exams; 1,896 immunizations; 4,455 physical health visits; and 1,796 mental health clinic visits. VSHC estimates that its services enabled the avoidance of more than 2,500 potential emergency room visits per academic year, associated with savings of about $375,000 per year (AAN, 2015).

IMPROVING THE QUALITY OF HEALTH CARE

Access to comprehensive health care services is a precursor to equitable, quality health care. Nurses are uniquely qualified to help improve the quality of health care by helping people navigate the health care system, providing close monitoring and follow-up across the care continuum, focusing care on the whole person, and providing care that is culturally respectful and appropriate. Nurses can help overcome barriers to quality care, including structural inequities and implicit bias, through care management, person-centered care, and cultural humility.

Care Management

In the current health care system, care is often disjointed, with processes varying between primary and specialty care and between traditional and emerging care sites. People may not understand the processes of the health care system, such as where they will receive care, how to make appointments, or the various providers with whom they may come into contact. Perhaps most important, patients may not understand why all the providers across settings where they receive care should be knowledgeable about the services they receive and the problems that have been identified to ensure seamless, continuous high-quality care. Social factors affecting people with complex health needs may also adversely affect their ability to receive optimal care. Care management, care coordination, and transitional care are activities that nurses perform as members of a health care team to decrease fragmentation, bolster communication, and improve care quality and safety. A care management approach is particularly important for people with complex health and social needs, who may require care from multiple providers, medical follow-up, medication management, and help in addressing their social needs.

Care management—a set of activities designed to "enhance coordination of care, eliminate duplication of services, reduce the need for expensive medical services, and increase patient engagement in self-care"—helps ensure seamless care (CHCS, 2007; Goodell et al., 2009). The components of care management include care coordination, transitional care, and social care.

Care coordination is defined as the "deliberate organization of patient care activities between two or more participants (including the patient) involved in a patient's care to facilitate the appropriate delivery of healthcare services." It is needed both to overcome obstacles of the health care system, such as fragmentation, communication, and billing/cost, and to increase access (McDonald et al., 2007, p. 4).

Transitional care entails coordinating care for people moving between various locations or levels of care, providing navigation, coordination, medication reconciliation, and education services (Storfjell et al., 2017). The Transitional Care Model, developed by Mary Naylor (see Box 4-2), and the Care Transitions Intervention, developed by Eric Coleman, are prominent nurse-centered care models focused on the often disjointed transition from an inpatient hospital stay to follow-up ambulatory care. Both models engage people with chronic illness from hospitalization to postdischarge, and employ a nursing coach or team "to manage clinical, psychosocial, rehabilitative, nutritional and pharmacy needs; teach or coach people about medications, self-care and symptom recognition and management; and encourage physician appointments" (Storfjell et al., 2017, p. 27). Both reduce readmissions and costs (Storfjell et al., 2017).

Health care delivery models that incorporate *social care* have created critical roles for nurses in coordinating care across providers and settings and collaborating with other professionals and community resources to improve the health of individuals with complex health and social needs. Chapter 5 provides examples of nurse-centered programs incorporating social care. Nurses are vital to carrying out these functions of care management. Common to nurses' roles are functions including providing care coordination, developing care plans based on a person's needs and preferences, educating people and families within care settings and during discharge, and facilitating continuity of care for people across settings and providers (ANA, n.d.).

Person-Centered Care

The person-centered care model embraces personal choice and autonomy and customizes care to an individual's abilities, needs, and preferences (Kogan et al., 2016; Van Haitsma et al., 2014). Through person-centered care, nurses collaborate with people, including the patient and other care team members, to deliver personalized quality care that addresses physical, mental, and social needs (CMS, 2012; Terada et al., 2013). Features of person-centered care include an emphasis on codesign of interventions, services, and policies that focus on what the person and

BOX 4-2
Transitional Care Model

The Transitional Care Model (TCM) is a rigorously tested nurse-led intervention targeting chronically ill older adults as they move across health care settings and between clinicians. TCM has multiple aims, such as improving care, reducing preventable hospital readmissions, reducing gaps in care, enhancing patient and family outcomes, and reducing costs. The intervention has been studied and refined over two decades. An assigned advanced practice registered nurse (APRN) works collaboratively with the person to develop health goals and to design and implement a care plan. That nurse maintains continuity of care across settings and between providers throughout episodes of acute illness. Care is both delivered and coordinated by the same APRN in collaboration with patients, their caregivers, physicians, and other health team members. The TCM nurse provides supplemental care if the person is hospitalized, and is responsible for care in the home (Hirschman et al., 2015).

TCM relies on a master's-level "transitional care nurse" who is trained in the care of people with chronic conditions. Upon hospitalization, the nurse

- conducts a comprehensive assessment of the patient's health status, health behaviors, level of social support, and goals;
- develops an individualized plan of care consistent with evidence-based guidelines, in collaboration with the patient and her doctors; and
- conducts daily patient visits, focused on optimizing patient health at discharge.

Following discharge, the nurse conducts periodic home visits and/or scheduled phone contacts with the patient based on a standard protocol. The postdischarge program varies in length from 1 to 3 months and includes an average of 4.5 to 12 home visits, with no scheduled phone contacts or weekly nurse-initiated phone contacts with patients or family caregivers. In both cases, the nurse is available to patients via telephone 7 days per week. The nurse home visits and phone contacts identify changes in the patient's health and help manage and/or prevent health problems, including making any adjustments in therapy in collaboration with the patient's physicians. The nurse also accompanies the patient to her first physician visit following hospital discharge to ensure effective communication. Each nurse handles a caseload of 18–20 patients.

Three randomized controlled trials found lower all-cause hospitalizations at 1 year postdischarge, resulting in cost savings as compared with a control group (Naylor et al., 1999, 2004, 2014). One study found lower readmission rates, a longer time period before death, and cost savings for people identified for the intervention through primary care settings as compared with those who received less intensive interventions (Naylor et al., 2014). Specifically, TCM resulted in a 30–50 percent reduction in rehospitalizations and net savings in health care expenditures of approximately $4,500 per patient within 5–12 months after patient discharge. TCM also replaces the hospital's usual discharge planning and postdischarge activities. Its cost ranges from $519 to $1,160 per patient, in 2017 dollars (Social Programs that Work, n.d.).

community want and need; respect for the beliefs and values of people; promotion of antidiscriminatory care; and attention to such issues as race, ethnicity, gender, sexual identity, religion, age, socioeconomic status, and differing ability status (Santana et al., 2018). And person-centered care focuses not only on the individual but also on families and caregivers, as well as prevention and health promotion. Integrating person-centered care that improves patient health literacy is necessary to ensure patient empowerment and engagement and maximize health outcomes. Health literacy ensures that "patients know what they must do after all health care encounters to self-manage their health" (Loan et al., 2018, p. 98).

Research has demonstrated the efficacy of person-centered care, for example, in reducing agitation, neuropsychiatric symptoms, and depression, as well as improving quality of life, for individuals with dementia (Kim and Park, 2017). In another example, people with acute coronary syndrome receiving person-centered care reported significantly higher self-efficacy (Pirhonen et al., 2017). Person-centered care is person-directed, such that people are provided with sufficient information to help them in making decisions about their care and increase their level of engagement in care (Pelzang, 2010; Scherger, 2009), and nurses who engage people in their care are less likely to make mistakes (Leiter and Laschinger, 2006; Prins et al., 2010; Shiparski, 2005). Person-centered care leads to better communication between patients and caregivers and improves quality of care, thereby increasing patient satisfaction, care adherence, and care outcomes (Hochman, 2017).

Cultural Humility

As discussed in Chapter 2, implicit bias can lead to discrimination against others. In particular, structural racism in health care compromises the ability to deliver culturally competent care (Evans et al., 2020).

> Historically, nursing has been at the forefront of advocacy, and there are many examples of how nurses have addressed, and are addressing, inequities in many aspects of our teaching, research, scholarship, and practice. Yet, there remain too many examples of structural racism throughout nursing and we must be open to continuing to examine, identify, and change these within our own profession. (Villaruel and Broome, 2020, p. 375)

Nurses may contribute to structural inequities in how they facilitate or hamper access to quality health care services since they are frequently the first point of contact for many individuals who need care. Cultural humility—"defined by flexibility; awareness of bias; a lifelong, learning-oriented approach to working with diversity; and a recognition of the role of power in health care interactions" (Agner, 2020, p. 1)—is therefore essential for nurses.

Cultural humility enables nurses to participate in more respectful partnerships with patients in order to advance health care equity. According to Foronda and colleagues (2016), cultural humility has been found to result in effective treatment, decision making, communication, and understanding; better quality of life; and improved care. In contrast, clinicians with implicit bias may show less compassion toward and spend less time and effort with certain patients, leading to adverse assessment and care (Narayan, 2019). Because implicit bias can negatively affect patient interactions and health outcomes, it is important for nurses to be aware of their bias and how it may directly or indirectly impact patient interactions and the quality of care they provide (Hall et al., 2015).

Multiple strategies exist to help nurses achieve cultural humility and manage implicit bias to ensure that they provide high-quality, equitable care. Chapter 7 details the importance of incorporating cultural humility in nursing education. Instead of focusing broadly on the general population, quality improvement interventions characterized by cultural humility focus on needs that are unique to people of color (POC) and tailor care to overcome cultural and linguistic barriers that cause disparities in care (Green et al., 2010). With this approach, data on disparities are used to assess an intervention, with an emphasis on addressing barriers that are specific to underrepresented groups (ANA, 2018; Green et al., 2010; Villarruel and Broome, 2020). Box 4-3 describes culturally and linguistically appropriate services, designed to equip nurses with the knowledge, skills, and awareness to provide high-quality care for all patients regardless of cultural or linguistic background.

BOX 4-3
Culturally and Linguistically Appropriate Services

Linguistic diversity is at record highs, making health care language barriers more prevalent. Nurses, often the first point of contact with patients in the health care system, can improve outcomes, including safety and satisfaction, through how they manage language barriers (Gerchow et al., 2021).

In some health care settings, resources exist to ensure that the organizations where nurses work are prepared to implement culturally and linguistically appropriate services (CLAS). The U.S. Department of Health and Human Services (HHS, n.d.) has national CLAS standards intended to promote health equity and improve quality. These include a principal standard that recognizes and respects diverse patient populations. Also included are governance, leadership, and workforce that support policy and practices focused on diverse leadership and governance and policies focused on CLAS and equity. Communication and language assistance is an area in which nurses can have the most direct impact because it aligns with nurses' charge to inform patients, receive their consent to treatment, and provide ongoing education in their care plan. These services should be extended to ensure that community health clinics, outpatient facilities, and public health partners also focus on CLAS in goals, policies, and management. Importantly, a community needs assessment would appropriately account for the community's demographics, changes in population, collaboration with stakeholders and constituencies, and the community's linguistic diversity to ensure services for equitable care (HHS, n.d.).

When nurses are educated and empowered to act at multiple levels—upstream, midstream, and downstream—they help reduce the effects of structural inequities generated by the health care system. This includes education about how structural inequities may affect their practice environments (as well as research and policy) and, by association, the people with whom they work in clinical and community-based settings (see the detailed discussion of nursing education in Chapter 7).

IMPLICATIONS OF COVID-19 FOR HEALTH CARE EQUITY

The COVID-19 pandemic has highlighted the pivotal role of nurses in addressing health care equity. During public health emergencies, nurses in hospitals and in public health and other community settings need to function collaboratively and seamlessly. The pandemic has heightened the need for team-based care, infection control, person-centered care, and other skills that capitalize on the strengths of nurses (LaFave, 2020). Broadening of scope-of-practice regulations and expansion of telehealth services during the COVID-19 pandemic have allowed nurses to practice to the full extent of their education and training, providing equitable care and increasing access to care.

The surge of critically ill people due to the pandemic created the need to rapidly increase the capacity of the health care workforce, especially to replenish workforce members who needed to quarantine or take time to care for sick family members or friends (Fraher et al., 2020). In response, multiple governors issued executive orders expanding the scope of practice for NPs. As of April 10, 2020, five states (Kentucky, Louisiana, New Jersey, New York, and Wisconsin) had temporarily suspended all practice agreement requirements, providing NPs with full practice authority (AANP, 2020). Thirteen states (Alabama, Arkansas, Indiana, Massachusetts, Michigan, Mississippi, Missouri, Oklahoma, Pennsylvania, South Carolina, Tennessee, Texas, and West Virginia) had enacted a temporary waiver of selected practice agreement requirements. By December 7, 2020, executive orders had expired for Kansas, Michigan, and Tennessee, and all practice agreement requirements had been temporarily suspended for Kentucky, Louisiana, New Jersey, New York, Virginia, and Wisconsin (AANP, 2020). Maintaining these broadened scopes of practice for nurses after the pandemic has ended would increase NPs' opportunities to increase access to quality health care for individuals with complex health and social needs.

Hospitals are also redeploying health care workers—physicians, NPs, nurses, and others—from areas with decreasing patient volumes (resulting from, for example, limitations on elective procedures) to higher-need intensive care unit (ICU), acute care, and emergency service areas. For example, nurse anesthetists have been redeployed from operating rooms to ICUs to intubate and place central lines for patients in the surge response to COVID-19 (Brickman et al., 2020). As of December 2020, CMS was finalizing changes that allow NPs to "supervise the performance of diagnostic tests within their scope of practice and state law, as they maintain required statutory relationships with supervising or collaborating physicians" (CMS, 2020a). These changes will help make permanent some of the workforce flexibilities that were allowed during the pandemic.

Although much attention has been paid to the dire need for health care supplies and hospital beds to treat patients with severe cases of COVID-19, less attention has been directed at impacts of the pandemic on communities; their ability to weather the crisis; and individuals' physical, mental, and social health. Nurses, including public health nurses, working in and with communities continue to be critical to efforts to contain the COVID-19 pandemic, as well as other pandemics that may occur in the future.

Older Adults

Older adults have been disproportionately affected by COVID-19, and older POC are even more likely to experience disproportionate morbidity and mortality. CMS data show that Black Medicare beneficiaries were hospitalized four times as often and contracted the virus nearly three times as often compared with Whites of similar age (CMS, 2020b; Godoy, 2020). According to the Centers for Disease Control and Prevention (CDC), 8 of 10 deaths from COVID-19 in the United States have been among adults 65 and older (Freed et al., 2020). Nursing homes have been particularly hard hit and faced multiple unique challenges in serving those most vulnerable to the virus.

The pandemic has had significant emotional, social, and mental health effects on older adults and their caregivers, and nurses and nursing assistants in nursing homes have borne a great burden in carrying out the front-line work of trying to keep residents healthy, care for recovered patients, and help mitigate isolation and its detrimental effects on residents. These tasks in many cases have been performed in the absence of residents' family members and friends, who have not been allowed to visit as part of efforts to prevent the spread of infection. Inside nursing homes, the nursing staff have had to act as both caregivers and confidants, carrying out their usual tasks while also supporting many residents through confusion, depression, and suicidal ideation. In multigenerational homes, additional steps have been required to mitigate COVID-19 risk for older adults, such as using separate bathrooms, wearing masks within the household if someone is sick, or avoiding visitors. Demand for home health nursing services, inclusive of following strict public health measures (masks, handwashing, quarantining), has increased during the pandemic.

Changes in Medicare policy during the COVID-19 pandemic have given older adults greater access to a variety of mental health services, including those provided in their homes. Access to telehealth has also been expanded to meet the urgent need to provide safe access to care. Medicare payment for telehealth visits in nursing homes was previously restricted to rural areas, but under the

1135 waiver and the Coronavirus Preparedness and Response Supplemental Appropriations Act, CMS temporarily broadened access to telehealth services to ensure that Medicare beneficiaries could access services from the safety of their homes (CMS, 2020b). Accordingly, NPs and other health care professionals have used telehealth to screen people for COVID-19 and treat noncritical illnesses that can be managed at home.

Telehealth also has helped address concerns about workforce capacity for adult health care due to the surging numbers of COVID-19 cases and reports of exposure among health care workers: "as many as 100 health care workers at a single institution have to be quarantined at home because of COVID-19" (Hollander and Carr, 2020). NPs who are quarantined because of exposure can provide telehealth services. It is important to note that the barriers discussed earlier due to restrictive scope-of-practice regulations may include limitations on providing telehealth services across state lines. Recognition of clinical licenses across states, such as through interstate agreements, could ease these barriers (NQF, 2020).

Children

Although CDC has reported that COVID-19 poses a relatively low risk for children, research on natural disasters has shown that, compared with adults, children are more vulnerable to the emotional impact of traumatic events that disrupt their daily lives. The pandemic has required that children make significant adjustments to their routines (e.g., because of school and child care closures and the need for social distancing and home confinement), disruptions that may interfere with a child's sense of structure, predictability, and security. Young people—even infants and toddlers—are keen observers of people and environments, and they notice and react to stress in their parents and other caregivers, peers, and community members (Bartlett et al., 2020). While most children eventually return to their typical functioning when they receive consistent support from sensitive and responsive caregivers, others are at risk of developing significant mental health problems, including trauma-related stress, anxiety, and depression. Children with prior trauma or preexisting mental, physical, or developmental problems, as well as those whose parents struggle with mental health disorders, substance misuse, or economic instability, are at especially high risk for emotional disturbance. Thus, in addition to keeping children physically safe during a public health emergency such as the COVID-19 pandemic, it is important to care for their emotional health (Bartlett et al., 2020).

Barriers to mental health care result in serious immediate and long-term disadvantages for young people, especially students of color. Mental health—a key component of children's healthy development—was already a growing concern prior to the pandemic and the concurrent nationwide protests in response to racial injustice and anti-Black racism, with the demand for mental health services among U.S. adolescents increasing in the past decade (Mojtabai et al., 2020). This concern has been fueled by increases in the incidence of anxiety and depression, as well as a trend in which victims of suicide have been younger. As noted earlier, programs such as Nurse-Family Partnership (see Box 4-1), as well as school nurses and school-based health centers, represent channels through which nurses can assist children and families with health care access to address mental health needs.

The health care system is being transformed by an increased focus on community-based coordinated care and the use of technology to improve communication so as to achieve better population health outcomes at lower cost. At the local level, providers in public health and school settings can collaborate strategically to increase their community's capacity to address the root causes of illness and improve overall population health by implementing broad social, cultural, and economic reforms that address SDOH. Such collaboration can benefit the entire health care system by leading to seamless care, reducing duplicative services, and lowering the costs of care.

CONCLUSIONS

Whether in an elementary school, a hospital, or a community health clinic, nurses work to address the root causes of poor health. As the largest and consistently most trusted members of the health care workforce, nurses practice in a wide range of settings. They have the ability to manage as well as collaborate within teams and connect clinical care, public health, and social services while building trust with communities. However, nurses are limited in realizing this potential by state and federal laws that prohibit them from working to the full extent of their education and training. The COVID-19 pandemic in particular has revealed that the United States needs to do a much better job of linking health and health care to social and economic needs, and nurses are well positioned to build that bridge.

Conclusion 4-1: Nurses have substantial and often untapped expertise to help individuals and communities access high-quality health care, particularly in providing care for people in underserved rural and urban areas. Improved telehealth technology and payment systems have the potential to increase access, allowing patients to obtain their care in their homes and neighborhoods. However, the ability of nurses to practice fully in these and other settings is limited by state and federal laws that prohibit them from working to the full extent of their education and training.

Conclusion 4-2: Nurses are uniquely qualified to improve the quality of health care by helping people navigate the health care system;

providing close monitoring, coordination, and follow-up across the care continuum; focusing care on the whole person; and providing care that is culturally respectful and appropriate. Through a team-based approach, nurses can partner with professionals and community members to lead and manage teams and connect clinical care, public health, and social services while building trust with communities and individuals.

REFERENCES

AAN (American Academy of Nursing). 2015. *Interprofessional practice at the Vine School Health Center: A school-based nurse-managed clinic*. American Academy of Nursing: Edge Runners. https://www.aannet.org/initiatives/edge-runners/profiles/edge-runners--interprofessional-practice-vine-school (accessed June 19, 2019).

AANP (American Association of Nurse Practitioners). 2020. *COVID-19 state emergency response: Suspended and waived practice agreement requirements*. https://www.aanp.org/advocacy/state/covid-19-state-emergency-response-temporarily-suspended-and-waived-practice-agreement-requirements (accessed April 13, 2020).

Agner, J. 2020. Moving from cultural competence to cultural humility in occupational therapy: A paradigm shift. *American Journal of Occupational Therapy* 74(4):7404347010.

ANA (American Nurses Association). 2015. *Code of ethics for nurses with interpretive statements*. Silver Spring, MD: American Nurses Association.

ANA. 2018. *The nurse's role in addressing discrimination: Protecting and promoting inclusive strategies in practice settings, policy, and advocacy*. Silver Spring, MD: American Nurses Association.

ANA. 2020. *Nurses, ethics and the response to the COVID–19 pandemic*. Silver Spring, MD: American Nurses Association.

ANA. n.d. *Care coordination and the essential role of nurses*. https://www.nursingworld.org/practice-policy/health-policy/care-coordination (accessed February 21, 2020).

Bachrach, D., and J. Frohlich. 2016. Retail clinics drive new health care utilization and that is a good thing. *Health Affairs* 35(3). doi: 10.1377/hlthaff.2015.0995.

Bartlett, J. D., J. Griffin, and D. Thomson. 2020. Resources for supporting children's emotional well-being during the COVID-19 pandemic. *Child Trends*. https://www.childtrends.org/publications/resources-for-supporting-childrens-emotional-well-being-during-the-covid-19-pandemic (accessed March 23, 2021).

Basch, C. E. 2011. Healthier students are better learners: A missing link in school reforms to close the achievement gap. *Journal of School Health* 81(10):593–598.

Beard, K. V., and W. A. Julion. 2016. Does race still matter in nursing? The narratives of African-American nursing faculty members. *Nursing Outlook* 64(6):583–596.

Bodenheimer, T., and D. Mason. 2016. Registered nurses: Partners in transforming primary care. In *Preparing registered nurses for enhanced roles in primary care*, chaired by T. Bodenheimer and D. Mason. Conference conducted in New York, sponsored by the Josiah Macy Jr. Foundation. https://macyfoundation.org/assets/reports/publications/macy_monograph_nurses_2016_webpdf.pdf (accessed March 23, 2021).

Bodenheimer, T., L. Bauer, S. Syer, and J. N. Olayiwola. 2015. *RN role reimagined: How empowering registered nurses can improve primary care*. Oakland, CA: California Health Care Foundation.

Brickman, D., A. Greenway, K. Sobocinski, H. Thai, A. Turick, K. Xuereb, D. Zambardino, P. S. Barie, and S. I. Liu. 2020. Rapid critical care training of nurses in the surge response to the coronavirus pandemic. *American Journal of Critical Care* 29(5):e104–e107.

Campaign for Action. n.d. *Issues*. https://campaignforaction.org/issues (accessed November 12, 2020).

Carthon, J., M. Brooks, T. Sammarco, D. Pancir, J. Chittams, and K. W. Nicely. 2017. Growth in retail-based clinics after nurse practitioner scope of practice reform. *Nursing Outlook* 65(2):195–201.

Castrucci, B., and J. Auerbach. 2019. Meeting individual social needs falls short of addressing social determinants of health. *Health Affairs Blog* 10.

CHCS (Center for Health Care Strategies). 2007. *Care management definition and framework*. https://www.chcs.org/media/Care_Management_Framework.pdf (accessed January 18, 2020).

Child and Family Research Partnership. 2015. *The top 5 benefits of home visiting programs*. https://childandfamilyresearch.utexas.edu/top-5-benefits-home-visiting-programs (accessed February 13, 2020).

CMS (Centers for Medicare & Medicaid Services). 2012. *2012 Nursing home action plan: Action plan for further improvement of nursing home quality*. Baltimore, MD: Centers for Medicare & Medicaid Services.

CMS. 2020a. *Trump administration finalizes permanent expansion of medicare telehealth services and improved payment for time doctors spend with patients*. https://www.cms.gov/newsroom/press-releases/trump-administration-finalizes-permanent-expansion-medicare-telehealth-services-and-improved-payment (accessed November 13, 2020).

CMS. 2020b. *Trump administration issues call to action based on new data detailing COVID-19 impacts on medicare beneficiaries*. https://www.cms.gov/newsroom/press-releases/trump-administration-issues-call-action-based-new-data-detailing-covid-19-impacts-medicare (accessed November 13, 2020).

Council on School Health. 2008. Role of the school nurse in providing school health services. *Pediatrics* 121(5):1052–1056. doi: 10.1542/peds.2008-0382.

Council on School Health. 2016. Role of the school nurse in providing school health services. *Pediatrics* 137(6):e20160852.

CPSTF (Community Preventive Services Task Force). 2015. *Vaccination programs: Standing orders*. https://www.thecommunityguide.org/findings/vaccination-programs-standing-orders (accessed September 3, 2020).

Davis, T. C., K. W. Hoover, S. Keller, and W. H. Replogle. 2020. Mississippi diabetes telehealth network: A collaborative approach to chronic care management. *Telemedicine and e-Health* 26(2):184–189.

Donelan, K., Y. Chang, J. Berrett-Abebe, J. Spetz, D. I. Auerbach, L. Norman, and P. I. Buerhaus. 2019. Care management for older adults: The roles of nurses, social workers, and physicians. *Health Affairs* 38(6):941–949.

Emanuel, E. J., E. Gudbranson, J. Van Parys, M. Gørtz, J. Helgeland, and J. Skinner. 2020. Comparing health outcomes of privileged US citizens with those of average residents of other developed countries. *JAMA Internal Medicine* 181(3):339–344. doi: 10.1001/jamainternmed.2020.7484.

Evans, M. K., L. Rosenbaum, D. Malina, S. Morrissey, and E. J. Rubin. 2020. Diagnosing and treating systemic racism. *The New England Journal of Medicine* 383:274–276.

Flinter, M., C. Hsu, D. Cromp, M. D. Ladden, and E. H. Wagner. 2017. Registered nurses in primary care: Emerging new roles and contributions to team-based care in high-performing practices. *Journal of Ambulatory Care Management* 40(4):287.

Foronda, C., D. L. Baptiste, M. M. Reinholdt, and K. Ousman. 2016. Cultural humility: A concept analysis. *Journal of Transcultural Nursing* 27(3):210–217.

Foster, S., M. Rollefson, T. Doksum, D. Noonan, G. Robinson, and J. Teich. 2005. *School Mental Health Services in the United States, 2002–2003*. Rockville, MD: Substance Abuse and Mental Health Services Administration.

Fraher, E., J. Spetz, and M. D. Naylor. 2015. *Nursing in a transformed health care system: New roles, new rules*. Philadelphia, PA: Leonard Davis Institute of Health Economics, University of Pennsylvania.

Fraher, E. P., P. Pittman, B. K. Frogner, J. Spetz, J. Moore, A. J. Beck, D. Armstrong, and P. I. Buerhaus. 2020. Ensuring and sustaining a pandemic workforce. *New England Journal of Medicine* 382(23):2181–2183.

Freed, M., J. Cubanski, T. Neuman, J. Kates, and J. Michaud. 2020. What share of people who have died of COVID-19 are 65 and older—and how does it vary by state? https://www.kff.org/coronavirus-covid-19/issue-brief/what-share-of-people-who-have-died-of-covid-19-are-65-and-older-and-how-does-it-vary-by-state/?utm_campaign=KFF-2020-Coronavirus&utm_medium=email&_hsmi=2&_hsenc=p2ANqtz-_U7Q7mXfWl1ySGkBOyS9wZp2ff8zbbxZycmAlJ0dVoHaHEJEriXDh5kBTFf6WHimqSHlyPNoqoaQnTdJu0fjLVEkmSPg&utm_content=2&utm_source=hs_email (accessed October 5, 2020).

Gaur, K. C., M. Sobhani, and L. A. Saxon. 2019. Retail healthcare update: Disrupting traditional care by focusing on patient needs. *The Journal of mHealth*. https://thejournalofmhealth.com/retail-healthcare-update-disrupting-traditional-care-by-focusing-on-patient-needs (accessed April 20, 2021).

Gerchow, L., L. R. Burka, S. Miner, and A. Squires. 2021. Language barriers between nurses and patients: A scoping review. *Patient Education and Counseling* 104(3):534–553.

Ghorob, A., and T. Bodenheimer. 2012. Share the care™: Building teams in primary care practices. *Journal of the American Board of Family Medicine* 25(2):143–145.

Godoy, M. 2020 (June 22). *Black Medicare patients with COVID-19 nearly 4 times as likely to end up in hospital*. National Public Radio. https://www.npr.org/sections/health-shots/2020/06/22/881886733/black-medicare-patients-with-covid-19-nearly-4-times-as-likely-to-end-up-in-hosp (accessed March 25, 2021).

Goodell, S., T. Bodenheimer, and R. Berry-Millett. 2009. *Care management of patients with complex health care needs*. Princeton, NJ: Robert Wood Johnson Foundation.

Hall, W. J., M. V. Chapman, K. M. Lee, Y. M. Merino, T. W. Thomas, B. K. Payneand, and T. Coyne-Beasley. 2015. Implicit racial/ethnic bias among health care professionals and its influence on health care outcomes: A systematic review. *American Journal of Public Health* 105(12):e60–e76.

Henderson, K., T. C. Davis, M. Smith, and M. King. 2014. Nurse practitioners in telehealth: Bridging the gaps in healthcare delivery. *Journal for Nurse Practitioners* 10(10):845–850.

HHS (U.S. Department of Health and Human Services). n.d. National Culturally and Linguistically Appropriate Services Standards. https://thinkculturalhealth.hhs.gov/clas/standards (accessed October 7, 2020).

Hirschman, K. B., E. Shaid, K. McCauley, M. V. Pauly, and M. D. Naylor. 2015. Continuity of care: The transitional care model. *Online Journal of Issues in Nursing* 20(3).

Hochman, O. 2017. Patient-centered care in healthcare and its implementation in nursing. *International Journal of Caring Sciences* 10(1):596.

Hollander, J. E., and B. G. Carr. 2020. Virtually perfect? Telemedicine for COVID-19. *New England Journal of Medicine* 382:1679–1681. doi: 10,1056/NEJMp2003539.

Holmes, B. W., M. Allison, R. Ancona, E. Attisha, N. Beers, C. De Pinto, and T. Young. 2016. Role of the school nurse in providing school health services. *Pediatrics* 137(6):e20160852.

Hood, C. M., K. P. Gennuso, G. R. Swain, and B. B. Catlin. 2016. County health rankings: Relationships between determinant factors and health outcomes. *American Journal of Preventive Medicine* 50(2):129–135.

HRSA (Health Resources and Services Administration). 2017. *School-based health centers*. https://www.hrsa.gov/our-stories/school-health-centers/index.html (accessed October 5, 2020).

IOM (Institute of Medicine). 1990. *Medicare: A strategy for quality assurance*. Vol. I. Washington, DC: National Academy Press.

IOM. 2001. *Crossing the quality chasm: A new health system for the 21st century*. Washington, DC: National Academy Press.

IOM. 2011. *The future of nursing: Leading change, advancing health*. Washington, DC: The National Academies Press.

Johnson, K. 2017. Healthy and ready to learn: School nurses improve equity and access. *Online Journal of Issues in Nursing* 22(3).

Kataoka, S. H., L. Zhang, and K. B. Wells. 2005. Unmet need for mental health care among US children: Variation by ethnicity and insurance status. *American Journal of Psychiatry* 159(9):1548–1555.

Kim, S. K., and M. Park. 2017. Effectiveness of person-centered care on people with dementia: A systematic review and meta-analysis. *Clinical Interventions in Aging* 12:381.

Kitzman, H., D. L. Olds, C. R. Henderson, Jr., C. Hanks, R. Cole, R. Tatelbaum, K. M. McConnochie, K. Sidora, D. W. Luckey, D. Shaver, K. Engelhardt, D. James, and K. Barnard. 1997. Effect of prenatal and infancy home visitation by nurses on pregnancy outcomes, childhood injuries, and repeated childbearing. A randomized controlled trial. *JAMA* 278(8):644–652.

Kogan, A. C., K. Wilber, and L. Mosqueda. 2016. Person-centered care for older adults with chronic conditions and functional impairment: A systematic literature review. *Journal of the American Geriatrics Society* 64(1):e1–e7.

Koschmann, K. S., N. K. Jeffers, and O. Heidari. 2020. "I can't breathe": A call for antiracist nursing practice. *Nursing Outlook* 68(5):P539–P541.

Ladden, M. D., T. Bodenheimer, N. W. Fishman, M. Flinter, C. Hsu, M. Parchman, and E. H. Wagner. 2013. The emerging primary care workforce: Preliminary observations from the primary care team: learning from effective ambulatory practices project. *Academic Medicine* 88(12):1830–1834.

LaFave, S. 2020 (May 13). Nurses are leading the COVID-19 response around the globe: Patricia Davidson discusses how the pandemic is highlighting work that nurses do during crisis situations and beyond. *Johns Hopkins Hub*. https://hub.jhu.edu/2020/05/13/patricia-davidson-nursing-covid-19 (accessed November 12, 2020).

Lamb, G., R. Newhouse, C. Beverly, D. Toney, S. Cropley, C. Weaver, E. Kurtzman, D. Zazworsky, M. Rantz, B. Zierler, M. Naylor, S. Reinhard, C. Sullivan, K. Czubaruk, M. Weston, M. Dailey, C. Peterson, and Task Force Members. 2015. Policy agenda for nurse-led care coordination. *Nursing Outlook* 63(4):521–530. doi: 10.106/j.outlook.2015.06.003.

Leeb, R. T., R. H. Bitsko, L. Radhakrishnan, P. Martinez, R. Njai, and K. M. Holland. 2020. *Mental health–related emergency department visits among children aged <18 years during the COVID-19 pandemic—United States, January 1–October 17, 2020*. https://www.cdc.gov/mmwr/volumes/69/wr/mm6945a3.htm (accessed December 3, 2020).

Leiter, M. P., and H. K. S. Laschinger. 2006. Relationships of work and practice environment to professional burnout: Testing a causal model. *Nursing Research* 55(2):137–146.

Levine, D. M., K. Ouchi, B. Blanchfield, A. Saenz, K. Burke, M. Paz, K. Diamond, C. Put, and J. L. Schnipper. 2020. Hospital-level care at home for acutely ill adults: A randomized controlled trial. *Annals of Internal Medicine* 172(2):77–85.

Lineberry, M. J., and M. J. Ickes. 2015. The role and impact of nurses in American elementary schools: A systematic review of the research. *The Journal of School Nursing* 31(1):22–33.

Lipson, S. K., A. Kern, D. Eisenberg, and A. M. Breland-Noble. 2018. Mental health disparities among college students of color. *Journal of Adolescent Health* 63(3):348–356.

Loan, L. A., T. A. Parnell, J. F. Stichler, D. K. Boyle, P. Allen, C. A. VanFosson, and A. J. Barton. 2018. Call for action: Nurses must play a critical role to enhance health literacy. *Nursing Outlook* 66(1):97–100.

Love, H. E., J. Schlitt, S. Soleimanpour, N. Panchal, and C. Behr. 2019. Twenty years of school-based health care growth and expansion. *Health Affairs* 38(5):755–764.

Maughan, E. D. 2018. School nurses: An investment in student achievement. *Phi Delta Kappan* 99(7):8–14.

McDonald, K. M., V. Sundaram, D. M. Bravata, R. Lewis, N. Lin, S. A. Kraft, and D. K. Owens. 2007. Closing the quality gap: A critical analysis of quality improvement strategies. In *AHRQ Technical Reviews and Summaries*. Vol. 7: Care Coordination. Rockville, MD: Agency for Healthcare Research and Quality.

Michalopoulos, C., S. S. Crowne, X. A. Portilla, H. Lee, J. H. Filene, A. Duggan, and V. Knox. 2019. *A summary of results from the MIHOPE and MIHOPE-strong start studies of evidence-based home visiting*. Washington, DC: Office of Planning, Research, and Evaluation, Administration for Children and Families, U.S. Department of Health and Human Services.

Miller, T. R. 2015. Projected outcomes of nurse-family partnership home visitation during 1996–2013, USA. *Prevention Science* 16(6):765–777.

Mojtabai R., and M. Olfson. 2020. National trends in mental health care for US adolescents. *JAMA Psychiatry* 77(7):703–714.

NACHC (National Association of Community Health Centers). 2019. *Community health center chartbook*. http://www.nachc.org/wp-content/uploads/2019/01/Community-Health-Center-Chartbook-FINAL-1.28.19.pdf (accessed March 21, 2020).

Narayan, M. C. 2019. CE: Addressing implicit bias in nursing: A review. *American Journal of Nursing* 119(7):36–43.

NASEM (National Academies of Sciences, Engineering, and Medicine). 2017. *Communities in action: Pathways to health equity*. Washington, DC: The National Academies Press.

NASEM. 2019. *Vibrant and healthy kids: Aligning science, practice, and policy to advance health equity*. Washington, DC: The National Academies Press.

NASN (National Association of School Nurses). 2020a. *School nurse workload: Staffing for safe care*. https://www.nasn.org/advocacy/professional-practice-documents/position-statements/ps-workload (accessed April 15, 2019).

NASN. 2020b. *NASN calls for 10,000 more school nurses*. https://schoolnursenet.nasn.org/nasn/blogs/nasn-profile/2020/04/22/nasn-calls-for-10000-more-school-nurses (accessed March 26, 2021).

Naylor, M. D., D. Brooten, R. Campbell, B. S. Jacobsen, M. D. Mezey, M. V. Pauly, and J. S. Schwartz. 1999. Comprehensive discharge planning and home follow-up of hospitalized elders: A randomized clinical trial. *Journal of the American Medical Association* 281(7):613–620.

Naylor, M. D., D. A. Brooten, R. L. Campbell, G. Maislin, K. M. McCauley, and J. S. Schwartz. 2004. Transitional care of older adults hospitalized with heart failure: A randomized, controlled trial. *Journal of the American Geriatrics Society* 52(5):675–684.

Naylor, M. D., K. B. Hirschman, A. L. Hanlon, K. H. Bowles, C. Bradway, K. M. McCauley, and M. V. Pauly. 2014. Comparison of evidence-based interventions on outcomes of hospitalized, cognitively impaired older adults. *Journal of Comparative Effectiveness Research* 3(3):245–257.

NQF (National Quality Forum). 2020. *The care we need: Driving better health outcomes for people and communities*. https://thecareweneed.org/wp-content/uploads/2020/08/Full-Report-The-Care-We-Need-Update-Aug-2020.pdf (accessed November 12, 2020).

ODPHP (Office of Disease Prevention and Health Promotion). 2020. Discrimination. *Healthy People 2020*. https://www.healthypeople.gov/2020/topics-objectives/topic/social-determinants-health/interventions-resources/discrimination (accessed April 13, 2020).

Olds, D. L., H. Kitzman, E. Anson, J. A. Smith, M. D. Knudtson, T. Miller, R. Cole, C. Hopfer, and G. Conti. 2019. Prenatal and infancy nurse home visiting effects on mothers: 18-year follow-up of a randomized trial. *Pediatrics* 144(6):e20183889.

OPRE (Office of Planning, Research and Evaluation). 2020. *Home visiting evidence of effectiveness review: Brief—December 2020*. Washington, DC: U.S. Department of Health and Human Services.

Patrick, S. W., L. E. Henkhaus, J. S. Zickafoose, K. Lovell, A. Halvorson, S. Loch, M. Letterie, and M. M. Davis. 2020. Well-being of parents and children during the COVID-19 pandemic: A national survey. *Pediatrics* 146(4):e2020016824.

Peikes, D. N., R. J. Reid, T. J. Day, D. D. F. Cornwell, S. B. Dale, R. J. Baron, R. S. Brown, and R. J. Shapiro. 2014. Staffing patterns of primary care practices in the comprehensive primary care initiative. *The Annals of Family Medicine* 12(2):142–149.

Pelzang, R. 2010. Time to learn: Understanding patient-centered care. *British Journal of Nursing* 19(14):912–917.

Pirhonen, L., E. H. Olofsson, A. Fors, I. Ekman, and K. Bolin. 2017. Effects of person-centered care on health outcomes—A randomized controlled trial in patients with acute coronary syndrome. *Health Policy* 121(2):169–179.

Pittman, P. 2019. Rising to the challenge: Re-embracing the Wald model of nursing. *The American Journal of Nursing* 119(7):46–52.

Prins, M. A., P. F. Verhaak, M. Smolders, M. G. Laurant, K. Van Der Meer, P. Spreeuwenberg, and J. M. Bensing. 2010. Patient factors associated with guideline-concordant treatment of anxiety and depression in primary care. *Journal of General Internal Medicine* 25(7):648–655.

RAND Corporation. 2016. *The evolving role of retail clinics*. Santa Monica, CA: RAND Corporation.

Remington, P. L., B. B. Catlin, and K. P. Gennuso. 2015. The county health rankings: Rationale and methods. *Population Health Metrics* 13(1):11.

RHI (Rural Health Information Hub). 2019. *Health-e-Schools*. https://www.ruralhealthinfo.org/project-examples/806 (accessed August 17, 2020).

Roth, M. 2018. *3 ways telehealth tackles aging-related needs*. https://www.healthleadersmedia.com/innovation/3-ways-telehealth-tackles-aging-related-needs (accessed December 3, 2020).

Santana, M. J., K. Manalili, R. J. Jolley, S. Zelinsky, H. Quan, and M. Lu. 2018. How to practice person-centered care: A conceptual framework. *Health Expectations* 21(2):429–440.

SBHA (School Based Health Alliance). 2018. *2016-17 national school-based health care census*. https://www.sbh4all.org/wp-content/uploads/2019/05/2016-17-Census-Report-Final.pdf (accessed September 3, 2020).

SBHA. n.d. *Core competencies*. http://www.sbh4all.org/resources/core-competencies (accessed September 3, 2020).

Scherger, J. E. 2009. Future vision: Is family medicine ready for patient-directed care. *Family Medicine* 41(4):285–288.

Shiparski, L. A. 2005. Engaging in shared decision making: Leveraging staff and management expertise. *Nurse Leader* 3(1):36–41.

Singh, S., D. Roy, K. Sinha, S. Parveen, G. Sharma, and G. Joshi. 2020. Impact of COVID-19 and lockdown on mental health of children and adolescents: A narrative review with recommendations. *Psychiatry Research* 293:113429.

Smolowitz, J., E. Speakman, D. Wojnar, E. M. Whelan, S. Ulrich, C. Hayes, and L. Wood. 2015. Role of the registered nurse in primary health care: Meeting health care needs in the 21st century. *Nursing Outlook* 63(2):130–136.

Social Programs that Work. n.d. *What works in social policy?* https://evidencebasedprograms.org (accessed December 1, 2020).

Sofaer, S., and J. Hibbard. 2010. *Best practices in public reporting No. 2: Maximizing consumer understanding of public comparative quality reports: Effective use of explanatory information*. Rockville, MD: Agency for Healthcare Research and Quality.

Spetz, J., L. Trupin, T. Bates, and J. M. Coffman. 2015. Future demand for long-term care workers will be influenced by demographic and utilization changes. *Health Affairs* 34(6):936–945.

Storfjell, J., B. Winslow, and J. Saunders. 2017. *Catalysts for change: Harnessing the power of nurses to build population health in the 21st century*. Princeton, NJ: Robert Wood Johnson Foundation.

Szanton, S. L., Q.-L. Xue, B. Leff, J. Guralnik, J. L. Wolff, E. K. Tanner, C. Boyd, R. J. Thorpe, Jr., D. Bishai, and L. N. Gitlin. 2019. Effect of a biobehavioral environmental approach on disability among low-income older adults: A randomized clinical trial. *JAMA Internal Medicine* 179(2):204–211.

Terada, S., E. Oshima, O. Yokota, C. Ikeda, S. Nagao, N. Takeda, and Y. Uchitomi. 2013. Person-centered care and quality of life of patients with dementia in long-term care facilities. *Psychiatry Research* 205(1–2):103–108.

United HealthCare. 2018. *United HealthCare House Calls: Together, we can help your patients achieve better health outcomes*. https://www.uhcprovider.com/content/dam/provider/docs/public/health-plans/HouseCalls-Program-Overview.pdf (accessed March 23, 2021).

Uscher-Pines, L., J. Sousa, M. Jones, C. Whaley, C. Perrone, C. McCullough, and A. J. Ober. 2021. Telehealth use among safety-net organizations in California during the COVID-19 pandemic. *JAMA* 325(11):1106–1107.

Van Haitsma, K., S. Crespy, S. Humes, A. Elliot, A. Mihelic, C. Scott, and A. R. Heid. 2014. New toolkit to measure quality of person-centered care: Development and pilot evaluation with nursing home communities. *Journal of the American Medical Directors Association* 15(9):671–680.

Villarruel, A. M., and M. E. Broome. 2020. Beyond the naming: Institutional racism in nursing. *Nursing Outlook* 68(4):375–376.

Walker, T. 2019. *Home healthcare market to expand in 2020*. Managed Healthcare Executive. https://www.managedhealthcareexecutive.com/article/home-healthcare-market-expand-2020 (accessed March 26, 2020).

Willgerodt, M. A. 2018. School nursing practice in the United States: An introduction to NASN infographics. *NASN School Nurse* 33(4):239–243.

Yao, N., J. B. Mutter, J. D. Berry, T. Yamanaka, D. T. Mohess, and T. Cornwell. 2021. In traditional Medicare, modest growth in the home care workforce largely driven by nurse practitioners. *Health Affairs* 40(3):478–486.

Zamosky, L. 2013. Chronic disease: A growing challenge for PCPs. *Medical Economics* 90(15):30–32, 35–36.

5

The Role of Nurses in Improving Health Equity

Being a nurse ... in 2020 must mean being aware of social injustices and the systemic racism that exist in much of nursing ... and having a personal and professional responsibility to challenge and help end them.

—Calvin Moorley, RN, and colleagues, "Dismantling Structural Racism: Nursing Must Not Be Caught on the Wrong Side of History"

Health equity is achieved when everyone has a fair and just opportunity to be as healthy as possible. Nurses are well positioned to play a major role in addressing the underlying causes of poor health by understanding and recognizing the wide range of factors that influence how well and long people live, helping to create individual- and community-targeted solutions, and facilitating and working with interdisciplinary and multisector teams and partners to implement those solutions. Nurses have the potential to reshape the landscape of health equity over the next decade by expanding their roles, working in new settings and in new ways, and markedly expanding efforts to partner with communities and other sectors. But for the United States to make substantial progress in achieving health equity, it will need to devote resources and attention to the conditions that affect people's health and make expanded investments in building nurse capacity. And nursing schools will need to shift education, training, and mindsets to support nurses' new and expanded roles.

When this study was envisioned in 2019, it was clear that the future of nursing would look different by 2030; however, no one could predict how rapidly and dramatically circumstances would shift before the end of 2020. Over the coming decade, the nursing profession will continue to be shaped by the pressing health, social, and ethical challenges facing the nation today. Having illuminated many of the health and social inequities affecting communities across the nation, the COVID-19 pandemic, along with other health crises, such as the opioid epidemic (Abellanoza et al., 2018), presents an opportunity to take a critical look at the nursing profession, and society at large, and work collaboratively to enable all individuals to have a fair and just opportunity for health and well-being, reflecting the concept of "social mission" described by Mullan (2017, p. 122) as "making health not only better but fairer." This chapter examines health equity and the role of nursing in its advancement in the United States.

As stated previously, health equity is defined as "the state in which everyone has the opportunity to attain full health potential and no one is disadvantaged from achieving this potential because of social position or any other socially defined circumstance" (NASEM, 2017a, p. 32). While access to equitable health care, discussed in Chapter 4, is an important part of achieving health equity, it is not sufficient. Health is affected by a wide range of other factors, including housing, transportation, nutrition, physical activity, education, income, laws and policies, and discrimination. Chapter 2 presents the Social Determinants of Health and Social Needs Model of Castrucci and Auerbach (2019), in which *upstream* factors represent the social determinants of health (SDOH) that affect individuals and communities in a broad and, today, inequitable way. Low educational status and opportunity, income disparities, discrimination, and social marginalization are examples of upstream factors that impede good health outcomes. *Midstream* factors comprise social needs, or the individual factors that may affect a person's health, such as homelessness, food insecurity, and trauma. Finally, *downstream* factors include disease treatment and chronic disease management.

Much of the focus on the education and training of nurses and the public perception of their role is on the treatment and management of disease. This chapter shifts that focus to nurses' role in addressing SDOH and social needs, including their potential future roles and responsibilities in this regard, and describes existing exemplars. First, the chapter provides a brief overview of nurses' role in addressing health equity. Next, it describes opportunities for nurses to improve health equity through four approaches: addressing social needs in clinical settings, addressing social needs and SDOH in the community, working across disciplines and sectors to meet multiple needs, and advocating for policy change. The chapter then details the opportunities and barriers associated with each of these approaches.

NURSES' ROLE IN ADDRESSING HEALTH EQUITY

As described in Chapter 1, the history of nursing is grounded in social justice and community health advocacy (Donley and Flaherty, 2002; Pittman, 2019; Rafferty, 2015; Tyson et al., 2018), and as noted in Chapter 2, the Code of Ethics for Nurses with Interpretive Statements, reiterated by American Nurses Association (ANA) President Ernest J. Grant in a public statement, "obligates nurses to be allies and to advocate and speak up against racism, discrimination, and injustice" (ANA, 2020).

Addressing social needs across the health system can improve health equity from the individual to the system level. The report *Integrating Social Care into the Delivery of Health Care* identifies activities in five complementary areas that can facilitate the integration of social care into health care: adjustment, assistance, alignment, advocacy, and awareness (NASEM, 2019) (see Figure 5-1 and Table 5-1). In

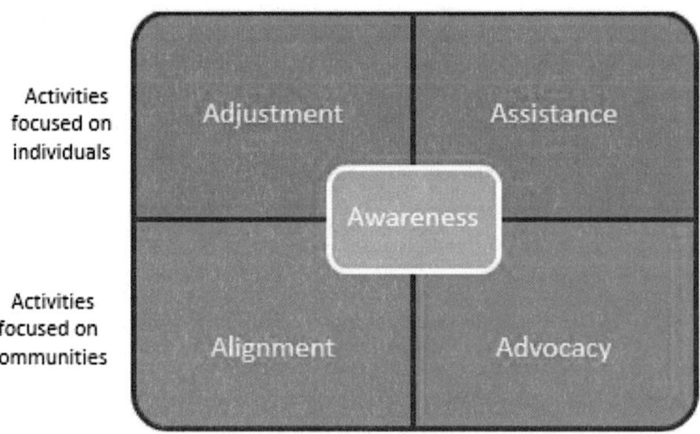

FIGURE 5-1 Areas of activity that strengthen integration of social care into health care.
SOURCE: NASEM, 2019.

TABLE 5-1 Definitions of Areas of Activities That Strengthen Integration of Social Care into Health Care

Activity	Definition	Transportation-Related Example
Awareness	Activities that identify the social risks and assets of defined patients and populations.	Ask people about their access to transportation.
Adjustment	Activities that focus on altering clinical care to accommodate identified social barriers.	Reduce the need for in-person health care appointments by using other options such as telehealth appointments.
Assistance	Activities that reduce social risk by providing assistance in connecting patients with relevant social care resources.	Provide transportation vouchers so that patients can travel to health care appointments. Vouchers can be used for ride-sharing services or public transit.
Alignment	Activities undertaken by health care systems to understand existing social care assets in the community, organize them to facilitate synergies, and invest in and deploy them to positively affect health outcomes.	Invest in community ride-sharing or time-bank programs.
Advocacy	Activities in which health care organizations work with partner social care organizations to promote policies that facilitate the creation and redeployment of assets or resources to address health and social needs.	Work to promote policies that fundamentally change the transportation infrastructure within the community.

SOURCE: NASEM, 2019.

the area of awareness, for example, clinical nurses in a hospital setting can identify the fall risks their patients might face upon discharge and the assets they can incorporate into their lives to improve their health. In the area of adjustment, telehealth and/or home health and home visiting nurses can alter clinical care to reduce the risk of falls by, for example, helping patients to adjust risks in their homes and learn to navigate their environment. And these activities can continue to the high level of system change through advocacy for health policies aimed at altering community infrastructure to help prevent falls.

In short, improving population health entails challenging and changing the factors and institutions that give rise to health inequity through interventions and reforms that influence the institutions, social systems, and public policies that drive health (Lantz, 2019). It is important to note, however, that there are shortcomings in how evaluations of health equity interventions are carried out (see Box 5-1).

BOX 5-1
Shortcomings of Evaluations of Health Equity Interventions

There is extensive literature on how to address health equity from the individual to the population level. To alleviate health inequities, interventions should intentionally target the needs of the most underresourced people or groups to help reduce the gaps in health outcomes as compared with less underresourced groups (Williams and Purdie-Vaughns, 2016). These interventions should occur at the individual, familial, community, and system levels (Agurs-Collins et al., 2019; Brown et al., 2019). Any potential intervention, however, should consider and/or address structural barriers to achieving health equity. When determining the impact of interventions on health equity metrics, the primary goal is the reduction and ultimate elimination of disparities in health and its determinants that adversely affect excluded or marginalized groups (Braveman et al., 2017).

The design and reporting of outcomes of evaluations of health equity interventions, however, have shortcomings. One frequent shortcoming of such evaluations is that they report improvements in health, or in a measure of health in a defined population, and implicitly assume that equity also has improved (Duran et al., 2019; Woolf et al., 2015). Intervention results can vary in how well the intervention has improved short-term outcomes (NASEM, 2017a) or long-term outcomes, or show that health in a defined group of people has improved enough to narrow the gaps in health status between groups (i.e., reduced disparities) (Krist et al., 2018).

For example, reporting aggregated data to describe the impact of interventions on distinct population subsets can be misleading. To illustrate, overall suicide trends in the United States for children aged 5–11 years remained stable between 1993 and 2012. However, analysis shows that suicide rates doubled for Black children, from 1.36 per million in 1993–1997 to 2.54 per million in 2008–2012 (period trend incidence rate ratio = 1.27; 95% confidence interval [CI] 1.11–1.45), but the rates significantly decreased among White children, from 1.14 per million in 1993–1997 to 0.77 per million in 2008–2012 (period trend incidence rate ratio=0.89; 95% CI 0.79–0.94). Suicide rates among Asian and Hispanic children remained relatively low and stable (Bridge et al., 2015).

Although it is valuable to show health improvements for disadvantaged groups, it is necessary to show that interventions targeting those groups actually reduced the disparities among groups to understand impacts on equity. Currently, research on health disparities has focused on identifying differences in health among groups and the underlying factors that contribute to those differences. To support effective change, evaluations need to focus both on cause and on how to effectively reduce the disparities (Dye et al., 2019; Jones et al., 2019).

ADDRESSING SOCIAL NEEDS IN CLINICAL SETTINGS

Although the provision of clinical care is a downstream determinant of health, the clinical setting presents an opportunity for nurses to address midstream determinants, or social needs, as well. Screening for social needs and making referrals to social services is becoming more commonplace in clinical settings as part of efforts to provide holistic care (Gottlieb et al., 2016; Makelarski et al., 2017; Thomas-Henkel and Schulman, 2017). Nurses may conduct screenings; review their results; create care plans based on social needs as indicated by those results; refer patients to appropriate professionals and social services; and coordinate care by interfacing with social workers, community health workers, and social services providers. Although the importance of screening people for social needs has led more providers to take on this role, it has yet to become a universal practice (CMS, 2020; NASEM, 2016), as most physician practices and hospitals do not perform screenings for the five key domains of social need[1]: food insecurity, housing instability, utility needs, transportation needs, and interpersonal violence (CMS, 2020; Fraze et al., 2019). As trusted professionals that spend significant time with patients and families, nurses are well equipped to conduct these screenings (AHA, 2019). Federally qualified health centers (FQHCs)—community-based health centers that receive funds from the Health Resources and Services Administration's (HRSA's) Health Center Program—often screen for social needs.

In many clinical settings, however, challenges arise with screening for social needs. Individuals may be hesitant to provide information about such issues as housing or food insecurity, and technology is required to collect social needs data and once obtained, to share these data across settings and incorporate them into

[1] These five domains of social needs are part of the Centers for Medicare & Medicaid Services' Accountable Health Communities Model (Fraze et al., 2019).

nursing practice in a meaningful way. While nurses have an educational foundation for building the skills needed to expand their role from assessing health issues to conducting assessments and incorporating findings related to social needs into care plans, this focus needs to be supported by policies where nurses are employed. As the incorporation of social needs into clinical consideration expands, nurses' education and training will need to ensure knowledge of the impact of social needs and SDOH on individual and population health (see Chapter 7). Communicating appropriately with people about social needs can be difficult, and training is required to ensure that people feel comfortable responding to personal questions related to such issues as housing instability, domestic violence, and financial insecurity (Thomas-Henkel and Schulman, 2017). Finally, the utility of social needs screening depends on networks of agencies that offer services and resources in the community. Without the ability to connect with relevant services, screenings and care plans can have little impact. Consequently, it is important for health care organizations to dedicate resources to ensuring that people are connected to appropriate resources, and to follow up by tracking those connections and offering other options as needed (Thomas-Henkel and Schulman, 2017).

ADDRESSING SOCIAL NEEDS AND SOCIAL DETERMINANTS OF HEALTH IN THE COMMUNITY

While interest in and action to address social needs in the clinical setting is rapidly expanding, nurse engagement in these issues in community settings has been long-standing. Nurses serving in the community often work directly to address social needs at the individual and family levels, and often work as well to address SDOH at the community and population levels. Public health nurses in particular have broad knowledge of health issues and the associated SDOH, as well as needs and resources, at the community level. Embedded within the community, they also are well positioned to build trust and are respected among community leaders. Also playing important roles in addressing social needs within the community are home visiting nurses. At the individual and family levels, home visiting nurses often represent the first line of health care providers with sustained engagement in addressing social needs for many individuals. They recognize and act on the limitations associated with social needs, such as the inability to afford transportation, or may work with an interdisciplinary team at the Special Supplemental Nutrition Program for Women, Infants, and Children (WIC) clinic to address food issues and other social needs. By connecting with individuals in their neighborhoods and homes, public health and other community-based nurses promote health and well-being for families within communities and engage in this work with partners from across social, health, and other services.

At the population health level, public health nurses work to achieve health equity within communities through both health promotion and disease prevention and control. They often work in municipal and state health departments and apply nursing, social, epidemiology, and other public health sciences in their contributions to population health (Bigbee and Issel, 2012; IOM, 2011 [see AARP, 2010]; Larsen et al., 2018). They offer a wide range of services to individuals and community members and are engaged in activities ranging from policy development and coalition building to health teaching and case management (Minnesota Department of Health, n.d.). Public health nurses serve populations that include those with complex health and social needs, frail elderly, homeless individuals, teenage mothers, and those at risk for a specific disease (Kulbok et al., 2012). Their interventions may target specific health risks, such as substance use disorder, HIV, and tobacco use, or populations at risk for health problems, such as individuals with complex health and social needs. Specific knowledge and skills they bring to communities include the ability to perform assessments of individual, family, and community health needs; use data and knowledge of environmental factors to plan for and respond to public health issues in their community; provide community and health department input in the development of policies and programs designed to improve the health of the community; implement evidence-based public health programs; and develop and manage program budgets (Minnesota Department of Health, n.d.).

Public health nursing roles are characterized by collaboration and partnerships with communities to address SDOH (Kulbok et al., 2012). Core to public health nursing is working across disciplines and sectors to advance the health of populations through community organizing, coalition building, policy analysis, involvement in local city and county meetings, collaboration with state health departments, and social marketing (Canales et al., 2018; Keller et al., 2004). Yet, while the work of public health nurses is foundational to the health of communities, their work is rarely visible. Additionally, regarding measurable reductions in health disparities, little research is available that connects directly and explicitly to public health nursing roles (Davies and Donovan, 2016; Schaffer et al., 2015; Swider et al., 2017).

Recent experiences with H1N1, Ebola, Zika, and COVID-19 underscore the importance of having strong, well-connected, well-resourced social services, public health, and health care systems, matched by an adequate supply of well-educated nurses. A 2017 report from the National Academies of Sciences, Engineering, and Medicine focused on global health notes that when infectious disease outbreaks occur, significant costs are often associated with fear and the worried-well seeking care (NASEM, 2017b). In their role as trusted professionals, and given their widespread presence in communities, incorporating public health nurses into community, state, and federal government strategies for health education and dissemination of information can help extend the reach and impact of messaging during infectious disease outbreaks and other public health emergencies. Nurses can serve as expert sources of information (e.g., on preventing infectious disease transmission within their communities) (Audain and Maher, 2017). In the United States, for example, as Zika infections were identified and spreading, one of the strategies used by the U.S. Department of Health and Human Services (HHS) was to work through nursing associations to reach nurses and through them, help reach the public with factual information and minimize unnecessary resource use (Minnesota Department of Health, 2019). Given their expertise in community engagement and knowledge of local and state government health and social services assets, public health nurses are well positioned to link to and share health-related information with community partners to help reach underresourced populations, including homeless individuals, non-English-speaking families, and others.

WORKING ACROSS DISCIPLINES AND SECTORS TO MEET MULTIPLE NEEDS

As nurses work in concert with other sectors and disciplines, interventions that address multiple and complex needs of individuals and communities can have far-reaching impacts on health outcomes and health care utilization. Through partnerships, community-based nurses work to address an array of health-related needs ranging from population-level diabetes management to community-based transportation to enable low-income families to access health care services.

Because multiple factors influence individual and population health, a multidisciplinary, multisectoral approach is necessary to improve health and reduce health inequity. While an approach focusing on only one SDOH may improve one dimension of health, such as food insecurity, intersectional approaches that simultaneously address complex, holistic needs of individuals, families, and communities are often required. Commonly found across underresourced communities are layers of intersecting challenges impacting health, ranging from adverse environmental exposures to food deserts. Health care systems, community-based organizations, government entitities, nurses, and others are increasingly working together to design interventions that reflect this complexity (NASEM, 2017a, 2019). Creative alliances are being built with for-profit and not-for-profit organizations, community groups, federal programs, hospitals, lending institutions, technology companies, and others (NASEM, 2019).

Work to prioritize and address health disparities and achieve health equity is predicated on meaningful, often multidimensional, assessments of community characteristics. One key opportunity to inform multisectoral efforts lies in community health needs assessments. The Patient Protection and Affordable Care Act requires nonprofit hospitals to conduct these assessments every 3 years, with input from local public health agencies. These assessments are then used to identify and prioritize significant health needs of the community served by the hospital while also identifying resources and plans for addressing these needs. Conducting a community health needs assessment is itself a multisectoral collaboration as it requires engaging community-based stakeholders (Heath, 2018). The results of the assessment present opportunities for multiple sectors to work together. For example, a hospital may partner with public health and area food banks to address food insecurity. Or it may partner with a health technology company and a local school board to address digital literacy for underserved youth and their families, and also extend the reach of broadband to support health care access through telehealth technology and strengthen digital literacy. In assessing the community's health needs, these hospitals are required to obtain and consider community-based input, including input from individuals or organizations with knowledge of or expertise in public health. The reports produced as part of this process are required to be publicly available (IRS, 2020).

These and other community engagement efforts can involve nurses from a variety of clinical and community-based settings in any and all steps of the process, from design to implementation and evaluation of the assessments themselves or the processes and programs established to address identified priorities. For example, the Magnet recognition program of the American Nurses Credentialing Center requires participating hospitals to involve nurses in their community health needs assessments (ANCC, 2017).

A variety of models feature nurses directly addressing health and social needs through multidisciplinary, multisectoral collaboration. Two illustrative programs are described below: the Camden Core Model and Edge Runner.

Camden Core Model

The Camden Coalition, based in Camden, New Jersey, is a multidisciplinary, nonprofit organization that works across sectors to address health and social needs. The Coalition's formation was based on the recognition that the U.S. health care system far too often fails people with complex health and social needs. These individuals cycle repeatedly through multiple health care, social services, and other systems without realizing lasting improvements in their health or well-being. The Coalition employs multiple approaches that include using faith-based partnerships to deliver health services and encourage healthy choices; sharing data among the criminal justice, health care, and housing sectors to identify points of intervention; and building local and national coalitions to support and educate others interested in implementing this model (Camden Coalition, n.d.). One of the Coalition's best-known programs is the Camden Core Model. This nationally recognized care management intervention is an example of a nurse-led care management program for people with complex medical and social needs. It applies the principles of trauma-informed care and harm reduction with the aim of empowering people with the skills and support they need to avoid preventable hospital use and improve their well-being (Finkelstein et al., 2020; Gawande, 2011). The model uses real-time data on hospital admissions to identify "super-utilizers," people with complex health issues who frequently use emergency care. An interprofessional team of registered nurses (RNs) and licensed practical nurses (LPNs), social workers, and community health workers engage in person with these individuals to help them navigate their care by connecting them with medical care, government benefits, and social services (Camden Coalition, n.d.; Finkelstein et al., 2020). With federal funding, similar versions of the model have been extended to cities outside of Camden (AF4Q, 2012; Crippen and Isasi, 2013; Mann, 2013).

Camden Coalition partnerships optimize the use of nurses in the community in several ways. An interprofessional team of nurses, social workers, and community health workers visits program participants, helps reconcile their medications, accompanies them to medical visits, and links them to social and legal services. Critical to the model's success is recruiting nurses who are from the local community, capitalizing on their cultural and systems-level knowledge to facilitate and improve access to and utilization of local health and social services. The culture of the Camden Coalition model has been key to its success. The uniform commitment of nurses, staff, and leadership to addressing people's complex needs has created a supportive work environment in which each team member's role is optimized. Care Team members have accompanied people to their meetings and appointments for primary care, helped with applications for such public benefits as food stamps, provided referrals to social services and housing agencies, arranged for medication delivery in partnership with local pharmacies, and coordinated care among providers.

The Camden Coalition focuses on "authentic healing relationships," defined as secure, genuine, and continuous partnerships between Care Team members and patients. This emphasis has evolved into a framework for patient engagement known as COACH, which stands for **C**onnect tasks with vision and priorities, **O**bserve the normal routine, **A**ssume a coaching style, **C**reate a backward plan, and **H**ighlight progress with data. An interprofessional team of nurses, social workers, and community health workers visits participants in the community. Team members are trained to problem solve with patients to achieve the program goals of helping them manage their chronic health conditions and reducing preventable hospital admissions.

Early evidence of the program's effect in a small sample showed a 56 percent reduction in monthly hospital charges, a roughly 40 percent reduction in monthly visits to hospitals and emergency departments, and an approximately 52 percent increase in rates of reimbursement to care providers (Green et al., 2010), although later evidence from a randomized controlled trial (RCT) indicated that the Camden Core Model did not reduce hospital readmissions (Finkelstein et al., 2020). Other RCTs, conducted in Philadelphia and Chicago, showed that similar social care programs using case management and community health workers can reduce hospital admissions and save money in addition to improving health and quality of health care. Kangovi and colleagues (2018) conducted an RCT in Philadelphia to assess Individualized Management for Patient-Centered Targets (IMPaCT), a standardized community health worker intervention addressing unmet social needs across three health systems (Kangovi et al., 2018). After 6 months, patients in the intervention group compared with controls were more likely to report the highest quality of care and spent fewer total days in the hospital (reduced by about two-thirds), saving $2.47 for each dollar invested by Medicaid annually (Kangovi et al., 2020). The RCT in Chicago assessed the effectiveness of a case management and housing program in reducing use of urgent medical services among homeless adults with chronic medical conditions and found a 29 percent reduction in hospitalizations and a 24 percent reduction in emergency department visits (Sadowski et al., 2009).

Edge Runner

The American Academy of Nurses' Edge Runner initiative identifies and promotes nurse-designed models of care and interventions that can improve health, increase health care access and quality, and/or reduce costs (AAN, n.d.a). As of February 2020, 59 such programs had been evaluated against a set of criteria and designated as part of this initiative. Many Edge Runner programs are built around the needs of underserved communities and seek to improve health through holistic care that addresses social needs and SDOH, including a range of upstream, midstream, and downstream determinants. Mason and colleagues (2015) assessed 30 Edge Runner models identified as of 2012, finding four main commonalities that illustrate these programs' broad and encompassing approach to health.

A holistic definition of health. Across the programs, health was defined broadly to include physical, psychological, social, spiritual, functional, quality-of-life, personal happiness, and well-being aspects. Additionally, the definition of health was based on the values of clients and shaped around their preferences. Typically, programs were grounded in SDOH to inform their design of individual- and community-level interventions.

Individual-, family-, and community-centric design. Most programs prioritized individual, family, and community goals over provider-defined goals through a "participant-led care environment" and "meeting people where they are." Thus, interventions were tailored to the values and culture present at each of these three levels.

Relationship-based care. The programs reflected the importance of building trusting relationships with individuals, families, and communities to help them engage in ways to create and sustain their own health.

Ongoing group and public health approaches to improving the health of underserved populations. The nurses who designed the programs viewed serving underserved populations as a moral imperative. Through peer-to-peer education, support groups, and public health approaches, they sought to empower clients, give them a sense of control, build self-care agency, and increase resilience.

An in-depth study of three Edge Runner programs (the Centering Pregnancy model, INSIGHTS, and the Family Practice and Counseling Network) revealed particular lessons: the essential role of collaboration and leaders who can collaborate with a wide range of stakeholders, the need for plans for scalability and financial sustainability, and the importance of social support and empowerment to help people (Martsolf et al., 2017). In these and other models, the capacity and knowledge associated with building meaningful, sustained partnerships across sectors is a key dimension of nursing practice that impacts health equity. The Edge Runner programs emphasize how, in the pursuit of improving care, lowering costs, and increasing satisfaction for people and families, nurses are actively working to achieve person-centered care that addresses social needs and SDOH and focusing on the needs of underserved populations to promote health equity (Martsolf et al., 2016, 2017; Mason et al., 2015). However, evidence directly linking the programs to decreases in disparities is generally not available. Two examples of Edge Runner programs are described in Box 5-2.

As models continue to evolve and be disseminated, it is critical to establish an evidence base that can help understand their impact on health and well-being and their contribution to achieving the broader aim of health equity. For care management programs incorporating social care, it is important to consider a broad array of both quantitative and qualitative measures beyond health care utilization (Noonan, 2020). Although RCTs generate the most reliable evidence, this evidence can be limited in scope. For example, the RCTs cited above assessed neither the multidimensional nature of care management/social care models that might be reflected in such outcomes as client self-efficacy, satisfaction, or long-term health outcomes nor their potential social impacts. Also important to note is that care management models incorporating social care are limited by the availability of resources in the community, such as behavioral health services, addiction treatment, housing, and transportation. Programs that connect clients to health and social

BOX 5-2
Examples of Edge Runner Programs

¡Cuídate! is an intervention aimed at sexual risk reduction. The program emphasizes the Latino cultural beliefs of familialism and gender-role expectations, and aims to increase knowledge about safer sex, HIV, and pregnancy while building skills for negotiating abstinence and safer sex practices (AAN, n.d.b).

INSIGHTS into Children's Temperament is a 10-week intervention developed in partnership with Hispanic and African American community members. The program provides parents, teachers, and caregivers with practical strategies tailored to the different temperaments of children in their care. It also gives children strategies for daily problem solving. The program has been shown to improve the behavior of children both with and without attention-deficit/hyperactivity disorder (ADHD) and to enhance engagement and performance in school (AAN, n.d.c).

services are unlikely to work if relevant services are unavailable (Noonan, 2020). Important to underscore in the context of this report is that multisector engagement, as well as health care teams that may involve social workers, community health workers, physicians, and others engaging alongside nurses, all are oriented to a shared agenda focused on improving health and advancing health equity.

ADVOCATING FOR POLICY CHANGE

Public policies have a major influence on health care providers, systems, and the populations they serve. Accordingly, nurses can help promote health equity by bringing a health lens to bear on public policies and decision making at the community, state, and federal levels. Informing health-related public policy can involve communicating about health disparities and SDOH with the public, policy makers, and organizational leaders, focusing on both challenges and solutions for addressing health through actions targeted to achieving health equity.

When nurses engage with policy change as an upstream determinant of health, they can have a powerful and far-reaching impact on the health of populations. In the National Academy of Medicine's *Vital Directions* series, Nancy Adler and colleagues (2016) note that "powerful drivers of health lie outside the conventional medical care delivery system.... Health policies need to expand to address factors outside the medical system that promote or damage health." Because health inequities and SDOH are based in social structures and policies, efforts to address them upstream as the root of poor health among certain populations and communities need to focus on policy change (NASEM, 2017a). Nurses alone cannot solve the problems associated with upstream SDOH that exist outside of health care systems. However, by engaging in efforts aimed at changing local, state, or federal policy with a Health in All Policies approach,[2] they can address SDOH that underlie poor health (IOM, 2011; NASEM, 2017a; Williams et al., 2018). Whether nurses engage in policy making full time or work to inform policy part time as a professional responsibility, their attention to policies that either create or eliminate health inequities can improve the underlying conditions that frame people's health. Nurses can bring a health and social justice lens to public policies and decision making at the community, state, and federal levels most effectively by serving in public- and private-sector leadership positions. Much of this work is discussed in Chapter 9 on nursing leadership, but it is noted in this chapter given the substantial

[2] Health in All Policies (HiAP) is a collaborative approach that integrates health considerations into policy making across sectors. It recognizes that health is created by a multitude of factors beyond health care and in many cases, beyond the scope of traditional public health activities. In accordance with HiAP, for example, decision makers in the health care sector should consider transportation, education, housing, commerce, and other sectors impacting communities. HiAP stresses the need to work across government agencies and with private partners from these different sectors to achieve healthy and safe communities. It also encourages partnerships between the health care sector and community developers, for example (CDC, 2016).

influence that policy decisions have on health equity. Nurses can and should use their expertise to promote policies that support health equity.

For example, a nurse in Delaware was influential in getting the state's legislature to pass legislation to implement a colorectal cancer screening program that has increased access to care and reduced disparities in morbidity and mortality from colorectal cancer (see Box 5-3). While individual nurses, often through their workplace and professional associations, engage in upstream efforts to impact health equity, there have been repeated calls from within the nursing community for more nurses to engage in informing public policy to improve health outcomes for individuals and populations.

BOX 5-3
Delaware Cancer Consortium

The Delaware Cancer Consortium is an example of how high-level policy can result in real, on-the-ground changes in health care access that markedly reduce large disparities in health outcomes. With regular screening, colorectal cancer can be prevented or treated at an early stage. However, there remain persistent disparities in incidence and survival rates between African Americans and Whites, even when screening is universally provided (Grubbs et al., 2013). The Delaware Cancer Consortium (formerly the Delaware Advisory Council on Cancer Incidence and Mortality) was created through state legislation in 2001; the drive to pass the legislation was led by a nurse who later entered the state legislature (Healthy Delaware, 2020). That nurse, Dr. Bethany Hall-Long, was trained as a community health nurse and currently serves as the lieutenant governor of Delaware.*

The Delaware Cancer Consortium supported a program that provided free colorectal cancer screening (colonoscopy) and treatment. African Americans received outreach through tailored, localized programs designed by nurse navigators (Grubbs et al., 2013). As a result of the program, more people were screened and treated for colorectal cancer than was the case prior to the program's inception. The Consortium's efforts relied on nurses to carry out several important aspects of the program. First, nurse navigators recruited participants into the program and promoted access to screening and timely follow-up care. Second, the nurses designed localized programs focused specifically on African American communities (Grubbs et al., 2013).

The program improved population health across the state and reduced disparities in access to colorectal cancer screening, treatment, and prevalence for African American populations (Grubbs et al., 2013). The disparity in incidence rates of colorectal cancer between Blacks and Whites were reduced, and the program created a greater degree of equity (Grubbs et al., 2013). Screening, nurse navigation, and care coordination helped achieve diagnosis of colorectal cancer among African Americans at an earlier, less-advanced stage of disease. Disparities in mortality rates between Whites and African Americans were reduced. This example shows components of both health equity, by reducing the disparity in population health, and health care equity, by extending access to screening and treatment.

* Personal communication, Bethany Hall-Long, email March 20, 2020.

CONCLUSIONS

In the coming decade, the United States will make substantial progress in achieving health equity only if it devotes resources and attention to addressing the adverse effects of SDOH on the health of underresourced populations. As 2030 approaches, numerous initiatives to address health equity are likely to be launched at the local, state, and national levels. Many of these initiatives will focus on health care equity. Yet, while expanding access to quality care is critical to reducing disparities and improving health outcomes, such efforts need to be accompanied by additional efforts to identify and change the social institutions, dynamics, and systems underlying health inequities from the local to the national level. Nurses can contribute to reshaping the landscape of health equity over the coming decade by serving in expanded roles, working in new settings and new ways, and partnering with communities and other sectors beyond health care. Some nurses are already working in roles and settings that support health equity and are engaged in educating about and advocating for health equity through their professional associations. Nonetheless, broader engagement as a core activity of every nurse will help advance health equity nationwide. To achieve this aim will require

- support for and the willingness of the nursing workforce to take on new roles in new settings in the community;
- consistency in nurses' preparation for engaging in downstream, midstream, and upstream strategies aimed at improving health equity by addressing issues that compromise health, such as geographic disparities, poverty, racism, homelessness, trauma, drug abuse, and behavioral health conditions;
- more experiential learning and opportunities to work in community settings throughout nursing education to ensure that nurses have skills and competencies to address individuals' complex needs and promote efforts to improve the well-being of communities;
- nursing education that goes beyond teaching the principles of diversity, equity, and inclusion to provide sustained student engagement in hands-on community and clinical experiences with these issues;
- funding to support new models of care and functions that address SDOH, health equity, and population health; and
- evaluation of models to build the evidence needed to scale programs and the policies and resources necessary to sustain them.

These issues are discussed in the chapters that follow. Programs described in this chapter, such as the Camden Coalition and the Edge Runner initiatives, are exemplars of the kind of multidisciplinary, multisector efforts that will be necessary to address the complex needs of individuals and communities and make a lasting impact by eliminating health disparities, with the goal of achieving health equity. Central to these future efforts, however, are parallel efforts that evaluate and provide the evidence base on which to determine the effectiveness of models. One of the greatest challenges this committee faced was finding evidence directly linking the efforts of nurses to address social needs and SDOH to reductions in health disparities that would signal improved population health outcomes and health equity. Such evidence is essential to informing payment policy decisions that can ensure the sustainability of and nurse engagement in these models (discussed further in Chapter 6). Through evidence, the nursing profession can leverage its own potential, and the public, other professionals, and other sectors can understand the impact and value of such nursing engagement.

> ***Conclusion 5-1: Nurses are in a position to improve outcomes for the underserved and can work to address the structural and institutional factors that produce health disparities in the first place.***

> ***Conclusion 5-2: Nurses can use their unique expertise and perspective to help develop and advocate for policies and programs that promote health equity.***

REFERENCES

AAN (American Academy of Nursing). n.d.a. *Transforming America's health system through nursing solutions*. https://www.aannet.org/initiatives/edge-runners (accessed November 3, 2020).

AAN. n.d.b. *¡Cuídate!: A culturally-based program to reduce sexual risk behavior among Latino youth*. https://www.aannet.org/initiatives/edge-runners/profiles/edge-runners--cuidate (accessed November 3, 2020).

AAN. n.d.c. *Insights into children's temperament: Supporting the development of low-income children*. https://www.aannet.org/initiatives/edge-runners/profiles/edge-runners--insights-into-childrens-temperament (accessed November 3, 2020).

AARP. 2010. *Preparation and roles of nursing care providers in America*. http://championnursing.org/resources/preparation-and-roles-nursing-care-providers-america (accessed June 3, 2021).

Abellanoza, A., N. Provenzano-Hass, and R. J. Gatchel. 2018. Burnout in ER nurses: Review of the literature and interview themes. *Journal of Applied Biobehavioral Research* 23(1):e12117.

Adler, N. E., M. M. Glymour, and J. Fielding. 2016. Addressing social determinants of health and health inequalities. *Journal of the American Medical Association* 316(16):1641–1642.

AF4Q (Aligning Forces for Quality). 2012. *Expanding "hot spotting" to new communities*. http://forces4quality.org/node/5182.html (accessed November 3, 2020).

Agurs-Collins, T., S. Persky, E. D. Paskett, S. L. Barkin, H. I. Meissner, T. R. Nansel, S. S. Arteaga, X. Zhang, R. Das, and T. Farhat. 2019. Designing and assessing multilevel interventions to improve minority health and reduce health disparities. *American Journal of Public Health* 109(S1):S86–S93.

AHA (American Hospital Association). 2019. *Screening for social needs: Guiding care teams to engage patients*. Chicago, IL: American Hospital Association.

ANA (American Nurses Association). 2020. *ANA president condemns racism, brutality and senseless violence against black communities*. https://www.nursingworld.org/news/news-releases/2020/ana-president-condemns-racism-brutality-and-senseless-violence-against-black-communities (accessed September 17, 2020).

ANCC (American Nurses Credentialing Center). 2017. *2019 Magnet®* application manual. Silver Spring, MD: American Nurses Credentialing Center.

Audain, G., and C. Maher. 2017. Prevention and control of worldwide mosquito-borne illnesses: Nurses as teachers. *Online Journal of Issues in Nursing* 22(1):5.

Bigbee, J. L., and L. M. Issel. 2012. Conceptual models for population-focused public health nursing interventions and outcomes: The state of the art. *Public Health Nursing* 29(4):370–379.

Braveman, P., E. Arkin, T. Orleans, D. Proctor, and A. Plough. 2017. *What is health equity? And what difference does a definition make?* Princeton, NJ: Robert Wood Johnson Foundation.

Bridge, J. A., L. Asti, L. M. Horowitz, J. B. Greenhouse, C. A. Fontanella, A. H. Sheftall, K. J. Kelleher, and J. V. Campo. 2015. Suicide trends among elementary school–aged children in the United States from 1993 to 2012. *JAMA Pediatrics* 169(7):673–677.

Brown, A. F., G. X. Ma, J. Miranda, E. Eng, D. Castille, T. Brockie, P. Jones, C. O. Airhihenbuwa, T. Farhat, L. Zhu, and C. Trinh-Shevrin. 2019. Structural interventions to reduce and eliminate health disparities. *American Journal of Public Health* 109(S1):S72–S78.

Camden Coalition. n.d. *Camden core model*. https://camdenhealth.org/care-interventions/camden-core-model (accessed November 4, 2020).

Canales, M. K., D. J. Drevdahl, and S. M. Kneipp. 2018. Letter to the editor: Public health nursing. *Nursing Outlook* 66(2):110–111.

Castrucci, B., and J. Auerbach. 2019. Meeting individual social needs falls short of addressing social determinants of health. *Health Affairs Blog*. doi: 10.1377/hblog20190115.234942.

CDC (Centers for Disease Control and Prevention). 2016. *Health in all policies*. https://www.cdc.gov/policy/hiap/index.html (accessed June 2, 2021).

CMS (Centers for Medicare & Medicaid Services). 2020. *Z codes utilization among Medicare fee-for-service (FFS) beneficiaries in 2017*. Baltimore, MD: Centers for Medicare & Medicaid Services Office of Minority Health.

Crippen, D., and F. Isasi. 2013. The untold story of 2013: Governors lead in health care transformation. *Health Affairs Blog*. https://www.healthaffairs.org/do/10.1377/hblog20131217.035878/full (accessed June 2, 2021).

Davies, N., and H. Donovan. 2016. National survey of commissioners' and service planners' views of public health nursing in the UK. *Public Health* 141:218–221.

Donley, R., and M. J. Flaherty. 2002. Revisiting the American Nurses Association's first position on education for nurses. *Online Journal of Issues in Nursing* 7(2):2.

Duran, D., Y. Asada, J. Millum, and M. Gezmu. 2019. Harmonizing health disparities measurement. *American Journal of Public Health* 109(S1):S25–S27.

Dye, B. A., D. G. Duran, D. M. Murray, J. W. Creswell, P. Richard, T. Farhat, N. Breen, and M. M. Engelgau. 2019. The importance of evaluating health disparities research. *American Journal of Public Health* 109(S1):S34–S40.

Finkelstein, A., A. Zhou, S. Taubman, and J. Doyle. 2020. Health care hotspotting—A randomized, controlled trial. *New England Journal of Medicine* 382(2):152–162.

Fraze, T. K., A. L. Brewster, V. A. Lewis, L. B. Beidler, G. F. Murray, and C. H. Colla. 2019. Prevalence of screening for food insecurity, housing instability, utility needs, transportation needs, and interpersonal violence by us physician practices and hospitals. *JAMA Network Open* 2(9):e1911514.

Gawande, A. 2011 (January 24). *The hot spotters*. https://www.newyorker.com/magazine/2011/01/24/the-hot-spotters (accessed October 14, 2020).

Gottlieb, L. M., D. Hessler, D. Long, E. Laves, A. R. Burns, A. Amaya, P. Sweeney, C. Schudel, and N. E. Adler. 2016. Effects of social needs screening and in-person service navigation on child health: A randomized clinical trial. *JAMA Pediatrics* 170(11):e162521.

Green, S. R., V. Singh, and W. O'Byrne. 2010. Hope for New Jersey's city hospitals: The Camden initiative. *Perspectives in Health Information Management* 7(Spring):1d.

Grubbs, S. S., B. N. Polite, J. Carney, Jr., W. Bowser, J. Rogers, N. Katurakes, P. Hess, and E. D. Paskett. 2013. Eliminating racial disparities in colorectal cancer in the real world: It took a village. *Journal of Clinical Oncology* 31(16):1928–1930.

Healthy Delaware. 2020. *Welcome Consortium Members and Partners*. https://www.healthydelaware.org/Consortium (accessed November 3, 2020).

Heath, S. 2018. *3 things to know to conduct a community health needs assessment*. https://patientengagementhit.com/news/3-things-to-know-to-conduct-a-community-health-needs-assessment (accessed October 6, 2020).

IOM (Institute of Medicine). 2011. *The future of nursing: Leading change, advancing health*. Washington, DC: The National Academies Press.

IRS (Internal Revenue Service). 2020. *Community health needs assessment for charitable hospital organizations-Section 501(r)(3)*. https://www.irs.gov/charities-non-profits/community-health-needs-assessment-for-charitable-hospital-organizations-section-501r3 (accessed June 2, 2021).

Jones, N. L., N. Breen, R. Das, T. Farhat, and R. Palmer. 2019. Cross-cutting themes to advance the science of minority health and health disparities. *American Journal of Public Health* 109(S1):S21–S24.

Kangovi, S., N. Mitra, L. Norton, R. Harte, X. Zhao, T. Carter, D. Grande, and J. A. Long. 2018. Effect of community health worker support on clinical outcomes of low-income patients across primary care facilities: A randomized clinical trial. *JAMA Internal Medicine* 178(12):1635–1643.

Kangovi, S., N. Mitra, D. Grande, J. Long, and D. Asch. 2020. Evidence-based community health worker program addresses unmet social needs and generates positive return on investment. *Health Affairs* 39(2). doi: 10.1377/hlthaff.2019.00981.

Keller, L. O., S. Strohschein, M. A. Schaffer, and B. Lia-Hoagberg. 2004. Population-based public health interventions: Innovations in practice, teaching, and management. Part II. *Public Health Nursing* 21(5):469–487.

Krist, A. H., T. A. Wolff, D. E. Jonas, R. P. Harris, M. L. LeFevre, A. R. Kemper, C. M. Mangione, C.-W. Tseng, and D. C. Grossman. 2018. Update on the methods of the U.S. Preventive Services task force: Methods for understanding certainty and net benefit when making recommendations. *American Journal of Preventive Medicine* 54(1 Suppl 1):S11–S18.

Kulbok, P. A., E. Thatcher, E. Park, and P. S. Meszaros. 2012. Evolving public health nursing roles: Focus on community participatory health promotion and prevention. *Online Journal of Issues in Nursing* 17(2):1.

Lantz, P. M. 2019. The medicalization of population health: Who will stay upstream? *Milbank Quarterly* 97(1):36–39.

Larsen, R., J. Ashley, T. Ellens, R. Frauendienst, K. Jorgensen-Royce, and M. Zelenak. 2018. Development of a new graduate public health nurse residency program using the core competencies of public health nursing. *Public Health Nursing* 35(6):606–612.

Makelarski, J. A., E. Abramsohn, J. H. Benjamin, S. Du, and S. T. Lindau. 2017. Diagnostic accuracy of two food insecurity screeners recommended for use in health care settings. *American Journal of Public Health* 107(11):1812–1817.

Mann, C. 2013. *CMCS informational bulletin: Targeting Medicaid super-utilizers to decrease costs and improve quality*. Baltimore, MD: Centers for Medicare & Medicaid Services.

Martsolf, G. R., T. Gordon, L. Warren May, D. Mason, C. Sullivan, and A. Villarruel. 2016. Innovative nursing care models and culture of health: Early evidence. *Nursing Outlook* 64(4):367–376.

Martsolf, G. R., D. J. Mason, J. Sloan, C. G. Sullivan, and A. M. Villarruel. 2017. *Nurse-designed care models: What can they tell us about advancing a culture of health?* Santa Monica, CA: RAND Corporation.

Mason, D. J., D. A. Jones, C. Roy, C. G. Sullivan, and L. J. Wood. 2015. Commonalities of nurse-designed models of health care. *Nursing Outlook* 63(5):540–553.

Minnesota Department of Health. 2019. *Public health interventions: Applications for public health nursing practice*, 2nd ed. St. Paul, MN: Minnesota Department of Health.

Minnesota Department of Health. n.d. *Public health nurse orientation and resource guide*. https://www.health.state.mn.us/communities/practice/ta/phnconsultants/guide-phn.html (accessed October 5, 2020).

Mullan, F. 2017. Social mission in health professions education: Beyond flexner. *Journal of the American Medical Association* 318(2):122–123.

NASEM (National Academies of Sciences, Engineering, and Medicine). 2016. *Accounting for social risk factors in Medicare payment: Identifying social risk factors*. Washington, DC: The National Academies Press.

NASEM. 2017a. *Communities in action: Pathways to health equity*. Washington, DC: The National Academies Press.

NASEM. 2017b. *Global health and the future role of the United States*. Washington, DC: The National Academies Press.

NASEM. 2019. *Integrating social care into the delivery of health care: Moving upstream to improve the nation's health*. Washington, DC: The National Academies Press.

Noonan, K. 2020. Disappointing randomized controlled trial results show a way forward on complex care in Camden and beyond. *Health Affairs Blog*. doi: 10.1377/hblog20200102.864819.

Pittman, P. 2019. Rising to the challenge: Re-embracing the Wald model of nursing. *American Journal of Nursing* 119(7):46–52.

Rafferty, A. M. 2015 (January 27). *Reinventing nursing's social mission*. Video. https://www.youtube.com/watch?v=8PjoiO8v-dE (accessed September 6, 2020).

Sadowski, L. S., R. A. Kee, T. J. VanderWeele, and D. Buchanan. 2009. Effect of a housing and case management program on emergency department visits and hospitalizations among chronically ill homeless adults: A randomized trial. *Journal of the American Medical Association* 301(17):1771–1778.

Schaffer, M. A., L. O. Keller, and D. Reckinger. 2015. Public health nursing activities: Visible or invisible? *Public Health Nursing* 32(6):711–720.

Swider, S. M., P. F. Levin, and V. Reising. 2017. Evidence of public health nursing effectiveness: A realist review. *Public Health Nursing* 34(4):324–334.

Thomas-Henkel, C., and M. Schulman. 2017. *Screening for social determinants of health in populations with complex needs: Implementation considerations*. Trenton, NJ: Center for Health Care Strategies.

Tyson, T., C. J. Kenon, Jr., and K. Nance. 2018. Nursing at historically black colleges and universities. *Journal of Professional Nursing* 34(3):167–170.

Williams, D. R., and V. Purdie-Vaughns. 2016. Needed interventions to reduce racial/ethnic disparities in health. *Journal of Health Politics, Policy and Law* 41(4):627–651.

Williams, S. D., J. M. Phillips, and K. Koyama. 2018. Nurse advocacy: Adopting a health in all policies approach. *Online Journal of Issues in Nursing* 23(3).

Woolf, S. H., J. Q. Purnell, S. M. Simon, E. B. Zimmerman, G. J. Camberos, A. Haley, and R. P. Fields. 2015. Translating evidence into population health improvement: Strategies and barriers. *Annual Review of Public Health* 36(1):463–482.

6

Paying for Equity in Health and Health Care

Health cannot be a question of income.
It is a fundamental human right.

—Nelson Mandela, social rights activist and politician

Maximizing the health of everyone needs to be a primary goal of the health care and health care payment systems. Payment systems today do little to improve health equity so that everyone has a fair and better chance of living a healthier life. To enable nurses to address the social factors that shape health and advance health equity, new and emerging payment models need to incentivize and support care management and team-based care, and expand nurses' scope of practice, community and school nursing, and telehealth. Payment models also need to be intentionally designed to foster a more diverse workforce that reflects the population and include improvements in experiential training to accelerate movement toward health equity.

Payment systems greatly impact whether and how health care systems use their resources, including nurses, to improve public health.[1] Nurses' ability to address an individual's social needs and the social determinants of health (SDOH) in the community, as well as to perform roles and implement interventions that can advance health equity, can be supported or inhibited by the payment systems that reimburse organizations and individual clinicians for the

[1] This chapter focuses on payment systems that pay health care organizations and clinicians for the care they provide to individuals and payment systems that support public health and school nursing. Health insurance also helps consumers access and afford health care.

care they provide. COVID-19 has revealed what many clinicians, policy makers, and patient organizations have known for years: that individuals with more health and social risk factors, such as people of color (POC) and those with low income, are more likely to suffer worse health outcomes, and the existing health and social safety nets are frequently unable to prevent these disparities because of a lack of a robust public health infrastructure. These disparities will only be exacerbated by the health, economic, and social disruptions caused by COVID-19, which will increase the number of persons with greater health and social risks, drive up costs and spending, and place further strain on health care and social services systems that are already inadequate. The feasibility and value of innovative reforms to improve the nation's health are highlighted by many of the temporary regulatory health care reforms enacted in response to COVID-19, such as increased flexibility and reimbursement for telehealth and expanded scopes of practice. Payment reform can help improve population health, address social needs and SDOH, and reduce health disparities, supporting the provision of effective, efficient, equitable, and accessible care for all across the care continuum instead of incentivizing the volume of care or low-value procedures and practices.

This chapter focuses on the relevance for nursing of general principles of payment systems that pay health care organizations and clinicians for the care they provide to individuals and payment systems that support public health and school nursing. The design of payment systems influences the health care provided to individuals and communities, where care is provided, and by whom. Removing such obstacles to health as poverty and discrimination and their consequences and tailoring health systems to meet the specific health and social needs of individuals will help reduce health inequity (Braveman et al., 2017). Payment systems can directly impact the ability of nurses to serve as change agents in bridging the health and social needs of individuals and communities. This chapter explains how existing and evolving payment systems present both challenges and opportunities for supporting and incentivizing nurses to address SDOH and advance health equity. To this end, it first summarizes the nursing roles and functions identified in the previous chapters. Next, the chapter outlines how the current predominant fee-for-service (FFS) and emerging value-based payment (VBP) and alternative payment models (APMs) could support these nursing roles and functions, and how it is essential for health care systems and policy makers to value, prioritize, and embrace these roles and functions if reforms are to occur. The chapter also reviews the potential roles of public health funding and social-sector resources in supporting nurses in addressing social factors and advancing health equity. The chapter then addresses the need for financial support to develop and advance mechanisms for further diversifying and preparing the nursing workforce. The final section presents conclusions.

ADDRESSING SOCIAL DETERMINANTS OF HEALTH AND ADVANCING HEALTH EQUITY BY EXPANDING NURSING ROLES AND FUNCTIONS

Chapters 4 and 5 identify major nursing roles and functions that can successfully address SDOH and advance health equity, all of which can be supported and incentivized through different payment models discussed in this chapter (FFS, VBP, and APMs). Payment models can support nurses' roles and functions to address SDOH and advance health equity in four key areas: care management and team-based care, expanded scope of practice, community nursing, and telehealth.

Care Management and Team-Based Care

Successful care management programs require a holistic view of the patient's health and social needs, and close monitoring and follow-up of patients to address these issues. For example, CareOregon, a Medicaid community care organization (CCO) health plan in which members receive managed physical, mental, and dental services, implemented a transitional care model and intervention called C-TRAIN (Englander and Kansagara, 2012). This program uses team-based care to assess patients during discharge to ensure that they receive appropriate follow-up care, focusing primarily on medically complex patients, people with newly identified or unmanaged chronic conditions, or those who face psychosocial barriers such as homelessness and food insecurity. Registered nurses (RNs) are essential members of the teams, and are paired with social workers for follow-ups. Typically, the care team follow-up occurs at up to 30 days, or longer in some cases. Interventions vary based on participants' needs, but nurses are available to assist with navigating the health care system; providing medication reconciliation, health coaching, and education; and identifying specific needs, such as food insecurity, homelessness, and insufficient clothing. The long-term goals are developing strong relationships between the care team and patient and connecting people to primary care, specialists, and behavioral health services.

Effective care management and team-based care screen patients for social needs and social risk. In Spartanburg County, South Carolina, AccessHealth Spartanburg (AHS) works with medically complex people who lack insurance and are high utilizers of the emergency department (Freundlich, 2018). With a screening questionnaire, AHS assesses people's needs and stratifies them into three categories of low, moderate, and high risk. People considered high risk are assigned to an RN case manager, those considered moderate risk are assigned to social workers, and those considered low risk are assigned to community health workers (Freundlich, 2018). These personnel help manage and coordinate care, and refer clients to a network of 10 local, county, and state organizations and programs for assistance with social needs.

Expanded Scope of Practice

A second area in which nursing roles and functions can be supported by and incentivized through different payment models to address SDOH and advance health equity involves regulations that control nurses' scope of practice. Such regulations control how advanced practice registered nurses (APRNs) provide primary care and impact how their services are paid. Sometimes private and public health systems constrain nurses working within their facilities, preventing them from practicing at full scope. Approximately 61.47 percent of health professional shortage areas (HPSAs) are rural (HRSA, 2021). As discussed in Chapter 2, many of these rural areas lack sufficient primary care and would benefit from increased access to APRNs (Auerbach et al., 2018). Studies have found that nurse practitioners (NPs) are more likely than physicians to practice in rural areas (Barnes et al., 2018; Buerhaus, 2018). As discussed in Chapter 3, the number of NPs is expected to grow 6.8 percent annually through 2030, compared with about 1 percent for physicians, whose numbers practicing in rural areas will fall through 2030. Additionally, several reviews have found little to no difference in the quality of care received by patients from NPs and physicians (DesRoches et al., 2017; McCleery et al., 2014), and in some cases found that patients perceived a more holistic approach to care from NPs (Moldestad et al., 2020).

Thus, the growing APRN and RN workforces have the potential to improve rural health disparities. It is as yet unknown, however, whether some states[2] may continue to impose restrictive scope-of-practice laws that limit the capacity of the nursing workforce once the COVID-19 pandemic has ended (Lai et al., 2020). There is strong evidence of the beneficial effect of NPs providing mental health care, primary care medication prescribing, and buprenorphine waivers for the treatment of patients with opioid use disorder. Evidence shows that broadening of prescriptive authority led to decreases in mental health–related mortality, and these improvements occurred specifically in underserved areas (Alexander and Shnell, 2019). NPs, along with physician assistants (PAs), obtaining the waiver have the potential to treat 15 percent more rural patients, increasing the number of people treated per 10,000 from 15.4 to 17.7 (Andrilla et al., 2020).

In late December 2016, the U.S. Department of Veterans Affairs (VA) loosened restrictions on scope of practice for three APRN nursing roles: certified nurse midwife, certified nurse specialist, and certified nurse practitioner. An evidence brief from the VA points to the need for large and robust studies that examine the difference in care between APRNs and physicians, providing an opportunity to continue tracking patient outcomes (McCleery et al., 2014).

---

[2] In March 2020, Florida passed House Bill 607: Direct Care Workers, which grants APRNs, beginning July 2020, the ability to work independently. This does not include certified nursing assistants.

Community Nursing

A third area in which nurses can address SDOH and advance health equity concerns their work in the community. Community nursing allows nurses to meet people in their homes, schools, and community sites, and address their medical and social needs in a timely, accessible manner. These nurses help bridge the gap between health care systems and communities, and their practice reflects the community needs. In 2016, the Josiah Macy Jr. Foundation called for the increased use of nurses in primary care and expansion of nurses' roles in community settings. The foundation also recommended that nursing educators include primary care in nurses' curriculum and provide students with increased clinical experiences in primary care and community settings (Bodenheimer and Mason, 2016).

Telehealth

Use of telehealth is a fourth area in which nurses can be supported and incentivized through different payment models to help address SDOH and advance health equity concerns. As discussed in Chapter 4, telehealth capitalizes on the proliferation of mobile devices and technology to connect with people. In 2016, the most common uses of telehealth were for physician office visits and mental health visits (MedPAC, 2018). The largest proportion of telehealth users were beneficiaries who lived in rural areas, had a disability, were dually eligible for Medicare and Medicaid (CMS, 2020b), or had a higher prevalence of chronic mental health conditions. NPs and other nurses caring for rural populations are prevented from being reimbursed for their telehealth services and from being supported by specialists located hundreds of miles away (Skinner et al., 2019). Paying for nursing telehealth services, mobile care, and remote diagnostic technology could increase access to care for rural populations and the homebound. Telehealth allows nurses the flexibility of being available during office hours and on call for symptom assessment and advice on treating minor issues or when to go to the emergency department, thereby reducing unnecessary emergency department visits.

PAYMENT SYSTEMS THAT SUPPORT AND INCENTIVIZE ADDRESSING SOCIAL DETERMINANTS OF HEALTH AND ADVANCING HEALTH EQUITY

Payment systems in the United States pay for health care based primarily on rewarding the volume of care rather than the value of care (Miller, 2009); treatment of illness rather than prevention and health promotion; and inpatient and specialty care rather than primary care, preventive care, and community/public health. Additionally, payment systems are directed predominantly toward directly reimbursing physician services while infrequently recognizing the explicit value of services of other clinicians, including nurses and advanced practice nurses working in a variety of settings. Nursing is part of labor costs for most employers of nurses and considered by Medicare to be part of "hospital services" (ANA, 2017), a position that underestimates nurses' work and impacts resource allocation. It is critical for payment systems to be better aligned with nurses' contributions to improving clinical performance and the quality of care, increasing revenues, and decreasing costs.

These payment designs have limited the ability of the current system to address social needs and SDOH. The inputs required to advance population health are diverse and include health care, education, housing, environmental safety, and employment. Yet, payment systems to advance population health have focused primarily on a single input: health care (Horner et al., 2019). Moreover, the main criterion for investing in interventions to address social factors has often been achieving cost savings rather than providing value or cost-effectiveness. For example, health care organizations often focus on the relatively few most resource-intensive, highest-cost patients (the "superutilizers") in their population health management programs instead of on the broader spectrum of patients who could benefit from such interventions. Even though health disparities across race, ethnicity, and socioeconomic status (SES) cost the nation trillions of dollars in direct medical costs, indirect costs such as lost productivity, and the costs of premature deaths (CDC, 2013; LaVeist et al., 2011), individual health care organizations have little incentive to reduce these disparities for underserved populations (Chin, 2016).

Nurses' roles in transitional care, care management, and care coordination also can reduce costs associated with chronic illness, complex patients, or dually eligible beneficiaries (NCSL, 2016) by helping to prevent hospital readmissions and emergency department visits (Naylor et al., 2012; NSCL, 2016; Ryan et al., 2019). Because health care delivery organizations employ the majority of the nation's nursing workforce (3.6 million nurses), incentives are needed to leverage nurses' expertise in novel ways to intervene in SDOH that block advances toward achieving health equity.

Increasingly, public and private policy makers, insurers, health associations, and health care delivery organizations are advocating for the states to remove scope-of-practice restrictions on APRNs (NGA, 2012). Team-based care is increasing, especially in primary care, and APRNs could further expand access to health care, particularly for important populations residing in rural and urban HPSAs (Gilman and Koslov, 2014; NGA, 2012; Shekelle and Begashaw, 2021).

New VBP and APM approaches theoretically can incentivize improved population health, prevention, higher performance, and better health outcomes. However, the total amount of payment at risk to health care organizations with these approaches has been modest, and the incentives provided have frequently been weak (Damberg et al., 2014). To date, therefore, the ability of VBP and APMs to improve population health and advance health equity has been limited, or close to nonexistent (Hsu et al., 2020). The financial incentives have frequently been insufficient to have a substantial effect on modifying the behavior of clinicians or inducing the operational changes within health care organizations required to address SDOH and advance health equity meaningfully, with sometimes worse health outcomes for safety-net hospitals (Damberg et al., 2014; Hsu et al., 2020). In addition, since most health care organizations have a diverse payer mix, financial incentives need to align across payers to create rewards sufficient to incentivize health care organizations to invest in health equity strategies, considering the complexity of the individuals being served in some facilities (Stone, 2020), and the staff needed to implement these strategies, such as nurses. Yet, too often health disparities are an afterthought for policy makers, neglected or seen as unintended negative consequences of health policy. In contrast, policies need to be designed proactively to advance health equity (Anderson et al., 2018; Chin et al., 2012; DeMeester et al., 2017; NASEM, 2017; NQF, 2017).

The most effective ways to design payment systems to address SDOH and advance health equity are areas of intense policy and research inquiry (DeMeester et al., 2017; NASEM, 2017; NQF, 2017). Key questions about payment functionality[3] to align incentives and behavior include the following (Gunter et al., 2021; Patel et al., 2021):

- What costs of care will a health care organization or health plan be held accountable for (e.g., primary care costs, specialty care costs, total cost of care)?
- How much money is at risk to the health care organization? For example, many existing VBP and APM programs provide relatively weak incentives for health care organizations, whereas putting more money at risk to health care organizations could have a greater influence on their behavior. (For example, will the incentive or penalty system affect 5 percent of the payment, 10 percent of the payment, or 50 percent of the payment?)
- Which patients/beneficiaries are attributed to the health care organization (e.g., accountable care organization, hospital) in determining quality performance and costs and subsequent payment based on those metrics?
- How can the data analytics capability needed by organizations to operate effectively in VBP and APM settings be ensured? For example, some safety-net providers, small practices, and rural clinics may lack robust

[3] For the purposes of this discussion, payment functionality is conceptualized as key operational issues for those mechanisms that pay for infrastructure (e.g., care management, care teams, nurse primary care functions, telehealth, workforce, and education) and those mechanisms that incentivize and reward specific processes of care and outcomes that advance health equity, such as those that address SDOH, improve population health, and reduce health disparities.

data infrastructure and analytical capability, placing them at a disadvantage in VBP and APM models.

- How do the cost and quality of care relate with respect to payment? For example, even if a health care organization saves money, does it need to meet quality metrics to receive its share of that saved money?
- How should performance reporting and payment be adjusted for populations' social risk in ways that neither mask disparities nor penalize health care organizations that provide care for patients with greater social risk (NASEM, 2017; NQF, 2017)?
- How will it be possible to ensure that the long-term societal benefits of improving public health are reflected in the short-term incentives provided to health care organizations to create a business case for them to address SDOH and improve health equity?
- How can the same services be paid for equitably regardless of the provider (e.g., normal delivery by certified nurse midwife [CNM] versus obstetrician-gynecologist physician; advanced practice nurse versus physician)?

The answers to these questions are evolving and will likely need to be tailored to different populations, markets, and policy contexts, and they can be informed by the input of nurses with experience in addressing SDOH and advancing health equity. Each question can also be asked from the perspective of how the payment system affects the role of nurses.

It is critical to ensure that the payment for health care services for both providers and health plans is adjusted appropriately for the complexity of the patient population. Current risk adjustment methodologies use primarily medical diagnosis and do not adequately take social risk factors into account (Ash et al., 2017; Meddings et al., 2017). The result can be underpayment to providers and plans that attract a disproportionate number of patients with social risk factors and can serve as a disincentive to innovation. For instance, if a health plan or provider develops a unique, novel, and effective program targeting complex patients experiencing homelessness and begins to attract more of these patients, it will be adversely impacted financially and could go out of business. Massachusetts has attempted to risk adjust using SDOH risk factors in its Medicaid premium payments to health plans (UMN, 2020). A key challenge to incorporating social factors is obtaining the relevant information from patients. Much work remains to refine these models and deploy them to various payer settings (Ash et al., 2017; Irvin et al., 2020).

Health care policy and payment systems are in flux as of this writing, as evidenced by the push for health systems to try new approaches through demonstration projects and grants to encourage innovative approaches. Thus, it is currently unclear what the predominant payment model will be in 2030. Accordingly, various possible mechanisms by which each of the predominant payment models (FFS, VBP, APMs) can support and incentivize health care organizations in enabling nurses to perform key nursing roles and functions are reviewed in this chapter. The committee suggests expanding the goal and purpose of payment systems beyond traditional health care and traditional government and private payers to explore how the public health and social sectors can support nurses in using their expertise to eliminate gaps and disparities in health and health care. This section is not meant to be an exhaustive exploration of the current payment system[4] but to give examples of the general principles by which current and future payment systems can be tailored to use nurses more wisely and effectively to improve population health and advance health equity.

Fee-for-Service

Historically, most health care providers in the United States have been paid through FFS payments, in which each individual service is billed separately (Berenson and Ginsberg, 2019). To bill for these FFS payments, all types of insurance (Medicare, Medicaid, and commercial) require that two components be submitted: a CPT (Current Procedure Terminology) code and one or more ICD-10 (*International Classification of Diseases, 10th Revision*) codes. The CPT code describes the service being provided, while the ICD-10 code describes the reason(s) that the service was provided.

There are more than 7,600 different CPT codes (Fuchs, 2013), and each insurance company has a unique fee schedule for each service. In negotiating with insurance companies, it would be overwhelming for providers to negotiate the price of all of the individual codes. In many instances, providers will negotiate their payment as a percentage of the Medicare fee schedule (Clemens and Gottlieb, 2017; Ginsburg, 2012; MedPAC, 2019). Medicare has a set, national fee schedule published and updated every year by the Centers for Medicare & Medicaid Services (CMS), a federal government agency. Thus, the Medicare fee schedule has become the relative baseline for much of the provider payment system in the United States. Researchers have demonstrated a link between the Medicare fee schedule and specialty choice, investment decisions, and innovation within health care (Clemens and Gottlieb, 2014, 2017).

Despite growing use of APMs, such as pay-for-quality and risk-based payment, the FFS payment structure underlies the calculation of many of these payments (Berenson and Ginsburg, 2019; Ginsburg, 2012). For instance, shared savings calculations are often based on the actual versus expected FFS expenditures. Additionally, within many health care organizations, providers are often paid using incentive compensation that is based on the volume and type of services being delivered (MGMA, 2020). Thus, providers may be financially

[4] For further information, see Needleman (2020).

incentivized to deliver a higher volume of expensive services if they have an incentive-based contract.

CPT codes are created, governed, and owned by the American Medical Association (AMA). The CPT codes are protected by copyright and are AMA's largest single source of revenue (Rosenthal, 2017). The federal government, states, and insurers license the CPT code set for use in their payment of providers (AMA, 2019b). The codes are overseen by an AMA-led CPT Editorial Panel with 17 members, 11 of whom must be physician members of AMA. Two members are required to be nonphysicians representing the CPT Health Care Professionals Advisory Committee, such as nurses.[5] The existence of a CPT code and the definition of the code have a critical impact on whether a service is reimbursed.

The valuation and ultimately relative prices paid for the CPT codes are based on the work of another AMA committee, the Relative Value Scale Update Committee (RUC) (AMA, 2019c). This committee makes recommendations to the federal government on the relative value and ultimately prices of services paid for by Medicare. Between 2011 and 2015, a U.S. Government Accountability Office (GAO) study found that 69 percent of RUC recommendations became Medicare payment policy (GAO, 2015). As previously described, these valuations then become the basis for the relative prices paid by all insurers in the United States. The RUC has 31 voting members who are all physicians; nurses serve in an advisory capacity.[6,7,8]

The prices in Medicare and for other insurers as well are based on a measurement called a relative value unit (RVU) consisting of three components: labor, overhead, and malpractice (Hsiao et al., 1987; MedPAC, 2020). Approximately 50 percent of the RVU measurement is based on the labor to deliver the health care service, which is called the work-RVU (Fuchs, 2013). This work-RVU is calculated by AMA's RUC through voluntary, unverified, and self-reported surveys from physicians themselves, which have been found to be inaccurate and overstated. Survey return rates can be quite low and data confidence intervals wide (Laugesen, 2014; MedPAC, 2019). The overhead-RVU component, the second-largest component of the calculation, is based on input from an RUC expert panel, which a GAO report also found to be inaccurate. According to that report, "officials sometimes price items on the basis of a single or small number of invoices" for the overhead report, ignoring normal economies of scale (GAO,

[5] Keepnews, D. J. 2020. Memo on Nursing, The Relative Value Scale Update Committee Process and Payment Policy. Sent by email and received on January 22, 2020.

[6] Keepnews, D. J. 2020. Memo on Nursing, The Relative Value Scale Update Committee Process and Payment Policy. Sent by email and received on January 22, 2020.

[7] Reinecke, P. 2019. Relative Value Scale Update Committtee Information. Memo from Peter Reinicke to Sue Hassmiller. Submitted by email from Sue Hassmiller on November 19, 2019.

[8] Sullivan, E. 2020. Memo on Comments Regarding Issues for Registered Nurses and Advanced Practice Registered Nurses and the Resource Based Relative Value System. Submitted by email and received on January 2, 2020.

2015). Also, as physicians get more efficient at delivering a service and the overhead drops from volume of service delivery, the data are not consistently recollected to recalculate the work- and overhead-RVUs. As a result of this system, the worth of 1 hour of provider time spent delivering a procedure can be three to five times higher than that of 1 hour spent talking to patients or coordinating care. According to Sinsky and Dugdale (2013), "Two common specialty procedures can generate more revenue in one to two hours of total time than a primary care physician receives for an entire day's work."

Through the CPT Editorial Panel and the RUC, AMA has had a singular and profound influence on both what gets paid and the relative value of those services in the American health care system (Laugesen, 2014). A 2015 GAO report requested by Congress states:

> GAO found that, in the majority of cases, CMS accepts the RUC's recommendations and participation by other stakeholders is limited. Given the process and data-related weaknesses associated with the RUC's recommendations, such heavy reliance on the RUC could result in inaccurate Medicare payment rates. (GAO, 2015, p. ii)

FFS pays for the transaction of health care services, which may often encourage reactive treatment, increasing the volume of services and procedures and resulting in overspending. FFS payment rate schedules tend to favor specialty and inpatient care and not to incentivize preventive and primary care (MedPAC, 2019; Shi, 2012).

The creation and valuation of codes for care coordination, patient assessment, end-of-life counseling, health education, and prevention services have lagged, with the focus given to highly paid, highly valued procedures. The former services, however, are especially important for patients experiencing significant SDOH risk factors. Even the choice of who may provide a service and therefore bill for that service is built into the definitions of the codes. Few codes allow for directly reimbursing for nurse-led services at the RN level. Instead, the codes attempt to value those services within the overhead-RVU component. The current system has long been criticized for undervaluing cognitive work, overvaluing procedural work, and inadequately capturing a range of nonprocedural work (Berenson and Goodson, 2016; Sullivan-Marx and Maislin, 2000; Sullivan-Marx et al., 2000). APRNs are reimbursed at 80–85 percent, compared with the full reimbursement physicians receive under the fee schedule (MLN, 2020).

Despite many weaknesses, it is possible to reform FFS payment to support key nursing roles—specifically, to allow nurses and health care organizations to bill and receive reimbursement for services that address SDOH and advance health equity at a level sufficient to support these interventions and incentivize organizations to persist in initiating and sustaining this work. Nonetheless, the committee recognizes that, while a shift away from the FFS model is under way, fully transitioning to another system may take years. Therefore, it will be necessary to support and incentivize nurses in taking on these roles and functions under the FFS system.

Attaching relative value to complex health care services is a challenging task. In the current system, the CPT codes and associated RVUs are a bottom-up estimate of cost, which is used by CMS and other insurers as measure of relative value in their payment of providers without reference to the overall societal value of the service, the availability/supply of the service, the evidence base for benefit from the service, the quality of the service delivered, and the outcome for the individual (Berenson and Lazaroff, 2019).

Possible approaches to reforming the process of creating, defining, and valuing health care services in an FFS environment could include such changes as (1) reforming the existing two committees (CPT Executive Panel and RUC) to include meaningful representation from nursing, or (2) the creation of a new multidisciplinary committee sponsored by CMS or an independent nonprofit. Given the ownership of the CPT codes and the complexity of developing codes and valuing services, no solution would be a simple undertaking. The committee recognizes the importance of this issue and highlights the potential for developing new approaches.

CPT Codes, Care Management, and Team-Based Care

CPT billing codes could be altered to include nursing-specific functions in care management and team-based care. As noted above, the FFS model frequently does not reimburse adequately or at all for time spent on cognitive activities and coordination services, such as screening people for social risk factors and connecting them to the appropriate social services (NASEM, 2019). Adding CPT codes for such services as care coordination could provide opportunities and financial incentives for care that supports social needs.

In some cases, billing codes have already been developed (e.g., for chronic care management) that allow care team members other than physicians to bill or allow for "incident-to" billing (NASEM, 2019, p. 118). Medicare reimburses nonphysicians in the category "incident to a physician's service," which requires working under a physician's supervision. Records log the physician as having provided the service (Rapsilber, 2019), and reimbursements thus credit the billing provider—the physician—and not the actual provider of service at the time. The result is undercounting of the services actually provided by NPs and PAs (Morgan et al., 2019). In 2019, the Medicare Payment Advisory Committee (MedPAC) found that NPs and PAs are increasingly providing more primary and some specialty services (Coldiron and Ratnarathorn, 2014; Muteanu et al., 2020) under "incident-to" billing, concluding and recommending that Congress eliminate the "incident-to" practice entirely so NPs and PAs can bill Medicare directly and the value of their services can be measured (MedPAC, 2019).

As described in Chapter 3, the degree to which a nonphysician can practice and bill varies by state practice laws (Larson et al., 2017), with differing impacts on the population. For instance, women in states where CNMs have practice autonomy and attend births have lower rates of low birthweight and preterm birth (NASEM, 2020a; Yang et al., 2016). These outcomes are also found in other countries where care is delivered by nurse midwives (Renfrew et al., 2014). Currently, Medicare reimburses APRNs for pre- and postdischarge care as part of transitional care management under the FFS model using CPT codes 99495 and 99496 (Fels et al., 2015); however, these billing codes have frequently been unwieldy to implement in practice.

While most health systems do not allow RNs or social workers to bill for care management or other team-based services (Dormond and Afayee, 2016), there is at least one example of innovators designing processes to allow such billing. CareOregon allows RNs and social workers to bill Medicaid for each episode of care management services with custom pricing using CPT codes 99368 and 99366, without requiring incident-to billing through a physician or APRN. Although the system was challenged by electronic health records not documenting services for people not engaged in primary care (i.e., "preprimary care"), collaboration among program staff, the billing department, and the information technology (IT) department resulted in a unique documentation and coding structure to support the program.[9]

Expanding Nurses' Scope of Practice

Nearly one-quarter of adults in the United States experience a behavioral health disorder, according to a 2018 survey by the Substance Abuse and Mental Health Services Administration (SAMHSA, 2018). A lack of behavioral health services has contributed to increased morbidity and mortality, with rural areas facing a particular burden compounded by health care provider shortages. Nearly half of rural areas were found to lack a physician with a U.S. Drug Enforcement Administration (DEA) waiver to prescribe buprenorphine (Andrilla et al., 2019), and there is a tremendous need for individuals with substance use disorder to be able to access a full array of treatment, including buprenorphine (Velander, 2018). Access to life-saving substance abuse disorder treatment could increase dramatically, particularly in rural areas, if more NPs were granted waivers to prescribe buprenorphine and other medications for treatment of substance abuse disorders (Barnett et al., 2019; Moore, 2019). Empowering and supporting NPs, APRNs, CNMs, and nurse anesthetists across all states to practice to the full extent of their license and training, especially in areas with maldistribution of health care providers, could expand access to an array of important health services for underserved populations (UM Behavioral Health Workforce Research Center, 2018).

---

[9] Personal communication with Jennifer Menisk Kennedy, January 29, 2020.

Reforms to the RUC's fee schedules to reflect current work values empirically would better support the work of NPs (Sullivan-Marx, 2008).

Expanded Funding for School Nursing Services

In 2014, the U.S. Department of Health and Human Services (HHS) rescinded a policy that prevented school nurses from billing Medicaid for their services (CMS, 2014; Maughan, 2018; Ollove, 2019; Wang, 2014). As of 2019, seven states had made changes to their Medicaid policies to allow school nurses to bill—an important policy change that affects how school nurses practice and extends their services to all children (see Chapter 4). Medical associations, nursing associations, and others have ongoing advocacy efforts for policies that allow all students to have access to health services (Council on School Health, 2016; Largent, 2019). Despite following an FFS model, implementation is irregular among states, and school districts and local counties will have to decide how to pay for health services rendered to students.

Telehealth

As part of the Bipartisan Budget Act of 2018, Medicare coverage of telehealth and eligible services was expanded; however, these services were limited to certain geographic areas (rural areas designated as HPSAs or outside of metropolitan statistical areas) or services provided as part of a CMS demonstration project (CMS, 2018). Historically, payment for telehealth services also has been limited by provider category, with limits on nurses and advanced practice nurses.

In March 2020, during the beginning of the COVID-19 pandemic, CMS issued temporary waivers to expand access to telehealth services so that beneficiaries could receive services without having to travel to a health care facility. As a result, beneficiaries can continue receiving routine services and maintain contact with their providers while sheltering in place (CMS, 2020a). The CMS policy encompasses telehealth reimbursement for a wide range of clinicians, including "physicians, nurse practitioners, physician assistants, nurse midwives, certified nurse anesthetists, clinical psychologists, clinical social workers, registered dietitians, and nutrition professionals, however, this is subject to state regulation of scope of practice" (CMS, 2020a). Some states have encouraged private payers to also cover telehealth services, but the legislative guidelines and implementation have varied across states (CCHP, 2017, 2019). Some telehealth laws aimed at private payers have required parity in covered services, meaning services that would be covered for in-person visits are also covered (CCHP, 2019). Ultimately, not all people receive the same services in all states.

Telehealth can maximize a care team's interaction with individuals and strengthen collaborative care in rural areas. One study found, for example, that nurse-led telehealth care management for children with medical complexities in an urban environment improved parents' understanding of how to care for their children's health issues (Cady et al., 2015). Project ECHO (Extension for Community Healthcare Outcomes) is another telehealth innovation designed to improve clinician collaboration by using video conferencing to connect specialists to primary care providers and care teams, which include nurses. While paying for a clinician's time to participate in teleECHO clinics is currently difficult under the FFS system, Project ECHO can assist nurses or intermediary providers with reimbursement through the collaborative care CPT code (Hager et al., 2018).

Value-Based Payment

Because payment based on FFS is the most important contributor to overutilization of services, inefficiency, and rising health care spending, both the Obama and Trump administrations, with bipartisan congressional support, have sought changes in federal payment systems to emphasize the value of health care services over the volume of services provided (CMS, 2019a). VBP, in contrast, links to both quality and value (Werner et al., 2021). Essentially, using VBP means paying providers more for delivering higher-quality care and achieving better patient outcomes, taking into account the cost of resources used to produce the outcomes. Similarly, providers are paid less for delivering lower-quality care and worse outcomes, again taking into account the cost of resources used to produce the outcomes. In this way, providers who produce better outcomes using less costly resources are rewarded compared with those who produce poorer outcomes at higher cost. A common example is pay-for-performance, in which providers and health care organizations receive more payment if they meet preestablished clinical performance accountability metrics.

In this context, it is important for performance metrics to incentivize nursing roles and functions that address SDOH and advance population health and health equity. Nurse-sensitive indicators could be developed using Donabedian's Structure-Process-Outcome framework for quality assessment (Gallagher and Rowell, 2003). A recommendation from the Nursing Knowledge: 2018 Big Data Science Conference included the creation of a national nurse identifier. A national nurse identifier would be useful because

> [H]ospitals and health systems need the ability to identify nurses in the EHR [electronic health record] enterprise resource planning system (ERP), and other health IT systems for documentation, education, research and training purposes; nursing documentation in the EHR, ERP, and other health IT systems can demonstrate nurses' value as healthcare transitions to a value-based reimbursement model; nursing documentation can demonstrate nurses' value and impact on improving patient/population outcomes, patient safety, operational efficiency and clinical effectiveness; nurses and employers need a mechanism to track nursing licensure across job and location changes; institutions need the ability to verify licensure status for their nurse employees. (UMN, 2018, p. 21)

Being able to track providers to patient outcomes would be beneficial overall to health systems, cost-effectiveness, and tracking of nurses' collective and individual contribution to outcomes (Sensmeier et al., 2019). A unique nurse identifier could also benefit research aimed at measuring and quantifying nursing care and inform future education and training for nurses (Sensmeier et al., 2019).

Measurement of health disparity indicators has been recommended as part of quality of care (IOM, 2015). Performance measures can illuminate existing gaps in access and disparities while assessing the effectiveness of interventions (NQF, 2017). The National Quality Forum (NQF) (2019) recommends creating measures that align SDOH measurement and activities across health care and clinical and community-based settings. Short- and long-term goals would build on these measures and aim to have half (50 percent) of health systems using aligned screening data with measurable SDOH improvements (NQF, 2020). Clinical performance metrics could be used to identify and track disparities by stratifying such risk factors as race, ethnicity, and measures of SES. It is critical for payers to reward reductions in health disparities in clinical and population health performance measures, improvements in measures for at-risk populations, and attainment of absolute target levels of high-quality performance.

Performance metrics that incorporate disparity-sensitive measures are key for assessing interventions. For example, metrics for care coordination and team-based care could incentivize investment in nurse-led care management programs that can reduce health disparities. Chronic diseases and ambulatory care–sensitive conditions—including asthma, diabetes, heart failure, hypertension, and depression—that are prevalent in POC and underserved populations and display disparities in outcomes compared with more advantaged populations often are well suited to nurse care management/team-based care programs (Davis et al., 2007; Lasater et al., 2016; Mose and Jones, 2018; Peek et al., 2007). Another disparity-sensitive measure relevant to nursing interventions is prevention of hospital admissions and readmissions for ambulatory care–sensitive conditions. Some transitional care models (TCMs) with an APRN leader have been found to reduce hospital admissions, and studies have found lower rates of hospital readmissions and avoidable hospitalizations among Medicare and Medicaid beneficiaries in states where NPs have full practice authority (Naylor, 2012; Oliver et al., 2014). For example, the Vermont Transitional Care Nurse program, led by nurses, is an established best practice (Fels et al., 2015). In this program, to support high-risk patients transferring from the hospital, an APRN designs and coordinates care with patients, their families and caregivers, physicians, and other health care professionals (Hirschman et al., 2015).

Measures of population health could reflect the impact of addressing SDOH. For example, the NQF recommended in 2019 that stakeholders such as public and private payers, social services providers, health care organizations, and community-based organizations improve the collection of data on SDOH in their community. The data collected should include key measures that prioritize local communities' needs, and are then used to create clinical and community outcome measures (NQF, 2012, 2019). In a 2019 report, the National Advisory Council on Nurse Education and Practice (NACNEP) strongly supported value-based care through funding measures or initiatives that develop nurse competencies (NACNEP, 2019); incentivize nurse care management and team-based care; and include population health measures, measures of the extent to which SDOH are identified and addressed, and measures to reward reductions in health disparities (NASEM, 2020b).

Alternative Payment Models

APMs are predominantly non-FFS models designed to promote value and cost-efficiency. APMs frequently incorporate VBP principles, such as taking on "substantial financial risk to deliver high quality care at lower cost" (Werner et al., 2021), and in practice many still use FFS models to distribute payment. APMs could provide effective mechanisms and incentives to fund nursing for addressing SDOH and advancing health equity (DeMeester et al., 2017). For example, various forms of capitated payment and global budgeting could provide up-front funding to support these key nursing roles and functions, as could payment systems that provide per member per month payments to health care organizations. The value argument for cost-efficiency of APMs and investments in nursing is that many of these nursing interventions prevent clinical deterioration and costly emergency department visits, inpatient care, and procedures.

APMs provide special opportunities and flexibility not present with FFS to reward high-value nursing activities. These payment mechanisms could support nurses in their SDOH-related work, such as increased home visits, health education, and care coordination ranging from prevention to chronic care and palliative care (Dahlin and Coyne, 2019).

Accountable Care Organizations

Some APMs are shared savings programs in which payers and health care organizations share any cost savings. An example of an APM that could incentivize value and cost-efficiency in care is accountable care organizations (ACOs) (Albright et al., 2016), many of which have rapidly expanded their use of NPs (Nyweide et al., 2020). ACOs are responsible for the health and costs of a predetermined population of patients. They frequently work with a fixed budget and often are required to meet clinical performance metrics to share with the payer in any cost savings. One of the earliest promising examples of ACOs' potential role in supporting nurses in addressing SDOH and advancing health equity comes from the state Medicaid programs in Oregon (see the description of the C-TRAIN transitional care model earlier in this chapter). ACOs are required to meet standard quality measures established by CMS (2019b), which are adjusted for high-risk beneficiaries (AMA, 2019a; CMS, 2019b). Overall, the Medicare Shared Savings Program has demonstrated cost savings with physician-group ACOs compared with hospital-integrated ACOs, which have not (McWilliams et al., 2018), along with high-average composite quality scores (Gonzalez-Smith et al., 2019).

Accountable Health Communities

Accountable health communities (AHCs), also known as accountable communities for health, accountable care communities, or community health innovation regions, are coalitions of partners from "health, social service, and other sectors working together to improve population health and clinical-community linkages within a geographic area" (Spencer and Freda, 2016, p. 2). AHC implementation requires a bridge organization that can operate as a hub to coordinate efforts across partners, conduct screenings, and make referrals to address health-related social needs for Medicare and Medicaid beneficiaries (CMS, 2019b).

Minnesota, considered one of CMS's pioneer states, created 15 AHCs—8 in urban areas, 6 in rural areas, and 1 with a presence in both urban and rural areas (Au-Yeung and Warell, 2018; Spencer and Freda, 2016). The AHCs in Minnesota use nurses in community care coordination and team-based care roles. At Morrison County Community-Based Care Coordination, a team consisting of a social worker, nurse, and doctor assists aging and other adults with mitigating overuse of prescription narcotics (Au-Yeung and Worrall, 2018). And another AHC used community health workers and medical assistants for less complex patients and tasks and employed RNs to care for more severe cases (Au-Yeung and Worrall, 2018). Nurses are present in community and health system settings, and their inclusion on these teams can potentially streamline complex cases from treatment to follow-up to referrals.

Medicare Advantage

Medicare Advantage plans, in which the federal government pays private insurance companies a fixed monthly amount to care for beneficiaries, have been available since 2000. These plans feature increased flexibility that allows funding to go beyond traditional Part A and B services to support such nonmedical benefits as transportation and home improvements for chronically ill beneficiaries, healthy meals, and other services (Green and Zook, 2019). Flexible funding allows health care organizations to adapt services that address SDOH and advance health equity to suit local contexts and beneficiaries (Thomas et al., 2019).

Program of All-Inclusive Care for the Elderly

Program of All-Inclusive Care for the Elderly (PACE), another alternative model, benefits elderly people who are dually eligible for Medicare and Medicaid, require long-term support services, and are eligible for nursing facility–based care. Medicare and Medicaid give providers capitation payments for enrollees.[10] Interdisciplinary teams, which often include a nurse, provide such comprehensive services (CMS, 2020b) as diet and nutrition counseling, social services, transportation, physical therapy, and personal care attendants (CMS, n.d.b; NPA, n.d.).

Health Insurance Contracting Requirements

Payers such as Medicare and Medicaid can incorporate incentives to address SDOH in their contracting requirements with insurance companies. For example, the Medical Loss Ratio provision of the Patient Protection and Affordable Care Act (ACA) requires most health insurance companies that cover individuals and small businesses to spend at least 80 percent of premiums on health care claims and quality improvement rather than on administration, marketing, and profit (KFF, 2012). Subsequent clarification of the regulations allows investments addressing SDOH to count toward required medical loss ratio spending (Machledt, 2017). A March 2020 review of 404 studies showed that Medicaid expansion under the ACA improved access to care, financial security, some health outcomes, and economic benefits to states (Guth et al., 2020). For example, Medicaid expansion was associated with lower rates of maternal and infant mortality (Searing and Ross, 2019). Thus, APMs can enable payers to incentivize addressing SDOH and support nursing infrastructure to this end.

SUPPORTING SCHOOL AND PUBLIC HEALTH NURSES TO ADDRESS SOCIAL DETERMINANTS OF HEALTH AND ADVANCE HEALTH EQUITY

School and public health nurses play crucial roles in improving the health of school-age children and their families, as well as the health of community members who are more likely to receive preventive care or treatment through community resources (APHN, 2016; Bogaert et al., 2020; NACCHO, 2020; NASN, 2016). These nurses provide direct care and advocacy, make referrals to partner organizations, and connect with nonhealth sectors related to the well-being of children and others. They regularly address individuals' social needs, promote health, and work to prevent illness. Therefore, school and public health nurses can reduce the demand for downstream treatment of individuals in costly health care

---

[10] See https://www.cms.gov/Medicare-Medicaid-Coordination/Medicare-and-Medicaid-Coordination/Medicare-Medicaid-Coordination-Office/FinancialAlignmentInitiative/CapitatedModel (accessed July 23, 2021).

delivery systems. The nursing workforce is a crucial component of Public Health 3.0,[11] providing health care and supporting the community (DeSalvo et al., 2017).

Some of the highest-value health and societal outcomes derive from the care received by children when they are very young. School and public health nurses are therefore valuable resources for addressing population health and health equity; however, they are underfunded (IOM, 2011; Sessions, 2012). In the United States, each locality has control over school and public health funds, and structural inequities exacerbate underfunding in many low-income and marginalized communities (Beitsch et al., 2015). Some states require school nurses, while others leave those decisions to local school districts, which are often faced with very limited funding. Those communities with the most complex health issues and social risks often cope with especially severe underfunding of often limited public health services (Welker-Hood, 2014).

Frequently, existing funding streams are insufficient to support school, public health department, and other community-based health efforts, the impact of which has been exacerbated by the COVID-19 pandemic. Indeed public health departments operate differently within each community and state (Beitsch et al., 2015). Thus, there exists a need to apportion more government general funds for these services or identify other dedicated revenue streams (Sessions, 2012). In the present context, creating consistent funding streams that support the health of children and communities by capitalizing on the expertise of school and public health nurses can be a key component of achieving health equity.

School Nurses

As described in Chapter 4, the average school nurse works simultaneously in three schools and is responsible for caring for diverse students with complex medical, health, and social needs (Willgerodt et al., 2018). The American Academy of Pediatrics (AAP), the American Nurses Association (ANA), and the National Association of School Nurses (NASN) recommend that all students have full access to a school nurse who can coordinate care, provide health education, administer medications, direct care, and help meet community and public health needs (ANA, 2007; Council on School Health, 2016; NASN, 2016). A cost/benefit study of the Massachusetts Essential School Health Services (ESHS) program found a net benefit of nurse health services. The study compared program costs, including the cost of nurse staffing and supplies, with program benefits, measured by savings related to avoided medical procedures, loss of teacher or instructor productivity, and parents' loss of productivity (Wang et al., 2014). The study ultimately found that each dollar invested in ESHS programs would yield $2.20 in savings per student.

[11] Public Health 3.0 refers to public health practices that include cross-sector collaboration and extends beyond traditional public departments (DeSalvo et al., 2017).

However, about 25 percent of schools do not employ a school nurse, and about 35 percent employ one only part-time (Willgerodt et al., 2018). On average, schools with more students who qualify for free or reduced-price lunches have less access to a school nurse (NCES, n.d.). The lack of school nurses in schools that serve disadvantaged communities reflects the larger association between school funding and school resources that adversely affects children from low-income families (Jackson et al., 2016). According to a 2015 NASN survey, moreover, the availability of school nurses varies greatly by region: the survey found that western states had the highest percentage of schools without a school nurse (Mangena and Maughan, 2015).

Additionally, there are inconsistencies in how school nurses are paid and in general oversight. School nursing remains underfunded as school district budgetary constraints force administrators to decide annually which resources to pare down or keep (Leachman et al., 2017). The NASN survey found that 85 percent of responding school nurses worked for public school districts; 90 percent of these respondents indicated that most of their funding came from public education department funds and the rest from special education funds (Mangena and Maughan, 2015). Outside of educational funding, public health departments and private or nonprofit hospitals are the major funders of school nurses (Becker and Maughan, 2017). In Massachusetts, for example, the ESHS program has been supported by the Department of Public Health since 1993 to support and fund nurse-managed health services and school-based health centers (Massachusetts Department of Health, 2012).

About 45 million children are enrolled in Medicaid. Since December 2014, federal law has allowed school nurses to bill Medicaid for services to beneficiaries (CMS, 2014), but only a handful of states have taken advantage of this opportunity (Ollove, 2019). Currently, only seven states allow students to receive free care under Medicaid (Ollove, 2019). In the NASN survey of school nurses, 57.6 percent of respondents affirmed that they or their employers billed Medicaid for reimbursement, but two-thirds did not know how the reimbursements were used (Mangena and Maughan, 2015). In a 2018 survey of school superintendents, 70 percent of respondents indicated that any revenue generated through Medicaid billing went toward salaries for health professionals. However, the administrative burden of billing poses a significant challenge for schools; the schools not taking advantage of Medicaid funding tend to be located in small rural school districts (AASA, 2019). Given the familiarity of rural hospitals with Medicaid billing, these institutions could explore partnering with their local small rural school districts to develop billing infrastructure.

Schools may need to take advantage of multiple funding sources to support robust school health programs and school nurses. For example, Grand Rapids Public Schools in Michigan partnered with Spectrum Health to improve student health outcomes and used for that purpose funds from the school district budget, Spectrum Health, the local intermediate school district, and the state department of education (Spectrum Health, n.d.; TFAH, n.d.). Grand Rapids Public Schools uses a model whereby 34 RNs direct licensed practical nurses (LPNs), health aides, and other health professionals in conducting health screenings and follow-up, administering immunizations, and connecting students to outside medical care through referrals (TFAH, n.d.).

More intensive work can be done in school settings to bridge social and health services and more broadly engage SDOH in communities. Nurses in the lowest salaried positions tend to be those working in community settings, and in contrast with Medicare and Medicaid, these are settings where funding streams are often tied to the local tax base and grant funding.

Public Health Nurses

Public health nurses address social issues through policy development, planning, and advocacy, as well as community involvement (APHA, 2013). As noted in Chapter 3, in the 2018 National Sample Survey of Registered Nurses, 1.7 percent of all responding RNs (n = 47,060) reported providing public/community health care. Public health nurses are funded by federal, state, and local public health budgets, as well as grants for specific programs. Current public health funding is complex, with sources including the federal government; all 50 states and Washington, DC; and several thousand local municipalities (IOM, 2012). Public health funding is discretionary spending that is often subject to reductions (TFAH, 2018a). Federal public health funding is a combination of funds from the Centers for Disease Control and Prevention (CDC), HHS, and the U.S. Department of Agriculture (USDA). Most federal funds flow through CDC, which saw a 10 percent decline in public health funding between 2010 and 2019, after adjusting for inflation (TFAH, 2019). State-level funding for public health has decreased over the past few years as well, with only 19 states and Washington, DC, maintaining their budgets. At the local level, the 2008 recession led to more than 55,000 staff positions being lost in local health departments as a result of layoffs or attrition, with most cuts not being restored (TFAH, 2018a). One of every five local health departments reported decreases in its public health budget during fiscal year 2017.

In the face of these reductions, the Public Health Leadership Forum estimates that "there is a $4.5 billion gap between current funding and what is needed to build a strong public health infrastructure nationwide" (DeSalvo et al., 2018; TFAH, 2019, p. 18). As of 2017, public health spending accounted for only 2.5 percent of health-related spending (about $274 per capita) (TFAH, 2019). In a survey of 377 state and local health departments, most public health nurses reported finding strengths in their departments. However, they also cited "barriers, such as a lack of promotion opportunities for RNs, job insecurity, lack of budget to hire vacant RN positions, and inability to offer a competitive salary to RNs" (Beck and Boulton, 2016, p. 149).

Sustaining public health infrastructure with continuous funding that supports the work of public health nurses is essential for healthy communities, particularly for communities of color and those of lower SES. By some estimates, moreover, the return on investment for public health dollars may be as high as 14 to 1 (TFAH, 2019).

ROLE OF THE HEALTH AND SOCIAL SECTORS IN SUPPORTING NURSES TO ADDRESS SOCIAL DETERMINANTS OF HEALTH AND ADVANCE HEALTH EQUITY

Historically, the health and social sectors (e.g., housing, transportation, food insecurity, employment, education, criminal justice) have had siloed funding streams and accountability metrics for judging and financially rewarding organizations. Policy makers, health care administrators, clinicians, social-sector leaders, and communities are increasingly recognizing the importance of coordinating the health and social sectors to address SDOH and advance health equity. Yet, efforts to increase communication, collaboration, and synergies between the two sectors raise difficult issues in such areas as governance (e.g., Who should be at the table? Who is in charge? Who has the power?). In addition, it has been challenging to devise suitable joint accountability metrics with which to align and reward desirable behaviors, and in the present context, to organize funding that supports nurses in addressing SDOH and advancing health equity.

Braiding and Blending Funding

Braiding and blending are two funding mechanisms that can support community interventions and services (TFAH, 2018b). Braiding coordinates two or more funding streams while imposing restrictions and regulations on the use of those funds. Activities and data, including expenses and performance measures, can be tracked and attributed to the original source of funding. Blending pools two or more funding sources into one funding stream and allows for more flexibility in the use of the funds because of fewer restrictions and regulations (Cabello, 2018). Through these mechanisms, the conjoined efforts of the health and nonmedical social sectors can support nurses working across settings and domains—community-based organizations, public health, education, health systems, and others (Clary and Riley, 2016).

Early Head Start, Head Start, and other child development programs are examples of such combined funding strategies that address community needs across public, private nonprofit, community-based, and faith-based organizations (OHS, 2020; Wallen and Hubbard, 2013). In a similar way, braiding and blending funding from the health and social sectors can support local public health departments in prioritizing health equity. The Bridging for Health Blueprint report from the Georgia Health Policy Center (2019) assesses a series of case studies to determine the kind of technical assistance local health departments and communities would need to sustain funding for health programs. A common characteristic identified in the case studies is pooling of community wellness funds, and a requirement for up-front capital and braiding and blending of funding from many sources.

In Rhode Island, a Health Equity Zone (HEZ) initiative was launched to capitalize on place-based community efforts to address local health needs (RIDOH, 2018) using braided funds from local, state, and federal sources. Eleven HEZ zones were established statewide, each focused on local priority issues and services, including providing psychological first aid, screening patients for depression and identifying patients at risk of suicide, developing safer roadways, banning smoking and vaping in town parks to ensure smoke-free areas, improving vacant or abandoned properties and addressing housing as a social determinant, building community linkages through the use of community health workers, and creating a community drop-in clinic for adults with substance abuse disorders (RIDOH, 2018). The initiative creates opportunities for people already living and working in their communities to improve health care access and health equity. Nurses can play critical roles in such community programs that braid funds to improve health equity (e.g., working at the front line to screen people in health care settings or schools, or serving as health care representatives to support housing policy).

Louisiana developed the Louisiana Permanent Supportive Housing (PSH) program following the devastation and destruction of Hurricane Katrina, which exacerbated the difficult circumstances of people already living with complex physical and behavioral health conditions. The PSH program recognizes stable and safe housing as an essential need that can support people's health. This cross-agency partnership between Medicaid and the state housing authority braided funding sources from disaster recovery funds, housing assistance programs such as Section 811, Medicaid, and SAMHSA. Nearly half of all beneficiaries were homeless before participating in the program (Clary and Kartika, 2017). Housing providers focused on housing needs, while Medicaid-enrolled clinicians provided health care to the tenants. Although roles and responsibilities of nurses are not called out as part of the PSH program, opportunities exist for nurses to provide transitional care that complements the social services people need, such as housing.

Pay-for-Success/Social Impact Bonds

Pay-for-success (PFS) models, sometimes referred to as social impact bonds (Galloway, 2014), allow private investors, rather than traditional investors such as government, to provide up-front capital for scaling social interventions that benefit the public sector—specifically, an underserved population (Iovan et al., 2018; Urban Institute, n.d.). PFS models have been used in such interventions as job training, criminal justice reform, reentry for formerly incarcerated people, and early education (Golden, 2014; NFF, n.d.). Interventions are considered successful when predetermined outcomes have been achieved, and investors are then repaid (Urban Institute, n.d.).

Iovan and colleagues (2018) evaluated more than 80 PFS interventions, several of which addressed multiple determinants of health and focused mainly on downstream and midstream factors. Most interventions were initially supported by a combination of public and private investors, and were implemented at the federal or the state or provincial level. In the United States, 11 interventions analyzed by Lantz and colleagues (2016) involved more than one investor, and several included banks and private foundations or philanthropic organizations.

One pay-for-success example is the Nurse-Family Partnership (NFP) in South Carolina. The NFP is a national public health intervention that allows nurses to build relationships with new mothers. The program has resulted in improved behavior and improved performance in school among young children (Karoly et al., 2005; Kitzman et al., 2019) and improved educational attainment and employment among mothers (Flowers et al., 2020), and has demonstrated cost-effectiveness (Dawley et al., 2007). The NFP focuses on first-time low-income mothers in 29 of the 46 state counties. Investors included BlueCross BlueShield of South Carolina Foundation, the Duke Endowment and other private funders, and the South Carolina Department of Health and Human Services (Urban Institute, 2016). Partnered with Social Finance, the focus on the NFP in South Carolina are outcomes that will yield payments include reducing preterm births, reducing child hospitalization, increasing birth spacing, and targeting first-time mothers in zip codes with high levels of poverty (SCDHHS, 2016).

WORKFORCE AND EDUCATION

Reforms in workforce development (see Chapter 3) and education (see Chapter 10) are required to support the nursing profession in markedly expanding and strengthening roles and functions needed to address SDOH and advance health equity. Achieving those reforms will require financial investment to incentivize and support nursing education programs responsible for educating nurses to make the necessary changes.

Diversifying the Nurse Workforce

As discussed in Chapter 3, a diverse workforce helps reduce health disparities. Nurses from diverse racial, ethnic, and socioeconomic backgrounds are more likely to work with diverse, underserved communities and provide culturally tailored care (IOM, 2004). This includes financial support to diversify the workforce and create opportunities for students who otherwise would not have the resources to fund their education.

Income share agreements (ISAs), a type of pay-for-success program, provide tuition assistance for the education and training of nurses to help diversify the workforce. ISAs are especially useful for low-income nursing students. For many individuals, the nursing workforce pipeline often begins in community colleges and in associate's degree in nursing (ADN) or LPN programs. Community colleges are frequently more affordable than 4-year public institutions[12] and serve a higher percentage of non-White students (Mann Levesque, 2018; NCES, 2020). However, students with large financial burdens often have difficulty bridging the gap between ADN or LPN programs and bachelor of science in nursing (BSN) education (NASEM, 2016). With ISAs, up-front costs of tuition are covered by private funders, and trainees are responsible for paying back the cost of their tuition based on their income. ISAs are predicated on students obtaining good jobs; when their income meets a minimum threshold, they begin paying back a fixed amount for a fixed term or until they reach a repayment cap (Social Finance, 2020).

Career impact bonds (CIBs) are a type of ISA specific to education investment that covers program costs and connects repayment to outcomes. As with ISAs, students are responsible for repayment only when they gain employment, at which point they begin repaying over a fixed duration or until they reach a repayment cap (Social Finance, 2020). Both ISAs and CIBs include such wraparound services as counseling and transportation subsidies.

Educating the Nursing Workforce About Social Determinants of Health and Health Equity

As noted in Chapter 10, RNs in public or community health or school health surveyed in the 2018 National Sample Survey of Registered Nurses said their performance in their roles would have benefited from more training in SDOH. For example, in addition to training in effective communication, shared decision making, and cultural humility when working with diverse populations (Foronda, 2020), nurses need training in screening for social risk factors, partnering with community-based organizations to address social needs, providing trauma-informed care, and understanding the underlying structural drivers of such inequities as structural racism and social privilege (Peek et al., 2020). Structural racism, for instance, is a reflection of the fact that inequities do not occur by chance but because of concrete decisions by government and private industry, as in the case of segregation of African Americans from Whites in housing, which resulted from zoning laws, the concentration of public housing, discrimination in mortgage loan practices, and preferential steering of clients to specific neighborhoods by real

---

[12] There was a higher percentage of non-White students enrolled at public 2-year institutions (52 percent) than at 4-year public institutions (45 percent) in 2018 (https://nces.ed.gov/programs/coe/indicator_csb.asp [accessed June 3, 2021]).

estate agents (Rothstein, 2017). As discussed in Chapter 7, the ability of nurses to understand and address this history and its complex legacy will depend on faculty development, academic–practice partnerships, and other investments to create a quality education that includes a substantive, sustained focus on issues of SDOH and health equity.

Federal Government Programs

For many decades, federal government agencies, including HHS, the Veterans Health Administration (VHA), and the U.S. Department of Defense have supported general graduate medical education (GME), and in recent years, CMS has provided modest support for graduate nurse education (GNE). The VHA has a transition-to-practice nurse residency program for all new nurses entering their first nursing role, including new graduates of ADN, BSN, and entry-level master's degree programs (VA, 2019). While the vast majority of HHS funding goes to physician medical training, HHS supports APRNs through a number of programs, including Advanced Nursing Education Residency, Nurse Faculty Loan, Advanced Nursing Education Workforce, and Nursing Workforce Diversity (GAO, 2019). The ACA supported a pilot program that funded residency training for APRNs, and CMS funded an evaluation of this program, but funding for this initiative was not continued. Additionally, training for nurses is hindered by a lack of preceptors and limited clinical placement sites that still persists (Copeland, 2020).

The 2016 National Academies report (NASEM, 2016) assessing progress toward the actions recommended in the 2011 *The Future of Nursing* report (IOM, 2011) does note an increase in diversity among younger nurses, a trend expected to continue into the current decade (NASEM, 2016) (see Chapter 3). Public and private payers can support diversification of the nursing workforce through focused recruitment and thoughtful hiring practices. The nursing pipeline can also be diversified through increased funding for educating nurses in SDOH and SDOH research, especially among nurse scientists from and with personal connections to underserved communities, and expanding nurses' roles in advancing health equity (BCBSIL, 2019; FNU, 2017; HHS, 2011; Jackson and Garcia, 2014; NQF, 2017). Training programs within HRSA could be adapted to further incentivize diversification of the nursing workforce and improve training in addressing SDOH and advancing health equity (Strickland et al., 2014). HRSA provides grants to fund multiple health professional programs, six of which are focused on nurses. One grant specifically targets diversifying the nurse pipeline and workforce, while others target professional development. Between 2015 and 2019, HRSA provided more than 180 grants focused on nursing diversity (HRSA, 2020).

HRSA administers and oversees the Nurse Corps Loan Repayment Program (LRP) and Scholarship Program (SP), which provide an incentive for nurses to work and serve in HPSAs. For the LRP, participants commit 2 service years to repay 60 percent of the outstanding principal and interest on their nursing education loans, with an additional 25 percent repayment for participants who work for a third year (HRSA, 2018a). However, the LRP and SP programs face challenges, such as a limited number of award recipients and low representation for some groups (HRSA, 2018a). In 2018, the number of applications for the LRP and SP programs was 7 times higher than the number of awards (7,833 applications versus 1,042 awards to residents of 49 states and the District of Columbia). In addition, only 7 American Indian/Alaska Native nurses, 40 Asian nurses, and 183 Black/African American nurses received LRP and SP awards, compared with 698 White nurses (HRSA, 2018a). Therefore, investing in similar programs is important for increasing the number of nurses with the proper education and training to provide care for underserved populations in critical shortage areas, including rural areas, and for people who need access to substance abuse disorder treatment (HRSA, 2018b).

The Indian Health Service (IHS) has resources that could potentially increase the diversity of the nursing workforce and the numbers of nurses working in rural areas, including Civil Service (IHS, n.d.), a 2-year post with the Commissioned Corps of the U.S. Public Health Service within IHS, and Direct Tribal Hire (IHS, n.d.). There are also programs that can award up to $20,000 per year toward health education loans, including the IHS Loan Repayment Program and Supplemental Loan Repayment Program, which can provide an incentive to enroll in nursing programs and complete nursing degrees.

One of the major factors limiting enrollment in advanced practice programs is the lack of preceptors, which is related to the paucity of federal funding for advanced nursing education relative to medical education. The GNE demonstration[13] project authorized CMS to fund five hospitals to partner with clinical education sites, schools of nursing, and community-based care settings (CCSs), such as FQHCs and rural health clinics, with the goal of expanding clinical education for APRN students (Hesgrove et al., 2019; HHS, 2018). CMS made reimbursements to the five GNE sites annually for 3 years between 2012 and 2015. Each site, including hospitals, schools of nursing, and CCSs, was designated as a "network" and used the funding in various ways, including hiring clinical placement coordinators; creating or supporting administrative databases to oversee the clinical placement process; and implementing innovative education

[13] The Center for Medicare & Medicaid Innovation (CMMI) is responsible for developing and evaluating new payment models in health care and new service delivery models with the aim of lowering costs, improving the quality of patient care, and aligning systems with patient-centered practice (CMS, n.d.a). The five hospitals chosen for the GNE demonstration were the Hospital of the University of Pennsylvania in Philadelphia, Pennsylvania; the Scottsdale Healthcare Medical Center in Scottsdale, Arizona; the Duke University Hospital in Durham, North Carolina; the Rush University Medical Center in Chicago, Illinois; and the Memorial Hermann-Texas Medical Center Hospital in Houston, Texas (CMS, 2012).

models, such as interprofessional education, which allowed the APRN students to work alongside pharmacy, medical, and psychology students. Interprofessional education, recommended in the 2011 *The Future of Nursing* report (IOM, 2011) and reviewed in the 2016 report assessing progress toward the 2011 report's recommendations (NASEM, 2016), improves medical students' perceptions of nurses, team-based care, self-efficacy, and patient-centered care (Butterworth et al., 2018; Homeyer et al., 2018; Nash et al., 2018). The GNE demonstration project strengthened relations between hospitals and schools of nursing, increased APRN student enrollment and graduation (HHS, 2018), increased clinical education hours for APRN students, and ensured that at least half of those hours were in CCS. The project gave APRN students holistic experiences in engaging in team collaboration and addressing SDOH.

Despite these successful outcomes, however, many networks described the challenge of sustaining the GNE activities without funding in the post-demonstration years. Finite financial support for nursing education can stimulate APRN student growth for only a limited time. Sustainable funding would benefit future APRN trainees and CCS. Spending on overall GME from public organizations and private funders amounted to about $15 billion annually between 2011 and 2013 (IOM, 2014); in contrast, the GNE demonstration allocated only $50 million per year from a single funder, CMS. Funding for GNE is crucial in building the APRN pipeline for HPSAs both as providers and alongside physicians in teams.

CONCLUSIONS

Improving the health of the nation's diverse population needs to be the primary goal of health care and its payment systems. Thus, payment systems need to be intentionally designed to support key nursing roles, including care management and team-based care, expanded scope of practice, community nursing, and telehealth, as well as diversification of the workforce and improved training in addressing SDOH and advancing health equity. Private insurers, governmental payers, policy makers, hospitals, health organizations, and social services agencies can incorporate health care and health equity into their fundamental goals and missions to help give all Americans the opportunity to attain better health and well-being. These important stakeholders can advance those vital goals by incorporating strategies that further leverage nursing, a powerful component of the health care workforce with expertise and presence across inpatient and community settings.

Nurses are critical to whole-person care. However, nurses cannot be utilized in new and developing roles if not supported by the health infrastructure at large. By supporting team-based care, improved communication, and proven interventions and strategies that can reduce health disparities (Chin et al., 2012; NASEM, 2016b), payment systems can enable nurses to make these essential contributions to improving care and outcomes for all individuals.

New payment models, such as ACOs, AHCs, and VBP strategies, can give health care organizations the flexibility to pursue these goals. For example, pay-for-performance strategies can reward successful efforts to address SDOH that impact population health, while capitation payments can support nurses who work with patients at social risk. Specific activities of nurses to address SDOH might include, for example, identification of social risks through routine screening; referral of individuals at social risk to community supports and services; regular communication and follow-up with individuals regarding their health; monitoring of individuals' adherence to treatment; facilitation and coordination among providers, patients, and support services; and education and advocacy directed at public policy makers from the community to the national level with respect to addressing social needs and SDOH. It is essential for nurses to help shape and use opportunities created by new payment models to sustain and replicate models of care that support them in addressing SDOH and advancing health equity.

The 2016 National Academies report (NASEM, 2016) assessing progress toward the recommendations in the 2011 *The Future of Nursing* report (IOM, 2011) includes the recommendation to "promote the involvement of nurses in the redesign of care delivery and payment systems." Nurses are strongly encouraged to collaborate with the public and private sectors to improve the health care delivery system. Other partners identified as facilitating redesign include retail clinics, insurance companies, professional groups and associations, and local government agencies. The present report strongly supports the recommendation that nurses participate in the redesign of care delivery and payment systems, particularly as they take on new functions and roles in health care and health equity.

> ***Conclusion 6-1: To enable nurses to more fully address social needs and social determinants of health, improve population health, and advance health equity, current payment structures and mechanisms need to be revised and strengthened and new payment models intentionally designed to serve those goals. The current health care system does not value addressing social determinants of health.***

School and public health nurses are valuable segments of the nursing workforce with great potential to help improve population health and health equity by intervening at early ages, focusing on prevention, and connecting with the community to understand and address social needs and SDOH. As content experts, schools and public health nurses are also valuable resources that can benefit nurses and other health care providers in other settings. *Yet, those nurses are inadequately supported by current funding mechanisms.*

> ***Conclusion 6-2: Underfunding limits the ability of school and public health nurses to extend health care services and create a bridge between health care and community health. Adequate funding would***

enable these nurses to expand their reach and help improve population health and health equity.

In addition, workforce and education policies greatly impact nurses' roles and capabilities.

Conclusion 6-3: Payment mechanisms need to be designed to support the nursing workforce and nursing education in addressing social needs and social determinants of health in order to improve population health and advance health equity.

The United States spends a very large and growing amount of money on health care (CMS, 2020c), and these funds pay for very few services addressing social factors that negatively affect health and well-being, and do little to improve health equity so that everyone can have a fairer and better chance of living a healthier life. Until current payment systems include payment for services to address upstream social needs and SDOH that negatively affect health, the nation will continue to spend more on costly health care, depleting resources available for other important social, economic, and environmental programs (Butler, 2020; Horwitz et al., 2020; Squires and Anderson, 2015).

Changing the way the nation pays for health care will cause discomfort among some, but will also stimulate those who seek innovative ways of maximizing the population's health.

REFERENCES

AASA (American Association of School Administrators). 2019. *Structural inefficiencies in the school-based Medicaid program disadvantage small and rural districts and students.* https://www.aasa.org/uploadedFiles/Policy_and_Advocacy/Resources/AASA_Medicaid_Report_FINAL.pdf (accessed April 6, 2021).

Albright, B. B., V. A. Lewis, J. S. Ross, and C. H. Colla. 2016. Preventive care quality of Medicare accountable care organizations: Associations of organizational characteristics with performance. *Medical Care* 54(3):326–335. doi: 10.1097/MLR.0000000000000477.

Alexander, D., and M. Schnell. 2019. Just what the nurse practitioner ordered: Independent prescriptive authority and population mental health. *Journal of Health Economics* 66:145–162.

AMA (American Medical Association). 2019a. *Summary of the 2018 accountable care organization (ACO) final rule*. https://www.ama-assn.org/system/files/2019-03/summary-2018-aco-final-rule.pdf (accessed April 6, 2021).

AMA. 2019b. *CPT® purpose & mission*. CPT Editorial Panel. https://www.ama-assn.org/about/cpt-editorial-panel/cpt-purpose-mission (accessed April 6, 2021).

AMA. 2019c. *RVS update committee (RUC)*. https://www.ama-assn.org/about/rvs-update-committee-ruc/rvs-update-committee-ruc (accessed April 6, 2021).

ANA (American Nurses Association). 2007. *ANA position statement: Assuring safe, high quality health care in pre-K through 12 educational settings*. https://www.nursingworld.org/practice-policy/nursing-excellence/official-position-statements/id/assuring-safe-high-quality-health-care (accessed April 6, 2021).

ANA. 2017. *Medicare payment for registered nurse services and care coordination*. Silver Spring, MD: American Nurses Association. https://www.nursingworld.org/~4983ef/globalassets/practiceandpolicy/health-policy/final_executivesummary_carecoordination.pdf (accessed April 6, 2021).

Anderson, A. C., E. O'Rourke, M. H. Chin, N. A. Ponce, S. M. Bernheim, and H. Burstin. 2018. Promoting health equity and eliminating disparities through performance measurement and payment. *Health Affairs* 37(3):371–377. doi: 10.1377/hlthaff.2017.1301.

Andrilla, C. H. A., T. Moore, D. Patterson, and E. Larson. 2019. Geographic distribution of providers with a DEA waiver to prescribe buprenorphine for the treatment of opioid use disorder: A 5-year update. *Journal of Rural Health* 35(1):108–112. doi: 10.1111/jrh.12307.

Andrilla, C. H. A., D. G. Patterson, T. E. Moore, C. Coulthard, and E. H. Larson. 2020. Projected contributions of nurse practitioners and physicians assistant to buprenorphine treatment services for opioid use disorder in rural areas. *Medical Care Research and Review* 77(2):208–216.

APHA (American Public Health Association). 2013. *The definition and practice of public health nursing*: A statement of the public health nursing section. Washington, DC: American Public Health Association. https://www.apha.org/-/media/files/pdf/membergroups/phn/nursingdefinition.ashx?la=en&hash=331DBEC4B79E0C0B8C644BF2BEA571249F8717A0 (accessed April 6, 2021).

APHN (Association of Public Health Nurses). 2016. *The public health nurse: Necessary partner for the future of healthy communities*. A position paper of the Association of Public Health Nurses. https://www.phnurse.org/assets/APHN-PHN%20Value-Position%20Paper%205%2030%20 2016.pdf (accessed April 6, 2021).

Ash, A. S., E. O. Mick, R. P. Ellis, C. I. Kiefe, J. J. Allison, and M. A. Clark. 2017. Social determinants of health in managed care payment formulas. *JAMA Internal Medicine* 177(10):1424–1430.

Au-Yeung, C., and C. Warell. 2018. *Minnesota's accountable communities for health: Context and core components*. State Health Access Data Assistance Center (SHADAC). https://www.shadac.org/sites/default/files/publications/MNSIM_ACH_brief_MARCH%20FINAL%20 FOR%20WEB.pdf (accessed April 6, 2021).

Auerbach, D. I., D. Staiger, and P. Buerhaus. 2018. Growing ranks of advanced practice clinicians—Implications for the physician workforce. *New England Journal of Medicine* 378(25):2358–2360. doi: 10.1056/NEJMp1801869.

Barnes, H., M. Richards, M. McHugh, and G. Martsolf. 2018. Rural And nonrural primary care physician practices increasingly rely on nurse practitioners. *Health Affairs* 37(6):908–914.

Barnett, M. L., D. Lee, and R. Frank. 2019. In rural areas, buprenorphine waiver adoption since 2017 driven by nurse practitioners and physician assistants. *Health Affairs (Millwood)* 38(12):2048–2056.

BCBSIL (Blue Cross and Blue Shield of Illinois). 2019. *AHA Institute for Diversity and Health Equity and Blue Cross and Blue Shield of Illinois announce collaboration and grant opportunity*. https://www.bcbsil.com/newsroom/news-releases/2019/aha-diversity-health-equity-collaboration (accessed April 6, 2021).

Beck, A. J., and M. L. Boulton 2016. The public health nurse workforce in U.S. state and local health departments, 2012. *Public Health Reports* 131(1):145–152. https://www.ncbi.nlm.nih.gov/pmc/articles/PMC4716482/pdf/phr131000145.pdf (accessed April 6, 2021).

Becker, S. I., and E. Maughan. 2017. A descriptive study of differing school health delivery models. *Journal of School Nursing* 33(6):415–425. doi: 10.1177/1059840517725788.

Beitsch, L. M., B. C. Castrucci, A. Dilley, J. P. Leider, C. Juliano, R. Nelson, S. Kaiman, and J. B. Sprague. 2015. From patchwork to package: Implementing foundational capabilities for state and local health departments. *American Journal of Public Health* 105(2):e7–e10. doi: 10.2105/AJPH.2014.302369.

Berenson, R. A., and P. B. Ginsburg. 2019. Improving the Medicare physician fee schedule: Make it part of value-based payment. *Health Affairs* 38(2):246–252. doi: 10.1377/hlthaff.2018.05411.

Berenson, R. A., and J. D. Goodson. 2016. Finding value in unexpected places—Fixing the Medicare physician fee schedule. *New England Journal of Medicine* 374(14):1306–1309. doi: 10.1056/NEJMp1600999.

Berenson, R. A., and A. E. Lazaroff. 2019. Time is of the essence: Solving office visit coding problems. *Journal of the American Geriatrics Society* 67(8):1552–1554.

Bodenheimer, T., and D. Mason. 2016. Registered nurses: Partners in transforming primary care. In *Preparing registered nurses for enhanced roles in primary care*, chaired by T. Bodenheimer and D. Mason. Conference conducted in New York, sponsored by the Josiah Macy Jr. Foundation. https://macyfoundation.org/assets/reports/publications/macy_monograph_nurses_2016_webpdf.pdf (accessed March 23, 2021).

Bogaert, K., B. C. Castrucci, E. Gould, K. Sellers, J. P. Leider, C. Whang, and V. Whitten. 2020. The public health workforce interests and needs survey (ph wins 2017): An expanded perspective on the state health agency workforce. *Journal of Public Health Management and Practice* 25:S16–S25.

Braveman, P., E. Arkin, T. Orleans, D. Proctor, and A. Plough. 2017. *What is health equity? And what difference does a definition make?* Princeton, NJ: Robert Wood Johnson Foundation.

Buerhaus, P. 2018. *Nurse practitioners: A solution to America's primary care crisis*. American Enterprise Institute. https://www.aei.org/research-products/report/nurse-practitioners-a-solution-to-americas-primary-care-crisis (accessed April 6, 2021).

Butler, S. 2020. *Achieving an equitable national health system for America*. Brookings Institution. https://www.brookings.edu/research/achieving-an-equitable-national-health-system-for-america (Accessed April 14, 2021).

Butterworth, K., R. Rajupadhya, R. Gongal, T. Manca, S. Ross, and D. Nichols. 2018. A clinical nursing rotation transforms medical students' interprofessional attitudes. *PLoS One* 13(5):e0197161. doi: 10.1371/journal.pone.0197161.

Cabello, M. 2018. *Braiding and blending: Managing multiple funds to improve health*. The Urban Institute. https://pfs.urban.org/pay-success/pfs-perspectives/braiding-and-blending-managing-multiple-funds-improve-health (accessed April 6, 2021).

Cady, R. G., M. Erickson, S. Lunos, S. Finkelstein, W. Looman, M. Celebreeze, and A. Garwick. 2015. Meeting the needs of children with medical complexity using a telehealth advanced practice registered nurse care coordination model. *Maternal and Child Health Journal* 19(7):1497–1506.

CCHP (Center for Connected Health Policy). 2017. *Telehealth private payer laws: Impact and issues*. Milbank Memorial Fund. https://www.milbank.org/wp-content/uploads/2017/08/MMF-Telehealth-Report-FINAL.pdf (accessed April 6, 2021).

CCHP. 2019. *Telehealth policy barriers*. Fact Sheet. https://www.cchpca.org/sites/default/files/2019-02/TELEHEALTH%20POLICY%20BARRIERS%202019%20FINAL.pdf (accessed April 6, 2021).

CDC (Centers for Disease Control and Prevention). 2013. CDC health disparities and inequalities report—United States, 2013. *Morbidity and Mortality Weekly Report* 62(3).

Chin, M. H. 2016. Creating the business case for achieving health equity. *Journal of General Internal Medicine* 31:792–796.

Chin, M. H., A. R. Clarke, R. S. Nocon, A. A. Casey, A. P. Goddu, N. M. Keesecker, and S. C. Cook. 2012. A roadmap and best practices for organizations to reduce racial and ethnic disparities in health care. *Journal of General Internal Medicine* 27:992–1000.

Clary, A. and T. Kartika. 2017. *Braiding funds to house complex Medicaid beneficiaries: Key policy lessons from Louisiana*. National Academy for State Health Policy. https://nashp.org/wp-content/uploads/2017/05/Braiding-Funds-Louisiana.pdf (accessed April 6, 2021).

Clary, A. and T. Riley. 2016. *Braiding and blending funding streams to meet the health-related social needs of low-income persons: Considerations for state health policymakers*. National Academy for State Health Policy. https://nashp.org/wp-content/uploads/2016/02/Jean1.pdf (accessed April 6, 2021).

Clemens, J., and J. D. Gottlieb. 2014. Do physicians' financial incentives affect medical treatment and patient health? *The American Economic Review* 104(4):1320–1349.

Clemens, J., and J. D. Gottlieb. 2017. In the shadow of a giant: Medicare's influence on private physician payments. *Journal of Political Economy* 125(1):1–39.

CMS (Centers for Medicare & Medicaid Services). 2012. *Graduate nurse education demonstration.* Fact Sheet. https://innovation.cms.gov/files/fact-sheet/gne-fact-sheet.pdf (accessed April 6, 2021).

CMS. 2014 (December 15). *Medicaid payment for services provided without charge (free care).* Letter to the State Medicaid Director. https://www.medicaid.gov/sites/default/files/federal-policy-guidance/downloads/smd-medicaid-payment-for-services-provided-without-charge-free-care.pdf (accessed April 6, 2021).

CMS. 2018. *Information on Medicare telehealth.* https://www.cms.gov/About-CMS/Agency-Information/OMH/Downloads/Information-on-Medicare-Telehealth-Report.pdf (accessed April 6, 2021).

CMS. 2019a (April 22). *HHS news: HHS to deliver value-based transformation in primary care.* Press Release. https://www.cms.gov/newsroom/press-releases/hhs-news-hhs-deliver-value-based-transformation-primary-care (accessed April 6, 2021).

CMS. 2019b. *Accountable health communities model.* https://innovation.cms.gov/initiatives/ahcm (accessed April 6, 2021).

CMS. 2020a. *People dually eligible for Medicare and Medicaid.* https://www.cms.gov/Medicare-Medicaid-Coordination/Medicare-and-Medicaid-Coordination/Medicare-Medicaid-Coordination-Office/Downloads/MMCO_Factsheet.pdf (accessed April 6, 2021).

CMS. 2020b. *Program of All-Inclusive Care for the Elderly (PACE).* https://www.cms.gov/Medicare-Medicaid-Coordination/Medicare-and-Medicaid-Coordination/Medicare-Medicaid-Coordination-Office/PACE/PACE (accessed April 6, 2021).

CMS. 2020c. *NHE Fact Sheet.* https://www.cms.gov/Research-Statistics-Data-and-Systems/Statistics-Trends-and-Reports/NationalHealthExpendData/NHE-Fact-Sheet (accessed April 4, 2021).

CMS. n.d.a. *About the CMS Innovation Center.* https://innovation.cms.gov/about (accessed April 6, 2021).

CMS. n.d.b. *Programs for All-Inclusive Care for the Elderly benefits.* https://www.medicaid.gov/medicaid/long-term-services-supports/pace/programs-all-inclusive-care-elderly-benefits/index.html (accessed April 6, 2021).

Coldiron, B., and M. Ratnarathorn. 2014. Scope of physician procedures independently billed by mid-level providers in the office setting. *JAMA Dermatology* 150(11):1153–1159.

Copeland, D. 2020. Paying for nursing student clinical placements, ethical considerations. *Journal of Professional Nursing* 36(5):330–333.

Council on School Health. 2016. Role of the school nurse in providing school health services. *Pediatrics* 137(6):e20160852. doi: 10.1542/peds.2016-0852.

Dahlin, C., and P. Coyne. 2019. The palliative APRN leader. *Annals of Palliative Medicine* 8(1). doi: 10.21037/apm.2018.06.03.

Damberg, C. L., M. E. Sorbero, S. L. Lovejoy, G. L. Martsolf, L. Raaen, and D. Mandel. 2014. Measuring success in value-based purchasing programs: Findings from an environmental scan, literature review, and expert panel discussions. *RAND Health Quarterly* 4(3):9.

Davis, A. M., L. M. Vinci, T. M. Okwuosa, A. R. Chase, and E. S. Huang. 2007. Cardiovascular health disparities: A systematic review of health care interventions. *Medical Care Research and Review* 64:29S–100S.

Dawley, K., J. Loch, and I. Bindrich. 2007. The nurse-family partnership. *American Journal of Nursing* 107(11):60–67; quiz 67–68.

DeMeester, R. H., L. J. Xu, R. S. Nocon, S. C. Cook, A. M. Ducas, and M. H. Chin. 2017. Solving disparities through payment and delivery system reform: A program to achieve health equity. *Health Affairs* 36:1133–1139.

DeSalvo, K. B., Y. C. Wang, A. Harris, J. Auerbach, D. Koo, and P. O'Carroll. 2017. Public health 3.0: A Call to action for public health to meet the challenges of the 21st century. *Preventing Chronic Disease* 14(170017). doi: 10.5888/pcd14.170017.

DeSalvo, K., Parekh, A., G. W. Hoagland, A. Dilley, S. Kaiman, M. Hines, and J. Levi. 2018. Developing a financing system to support public health infrastructure. *American Journal of Public Health* 109(10):1358–1361.

DesRoches, C. M., S. Clarke, J. Perloff, M. O'Reilly-Jacob, and P. Buerhaus. 2017. The quality of primary care provided by nurse practitioners to vulnerable Medicare beneficiaries. *Nursing Outlook* 65(6):679–688. doi: 10.1016/j.outlook.2017.06.007.

Dormond, M., and S. Ayafee. 2016. *Understanding billing restrictions for behavioral health providers*. Behavioral Health Workforce Research Center. http://www.behavioralhealthworkforce.org/wp-content/uploads/2017/01/FA3P4_Billing-Restrictions_Full-Report.pdf (accessed April 6, 2021).

Englander, H., and D. Kansagara. 2012. Planning and designing the care transitions innovation (C-TRAIN) for uninsured and Medicaid patients. *Journal of Hospital Medicine* 7(7):524–529. doi: 10.1002/jhm.1926.re.

Fels, J., B. L. Allard, K. Coppin, K. Hewson, and B. Richardson. 2015. Evolving role of the transitional care nurse in a small rural community. *Home Healthcare Now* 33(4):215–221. doi: 10.1097/nhh.0000000000000219.

Flowers, M., S. Sainer, A. Stoneburner, and W. Thorland. 2020. Education and employment outcomes in clients of the Nurse-Family Partnership. *Public Health Nursing* 37(2):206–214.

FNU (Frontier Nursing University). 2017. *Frontier Nursing University awarded $1,998,000 nursing workforce diversity grant*. https://frontier.edu/news/frontier-nursing-university-awarded-1998000-nursing-workforce-diversity-grant (accessed April 6, 2021).

Foronda, C. 2020. A theory of cultural humility. *Journal of Transcultural Nursing* 31(1):7–12.

Freundlich, N. 2018. *AccessHealth Spartanburg: Wrap-around community support for South Carolina's most vulnerable patients: Connecting the uninsured to primary care and a network of resources*. Center for Health Care Strategies, Inc. https://www.chcs.org/media/AHS-TCC-profile_050318.pdf (accessed April 6, 2021).

Fuchs, D. 2013. Medicare price problems and the RUC: Wagging the dog. *St. Louis University Journal of Health Law & Policy* 7:175. https://ssrn.com/abstract=2418824 (accessed April 6, 2021).

Gallagher, R. M., and P. A. Rowell. 2003. Claiming the future of nursing through nursing-sensitive quality indicators. *Nursing Administration Quarterly* 27(4):273–284. doi: 10.1097/00006216-200310000-00004.

Galloway, I. 2014. Using pay-for-success to increase investment in the nonmedical determinants of health. *Health Affairs* 33(11):1897–1904.

GAO (U.S. Government Accountability Office). 2015. *Medicare physician payment rates: Better data and greater transparency could improve accuracy*. GAO-14-434. https://www.gao.gov/products/GAO-15-434 (accessed April 6, 2021).

GAO. 2019. *Health care workforce: Views on expanding Medicare graduate medical education funding to nurse practitioners and physician assistants*. GAO-20-162. https://www.gao.gov/products/gao-20-162 (accessed April 6, 2021).

Georgia Health Policy Center. 2019. *Bridging for health*. GHPC Books. 8. https://scholarworks.gsu.edu/ghpc_books/8.

Gilman, D. J., and T. I. Koslov. 2014. Policy perspectives competition and the regulation of advanced practice nurses. Federal Trade Commission.

Ginsburg, P. B. 2012. Fee-for-service will remain a feature of major payment reforms, requiring more changes in Medicare physician payment. *Health Affairs* 31(9):1977–1983.

Golden, M. 2014. Pay-for-success financing: A new vehicle for improving population health? *Population Health News* 1(1):1–3.

Gonzalez-Smith, J., W. Bleser, D. Muhlestein, R. Richards, M. McClellan, and R. Saunders. 2019 (October 25). Medicare ACO results for 2018: More downside risk adoption, more savings, and all ACO types now averaging savings. *Health Affairs Blog*. doi: 10.1377/hblog20191024.65681/full.

Green, K., and M. Zook. 2019. When talking about social determinants of health, precision matters. *Health Affairs Blog*. doi: 10.1377/hblog20191025.776011.

Gunter, K. E., M. E. Peek, J. P. Tanumihardjo, E. Loehmer, E. Cabrey, R. Crespo, T. Johnson, B. R. Yamashita, E. I. Schwartz, C. Sol, C. Wilkinson, J. Wilson, and M. H. Chin. 2021. Population health innovations and payment to address social needs of patients and communities with diabetes. *Milbank Quarterly*.

Guth, M., R. Garfield, and R. Rudowitz. 2020. *The effects of Medicaid expansion under the ACA: Updated findings from a literature review*. Kaiser Family Foundation. http://files.kff.org/attachment/Report-The-Effects-of-Medicaid-Expansion-under-the-ACA-Updated-Findings-from-a-Literature-Review.pdf (accessed June 22, 2020).

Hager, B., M. Hasselberg, E. Arzubi, J. Betlinski, M. Duncan, J. Richman, and L. Raney. 2018. Leveraging behavioral health expertise: Practices and potential of the Project ECHO approach to virtually integrating care in underserved areas. *Psychiatric Services* 69(4):366–369. doi: 10.1176/appi.ps.201700211.

Hesgrove, B., D. Zapata, C. Bertane, C. Corea, L. Weinmann, S. Liu, B. Feng, and K. Kauffman. 2019. *The graduate nurse education demonstration: Final evaluation report*. Columbia, MD: IMPAQ International.

HHS (U.S. Department of Health and Human Services). 2011. *HHS action plan to reduce racial and ethnic health disparities: A nation free of disparities in health and health care*. https://www.minorityhealth.hhs.gov/npa/files/Plans/HHS/HHS_Plan_complete.pdf (accessed April 6, 2021).

HHS. 2018. *Evaluation of the graduate nurse education demonstration project: Report to Congress*. https://innovation.cms.gov/files/reports/gne-rtc.pdf (accessed April 6, 2021).

Hirschman, K., E. Shaid, K. McCauley, M. Pauly, and M. Naylor. 2015. Continuity of care: The transitional care model. *Online Journal of Issues in Nursing* 20(3). doi: 10.3912/OJIN.Vol20No03Man01.

Homeyer, S., W. Hoffman, P. Hingst, R. Oppermann, and A. Dreier-Wolfgramm. 2018. Effects of interprofessional education for medical and nursing students: Enablers, barriers and expectations for optimizing future interprofessional collaboration—A qualitative study. *BMC Nursing* 17:13. doi: 10.1186/s12912-018-0279-x.

Horner, B., W. van Leeuwem, M. Larkin, J. Baker, and S. Larsson. 2019. *Paying for value in health care*. Boston Consulting Group. https://www.bcg.com/publications/2019/paying-value-health-care (accessed April 6, 2021).

Horwitz, L. I., C. Chang, H. N. Arcilla, and J. R. Knickman,. 2020. Quantifying health systems' investment in social determinants of health, by sector, 2017–19. *Health Affairs* 39(2):192–198.

HRSA (Health Resources and Services Administration). 2018a. *Report to Congress Nurse Corps Loan Repayment and Scholarship Programs Fiscal Year 2019*. Rockville, MD: Health Resources and Services Administration.

HRSA. 2018b. *FY 2018 Nurse Corps Participant Satisfaction Survey*. Rockville, MD: Health Resources and Services Administration.

HRSA. 2020. *Find grants*. https://data.hrsa.gov/tools/find-grants (accessed on May 12, 2020).

Hsiao, W. C., P. Braun, E. R. Becker, and S. R. Thomas. 1987. The resource-based relative value scale. Toward the development of an alternative physician payment system. *Journal of the American Medical Association* 258(6):799–802.

Hsu, H. E., R. Wang, C. Broadwell, K. Horan, R. Jin, C. Rhee, and G. M. Lee. 2020. Association between federal value-based incentive programs and health care–associated infection rates in safety-net and non–safety-net hospitals. *JAMA Network Open* 3(7):e209700.

IHS (Indian Health Service). n.d. *Commissioned Corps*. https://www.ihs.gov/nursing/careerpaths/commissionedcorps (accessed September 22, 2020).

IOM (Institute of Medicine). 2004. *In the nation's compelling interest: Ensuring diversity in the health-care workforce*. Washington, DC: The National Academies Press.

IOM. 2011. *The future of nursing: Leading change, advancing health*. Washington, DC: The National Academies Press.

IOM. 2012. *For the public's health: Investing in a healthier future*. Washington, DC: The National Academies Press.

IOM. 2014. *Graduate medical education that meets the nation's health needs*. Washington, DC: The National Academies Press.

IOM. 2015. *Vital signs: Core metrics for health and health care progress*. Washington, DC: The National Academies Press.

Iovan, S., P. M. Lantz, and S. Shapiro. 2018. "Pay for success" projects: Financing interventions that address social determinants of health in 20 countries. *American Journal of Public Health* 108(11):1473–1477. doi: 10.2105/AJPH.2018.304651.

Irvin, J. A., A. A. Kondrich, M. Ko, P. Rajpurkar, B. Haghgoo, B. E. Landon, R. L. Phillips, S. Petterson, A. Y. Ng, and S. Basu. 2020. Incorporating machine learning and social determinants of health indicators into prospective risk adjustment for health plan payments. *BMC Public Health* 20(1):608.

Jackson, C. S., and J. N. Gracia. 2014. Addressing health and health-care disparities: The role of a diverse workforce and the social determinants of health. *Public Health Reports* 129(Suppl 2):57–61.

Jackson, C. K., R. Johnson, and C. Persico. 2016. The effects of school spending on educational and economic outcomes: Evidence from school finance reforms. *Quarterly Journal of Economics* 131(1):157–218. doi: 10./1093/qje/qjv036.

Karoly, L., M. R. Kilburn, and J. Cannon. 2005. *Early childhood interventions: Proven results, future promise*. Santa Monica, CA: RAND Corporation.

KFF (Kaiser Family Foundation). 2012. *Explaining health care reform: Medical loss ratio (MLR)*. https://www.kff.org/health-reform/fact-sheet/explaining-health-care-reform-medical-loss-ratio-mlr (accessed April 6, 2021).

Kitzman, H., D. L. Olds, M. D. Knudtson, R. Cole, E. Anson, J. A. Smith, D. Fishbein, R. DiClemente, G. Wingood, A. M. Caliendo, C. Hopfer, T. Miller, and G. Conti. 2019. Prenatal and infancy nurse home visiting and 18-year outcomes of a randomized trial. *Pediatrics* 144(6):e20183876. doi: 10.1542/peds.2018-3876.

Lai, A. Y., S. Skillman, and B. Frogner. 2020 (June 29). Is it fair? How to approach professional scope-of-practice policy after the COVID-19 pandemic. *Health Affairs Blog*. doi: 10.1377/hblog20200624.983306.

Lantz, P. M., S. Rosenbaum, L. Ku, and S. Iovan. 2016. Pay for success and population health: Early results from eleven projects reveal challenges and promise. *Health Affairs (Millwood)* 35(11):2053–2061. doi: 10.1377/hlthaff.2016.0713.

Largent, P. 2019. The nurse act. *NASN School Nurse* 34(4):210.

Larson, E. L., Cohen, B., Liu, J., Zachariah, P., Yao, D., and Shang, J. 2017. Assessing intensity of nursing care needs using electronically available data. *Computers, Informatics, Nursing* 35(12):617–623. doi: 10.1097/CIN.0000000000000375.

Lasater, K. B., H. D. Germack, D. S. Small, and M. D. McHugh. 2016. Hospitals known for nursing excellence perform better on value based purchasing measures. *Policy, Politics & Nursing Practice* 17(4):177–186. doi: 10.1177/1527154417698144.

Laugesen, M. 2014. The resource-based relative value scale and physician reimbursement policy. *Chest* 146(5):1413–1419.

LaVeist, T. A., D. Gaskin, and P. Richard. 2011. Estimating the economic burden of racial health inequalities in the United States. *International Journal of Health Services* 41(2):231–238.

Leachman, M., K. Masterson, and E. Figueroa. 2017 (November 29). *A punishing decade for school funding*. Center on Budget and Policy Priorities. https://www.cbpp.org/research/state-budget-and-tax/a-punishing-decade-for-school-funding (accessed April 6, 2021).

Machledt. 2017. *Addressing the social determinants of health through Medicaid managed care*. Issue Brief. https://www.commonwealthfund.org/publications/issue-briefs/2017/nov/addressing-social-determinants-health-through-medicaid-managed (accessed April 6, 2021).

Mangena, A. S., and E. Maughan. 2015. The 2015 NASN school nurse survey: Developing and providing leadership to advance school nursing practice. *NASN School Nurse* 30(6):328–335. doi: 10.1177/1942602X15608183.

Mann Levesque, E. 2018. *Improving community college completion rates by addressing structural and motivational barriers*. Brookings Institution. https://www.brookings.edu/research/community-college-completion-rates-structural-and-motivational-barriers (accessed April 6, 2021).

Massachusetts Department of Health. 2012. *2012 program update: Essential school health services*. https://archives.lib.state.ma.us/bitstream/handle/2452/684841/ocn984131182-2012.pdf (accessed April 6, 2021).

Maughan, E. D. 2018. School nurses: An investment in student achievement. *Phi Delta Kappan* 99(7):8–14. doi: 10.1177/0031721718767853.

McCleery, E., V. Christensen, K. Peterson, L. Humphrey, and M. Helfand. 2014. Evidence brief: The quality of care provided by advanced practice nurses. In *VA evidence synthesis program evidence briefs*. Washington, DC: U.S. Department of Veterans Affairs. https://www.ncbi.nlm.nih.gov/books/NBK384613 (accessed April 6, 2021).

McWilliams, J. M., L, Hatfield, B. Landon, and P. Hamed. 2018. Medicare spending after 3 years of the Medicare shared savings program. *New England Journal of Medicine* 379(12):1139–1149.

Meddings, J., H. Reichert, S. N. Smith, T. J. Iwashyna, K. M. Langa, T. P. Hofer, and L. McMahon. 2017. The impact of disability and social determinants of health on condition-specific readmissions beyond Medicare risk adjustments: A cohort study. *Journal of General Internal Medicine* 32(1):71–80.

MedPAC (Medicare Payment Advisory Commission). 2018. *Medicare and the health care delivery system: Report to the Congress*. http://MedPAC.gov/docs/default-source/reports/jun18_MedPACreporttocongress_sec.pdf (accessed April 6, 2021).

MedPAC. 2019. *Medicare and the health care delivery system: Report to the Congress*. http://www.MedPAC.gov/docs/default-source/reports/jun19_MedPAC_reporttocongress_sec.pdf?sfvrsn=0 (accessed April 6, 2021).

MedPAC. 2020. *Physician and other health professional payment system: Payment basics*. http://MedPAC.gov/docs/default-source/payment-basics/MedPAC_payment_basics_20_physician_final_sec.pdf?sfvrsn=0 (accessed April 6, 2021).

MGMA (Medical Group Management Association). 2020 (May 20). *New MGMA research finds physician compensation increased in 2019*. Press Release. https://www.mgma.com/news-insights/press/new-mgma-research-finds-physician-compensation-inc (accessed April 6, 2021).

Miller, H. D. 2009. From volume to value: Better ways to pay for health care. *Health Affairs* 28(5):1418–1428.

MLN (Medicare Learning Network). 2020. *Advanced practice registered nurses, anesthesiologist assistants, and physician assistants*. Baltimore, MD: Centers for Medicare & Medicaid Services.

Moldestad, M., P. Greene, G. Sayre, E. Neely, C. Sulc, A. Sales, A. Reddy, E. Wong, and C-F. Liu. 2020. Comparable, but distinct: Perceptions of primary care provided by physicians and nurse practitioners in full and restricted practice authority states. *Journal of Advanced Nursing* 76(11):3092–3103.

Moore, D. J. 2019. Nurse practitioners' pivotal role in ending the opioid epidemic. *Journal for Nurse Practitioners* 15(5):323–327.

Morgan, P. A., V. A. Smith, T. S. Berkowitz, D. Edelman, C. Van Houtven, S. L. Woolson, C. C. Hendrix, C. M. Everett, B. S. White, and G. L. Jackson. 2019. Impact of physicians, nurse practitioners, and physician assistants on utilization and costs for complex patients. *Health Affairs* 38(6):1028–1036.

Mose, J., and C. Jones. 2018. Alternative payment models and team-based care. *North Carolina Medical Journal* 79(4):231–234. https://www.ncmedicaljournal.com/content/ncm/79/4/231.full.pdf (accessed April 6, 2021).

Munteanu, T., E. H. Ference, A. Danielian, V. M. Talati, R. C. Kern, J. A. Eloy, and S. S. Smith. 2020. Analysis of sinus balloon catheter dilation providers based on medicare provider utilization and payment data. *The American Journal of Rhinology & Allergy* 34(4):463–470.

NACCHO (National Association of County and City Health Officials). 2020. *Statement of policy: Public health nurses*. https://www.naccho.org/uploads/downloadable-resources/05-08-Public-Health-Nurses.pdf (accessed April 6, 2021).

NACNEP (National Advisory Council on Nurse Education and Practice). 2019. Promoting nursing leadership in the transition to value-based care. Fifteenth Report to the Secretary of Health and Human Services and the U.S. Congress. National Advisory Council on Nurse Education and Practice (NACNEP). Based on the 134th and 135th Meetings of NACNEP.

NASEM (National Academies of Sciences, Engineering, and Medicine). 2016. *Assessing progress on the Institute of Medicine report* The Future of Nursing. Washington, DC: The National Academies Press.

NASEM. 2017. *Accounting for social risk factors in Medicare payment*. Washington, DC: The National Academies Press.

NASEM. 2019. *Integrating social care in the delivery of health care: Moving upstream to improve the nation's health*. Washington, DC: The National Academies Press.

NASEM. 2020a. *Birth settings in America: Improving outcomes, quality, access, and choice*. Washington, DC: The National Academies Press.

NASEM. 2020b. *Leading health indicators 2030: Advancing health, equity, and well-being*. Washington, DC: The National Academies Press.

Nash, W., L. Hall, S. L. Ridner, D. Hayden, T. Mayfield, J. Firriolo, W. Hupp, C. Weathers, and T. Crawford. 2018. Evaluation of an interprofessional education program for advanced practice nursing and dental students: The oral-systemic health connection. *Nursing Education Today* 66:25–32.

NASN (National Association of School Nurses). 2016. *The role of the 21st century school nurse: Position statement*. https://www.nasn.org/advocacy/professional-practice-documents/position-statements/ps-role (accessed April 6, 2021).

Naylor, M. D., E. T. Kurtzman, D. C. Grabowski, C. Harrington, M. McClellan, and S. C. Reinhard. 2012. Unintended consequences of steps to cut readmissions and reform payment may threaten care of vulnerable older adults. *Health Affairs (Millwood)* 31(7):1623–1632.

NCES (National Center for Education Statistics). 2020. Characteristics of postsecondary students. *The Condition of Education: A Letter from the Commissioner*. https://nces.ed.gov/programs/coe/indicator_csb.asp (accessed June 26, 2020).

NCES. n.d. Average FTE nurses in schools and ratio of students to FTE nurses with at least one nurse, by school type and selected school characteristics: 2007-08 and 2011-12. *Schools and Staffing Survey (SASS)*. https://nces.ed.gov/surveys/sass/tables/sass1112_20161115001_s12n.asp (accessed April 6, 2021).

NCSL (National Conference of State Legislators). 2016. *Health cost containment and efficiencies, NCSL briefs for state legislators*. Denver, CO: NCSL. https://www.ncsl.org/documents/health/IntroandBriefsCC-16.pdf (accessed July 23, 2021).

Needleman, J. 2020. *Paying for nursing care in fee-for-service and value-based symptoms*. Paper commissioned by the Committee on the Future of Nursing 2020–2030.

NFF (Nonprofit Finance Fund). n.d. *Invest in results: Pay for success and other outcomes funding.* https://nff.org/invest-in-results (accessed April 6, 2021).

NGA (National Governors Associations). 2012. *The role of nurse practitioners in meeting increasing demand for primary care.* https://www.nga.org/center/publications/the-role-of-nurse-practitioners-in-meeting-increasing-demand-for-primary-care-2 (accessed April 6, 2021).

NPA (National PACE Association). n.d. *Core differences between PACE and MA plans.* https://www.npaonline.org/sites/default/files/PDFs/Core%20Differences%20Between%20PACE%20and%20MA%20Plans.pdf (accessed April 6, 2021).

NQF (National Quality Forum). 2012. *Changing healthcare by the numbers: NQF report to Congress.* http://www.qualityforum.org/Publications/2012/03/2012_NQF_Report_to_Congress_Document.aspx (accessed April 6, 2021).

NQF. 2017. *A roadmap for promoting health equity and eliminating disparities: The four I's for health equity.* http://www.qualityforum.org/Publications/2017/09/A_Roadmap_for_Promoting_Health_Equity_and_Eliminating_Disparities__The_Four_I_s_for_Health_Equity.aspx (accessed April 6, 2021).

NQF. 2019. *A national call to action: Quality and payment innovation in social determinants of health.* Washington, DC: National Quality Forum.

Nyweide, D. J., W. Lee, and C. H. Colla. 2020. Accountable care organizations' increase in nonphysician practitioners may signal shift for health care workforce. *Health Affairs* 39(6):1080–1086.

OHS (Office of Head Start). 2020. *Funding opportunities announcement (FOA) locator.* https://www.acf.hhs.gov/ohs/funding (accessed April 6, 2021).

Oliver, G. M., L. Pennington, S. Revelle, and M. Rantz. 2014. Impact of nurse practitioners on health outcomes of Medicare and Medicaid patients. *Nursing Outlook* 62(6):440–447.

Ollove, M. 2019. *More kids on Medicaid to get health care in school.* The Pew Charitable Trusts. https://www.pewtrusts.org/en/research-and-analysis/blogs/stateline/2019/11/27/more-kids-on-medicaid-to-get-health-care-in-school (accessed April 6, 2021).

Patel, S., A. Smithey, K. Tuck, and T. McGinnis. 2021. *Leveraging value-based payment approaches to promote health equity: Key strategies for health care payers.* https://www.chcs.org/resource/leveraging-value-based-payment-approaches-to-promote-health-equity-key-strategies-for-health-care-payers (accessed February 27, 2021).

Peek, M. E., A. Cargill, and E. S. Huang. 2007. Diabetes health disparities: A systematic review of health care interventions. *Medical Care Research and Review* 64:101S–156S.

Peek, M. E., M. B. Vela, and M. H. Chin. 2020. Practical lessons for teaching about race and racism: Successfully leading free, frank, and fearless discussions. *Academic Medicine* 95(12S):S139–S144. doi: 10.1097/ACM.0000000000003710.

Rapsilber, L. 2019. Incident to billing in a value-based reimbursement world. *Nurse Practitioner* 44(2):15–17.

Renfrew, M. J., A. McFadden, M. Bastos, J. Campbell, A. Channon, n. Cheung, D. Silva, S. Downe, H. Kennedy, A. Malata, F. McCormick, L. Wick, and E. Declerq. 2014. Midwifery and quality care: Findings from a new evidence-informed framework for maternal and newborn care. *Lancet* 384(9948):1129–1145.

RIDOH (Rhode Island Department of Health). 2018. *Health equity zones.* https://health.ri.gov/publications/brochures/HealthEquityZones.pdf (accessed April 6, 2021).

Rosenthal, E. 2017 (March 29). Those indecipherable medical bills? They're one reason health care costs so much. *The New York Times.* https://www.nytimes.com/2017/03/29/magazine/those-indecipherable-medical-bills-theyre-one-reason-health-care-costs-so-much.html (accessed April 6, 2021).

Rothstein, R. 2017. *The color of law: A forgotten history of how our government segregated America.* New York: Liveright.

Ryan, C. J., R. Bierle, and K. Vuckovic. 2019. The three Rs for preventing heart failure readmission: Review, reassess, and reeducate. *Critical Care Nurse* 39(2):85–93.

SAMHSA (Substance Abuse and Mental Health Services Administration). 2018. *Key substance use and mental health indicators in the United States: Results from the 2018 National Survey on Drug Use and Health*. https://www.samhsa.gov/data/sites/default/files/cbhsq-reports/NSDUHNationalFindingsReport2018/NSDUHNationalFindingsReport2018.pdf (accessed April 6, 2021).

SCDHHS (South Carolina Department of Health and Human Services). 2016. *South Carolina Nurse-Family Partnership pay for success project*. Fact Sheet. https://www.scdhhs.gov/sites/default/files/2-16-16-SC-NFP-PFS-Fact-Sheet_3.pdf (accessed April 6, 2021).

Searing, A., and D. C. Ross. 2019. *Medicaid expansion fills gaps in maternal health coverage leading to healthier mothers and babies*. Georgetown University Health Policy Institute Center for Children and Families. https://ccf.georgetown.edu/wp-content/uploads/2019/05/Maternal-Health-3a.pdf (accessed April 6, 2021).

Sensmeier, J., I. Androwich, M. Baernholdt, W. Carroll, W. Fields, V. Fong, J. Murphy, A. Omery, and N. Rajwany. 2019. Demonstrating the value of nursing care through a unique nurse identifier. *Online Journal of Nursing Informatics* 23(2).

Sessions, S. Y. 2012. *Financing state and local public health departments: A problem of chronic illness*. Paper commissioned by the Committee on the Future of Nursing (see Appendix D).

Shekelle, P. G., and M. Begashaw. 2021. What are the effects of different team-based primary care structures on the quadruple aim of care?: A rapid review. Los Angeles, CA: Evidence Synthesis Program, Health Services Research and Development Service, Office of Research and Development, U.S. Department of Veterans Affairs. VA ESP Project #05-226; 2021. https://www.hsrd.research.va.gov/publications/esp/reports.cfm (accessed July 23, 2021).

Shi, L. 2012. The impact of primary care: A focused review. *Scientifica* 432892.

Sinsky, C., and D. Dugdale. 2013. Medicare payment for cognitive vs procedural care: Minding the gap. *JAMA Internal Medicine* 173(18):1733–1737.

Skinner, L., D. Staiger, D. Auerbach, and P. Buerhaus. 2019. Implications of an aging rural physician workforce. *New England Journal of Medicine* 381(4):299–301.

Social Finance. 2020. *Increasing access to nursing education: Student-centered income share agreements as a potential solution*. https://socialfinance.org/wp-content/uploads/2020.05_Income-Share-Agreements-for-Nursing_SENT.pdf (accessed April 6, 2021).

Spectrum Health. n.d. *School health program*. https://www.spectrumhealth.org/healthier-communities/our-programs/school-health-program (accessed April 6, 2021).

Spencer, A., and B. Freda. 2016. Advancing state innovation model goals through accountable communities for health. Center for Health Care Strategies, Inc. https://www.chcs.org/media/SIM-ACH-Brief_101316_final.pdf (accessed April 6, 2021).

Squires, D., and C. Anderson, 2015. U.S. health care from a global perspective: spending, use of services, prices, and health in 13 countries. The Commonwealth Fund. https://www.commonwealthfund.org/sites/default/files/documents/___media_files_publications_issue_brief_2015_oct_1819_squires_us_hlt_care_global_perspective_oecd_intl_brief_v3.pdf (accessed April 14, 2021).

Stone, P. W. 2020. Value-based incentive programs and health disparities. *JAMA Network Open* 3(7):e2010231.

Strickland, C. J., R. Logsdon, B. Hoffman, and T. Garrett Hill. 2014. Developing an academic and American Indian tribal partnership in education: A model of community health nursing clinical education. *Nurse Educator* 39(4):188–192. doi: 10.1097/NNE.0000000000000048.

Sullivan-Marx, E. M. 2008. Lessons learned from advanced practice nursing payment. *Policy, Politics, & Nursing Practice* 9(2):121–126.

Sullivan-Marx, E. M., and G. Maislin. 2000. Comparison of nurse practitioner and family physician relative work values. *Journal of Nursing Scholarship* 32(1):71–76.

Sullivan-Marx, E. M., M. B. Happ, K. Bradley, and G. Maislin. 2000. Nurse practitioner services: Content and relative work value. *Nursing Outlook* (48):269–275.

TFAH (Trust for America's Health). 2018a. *A funding crisis for public health and safety: State-by-state public health funding and key health facts*. https://www.tfah.org/wp-content/uploads/2019/03/InvestInAmericaRpt-FINAL.pdf (accessed April 6, 2021).

TFAH. 2018b. *Braiding and blending funds to support community health improvement: A compendium of resources and examples*. https://www.tfah.org/wp-content/uploads/2018/01/TFAH-Braiding-Blending-Compendium-FINAL.pdf (accessed April 6, 2021).

TFAH. 2019. The impact of chronic underfunding on America's public health system: Trends, risks, and recommendations, 2019. https://www.tfah.org/report-details/2019-funding-report (accessed February 13, 2020).

TFAH. n.d. *How embedding health access and nurses in schools improves health in Grand Rapids, Michigan*. https://www.tfah.org/story/how-embedding-health-access-and-nurses-in-schools-improves-health-in-grand-rapids-michigan (accessed April 6, 2021).

Thomas, S. Durfey, E. Gadbois, D. Meyers, J. Brazier, E. McCreedy, S. Fashaw, and T. Wetle. 2019. Perspectives of Medicare Advantage Plan representatives on addressing social determinants of health in response to the CHRONIC Care Act. *JAMA Network Open* 2(7):e196923. doi: 10.1001/jamanetworkopen.2019.6923.

UM (University of Michigan) Behavioral Health Workforce Research Center. 2018. *Characteristics of the Rural Behavioral Health Workforce: A survey of Medicaid/Medicare reimbursed providers*. Ann Arbor, MI: University of Michigan School of Public Health. http://www.behavioralhealthworkforce.org/wp-content/uploads/2019/01/Y3-FA2-P1-Rural-Pop_Full-Report.pdf (accessed April 6, 2021).

UMN (University of Minnesota). 2018. *Nursing knowledge: 2018 big data science*. Conference conducted at the University of Minnesota, June 13–15, 2018. https://www.nursing.umn.edu/sites/nursing.umn.edu/files/nkbds_proceedings_2018.pdf (accessed April 6, 2021).

UMN. 2020. *Risk adjustment based on social factors and strategies for filling data gaps*. https://www.shadac.org/sites/default/files/FINAL_SHVS-Risk-Adjustment-Brief.pdf (accessed November 16, 2020).

Urban Institute. 2016. *South Carolina Nurse-Family Partnership project*. Fact Sheet. https://pfs.urban.org/pfs-project-fact-sheets/content/south-carolina-nurse-family-partnership-project (accessed April 6, 2021).

Urban Institute. n.d. *What is PSF?* https://pfs.urban.org/what-pfs (accessed April 6, 2021).

VA (U.S. Department of Veterans Affairs). 2019. *RN transition-to-practice (TTP)*. Office of Nursing Services. https://www.va.gov/nursing/workforce/RNTTP.asp (accessed April 6, 2021).

Velander, J. R. 2018. Suboxone: Rationale, science, misconceptions. *Ochsner Journal* 18(1):23–29.

Wallen, M., and A. Hubbard. 2013. *Blending and braiding early childhood program funding streams toolkit: Enhancing financing for high-quality early learning programs*. https://www.buildinitiative.org/Portals/0/Uploads/Documents/resource-center/community-systems-development/3E%202%20Blended-Funding-Toolkit.pdf (accessed April 6, 2021).

Wang, L. Y., M. Vernon-Smiley, M. A. Gapinski, M. Desisto, E. Maughan, and A. Sheetz. 2014. Cost-benefit study of school nursing services. *JAMA Pediatrics* 168(7):642–648.

Welker-Hood, K. 2014. Underfunding and undervaluing the public health infrastructure: Reinforcing the haves and the have-nots in health. *Public Health Nursing* 31(6):481–483. doi: 10.1111/phn.12165.

Werner, R. M., E. J. Emanuel, H. H. Pham, and A. S. Navanthe. 2021. *The future of value-based payment: A road map to 2030*. Philadelphia, PA: University of Pennsylvania, Leonard Davis Institute of Health Economics.

Willgerodt, M. A., D. Brock, and E. Maughan. 2018. Public school nursing practice in the United States. *Journal of School Nursing* 34(3):232–244.

Yang, Y. T., L. B. Attanasio, and K. B. Kozhimannil. 2016. State scope of practice laws, nurse-midwifery workforce, and childbirth procedures and outcomes. *Women's Health Issues* 26(3):262–267. doi: 10.1016/j.whi.2016.02.003.

7

Educating Nurses for the Future

You cannot transmit wisdom and insight to another person. The seed is already there. A good teacher touches the seed, allowing it to wake up, to sprout, and to grow.

—Thich Nhat Hanh, global spiritual leader and peace activist

By 2030, the nursing profession will look vastly different and will be caring for a changing America. Nursing school curricula need to be strengthened so that nurses are prepared to help promote health equity, reduce health disparities, and improve the health and well-being of everyone. Nursing schools will need to ensure that nurses are prepared to understand and identify the social determinants of health, have expanded learning experiences in the community so they can work with different people with varied life experiences and cultural values, have the competencies to care for an aging and more diverse population, can engage in new professional roles, are nimble enough to adapt continually to new technologies, and can lead and collaborate with other professions and sectors. And nursing students—and faculty—not only need to reflect the diversity of the population, but also need to help break down barriers of structural racism prevalent in today's nursing education.

Throughout the coming decade, it will be essential for nursing education to evolve rapidly in order to prepare nurses who can meet the challenges articulated in this report with respect to addressing social determinants of health (SDOH), improving population health, and promoting health equity. Nurses will need to be educated to care for a population that is both aging, with declining mental and physical health, and becoming increasingly diverse; to engage in new professional roles; to adapt to new technologies; to function in a changing policy environment;

and to lead and collaborate with professionals from other sectors and professions. As part of their education, aspiring nurses will need new competencies and different types of learning experiences to be prepared for these new and expanded roles. Also essential will be recruiting and supporting diverse students and faculty to create a workforce that more closely resembles the population it serves. Given the growing focus on SDOH, population health, and health equity within the public health and health care systems, the need to make these changes to nursing education is clear. Nurses' close connection with patients and communities, their role as advocates for well-being, and their placement across multiple types of settings make them well positioned to address SDOH and health equity. For future nurses to capitalize on this potential, however, SDOH and equity must be integrated throughout their educational experience to build the competencies and skills they will need.

The committee's charge included examining whether nursing education provides the competencies and skills nurses will need—the capacity to acquire new competencies, to work outside of acute care settings, and to lead efforts to build a culture of health and health equity—as they enter the workforce and throughout their careers. A thorough review of the current status and future needs of nursing education in the United States was beyond the scope of this study, but in this chapter, the committee identifies priorities for the content and nature of the education nurses will need to meet the challenge of addressing SDOH, advancing health equity, and improving population health. Nursing education is a lifelong pursuit; nurses gain knowledge and skills in the classroom, at work, through continuing professional development, and through other formal and informal mechanisms (IOM, 2016b). While the scope of this study precluded a thorough discussion of learning outside of nursing education programs, readers can find further discussion of lifelong learning in *A Framework for Educating Health Professionals to Address the Social Determinants of Health* (IOM, 2016b), *Redesigning Continuing Education in the Health Professions* (IOM, 2010), and *Exploring a Business Case for High-Value Continuing Professional Development: Proceedings of a Workshop* (NASEM, 2018a).

To change nursing education meaningfully so as to produce nurses who are prepared to meet the above challenges in the decade ahead will require changes in four areas: what is taught, how it is taught, who the students are, and who teaches them. This chapter opens with a description of the nursing education system and the need for integrating equity into education, and then examines each of these four areas in turn:

- domains and competencies for equity,
- expanded learning opportunities,
- recruitment of and support for diverse prospective nurses, and
- strengthening and diversification of the nursing faculty.

In addition to changes in these specific areas, there is a need for a fundamental shift in the idea of what constitutes a "quality" nursing education. Currently, National Council Licensure Examination (NCLEX) pass rates are used as the primary indicator of quality, along with graduation and employment rates (NCSBN, 2020a; O'Lynn, 2017). This narrow focus on pass rates has been criticized for diverting time and attention away from other goals, such as developing student competencies, investing in faculty, and implementing innovative curricula (Giddens, 2009; O'Lynn, 2017; Taylor et al., 2014). In addition, the NCLEX is heavily focused on acute care rather than on such areas of nursing as primary care, disease prevention, SDOH, and health equity (NCSBN, 2019). In response to such concerns about the NCLEX, the National Council of State Boards of Nursing (NCSBN) conducted a study to identify additional quality indicators for nursing education programs; indicators were identified in the areas of administration, program director, faculty, students, curriculum and clinical experiences, and teaching and learning resources (Spector et al., 2020). To realize the committee's vision for nursing education, it will be necessary for nursing schools, accreditors, employers, and students to look beyond NCLEX pass rates and include these types of indicators in the assessment of a quality nursing education.

OVERVIEW OF NURSING EDUCATION

Nurses are educated at universities, colleges, hospitals, and community colleges and can follow a number of educational pathways. Table 7-1 identifies the various degrees that nurses can hold, and describes the programs that lead to each degree and the usual amount of time required to complete them. In 2019, there were more than 200,000 graduates from baccalaureate, master's, and doctoral nursing programs in the United States and its territories, including 144,659 who received a baccalaureate degree (AACN, 2020a) (see Table 7-2).

Nursing programs are nationally accredited by the Accreditation Commission for Education in Nursing (ACEN); the Commission on Collegiate Nursing Education (CCNE); the Commission for Nursing Education and Accreditation (CNEA); and other bodies focused on specialty areas of nursing, such as midwifery. Graduating registered nurses (RNs) seek licensure as nurses through state boards, and take examinations administered by the NCSBN as graduates with their first professional degree and then as specialists with certification exams offered through specialty organizations. These bodies set minimum standards for nursing programs and establish criteria for certification and licensing, faculty qualifications, course offerings, and other features of nursing programs (Gaines, n.d.).

TABLE 7-1 Pathways in Nursing Education

Type of Degree	Description of Program
Doctor of Philosophy in Nursing (PhD) and Doctor of Nursing Practice (DNP)	PhD programs are research focused, and graduates typically teach and conduct research, although these roles are expanding. DNP programs are practice focused, and graduates typically serve in advanced practice registered nurse (APRN) roles and other advanced clinical positions, including faculty positions. Time to completion: 3–5 years. Bachelor of science in nursing (BSN)- or master of science in nursing (MSN)-to-nursing doctorate options available.
Master's Degree in Nursing (MSN/MS)	Prepares APRNs: nurse practitioners, clinical nurse specialists, nurse midwives, and nurse anesthetists, as well as clinical nurse leaders, educators, administrators, and other areas or roles. Time to completion: 18–24 months. Three years for associate's degree in nursing (ADN)-to-MSN option.
Accelerated BSN or Master's Degree in Nursing	Designed for students with a baccalaureate degree in another field. Time to completion: 12–18 months for BSN and 3 years for MSN, depending on prerequisite requirements.
Bachelor of Science in Nursing (BSN) Registered Nurse (RN)	Educates nurses to practice the full scope of nursing responsibilities across all health care settings. Curriculum provides additional content in physical and social sciences, leadership, research, and public health. Time to completion: 4 years or up to 2 years for ADN/diploma RNs and 3 years for licensed practical nurses (LPNs), depending on prerequisite requirements.
Associate's Degree in Nursing (ADN) (RN) and Diploma in Nursing (RN)	Prepares nurses to provide direct patient care and practice within the legal scope of nursing responsibilities in a variety of health care settings. Offered through community colleges and hospitals. Time to completion: 2 to 3 years for ADN (less in the case of LPN entry) and 3 years for diploma (all hospital-based training programs), depending on prerequisite requirements.
Licensed Practical Nurse (LPN)/Licensed Vocational Nurse (LVN)	Trains nurses to provide basic care (e.g., take vital signs, administer medications, monitor catheters, and apply dressings). LPN/LVNs work under the supervision of physicians and RNs. Offered by technical/vocational schools and community colleges. Time to completion: 12–18 months.

SOURCES: Adapted from IOM, 2011 (AARP, 2010. Courtesy of AARP. All rights reserved).

The Need for Nursing Education on Social Determinants of Health and Health Equity

A report of the Institute of Medicine (IOM) from nearly two decades ago asserts that all health professionals, including nurses, need to "understand determinants of health, the link between medical care and healthy populations, and professional responsibilities" (IOM, 2003, p. 209). The literature is replete with calls for all nurses to understand concepts associated with health equity, such as disparities, culturally competent care, equity, and social justice. For example, Morton and colleagues (2019) identify essential content to prepare nurses for

TABLE 7-2 Number of Graduates from Nursing Programs in the United States and Territories, 2019

Type of Degree or Certificate	Number of Graduates
Licensed practical nurse (LPN)/licensed vocational nurse (LVN)[a]	48,234
Associate's degree in nursing (ADN)[a]	84,794
Generic entry-level baccalaureate (includes accelerated BSN and LPN-to-BSN)	78,394
RN-to-baccalaureate programs	66,265
Master's	49,895
Doctor of nursing practice (DNP)	7,944
PhD	804
Postdoctoral	57

[a] Number of first-time NCLEX test takers, which is proxy for new graduates (NCSBN, 2020a).
SOURCE: AACN, 2020a.

community-based practice, including SDOH, health disparities/health equity, cultural competency, epidemiology, community leadership, and the development of enhanced skills in community-based settings. O'Connor and colleagues (2019) call for an inclusive educational environment that prepares nurses to care for diverse patient populations, including the study of racism's impacts on health from the genetic to the societal level, systems of marginalization and oppression, critical self-reflection, and preparation for lifelong learning in these areas. And Thornton and Persaud (2018) state that the content of nursing education should include instruction in cultural sensitivity and culturally competent care, trauma-informed care and motivational interviewing, screening for social needs, and referring for services. These calls align with the Health Resources and Services Administration's (HRSA's) most recent strategic plan, which prioritizes the development of a health care workforce that is able to address current and emerging needs for improving equity and access (HRSA, 2019). Additionally, recommendations of the National Advisory Council on Nurse Education and Practice (NACNEP) (2016) include that population health concepts be incorporated into nursing curriculum and that undergraduate programs create partnerships with HRSA, the U.S. Department of Veterans Affairs (VA), and the Indian Health Service (IHS), agencies that serve rural and frontier areas, to increase students' exposure to different competencies, experiences, and environments.

In concert with these perspectives and recommendations, nursing organizations have developed guidelines for how nursing education should prepare nurses to work on health equity issues and address SDOH. In 2019, the National League for Nursing (NLN) issued a *Vision for Integration of the Social Determinants of Health into Nursing Education Curricula*, which describes the importance of SDOH to the mission of nursing and makes recommendations for how SDOH should be integrated into nursing education (see Box 7-1).

BOX 7-1
National League for Nursing's (NLN's) Vision for Integration of the Social Determinants of Health into Nursing Education Curricula

For Faculty

- Utilize the NLN toolkit to provide evidence-based approaches to teaching/learning strategies related to the SDH [social determinants of health].
- Raise students' consciousness about SDH, how to develop an inclusive understanding of the SDH, and how recognizing the shared impact of the SDH on health and wellness leads to new perspectives related to differences and mitigates bias and racism.
- Create partnerships with community agencies to provide experiences that intentionally expose students to address the impact of SDH on patients, families and communities.
- Thread SDH education throughout the program of learning in varied educational settings (e.g., classroom, clinical settings, and simulation-learning environments).
- Be intentional about providing opportunities for students to assess and implement actions to address SDH in a variety of health care settings.
- Develop curricula that strengthen the links between SDH, health equity, and nursing's social mission.

For Leadership in Nursing Programs

- Engage faculty and staff in conversations directed toward addressing explicit and implicit bias related to SDH to foster a more inclusive understanding of the SDH and their effects on health and wellness.
- Encourage faculty to co-create new narratives around health and wellness, to include dialogue that makes the case, for example, for the link between housing and health, livable wages and health equity, and access to resources and health disparities.
- Provide faculty development opportunities to prepare faculty to co-create and implement educational experiences related to assessment and intervention to decrease the impact of SDH.
- Maximize educational capacity by establishing partnerships with practice colleagues and the community around innovative curriculum design to build collaborative initiatives that address SDH.
- Support institutional and faculty research that examines the effect of the SDH on patient outcomes and the way students link the SDH to nursing's social mission and health equity.

SOURCE: Excerpted from NLN, 2019.

As described in Chapter 9, the American Association of Colleges of Nursing's (AACN's) *Essentials*[1] provides an outline for the necessary curriculum content and expected competencies for graduates of baccalaureate, master's, and doctor of nursing practice (DNP) programs. *Essentials* identifies "Clinical Prevention and Population Health" as one of the nine essential areas of baccalaureate nursing education. Among other areas of focus, *Essentials* calls for baccalaureate programs to prepare nurses to

- collaborate with other health care professionals and patients to provide spiritually and culturally appropriate health promotion and disease and injury prevention interventions;
- assess the health, health care, and emergency preparedness needs of a defined population;
- collaborate with others to develop an intervention plan that takes into account determinants of health, available resources, and the range of activities that contribute to health and the prevention of illness, injury, disability, and premature death;
- participate in clinical prevention and population-focused interventions with attention to effectiveness, efficiency, cost-effectiveness, and equity; and
- advocate for social justice, including a commitment to the health of vulnerable populations and the elimination of health disparities.

Curriculum content and expected competencies laid out in *Essentials* for master's- and DNP-level nursing education also address SDOH, disparities, equity, and social justice (AACN, 2006, 2011). While *Essentials* only guides baccalaureate, master's, and DNP programs, the document's emphasis on health equity and SDOH demonstrates the importance of these topics to the nursing profession as a whole.

As of 2020, AACN has been shifting toward a competency-based curriculum. As part of this effort, AACN published a draft update to *Essentials* that identifies 10 domains for nursing education: knowledge for nursing practice; person-centered care; population health; scholarship for nursing discipline; quality and safety; interprofessional partnerships; systems-based practice; informatics and health care technologies; professionalism; and personal, professional, and leadership development. Within these 10 domains are specific competencies that AACN believes are essential for nursing practice (AACN, 2020b), including

- engage in effective partnerships,
- advance equitable population health policy,
- demonstrate advocacy strategies,

---

[1] See https://www.aacnnursing.org/Education-Resources/AACN-Essentials (accessed April 13, 2021).

- use information and communication technologies and informatics processes to deliver safe nursing care to diverse populations in a variety of settings, and
- use knowledge of nursing and other professions to address the health care needs of patients and populations.

Nurses themselves have also indicated the need for more education and training on these topics. The 2018 National Sample Survey of Registered Nurses (NSSRN) asked the question, "As of December 31, 2017, what training topics would have helped you do your job better?" Figure 7-1 shows the percentage of six different training topics that RNs said would help them do their job better. Overall, RNs working in schools, public health, community health, and emergency and urgent care were more likely than RNs working in all other employment settings listed in Figure 7-1 to indicate that they could have done their job better if they had received training in SDOH, population health, working in underserved communities, caring for individuals with complex health and social needs, and especially mental health. These results could reflect RNs encountering increasingly complex individuals and populations, rising numbers of visits and caseloads, the fact that the RNs working in these settings frequently provide

RN Training Topics

Social determinants of health (e.g., impact of race and social-economic status)		
	Average	Range
All nurses	18.7%	10.0–38.0%
Grad after 2010	21.5%	12.9–56.8%
Grad before 2010	17.3%	7.8–36.7%

Top 3 types of work performed by RNs	
Type	Overall average
School nurse	38.0%
Public health/Community health	38.0%
Urgent care	23.9%

Population-based health		
	Average	Range
All nurses	14.5%	5.3–36.5%
Grad after 2010	15.8%	0.0–42.1%
Grad before 2010	13.9%	5.5–38.7%

Top 3 types of work performed by RNs	
Type	Overall average
School nurse	23.7%
Public health/Community health	36.5%
Health care management/Administration	22.1%

Mental health		
	Average	Range
All nurses	24.5%	8.9–51.2%
Grad after 2010	30.6%	0.0–51.9%
Grad before 2010	21.7%	5.3–51.1%

Top 3 types of work performed by RNs	
Type	Overall average
School nurse	51.2%
Emergency	44.2%
Public health/Community health	38.0%

Working in underserved communities		
	Average	Range
All nurses	14.1%	6.9–37.5%
Grad after 2010	16.7%	5.9–47.3%
Grad before 2010	12.9%	2.7–38.1%

Top 3 types of work performed by RNs	
Type	Overall average
School nurse	28.0%
Public health/Community health	37.5%
Emergency	22.6%

Caring for medically complex/special needs patients		
	Average	Range
All nurses	28.7%	9.7–39.8%
Grad after 2010	34.2%	7.5–52.0%
Grad before 2010	26.1%	9.9–37.4%

Top 3 types of work performed by RNs	
Type	Overall average
Sub-acute care	39.8%
Public health/Community health	38.1%
Step-down/transitional	37.2%

Value-based care		
	Average	Range
All nurses	15.3%	5.9–24.4%
Grad after 2010	15.2%	1.4–30.0%
Grad before 2010	15.3%	6.3–25.3%

Top 3 types of work performed by RNs	
Type	Overall average
Informatics	24.4%
Health care management/Administration	24.3%
Education	16.7%

FIGURE 7-1 Training topics that would have helped registered nurses do their jobs better, by type of work performed and graduation from their nursing program, 2018.
SOURCE: Calculations based on the 2018 National Sample Survey of Registered Nurses (HRSA, 2020).

care for people facing multiple social risk factors that harm their health and well-being, or inadequacy of the training in these areas that RNs had received. RNs—particularly those working in informatics, health care management and administration, and education—also indicated that training in value-based care would have been helpful. Additionally, RNs who had graduated after 2010 were more likely than those who had graduated before then to indicate that they could have done their job better with training across all of these topics.

Nurse practitioners (NPs) have also indicated the need for more training in SDOH. In response to the 2018 NSSRN question described above, NPs working in public health and community health, emergency and urgent care, education, and long-term care reported that they could have done their job better if they had received training in SDOH, mental health, working in underserved communities, and providing care for medically complex/special needs. Across all types of practice settings, one-third felt that training in mental health issues would have helped them do their job better, while very few NPs indicated that training in value-based care would have been helpful. Additionally, NPs who had graduated since 2010 were more likely than those who had graduated before then to indicate that they would have benefited from training in these topics. Figure 7-2 shows the percentage of six different training topics that NPs mentioned would have helped them do their job better.

APRN Training Topics

Social determinants of health (e.g., impact of race and social-economic status)		
	Average	Range
All nurses	20.2%	11.9–30.3%
Grad after 2010	21.1%	11.8–28.4%
Grad before 2010	19.1%	12.1–33.4%

Top 3 types of work performed by NPs	
Type	Overall average
Public health/Community health	30.3%
Home health/hospice	27.8%
Education	23.1%

Population-based health		
	Average	Range
All nurses	14.4%	7.5–30.1%
Grad after 2010	15.4%	7.7–35.2%
Grad before 2010	13.1%	7.2–29.8%

Top 3 types of work performed by NPs	
Type	Overall average
Public health/Community health	30.1%
Education	31.7%
Home health/hospice	19.9%

Mental health		
	Average	Range
All nurses	33.4%	10.7–44.9%
Grad after 2010	35.3%	13.2–52.1%
Grad before 2010	31.1%	8.0–39.4%

Top 3 types of work performed by NPs	
Type	Overall average
Public health/Community health	44.9%
Ambulatory care	39.4%
Long-term care/nursing care	39.3%

Working in underserved communities		
	Average	Range
All nurses	17.0%	6.5–43.0%
Grad after 2010	19.4%	8.1–44.7%
Grad before 2010	14.0%	4.2–40.1%

Top 3 types of work performed by NPs	
Type	Overall average
Home health/hospice	43.0%
Public health/Community health	28.8%
Education	24.9%

Caring for medically complex/special needs patients		
	Average	Range
All nurses	36.3%	26.1–49.7%
Grad after 2010	38.4%	28.1–47.1%
Grad before 2010	33.6%	21.3–53.0%

Top 3 types of work performed by NPs	
Type	Overall average
Home health/hospice	46.9%
Long-term care/nursing care	49.7%
Emergency	39.5%

Value-based care		
	Average	Range
All nurses	14.9%	11.8–20.9%
Grad after 2010	15.8%	11.9–21.3%
Grad before 2010	13.9%	10.5–24.3%

Top 3 types of work performed by NPs	
Type	Overall average
Urgent care	20.9%
Education	20.8%
Long-term care/nursing care	16.5%

FIGURE 7-2 Training topics that would have helped nurse practitioners do their jobs better, by type of work performed and graduation from their nursing education program, 2018.
SOURCE: Calculations based on the 2018 National Sample Survey of Registered Nurses (HRSA, 2020).

The Need for Integration of Social Determinants of Health and Health Equity into Nursing Education

Despite guidelines from both the American Association of Colleges of Nursing (AACN) and the National League for Nursing (NLN) and numerous calls for including equity, population health, and SDOH in nursing education, SDOH and related concepts are not currently well integrated into undergraduate and graduate nursing education. Nor has the degree to which nurses are prepared and educated in these areas been studied systematically (NACNEP, 2019; Tilden et al., 2018). The committee was unable to locate a central repository of information about the coursework and other educational experiences available to nursing students across types of programs and institutions, or any other source of systematic analysis of nursing curricula. This lack of information about nursing preparation programs limits the conclusions that can be drawn about them. Thus, the discussion in this chapter is based on the assumption that some nursing programs are likely already pursuing many of the goals identified herein, but that this critically important content is not yet standard practice throughout nursing education.

One way to explore whether and how health equity and related concepts are currently integrated into nursing education is to look at accreditation standards. While the standards do not detail every specific topic to be covered in nursing curricula, they do set expectations, convey priorities, and identify important areas of study. For example, the accreditation standards of the CCNE state that advanced practice registered nurse (APRN) programs must include study of advanced physiology, advanced health assessment, and advanced pharmacology (CCNE, 2018). Accreditation standards could be used to prioritize the inclusion of health equity and SDOH in nursing curriculum; however, this is not currently the case. The CCNE standards state that accredited programs must incorporate the AACN *Essentials* into their curricula, and while these standards do not specifically mention equity, SDOH, or other relevant concepts (CCNE, 2018), that is expected to change to correspond with the updates to the *Essentials* described previously (see Box 7-1). CNEA's accreditation standards likewise include no mention of population health, SDOH, or health equity (NLN, 2016), although a more recent document from NLN makes a strong case for the integration of SDOH into nursing education curricula (NLN, 2019). ACEN's associate's and baccalaureate standards call for inclusion of "cultural, ethnic, and socially diverse concepts" in the curriculum; the master's and doctoral standards require that curriculum be "designed so that graduates of the program are able to practice in a culturally and ethnically diverse global society," but do not address health equity, population health, or SDOH.

Another approach for examining the inclusion of these concepts in nursing education is to look at exemplar programs. As part of the Future of Nursing: Campaign for Action, the Robert Wood Johnson Foundation commissioned a study of best practices in nursing education to support population health (Campaign for

Action, 2019b). That report notes that although many nursing programs reported including population health content in their curriculum, few incorporated the topic substantially. However, the report also identifies exemplars of programs with promising population health models. These exemplars include Oregon Health & Science University, which incorporates population health throughout the curriculum as a key competency; Rush University, which incorporates cultural competence throughout the curriculum; and Thomas Jefferson University, which offers courses in health promotion, population health, health disparities, and SDOH. NACNEP has also examined exemplars of nursing programs that incorporate health equity and SDOH into their curricula (NACNEP, 2019). The programs highlighted include the University of Pennsylvania School of Nursing, which has a course called Case Study—Addressing the Social Determinants of Health: Community Engagement Immersion (Schroeder et al., 2019). This course offers experiential learning opportunities that focus on SDOH in vulnerable and underserved populations and helps students design health promotion programs for these communities. The school also offers faculty education in SDOH.

As far as the committee was able to determine, most programs include content on SDOH in community or public health nursing courses. However, this material does not appear to be integrated thoroughly into the curriculum in the majority of programs, nor could the committee identify well-established designs for curricula that address this content outside of community health rotations (Campaign for Action, 2019b; Storfjell et al., 2017; Thornton and Persaud, 2018). In the committee's view, a single course in community and/or public health nursing is insufficient preparation for creating a foundational understanding of health equity and for preparing nurses to work in the wide variety of settings and roles envisioned in this report. Ideally, education in these concepts would be integrated throughout the curriculum to give nurses a comprehensive understanding of the social determinants that contribute to health inequities (NACNEP, 2019; NLN, 2019; Siegel et al., 2018). Moreover, academic content alone is insufficient to provide students with the knowledge, skills, and abilities they need to advance health equity; rather, expanded opportunities for experiential and community learning are critical for building the necessary competencies (Buhler-Wilkerson, 1993; Fee and Bu, 2010; NACNEP, 2016; Sharma et al., 2018). All those involved in nursing education—administrators, faculty, accreditors, and students—need to understand that health equity is a core component of nursing, no less important than alleviating pain or caring for individuals with acute illness. Graduating students need to understand and apply knowledge of the impact of such issues as classism, racism, sexism, ageism, and discrimination and to be empowered to advocate on these issues for people who they care for and communities.

As currently constituted, then, nursing education programs fall short of conveying this information sufficiently in the curriculum or through experiential learning opportunities. Yet, the existing evidence on what nursing education programs offer is scant. Research is therefore needed to assess whether and how many nursing programs are offering sufficient coursework and learning opportunities related to SDOH and health equity and to examine the extent to which graduating nurses have the competencies necessary to address these issues in practice.

The Need for BSN-Prepared Nurses

The 2011 *The Future of Nursing* report includes the recommendation that the percentage of nurses who hold a baccalaureate degree or higher be increased to 80 percent by 2020. The report gives several reasons for this goal, including that baccalaureate-prepared nurses are exposed to competencies including health policy, leadership, and systems thinking; they have skills in research, teamwork, and collaboration; and they are better equipped to meet the increasingly complex demands of care both inside and outside the hospital (IOM, 2011, p. 170). In 2011, 50 percent of employed nurses held a baccalaureate degree or higher; as of 2019, that proportion had increased to 59 percent (Campaign for Action, 2020). Both the number of baccalaureate programs and program enrollment have increased substantially since 2011[2] (AACN, 2019a), and the number of RNs who went on to receive BSNs in RN-to-BSN programs increased 236 percent between 2009 and 2019 (Campaign for Action, n.d.). However, the goal of 80 percent of nurses holding a BSN was still not achieved by 2020, for a number of reasons. Although the proportion of new graduates with a BSN is higher than the proportion of existing nurses with a BSN, the percentage of new graduates joining the nursing workforce each year is small. Given this ratio, it would have been "extraordinarily difficult" to achieve the goal of 80 percent by 2020 (IOM, 2016a; McMenamin, 2015). Nurses already in the workforce face barriers to pursuing a BSN, including time, money, work–life balance, and a perception that additional postlicense education is not worth the effort (Duffy et al., 2014; Spetz, 2018). Moreover, schools and programs have limited capacity for first-time nursing students and ADN, LPN nurses, or RNs without BSN degrees (Spetz, 2018).

Nonetheless, the goal of achieving a nursing workforce in which 80 percent of nurses hold a baccalaureate degree or higher remains relevant, and continuing efforts to increase the number of nurses with a BSN are needed. Across the globe, the proportion of BSN-educated nurses is correlated with better health outcomes (Aiken et al., 2017; Baker et al., 2020), and there are clear differences as well as similarities between associate's degree in nursing (ADN) programs and BSN programs. In particular, BSN programs are more likely to cover topics relevant to liberal education, organizational and systems leadership, evidence-based practice, health care policy, finance and regulatory environments, interprofessional collaboration, and population health (Kumm et al., 2014). Accelerated, nontraditional, and other pathways to the BSN degree are discussed later in this chapter.

---

[2] See Chapter 3 for demographic information on employed nurses in the United States.

The Need for PhD-Prepared Nurses

There are two types of doctoral degrees in nursing: the PhD and the DNP. The former is designed to prepare nurse scientists to conduct research, whereas the latter is a clinically focused doctoral degree designed to prepare graduates with advanced competencies in leadership and management, quality improvement, evidence-based practice, and a variety of specialties. PhD-prepared nurses are essential to the development of the research base required to support evidence-based practice and add to the body of nursing knowledge, and DNP-educated nurses play a key role in translating evidence into practice and in educating nursing students in practice fundamentals (Tyczkowski and Reilly, 2017) (see Chapter 3 for further discussion of the role of DNPs).

The number of nurses with doctoral degrees has grown rapidly since the 2011 *The Future of Nursing* report was published (IOM, 2011). As a proportion of doctorally educated nurses, however, the number of PhD graduates has remained nearly flat. In 2010, there were 1,282 graduates from DNP programs and 532 graduates receiving a PhD in nursing. By 2019, the number of DNP graduates had grown more than 500 percent to 7,944, while the number of PhD graduates had grown about 50 percent to 804 (AACN, 2011, 2020a).

The slow growth in PhD-prepared nurses is a major concern for the profession and for the nation, because it is these nurses who serve as faculty at many universities and who systematically study issues related to health and health care, including the impact of SDOH on health outcomes, health disparities, and health equity. PhD-prepared nurses conduct research on a wide variety of issues relating to SDOH, including the effect of class on children's health; linguistic, cultural, and educational barriers to care; models of care for older adults aging in place; and gun violence (Richmond and Foman, 2018; RWJF, 2020; Szanton et al., 2014). Nurse-led research provided evidence-based solutions in the early days of the COVID-19 pandemic for such challenges as the shift to telehealth care, expanding demand for health care workers, and increased moral distress (Lake, 2020). However, Castro-Sánchez and colleagues (2021) note a dearth of nurse-led research specifically related to COVID-19; they posit that this gap can be attributed to workforce shortages, a lack of investment in clinical academic leadership, and the redeployment of nurses into clinical roles. More PhD-prepared nurses are needed to conduct research aimed at improving clinical and community health, as well as to serve as faculty to educate the next generation of nurses (Broome and Fairman, 2018; Fairman et al., 2020; Greene et al., 2017).

Nursing practice is dependent on a robust pipeline of research to advance evidence-based care, inform policy, and address the health needs of people and communities (Bednash et al., 2014). The creation of the BSN-to-PhD direct entry option has helped produce more research-oriented nurse faculty (Greene et al., 2017), but time, adequate faculty mentorship, mental health issues, and financial hardships, including the cost of tuition, are barriers for nurses pursuing these advanced degrees (Broome and Fairman, 2018; Fairman et al., 2020; Squires et al., 2013). One approach for increasing the number of PhD-prepared nurses is the Future of Nursing Scholars program, which successfully graduated approximately 200 PhD students through an innovative accelerated 3-year program (RWJF, 2021). Similar programs have been funded by such foundations as the Hillman Foundation and Jonas Philanthropies to help stimulate the pipeline, build capacity (especially in health policy) among graduates, and model innovative curricular approaches (Broome and Fairman, 2018; Fairman et al., 2020).

DOMAINS AND COMPETENCIES FOR EQUITY

As noted earlier, a number of existing recommendations specify what nurses need to know to address SDOH and health inequity in a meaningful way. In addition, the Future of Nursing: Campaign for Action surveyed and interviewed faculty and leaders in nursing and public health, asking about core content and competencies for all nurses (Campaign for Action, 2019b). Respondents specifically recommended that nursing education cover seven areas:

- policy and its impact on health outcomes;
- epidemiology and biostatistics;
- a basic understanding of SDOH and illness across populations and how to assess and intervene to improve health and well-being;
- health equity as an overall goal of health care;
- interprofessional team building as a key mechanism for improving population health;
- the economics of health care, including an understanding of basic payment models and their impact on services delivered and outcomes achieved; and
- systems thinking, including the ability to understand complex demands, develop solutions, and manage change at the micro and macro system levels.

Drawing on all of these recommendations, guidelines, and perspectives, as well as looking at the anticipated roles and responsibilities outlined in other chapters of this report, the committee identified the core concepts pertaining to SDOH, health equity, and population health that need to be covered in nursing school and the core knowledge and skills that nurses need to have upon graduation. For consistency with the language used by the AACN, these are referred to, respectively, as "domains" (see Box 7-2) and "competencies" (see Box 7-3). The domains in Box 7-2 are fundamental content that the committee believes can no longer be covered in public health courses alone, but need to be incorporated and applied by nursing students throughout nursing curricula. All nurses, regardless of setting or type of nursing, need to understand and be prepared to address the underlying barriers to better health in their practice.

BOX 7-2
Domains for Nursing Education

- Health equity and health care equity
- Social determinants of health
- Social needs
- Social justice
- Racism, ageism, classism, sexism
- Implicit bias
- Ethics
- Population health
- Environmental health
- Disasters/public health emergencies
- Nurse well-being

BOX 7-3
Competencies for Nursing Education, Depending on Preparation Level

- Population health
  - Aging competencies
  - Mental and behavioral health competencies
  - Community/public health nursing competencies
- Health systems (domestic and international)
  - Health economics
- Human-centered design thinking
  - Innovation mindset
  - Developing, implementing, and scaling interventions
- Continually adapting to new technologies
  - Using digital health tools
- Delivering person-centered care to diverse populations
  - Cultural humility
  - Awareness of implicit bias
  - Trauma-informed care
  - Motivational interviewing
- Collaborating across professions, disciplines, and sectors
  - Teamwork among health care providers and community partners
  - Interpersonal communication skills
  - Conflict resolution skills
  - Partnership development (interprofessional and multisector)
- Health policy and advocacy
- Preparedness for and response to natural disasters and public health emergencies
- Nurse well-being

The committee believes that incorporation of these domains and competencies can guide expeditious and meaningful changes in nursing education. The committee acknowledges that making room for these concepts will inevitably require eliminating some existing material in nursing education. The committee does not believe that it is the appropriate entity to identify what specific curriculum changes should be made; a nationwide evaluation will be needed to ensure that nursing curricula are preparing the future workforce with the skills and competencies they will need. The committee also acknowledges that nursing programs differ in length, and that an ADN program cannot cover SDOH equity to the same extent as a BSN program. The specific knowledge and skills a nurse will need will vary depending on her or his level of nursing education. For example, a nurse with a BSN may need to understand and be able to use the technologies that are relevant to his or her area of work (e.g., telehealth applications, electronic health records [EHRs], home monitors), while an APRN may need a deeper understanding of how to analyze health records in order to provide care and monitor health status for populations outside clinical settings.

Nonetheless, nursing education at all levels—from licensed practical nurse (LPN) to ADN to BSN and beyond—needs to incorporate and integrate the domains and competencies in Boxes 7-2 and 7-3 to the extent possible so as to develop knowledge and skills that will be relevant and useful to nurses and essential to achieving equity in health and health care. Given the relationship among SDOH, social needs, and health outcomes and the increasing focus of health care systems on addressing these community and individual needs, the domains and competencies identified here are essential to ensure that all nurses understand and can apply concepts related to these issues; work effectively with people, families, and communities across the spectrum of SDOH; promote physical, mental, and social health; and assume leadership and entrepreneurial roles to create solutions, such as by fostering partnerships in the health and social sectors, scaling successful interventions, and engaging in policy development. While none of the domains listed in Box 7-2 are new to nursing, the health inequities that have become increasingly visible—especially as a result of the COVID-19 pandemic—demand that these domains now be substantively integrated into the fabric of nursing education and practice.

Many sources highlight both the challenges faced by front-line graduates when confronted with these issues, and the reality that many nursing schools lack faculty members with the knowledge and competencies to educate nurses effectively on these issues (Befus et al., 2019; Effland et al., 2020; Hermer et al., 2020; Levine et al., 2020; Porter et al., 2020; Rosa et al., 2019; Valderama-Wallace and Apesoa-Varano, 2019). To remedy the latter gap, educators need to have a clear understanding of these issues and their links to both educational and patient outcomes (see the section below on strengthening and diversifying the nursing faculty). It is important to note as well that some of these topics, including the connections among implicit biases, structural racism, and health equity, may be difficult for educators and students to discuss (see Box 7-4).

BOX 7-4
Discussing Difficult Topics

Educators and students may find it uncomfortable or difficult to grapple with some of the health equity–related domains listed in Box 7-2. For example, discussions about the impact of racism on health and health care or about individual biases could lead to discomfort, guilt, anger, or feelings of helplessness. White students may experience heightened sensitivity when faced with discussions on racism; the term "White privilege" in particular may induce anger, defensiveness, and resistance (Burnett et al., 2020). This "White fragility" has been recognized as a substantial barrier to open discussions about the causes of and solutions for social inequity (DiAngelo, 2011, 2018; Peek et al., 2020). Students from underserved racial and ethnic groups, who are likely to be underrepresented in the classroom, may also feel uncomfortable discussing these issues or feel the burden of speaking for their entire group (Ackerman-Barger et al., 2020; Peek et al., 2020).

Peek and colleagues (2020) offer recommendations for successfully teaching about race and racism by balancing "emotional safety and honest truth-telling." Their recommendations include the following:

- Create a psychologically safe learning space, and create expectations for civil discourse.
- Take the individual blame out of the conversation about bias and racism.
- Talk about race as a social construct before talking about racism.
- Engage in "free, frank, and fearless discussions" about structural racism, colonialism, and White privilege.
- Teach about systems, not just interpersonal cultural humility.
- Teach about solutions and how to be a leader and an advocate.

Given the limited scope of this report, the committee has chosen to highlight three of the competencies from Box 7-3 in this section.[3] The first is delivering person-centered care to diverse populations. As the United States becomes increasingly diverse, nurses will need to be aware of their own implicit biases and be able to interact with diverse patients, families, and communities with empathy and humility. The second is learning to collaborate across professions, disciplines, and sectors. As discussed previously in this report, addressing SDOH is necessarily a multisectoral endeavor given that these determinants go beyond health to include such issues as housing, education, justice, and the environment. The third is continually adapting to new technologies. Advances in technology are reshaping both health care and education, and making it possible for both to

[3] For further discussion of domains and competencies, see AACN, 2020b; Campaign for Action, 2019b; IOM, 2016b; NACNEP, 2019; NLN, 2019; Thornton and Persaud, 2018.

be delivered in nontraditional settings and nontraditional ways. In the present context, technology can expand access to underserved populations of patients and students—for example, telehealth and online platforms can be used to connect with those living in rural areas—but it can also exacerbate existing disparities and inequities. Nurses need to understand both the promises and perils of technology, and be able to adapt their practice and learning accordingly.

Delivering Person-Centered Care and Education to Diverse Populations

As discussed in Chapter 2, people's family and cultural background, community, and other experiences may have profound impacts on their health. Given the increasing diversity of the U.S. population, it is critical that nurses understand the impact of these factors on health, can communicate and connect with people of different backgrounds, and can be self-reflective about how their own beliefs and biases may affect the care they provide. To this end, the committee believes it is essential that nursing education include the concepts of cultural humility and implicit bias as a thread throughout the curriculum.

An integral part of learning about these concepts is an opportunity to reflect on what one is learning and to draw connections with past learning and experiences. Researchers have established that instruction that guides students in reflection helps reinforce skills and competencies (see, e.g., NASEM, 2018c). This idea has been explored in the context of education in health professions and has been identified as a valuable way to foster understanding of health equity and SDOH (IOM, 2016b; Mann et al., 2007). While the strategies, goals, and structure of such reflection may vary, the process in general helps learners in health care settings examine their own values, assumptions, and beliefs (El-Sayed and El-Sayed, 2014; Scheel et al., 2017). In the course of structured reflection, for example, students might consider how such issues as racism, implicit bias, trauma, and policy affect the care people receive and create conditions for poor health, or how their own experiences and identities influence the care they provide.

Cultural Humility

In recent years, the focus in discussions of patient care has shifted from *cultural competency* to *cultural humility* (Barton et al., 2020; Brennan et al., 2012; Kamau-Small et al., 2015; Periyakoil, 2019; Purnell et al., 2018; Walker et al., 2016). The concept of cultural competency has been interpreted by some as limited for a number of reasons. First, it implies that "culture" is a technical skill in which clinicians can develop expertise, and it can become a series of static dos and don'ts (Kleinman and Benson, 2006). Second, the concept of cultural competency tends to promote a colorblind mentality that ignores the role of power, privilege, and racism in health care (Waite and Nardi, 2017). Third, cultural competency is not actively antiracist but instead leaves institutionalized structures of White privilege and racism intact (Schroeder and DiAngelo, 2010).

In contrast, cultural humility is defined by flexibility, a lifelong approach to learning about diversity, and a recognition of the role of individual bias and systemic power in health care interactions (Agner, 2020). Cultural humility is considered a self-evaluating process that recognizes the self within the context of culture (Campinha-Bacote, 2018). The concept of cultural humility can be woven into most aspects of nursing and interprofessional education. For example, case studies in which students learn about the experience of a particular disease or strategies for disease prevention can be designed to model culturally humble approaches in the provision of nursing care and the avoidance of stereotypical thinking (Foronda et al., 2016; Mosher et al., 2017). One effective approach to cultivating cultural humility is to accompany experiential learning opportunities or case studies with reflection that expands learning beyond skills and knowledge. This includes questioning current practices and proposing changes to improve the efficiency and quality of care, equality, and social justice (Barton et al., 2020; Foronda et al., 2013). Programs designed to develop nurses' cultural sensitivity and humility, as well as cultural immersion programs, have been developed, and research suggests that such programs can effectively develop skills that strengthen nurses' confidence in treating diverse populations, improve patient and provider relationships, and increase nurses' compassion (Allen, 2010; Gallagher and Polanin, 2015; Sanner et al., 2010).

Implicit Bias

Implicit bias is an unconscious or automatic mental association made between members of a group and an attribute or evaluation (FitzGerald and Hurst, 2017). For example, a clinician may unconsciously view White patients as more medically compliant than Black patients (Sabin et al., 2008). These types of biases not only can have consequences for individual health outcomes (Aaberg, 2012; Linden and Redpath, 2011) but also may play a role in maintaining or exacerbating health disparities (Blair et al., 2011). There are many resources available for implicit bias awareness and training; for example, Harvard University offers a number of Implicit Association Tests (IATs), the Institute for Healthcare Improvement offers free online resources to address implicit bias, and the AACN offers implicit bias workshops for nurses (AACN, n.d.; Foronda et al., 2018).

Evidence on the use of implicit bias training is limited. One review of the use of an IAT in health professions education found that the test had contrasting uses, with some curricula using it as a measure of implicit bias and others using it to initiate discussions and reflection. The review found a dearth of research on the use of IATs; the authors note that the nature of implicit bias is highly complex and cannot necessarily be reduced to the "time-limited" use of an IAT (Sukhera et al., 2019). A systematic review of interventions designed to reduce implicit bias found that many such interventions are ineffective, and some may even increase implicit biases. The authors note that while there is no clear path for reducing biases, the lack of evidence does not weaken the case for "implementing widespread structural and institutional changes that are likely to reduce implicit biases" (FitzGerald et al., 2019). One promising model is an intervention that helps participants break the "prejudice habit" (Devine et al., 2012). This multifaceted intervention, which includes situational awareness of bias, education about the consequences of bias, strategies for reducing bias, and self-reflection, has been shown to reduce implicit racial bias for at least 2 months (Devine et al., 2012). Clearly, more research is needed in this area.

Learning to Collaborate Across Professions, Disciplines, and Sectors

As discussed in Chapter 9, eliminating health disparities will require the active engagement and advocacy of a broad range of stakeholders working in partnership to address the drivers of structural inequities in health and health care (NASEM, 2017). In these efforts, nurses may lead or work with people from a variety of professions, disciplines, and sectors, including, for example, physicians, social workers, educators, policy makers, lawyers, faith leaders, government employees, community advocates, and community members. Working across sectors, especially as they relate to SDOH (food insecurity, transportation barriers, housing, etc.), is a critical competence. Collaboration among these types of stakeholders has multiple benefits, including broader expertise and perspective, the capacity to address wide-ranging social needs, the ability to reach underserved populations, and sustainability and alignment of efforts (see Chapter 9 for further discussion). A traditional nursing education, which focuses on what is taught rather than on building competencies, is unlikely to give students the understanding of broader social, political, and environmental contexts that is necessary for working in these types of strategic partnerships (IOM, 2016b). If nursing students are to be prepared to practice interprofessionally after graduation, they must be given opportunities to collaborate with others before graduation (IOM, 2013) and to build the competencies they will need for collaborative practice. The Interprofessional Education Collaborative (IPEC) identified four core competencies for interprofessional collaborative practice (IPEC, 2016). While these competencies were developed specifically to prepare students for interprofessional practice within health care, they are also applicable to broader collaborations among other professions, disciplines, and sectors both within and outside of health care:

- Work with individuals of other professions to maintain a climate of mutual respect and shared values.
- Use the knowledge of one's own role and those of other professionals to appropriately assess and address the health care needs of patients and to promote and advance the health of populations.

- Communicate with patients, families, communities, and professionals in health and other fields in a responsive and responsible manner that supports a team approach to the promotion and maintenance of health and the prevention and treatment of disease.
- Apply relationship-building values and the principles of team dynamics to perform effectively in different team roles in planning, delivering, and evaluating patient/population-centered care and population health programs and policies that are safe, timely, efficient, effective, and equitable.

There are opportunities for nursing students to gain interprofessional and multisector collaborative competencies through both experiential learning in the community (discussed in detail below) and classroom work. Increasingly, nursing schools are working with other institutions to offer students classes in which they learn with or from students and professionals in other disciplines. For example, the University of Michigan Center for Interprofessional Education offers courses in such topics as health care delivery in low- and middle-income countries, social justice, trauma-informed practice, interprofessional communication, and teamwork. Courses are open to students from the schools of social work, pharmacy, medicine, nursing, dentistry, physical therapy, public health, and business.[4]

Despite the benefits of interprofessional education, however, there are barriers that affect the implementation of such programs in health professions education, including different schedules, lack of meeting space, incongruent curricula plans, faculty not trained to teach interprofessionally, faculty overload, and the challenge of providing adequate opportunities for all levels of students (NLN, 2015a). The use of simulation has been proposed as a vehicle for overcoming such barriers to impart interprofessional collaborative competencies (NLN, 2013); a systematic review of the evidence found that this approach can be effective (Marion-Martins and Pinho, 2020). Nurses can also gain interprofessional experience by pursuing dual degrees. For example, the University of Pennsylvania offers dual degrees that combine nursing with health care management, bioethics, public health, law, or business administration.

Continually Adapting to New Technologies

Nurses can use a wide variety of existing and emerging technologies and tools to address SDOH and provide high-quality care to all patients (see Box 7-5). Broadly speaking, these technologies and tools fall into three categories: patient-facing, clinician-facing, and data analytics. Patient- and clinician-facing tools collect data and help providers and patients connect and make decisions

[4] Not all courses are open to students from all schools.

BOX 7-5
Highlights from the Seattle Townhall on Technology and Health Equity and Implications for Nursing Education

At a town hall information-gathering session convened by the committee in Seattle, Washington, on August 7, 2019, the dean of nursing and health sciences at Nassau Community College, Dr. Kenya Beard, discussed opportunities and challenges associated with advancing health equity. She observed that although all individuals should have the right to achieve their highest level of health, every day that fundamental right is denied to more than a few individuals. Discussing technology that can help improve health equity, she described the benefits of apps that help manage a patient's condition, inform patients whether their symptoms warrant a visit to the emergency room, and allow patients to confirm appointments and view test results. However, she also stressed that nurses must become more "tech literate" and "ask critical questions and consider how high-tech tools could amplify existing inequities, harming the vulnerable populations we seek to help." Beard shared an example of a patient who spoke limited English and sought a doctor's appointment. She was told her appointment had been canceled since she had failed to confirm it when contacted by phone and text. Although the patient communicated that she had not understood the message, she was still sent home.

Dr. Molly Coye, executive-in-residence at Advancing Health Care Equity in the Digital Age, discussed the emerging patterns of digitally enabled care that will profoundly change the roles and responsibilities of nurses and other clinicians. She shared several examples of technological tools, including text-based primary care; a virtual triage app that uses a chatbot; and a program in which poor, dual-eligible women were given smartphones and asked to take pictures of their medications each day in exchange for cash payments. This medication adherence program was very successful in decreasing emergency room visits and hospitalizations, said Coye.

about care. Data analytics uses data, collected from patients or other sources, to analyze trends, identify disparities, and guide policy decisions. Beginning as students, all nurses need to be familiar with these technologies, be able to engage with patients or other professionals around their appropriate use, and understand how their use has the potential to exacerbate inequalities.

Patient-facing technologies include apps and software, such as mobile and wearable health devices, as well as telehealth and virtual visit technologies (FDA, 2020). These tools allow nurses and other health care providers to expand their reach to those who might otherwise not have access because of geography, transportation, social support, or other challenges. For example, telehealth and mobile apps allow providers to see people in their homes, mitigating such barriers to care as transportation while also helping providers understand people in the context of their everyday lives. Essential skills for nurses using these new tools will include the ability to project a caring relationship through technology (Massachusetts Department of Higher Nursing Education Initiative, 2016) and to use technology to personalize care based on patient preferences, technology access, and individual needs (NLN, 2015b). The role of telehealth and the importance of training nurses in this technology have been recognized for several years (NONPF, 2018; Rutledge et al., 2017), but the urgent need for telehealth services during the COVID-19 pandemic has made it "imperative" to include telehealth training in nursing curricula (Love and Carrington, 2020). Moreover, it is anticipated that the shift to telehealth for some types of care will become a permanent feature of the health care system in the future (Bestsennyy et al., 2020).

Clinician-facing technologies include EHRs, clinical decision support tools, mobile apps, and screening and referral tools (Bresnick, 2017; CDC, 2018; Heath, 2019). A number of available digital technologies can facilitate the collection and integration of data on social needs and SDOH and help clinicians hold compassionate and empathetic conversations about those needs (AHA, 2019; Giovenco and Spillane, 2019). In 2019, for example, Kaiser Permanente launched its Thrive Local network (Kaiser Permanente, 2019), which can be used to screen for social needs and connect people with community resources that can meet these needs. The system is integrated with the EHR, and it is capable of tracking referrals and outcomes to measure whether needs are being met; these data can then be used to continuously improve the network.

Nurses will need to understand how and when to use these types of tools, and can leverage their unique understanding of patient and community needs to improve and expand them. As described in Chapter 10, such technologies as EHRs and clinical alarms can burden nurses and contribute to workplace stress. However, nurses have largely been left out of conversations about how to design and use these systems. For example, although nurses are one of the primary users of EHR systems, little research has been conducted to understand their experiences with and perceptions of these systems, which may be different from those of other health care professionals (Cho et al., 2016; Higgins et al., 2017). Out of 346 usability studies on health care technologies conducted between 2003 and 2009, only 2 examined use by nurses (Yen and Bakken, 2012). Educating nurses to understand and assess the benefits and drawbacks of health care technologies and have the capacity to help shape and revamp them can ultimately improve patient care and the well-being of health professionals.

Tools for *data analytics* are increasingly important for improving patient care and the health of populations (Ibrahim et al., 2020; NEJM Catalyst, 2018). Analysis of large amounts of data from such sources as EHRs, wearable monitors, and surveys can help in detecting and tracking disease trends, identifying disparities, and finding patterns of correlation (Breen et al., 2019; NASEM, 2016a; Shiffrin, 2016). The North Carolina Institute for Public Health, for example, collaborated with a local health system in analyzing data to inform a community health improvement plan (Wallace et al., 2019). Data on 12 SDOH indicators were sourced from the American Community Survey and mapped by census tract. The mapping provided a visualization of the disparities in the community and allowed the health system to focus its efforts strategically to improve community health. The North Carolina Department of Health and Human Services later replicated this strategy across the entire state (NCDHHS, 2020).

There are opportunities for nurses to specialize in this type of work. For example, nursing informatics is a specialized area of practice in which nurses with expertise in such disciplines as information science, management, and analytical sciences use their skills to assess patient care and organizational procedures and identify ways to improve the quality and efficiency of care. In the context of SDOH, nursing informaticists will be needed to leverage artificial intelligence and advanced visualization methods to summarize and contextualize SDOH data in a way that provides actionable insights while also eliminating bias and not overwhelming nurses with extraneous information. Big data are increasingly prevalent in health care, and nurses need the skills and competencies to capitalize on its potential (Topaz and Pruinelli, 2017). Even nurses who do not specialize in informatics will need to understand how the analysis of massive datasets can impact health (Forman et al., 2020; NLN, 2015b). Investments in expanding program offerings, certifications, and student enrollment will be needed to meet the demand for nurses with such skills.

As noted, however, despite its promise for improving patient care and community health, technology can also exacerbate existing disparities (Ibrahim et al., 2020). For example, people who lack access to broadband Internet and/or devices are unable to take advantage of such technologies as remote monitoring and telehealth appointments (Wise, 2012). Older adults, people with limited formal education, those living in rural and remote areas, and the poor are less likely to have access to the Internet. As health care becomes more reliant on technology, these groups are likely to fall behind (Arcaya and Figueroa, 2017). In addition, such technologies as artificial intelligence and algorithmic decision-making tools may exacerbate inequities by reflecting existing biases (Ibrahim et al., 2020). Nursing education needs to prepare nurses to understand these potential downsides of technology in order to prevent and mitigate them. This has become a particularly critical issue during the COVID-19 pandemic, with the rapid shift to telehealth potentially having consequences for those with low digital literacy, limited English proficiency, and a lack of access to the Internet (Velasquez and Mehrotra, 2020).

Not all nurses will need to acquire all of the key technological competencies; curricula can be developed according to the likely needs of nurses working at different levels. For example, most nurses will need the knowledge and skills to use telehealth, digital health tools, and data-driven clinical decision-making skills in practice, whereas nurse informaticians and some doctoral-level nurses will need to be versed in device design, bias assessment in algorithms, and big data analysis.

EXPANDING LEARNING OPPORTUNITIES

As stated previously, the domains and competencies enumerated above cannot be conveyed to nursing students through traditional lectures alone. Building the competencies to address population health, SDOH, and health inequities will require substantive experiential learning, collaborative learning, an integrated curriculum, and continuing professional development throughout nurses' careers (IOM, 2016b). The 2019 Campaign for Action survey of nursing educators and leaders found that a majority of respondents identified "innovative community clinical experiences" and "interprofessional education experiences" as the top methods for teaching population health (Campaign for Action, 2019b). A recurrent theme in interviews with respondents was the importance of active and experiential learning, with opportunities for partnering with nontraditional agencies (Campaign for Action, 2019b). These types of community-based educational opportunities, particularly when they involve partnerships with others, are critical for nursing education for multiple reasons.

First, experience in the community is essential to understanding SDOH and gaining the competencies necessary to advance health equity (IOM, 2016b). In fact, restricting education in SDOH to the classroom may even be harmful, given the finding of a 2016 study that medical students who learned about SDOH in the classroom rather than through experiential learning demonstrated an increase in negative attitudes toward medically underserved populations (Schmidt et al., 2016).

Second, community-based education offers opportunities for students to engage with community partners from other sectors, such as government offices of housing and transportation or community organizations, preparing them for the essential work of participating in and leading partnerships to address SDOH. An example is a pilot interdisciplinary partnership between a school of nursing and a city fire department in the Pacific Northwest that allows students to practice such skills as motivational interviewing to identify the range of problems (e.g., transportation issues, difficulty accessing insurance or providers, lack of caregiving support) faced by people calling emergency services (Yoder and Pesch, 2020).

Third, nursing is increasingly practiced in community settings, such as schools and workplaces, as well as through home health care (WHO, 2015). Nursing students are prepared to practice in hospitals, but do not necessarily receive the same training and preparation for these other environments (Bjørk et al., 2014). Education in the community allows nursing students to learn about the broad range of care environments and to work collaboratively with other professionals who work in these environments. For example, students may work in a team with community health workers, social workers, and those from other sectors (e.g., housing and transportation), work that both enriches the experience of student nurses and creates bridges between nursing and other fields (Zandee et al., 2010). Nurses who have these experiences during school may then be more prepared to lead and participate in multisector efforts to address SDOH—the importance of which is emphasized throughout this report—once they enter practice. Evidence suggests that graduating students are more likely to seek work in areas that are familiar to them from their education, clinical experience, and theoretical training (Jamshidi et al., 2016); thus, these nontraditional educational experiences may increase the number of nurses interested in working in the community. Moreover, while training in acute care settings has often been regarded as more valuable than that provided in community settings, evidence indicates that the two offer comparable opportunities for learning clinical skills (Morton et al., 2019). In fact, clinical care in community-based settings can present greater complexity relative to that in the hospital, and some technical skills (e.g., epidemiologic disease tracking, tuberculosis assessment and management, immunizations) are more available in community than in acute care settings (Morton et al., 2019).

Some nursing programs have incorporated community-based experiential learning into their programs. At community colleges and universities, schools have implemented nurse-managed clinics that serve the local population and their own students while also giving students technical skills and experience in interacting with the community. Lewis and Clark Community College, for example, operates a mobile health unit that brings health and dental care to six counties in southern Illinois (Lewis and Clark, n.d.), while nursing students at Alleghany College of Maryland can gain experience in the Nurse Managed Wellness Clinic, which offers such services as immunizations, screenings, and physicals (Alleghany College, 2020). At the baccalaureate and master's level, a number of schools offer longitudinal, integrated experiences in settings as varied as federally qualified health centers (FQHCs), public health departments, homeless shelters, public housing sites, public libraries, and residential addiction programs (AACN, 2020c). Students and faculty at the University of Washington School of Nursing, for example, support community-oriented projects in partnership with three underserved communities in the Seattle area. Graduate students work for 1 year on grassroots projects (e.g., food banks, school health) and then reinforce this experience with 1 year of work at the policy level (AACN, 2020c). At the doctoral level, Washburn University transformed its DNP curriculum to incorporate SDOH and reinforce that instruction through experiential learning in the community (see Box 7-6). In addition to clinical education, nursing students can participate in nontraditional clinical community engagement and service learning opportunities, such as volunteering at a homeless shelter or working in a service internship for a community organization. These opportunities get students into the community, help them build relationships with people from health care and other sectors, and promote understanding of and engagement with SDOH (Bandy, 2011).

BOX 7-6
Pine Ridge Family Health Center

In 2017, the Pine Ridge Family Health Center opened in Topeka, Kansas. The center was the result of a collaboration between Washburn University and the Topeka Housing Authority, and was aimed at serving individuals and families in the Topeka area, many of whom are poor, lack transportation, and do not have access to care elsewhere. The goal of the center is to meet the needs of community members and to address multiple social determinants of health. The center was built from the ground up through a collaboration among the university, the housing authority, the local community, local organizations, and residents of the public housing neighborhood in which the center is situated.

The center was envisioned as a place that would not only meet the health and social needs of community members but also serve as an educational opportunity for students from Washburn University. An interprofessional and interdisciplinary team of faculty from the School of Nursing, School of Business, Department of Communication Studies, Small Business Development Center, and Office of Sponsored Projects worked together to create a curriculum and develop the center. The curriculum included instruction in social justice, motivational interviewing, business ethics, leadership of self, crisis communication, and trauma-informed care, and students from the various departments and schools helped plan and organize the creation of the center. The team used a community-based participatory research model to engage community members at every step of development and ensure a focus on their needs.

The center is led by a nurse practitioner (NP) and is a dedicated training site for NP students at Washburn. In addition, a registered nurse (RN) was added to the team in 2019 to serve as a preceptor for bachelor of science in nursing (BSN) students, and the curriculum is being expanded to give students rotations in the center with a focus on social determinants of health.

SOURCES: NASEM, 2019; Personal communication between National Academies staff and Shirley Dinkel, Washburn University, November 2020.

Simulation-Based Education

Simulation-based education is another useful tool for teaching nursing concepts and developing competencies and skills (Kononowicz et al., 2019; Poore et al., 2014; Shin et al., 2015). It can range from very low-tech (e.g., using oranges to practice injections) to very high-tech (e.g., a virtual reality emergency room "game"), but all simulations share the ability to bridge the gap between education and practice by imparting skills in a low-risk environment (SSIH, n.d.).

Simulations give students an opportunity to make real-time decisions and interact with virtual patients without having to face many of the challenges of traditional clinical education (Hayden et al., 2014). They can be used to enhance many types of skills, including communication (NASEM, 2018b), cultural sensitivity (Lau et al., 2016), and screening for SDOH (Thornton and Persaud, 2018). Several simulation-based tools are available for learning about the realities of poverty, such as the Community Action Poverty Simulation (see Box 7-7) and the Cost of Poverty Experience (ThinkTank, n.d.). Such tools can help nurses identify ways in which their practice could directly mitigate the effects of poverty on individuals, families, and communities. Evaluations of poverty simulations have found that they can positively impact attitudes toward poverty and empathy among nurses and nursing students (Phillips et al., 2020; Turk and Colbert, 2018), although one study noted that the simulations should be accompanied by the inclusion of social justice concepts throughout the curriculum to achieve lasting change (Menzel et al., 2014).

Individual schools may or may not have the resources or faculty to support some types of simulation activities. For those that do not, simulation centers shared by schools of multiple professions and hospitals can provide access (Marken et al., 2010). For example, the New York Simulation (NYSIM) Center was created through a public–private partnership to manage interprofessional, simulation-based education for students and hospital employees across multiple sites (NYSIM, 2017). The opportunity to take part in simulation experiences with students from other health professions can also improve collaboration and teamwork and prepare nurses for practicing interprofessionally in the workplace (von Wendt and Niemi-Murola, 2018).

Limitations on in-person clinical training during the COVID-19 pandemic conditions have demonstrated the promise of simulation-based education as

BOX 7-7
The Community Action Poverty Simulation

This poverty simulation is intended to break down stereotypes by allowing students to experience real-life situations, allowing them to consider the perspectives of actual individuals (clients of the developing organization) facing the complex and interconnected effects of poverty. In this simulation, groups of students take on the roles of individuals who are members of families facing a variety of challenging but typical circumstances. Each student group participates as a family; they are given a card explaining their family's unique circumstances. The families are then tasked with providing food, shelter, and other basic necessities by accessing various community resources during the course of four 15-minute "weeks," which represent 1 month in the life of someone living in poverty. In addition to improving understanding of the challenges of living in poverty, the exposure to multiple agencies through the simulation introduces students to many of the sectors that work collaboratively to create health equity.

SOURCE: The Poverty Simulation, n.d.

a way to supplement traditional nursing education, allowing students to complete their education and sustaining the nursing workforce pipeline (Horn, 2020; Jiménez-Rodríguez et al., 2020; Yale, 2020). Before the pandemic, the NCSBN conducted a longitudinal, randomized controlled trial of the use of simulation and concluded that substituting simulation-based education for up to half of a nursing student's clinical hours produces comparable educational outcomes and students who are ready to practice (Hayden et al., 2014). The COVID-19 pandemic has necessitated and accelerated the use of simulation to replace direct care experience in nursing schools, and state boards of nursing have loosened previous restrictions on its use (NCSBN, 2020b). Evaluation of this expanded use of simulation and other virtual experiences during the pandemic is needed, both in preparation for future emergencies and for use in nursing education generally.

RECRUITING AND SUPPORTING DIVERSE PROSPECTIVE NURSES

The composition of the population of prospective nurses and the ways they are supported throughout their education are important factors in how prepared the future nursing workforce will be to address SDOH and health equity. As discussed in prior chapters, developing a more diverse nursing workforce will be key to achieving the goals of reducing health disparities, providing culturally relevant care for all populations, and fostering health equity (Center for Health Affairs, 2018; IOM, 2011, 2016; Williams et al., 2014). A diverse workforce is one that reflects the variations in the nation's population in such characteristics as socioeconomic status, religion, sexual orientation, gender, race, ethnicity, and geographic origin.

The nursing workforce has historically been overwhelmingly White and female, although it is steadily becoming more diverse (see Chapter 3). The 2016 IOM report assessing progress on the 2011 *The Future of Nursing* report notes that shifting the demographics of the overall workforce is inevitably a slow process since only a small percentage of the workforce leaves and enters each year (IOM, 2016a). The pipeline of students entering the field, on the other hand, can respond much more rapidly to efforts to increase diversity (IOM, 2016a). Since the 2011 report was published, significant gains have been realized in the diversity of nursing students. The number of graduates from historically underrepresented ethnic and racial groups more than doubled for BSN programs, more than tripled for entry-level master's programs, and more than doubled for PhD programs (AACN, 2020a). The number of underrepresented students graduating from DNP programs grew by more than 1,000 percent, although this gain was due in large part to rapid growth in these programs generally. Yet, despite these gains, nursing students remain largely female and White: in 2019, 85–90 percent of students were female, and around 60 percent were White. The percentages of ADN, BSN, entry-level master's, PhD, and DNP graduates in 2019 by race/ethnicity and gender are shown in Tables 7-3 and 7-4, respectively. For example, the proportion of Hispanic or Latino nurses is highest among ADN graduates (12.8 percent) and lowest among PhD (5.5 percent) and DNP (6 percent) graduates, while the proportion of Asian nurses is highest among MSN graduates (11.2 percent) and lower among graduates with all other degrees. The proportion of PhD graduates who are male (9.9 percent) is significantly lower than the proportion of graduates with other degrees who are male.

Diversifying and strengthening the nursing student body—and eventually, the nursing workforce—requires cultivating an inclusive environment, recruiting and admitting a diverse group of students, and providing students with support and addressing barriers to their success throughout their academic career and into practice. In addition, it is essential to make available information that will enable prospective students to make informed decisions about their education and give them multiple pathways for completing their education (e.g., distance learning, accelerated programs). Accrediting bodies can play a role in advancing diversity and inclusion in nursing schools by requiring certain policies, practices, or systems. For example, the accreditation standards for medical schools of the Liaison Committee on Medical Education (LCME) include the following expectation (LCME, 2018):

TABLE 7-3 Nursing Program Graduates by Degree Type[a] and by Race/Ethnicity, 2019

Race/Ethnicity	ADN[b]	BSN	MSN[c]	PhD	DNP
Total number of degrees	75,470	77,363	3,254	801	7,944
Native Hawaiian or other Pacific Islander	0.3%	0.5%	0.4%	1.2%	0.3%
American Indian or Alaska Native	0.7%	0.4%	0.6%	0.6%	0.5%
Asian	4.6%	7.9%	11.2%	6.6%	6.9%
Hispanic or Latino	12.8%	10.2%	11.3%	5.5%	6.0%
Black or African American	12.1%	8.7%	8.7%	12.1%	15.0%
White	63.2%	63.6%	59.4%	59.2%	63.7%
Two or more races	2.5%	2.8%	2.5%	1.4%	2.4%
Non-U.S. residents (International)	0.6%	1.0%	0.5%	9.1%	0.6%
Unknown	n/a	5.0%	5.5%	4.2%	4.6%

NOTE: ADN = associate degree in nursing; BSN = bachelor of science in nursing; DNP = doctor of nursing practice; LPN/LVN = licensed practical/vocational nurse; MSN = master of science in nursing.

[a] Data not available for LPN/LVN.

[b] ADN data are from 2018.

[c] Entry-level master's degree.

SOURCE: American Association of Colleges of Nursing, Enrollment & Graduations in Baccalaureate and Graduate Programs in Nursing (series); Integrated Postsecondary Education Data System (IPEDS), Completions Survey (series) for ADN data.

TABLE 7-4 Nursing Program Graduates by Degree Type[a] and Gender, 2019

Gender	ADN[b]	BSN	MSN[c]	PhD	DNP
Total number of degrees	77,993	77,363	3,254	801	7,944
Male	14.4%	13.6%	15.2%	9.9%	13.1%
Female	85.6%	85.1%	84.7%	89.9%	86.6%
Unknown	n/a	1.4%	0.1%	0.2%	0.3%

NOTE: ADN = associate degree in nursing; BSN = bachelor of science in nursing; DNP = doctor of nursing practice; LPN/LVN = licensed practical/vocational nurse; MSN = master of science in nursing.

[a] Data not available for LPN/LVN.

[b] ADN data are from 2018.

[c] Entry-level master's degree.

SOURCE: American Association of Colleges of Nursing, Enrollment & Graduations in Baccalaureate and Graduate Programs in Nursing (series); Integrated Postsecondary Education Data System (IPEDS), Completions Survey (series) for ADN data.

> A medical school has effective policies and practices in place, and engages in ongoing, systematic, and focused recruitment and retention activities, to achieve mission appropriate diversity outcomes among its students, faculty, senior administrative staff, and other relevant members of its academic community. These activities include the use of programs and/or partnerships aimed at achieving diversity among qualified applicants for medical school admission and the evaluation of program and partnership outcomes.

Currently, none of the major nursing accreditors (ACEN, CCNE, CNEA) includes similar language in its accreditation standards. As shown in Table 7-5, of six possible areas for standards on diversity and inclusion, ACEN and CCEN have standards only for student training, while CNEA has standards for student training and faculty diversity. No nursing accreditors have standards for student diversity; in comparison, accrediting bodies for pharmacy, physician assistant, medical, and dental schools all have such standards.

Cultivating an Inclusive Environment

Efforts to recruit and educate prospective nurses to serve a diverse population and advance health equity will be fruitless unless accompanied by efforts to acknowledge and dismantle racism within nursing education and nursing practice (Burnett et al., 2020; Schroeder and DiAngelo, 2010; Villaruel and Broome, 2020; Waite and Nardi, 2019). The structural, individual, and ideological racism that exists in nursing is rarely called out, and this silence further entrenches the idea of Whiteness as the norm within nursing while marginalizing and silencing other groups and their perspectives (Burnett et al., 2020; Iheduru-Anderson, 2020; Schroeder and DiAngelo, 2010). Non-White students report a wide variety of negative experiences in nursing school, including unsupportive faculty, discrim-

TABLE 7-5 Diversity and Inclusion in Accreditation Standards

Accrediting Body	Student Diversity	Faculty Diversity	Academic Leadership Diversity	Pipeline Programs	Student Training	Faculty Training
Accreditation Commission for Education in Nursing (ACEN)	—	—	—	—	Yes	—
Accreditation Council for Pharmacy Education (ACPE)	Yes	—	—	—	Yes	—
Accreditation Review Commission on Education for the Physician Assistant, Inc. (ARC-PA)	Yes	Yes	—	—	Yes	—
Commission for Nursing Education Accreditation (CNEA)	—	Yes	—	—	Yes	—
Commission on Collegiate Nursing Education (CCNE)	—	—	—	—	Yes	—
Commission on Dental Accreditation (CODA)	Yes	Yes	—	—	Yes	—
Commission on Osteopathic College Accreditation (COCA)	Yes	Yes	Yes	—	Yes	Yes
Committee on Accreditation of Canadian Medical Schools (CACMS)	Yes	Yes	Yes	—	Yes	—
Liaison Committee on Medical Education (LCME)	Yes	Yes	Yes	Yes	Yes	—

SOURCE: Batra and Orban, 2020.

ination and microaggressions[5] on the part of faculty and peers, bias in grading, loneliness and social isolation, feeling unwelcome and excluded, being viewed as a homogeneous population despite being from varying racial/ethnic groups, lack of support for career choices, and a lack of mentors (Ackerman-Barger et al., 2020; Graham et al., 2016; Johansson et al., 2011; Loftin et al., 2012; Metzger et al., 2020). These experiences are associated with adverse outcomes that include disengagement from education, loss of "self," negative perceptions of inclusivity and diversity at the institution, and institutions' inability to recruit and retain a diversity of students (Metzger et al., 2020). By contrast, when students characterize the learning environment as inclusive, they are more satisfied and confident in their learning and rate themselves higher on clinical self-efficacy and clinical belongingness (Metzger and Taggart, 2020).

Notably, however, underrepresented and majority students describe inclusive environments differently. In a study of fourth-year baccalaureate nursing students, both groups described an inclusive classroom as one where they felt comfortable and respected and had a sense of belonging, but underrepresented minority students also noted the importance of feeling safe, feeling free from hostility, and being seen as themselves and not a representative of their group (Metzger and Taggart, 2020). Both groups agreed that inclusivity requires a top-down approach, and that faculty are particularly influential in creating an inclusive environment, yet underrepresented students shared many experiences in which faculty either disrupted the sense of belonging or did not intervene when someone else did (Metzger and Taggart, 2020).

While increased attention has recently been focused on increasing diversity in nursing education, the pervasiveness of racism requires more open acknowledgment and discussion and a systematic and intentional approach that may, as discussed earlier, be uncomfortable for some (Ackerman-Barger et al., 2020; Villaruel and Broome, 2020). Cultivating an inclusive environment requires acknowledging and challenging racism in all aspects of the educational experience, including curricula, institutional policies and structures, pedagogical strategies, and the formal and informal distribution of resources and power (Iheduru-Anderson, 2020; Koschmann et al., 2020; Metzger and Taggart, 2020; Schroeder and DiAngelo, 2010; Villaruel and Broome, 2020; Waite and Nardi, 2019). Nursing school curricula have historically focused on the contributions of White and female nurses (Waite and Nardi, 2019). The weight given to this curricular content sends a message to students—both White students and students of color—about what faculty consider important (Villaruel and Broome, 2020). Moving forward, curricula need to include a critical examination of the history of racism within nursing and an acknowledgment and celebration of the contribution of nurses of color (Waite and Nardi, 2019). Such efforts need to be led by a broad group of individuals from all levels within an institution; racism in institutional practices

[5] Brief and commonplace daily indignities (see Chapter 10).

can be so ingrained that it is difficult for those with power to recognize (Villaruel and Broome, 2020). Faculty often understand the importance of an inclusive learning environment, but struggle with moving from intention to action (Beard, 2013, 2014; Metzger et al., 2020).

While institutional efforts to change organizational culture are thoroughly described in the literature, they remain too rare to address the problems described above effectively (Breslin et al., 2018). In the early 2000s, the University of Washington School of Nursing implemented a project designed to change the "climate of whiteness" at the school (Schroeder and DiAngelo, 2010). The project involved many facets, including year-long antiracist workshops; a comprehensive and institutionalized diversity statement; and action plans for addressing admission barriers, encouraging ongoing education for faculty, and disseminating antiracist information to the entire campus. The authors of an evaluation of the project note that while initial feedback was positive, changing the sociopolitical climate of a school is a long-term process that requires institutional commitment, innovative leadership, long- and short-term strategies, and patience (Schroeder and DiAngelo, 2010). Unfortunately, many administrators and leaders may hesitate to initiate dialogues about these issues or may lack knowledge of how to address the challenges, and in many institutions, faculty and administrators from underserved groups have been expected to carry this burden, which can allow their colleagues to remain passive (Lim et al., 2015). The committee stresses that addressing racism and discrimination within the nursing profession requires more than mere programs or statements; it requires developing action-oriented strategies, holding difficult conversations about privilege, dismantling long-standing structures and traditions, conducting curricular reviews to detect biases and correct as necessary, and exploring how interpersonal and structural racism shapes the student experience both consciously and unconsciously (Burnett et al., 2020; Iheduru-Anderson, 2020; Waite and Nardi, 2019).

Recruitment and Admissions

Many social and structural barriers impede the entry of underrepresented students into the nursing profession (NACNEP, 2019). Several approaches can be taken to improve access for prospective underrepresented students and, by extension, increase the diversity of the nursing workforce. Recruitment of underrepresented students can start years before nursing school through such approaches as improved K–12 science education (AAPCHO, 2009) and outreach to junior high and high school students, such as through summer pipeline programs (Katz et al., 2016) or health career clubs (Murray et al., 2016). K–12 education is particularly important for sparking students' interest in the health professions, as well as for giving them the foundational knowledge necessary for success (NASEM, 2016b). One innovative approach to preparing young people for a career in nursing is the Rhode Island Nurses Institute Middle College Charter High School (RINIMC).

RINIMC offers a free, 4-year, nursing-focused, high school education open to any student in Rhode Island; students graduate with experience in health care as well as up to 20 college credits. Nearly half of the program's students are Latinx, and more than one-third are Black (RINIMC, n.d.). Establishing a pathway to nursing education for diverse students well before undergraduate school is important, particularly for first-generation students (Katz et al., 2016; McCue, 2017). Some states offer dual enrollment programs. An example is Ohio's College Credit Plus program, in which students in grades 7 to 12 have the opportunity to earn college and high school credits simultaneously, thus preparing them for postsecondary success.[6]

Once students have applied to nursing school, a system of holistic admissions can improve the diversity of the incoming class (Glazer et al., 2016, 2020). A holistic admissions system involves evaluating an applicant based not only on academic achievement but also on experiences, attributes, potential contributions, and the fit between the applicant and the institutional mission (DeWitty, 2018; NACNEP, 2019). Schools that have implemented such a system have seen an increase in the diversity of their student body (Glazer et al., 2016, 2018). Academic measures (e.g., graduation and exam pass rates) have remained unchanged or improved, and schools have reported increases in such measures as student engagement, cooperation and teamwork, and openness to different perspectives (Artinian et al., 2017; Glazer et al., 2016, 2020). In a recent paper published by AACN (2020d), the following promising practices in holistic admissions were identified: (1) review institutional mission, vision, and values statements to ensure that they value diversity and inclusion; (2) create an "experience, attributes, and metrics (E-A-M) model" (p. 16) that connects back to the institution's mission statement; (3) identify recruitment practices that align with the E-A-M model; (4) design rubrics to be used by admissions committees that are reflective of the E-A-M model; (5) engage faculty and staff in the holistic admissions review process; (6) use technology resources such as a centralized application system to maintain efficiencies; (7) develop tailored support services for underrepresented students; and (8) engage in a review and assessment of the entire process.

Addressing Barriers to Success

Part of cultivating an inclusive educational environment is acknowledging and addressing barriers that may prevent students from achieving their potential. As noted previously, some students—particularly those from underrepresented groups—may need support in a number of areas, including economic, social and emotional, and academic and career progression. Attention to the barriers faced by students is essential at each step along the pathway from high school preparation; to recruitment, admission, retention, and academic success in nurs-

---

[6] See https://www.ohiohighered.org/collegecreditplus (accessed April 13, 2021).

ing school; to graduation and placement in a job; to retention and advancement within a nursing career (IOM, 2016b).

Providing Economic Supports

Cost is a key factor in decisions about nursing education for most students, and is particularly salient for those from underrepresented groups, who come disproportionately from families with comparatively low incomes and levels of wealth (Diefenbeck et al., 2016; Graham et al., 2016; Sullivan, 2004). Sabio and Petges (2020) interviewed associate's degree nursing students in a Midwestern state and found that the total cost of a baccalaureate degree and student debt was the greatest barrier to pursuing a degree, followed by family and personal, such as head-of-household, responsibilities. This challenge is pervasive in higher education, and there are indications that the problem is growing (Advisory Committee on Student Financial Assistance, 2013). Students need to have the financial resources not only for tuition but also for an array of education-related expenses, including housing, food, work attire, books, and supplies.

Providing clear information about the costs of nursing education and available financial supports early in the recruitment and admission process is key to identifying those who need help and encouraging them to enroll (Pritchard et al., 2016). Recruitment and admission practices need to take into account student finances and how future salaries affect choices, particularly for certain groups of students. Most health care systems provide some level of tuition reimbursement for baccalaureate and higher education, and this support may lead students toward certain settings (e.g., acute care) and away from others (e.g., public health, primary care) (Larsen, 2012). Other financial support options are available, including the Public Service Loan Forgiveness program, which offers full forgiveness after 10 years for employees of nonprofit or government organizations (U.S. Department of Education, n.d.b), and programs through HRSA that award loan repayment to RNs and advanced practice nurses who work in health professions shortage areas for at least 2 years (HRSA, 2021).

State policy reform can help remove some of the structural barriers to education. For example, New York State has implemented a program that allows New York households earning less than $125,000 annually to qualify for free in-state tuition at state public universities (New York State, n.d.). New nurses who complete an associate's degree in New York are required to complete a bachelor's degree within 10 years of graduation; free in-state tuition could make a considerable difference for these nurses in pursuing their next degree. While it is too early to assess the effects on the composition of the nursing workforce, this approach bears further evaluation. Certainly it is critical for state policies to facilitate the financing of nursing education using models other than additional student loans. There are demonstrated disparities in the burden of student debt between Black and White students (Brookings Institution, 2016), and the risk of assuming large amounts of debt for students from disadvantaged backgrounds may be one they cannot afford to take. Therefore, innovative financing models are necessary to ensure that all nurses can pursue educational opportunities.

It is also important to note that as they progress in their education, students of many backgrounds may experience food insecurity, struggles with housing, or issues with transportation that affect their ability to perform (AAC&U, 2019; Laterman, 2019; Strauss, 2020). Institutions need to ensure that students' basic needs are met during their studies through sustained, multiyear funding and resources to support students facing financial emergencies.

Social and Academic Supports

Once students have been admitted, some nursing schools offer programs, such as summer programs that bridge high school and college, designed to prepare them academically and socially for the rigors of nursing education. Some of these programs are designed specifically for underrepresented and/or first-generation college students (Pritchard et al., 2016), who may lack adequate family, emotional, and moral support; mentorship opportunities; professional socialization; and academic support (Banister et al., 2014; Loftin et al., 2012). A study at the University of Cincinnati College of Nursing found that the impact of its summer bridge program lasted throughout the first year of school, and that grade point averages and retention were similar between underrepresented and majority students (Pritchard et al., 2016). The Recruitment & Retention of American Indians into Nursing (RAIN) program at the University of North Dakota conducts a "No Excuses Orientation" workshop to give incoming American Indian students an opportunity to create connections and become acquainted with people and resources at the university (UND, 2020). Tribal leaders are included in the orientation, along with discussions of cultural and family values and issues.

Another approach for supporting students is through mentoring programs. As discussed in Chapter 9, these programs create supportive environments by providing peer and faculty role modeling, academic guidance, and support (Wilson et al., 2010). Evidence indicates that mentoring programs for students from underrepresented groups are more effective when they include nurses and faculty from those groups, who have firsthand understanding of the unique challenges these students and nurses regularly confront (Banister et al., 2014). This observation underscores the need for diverse faculty, mentors, and preceptors with the availability and willingness to guide these students and teach them leadership. For example, the RAIN program provides mentoring to American Indian students; staff and leaders are heavily involved in the local American Indian communities, and many are tribal members themselves (Minority Nurse, 2013).

Students who represent the first generation in their families to enter a postsecondary institution may face challenges other students do not, and are more likely to graduate if they receive support (Costello et al., 2018). Parents and significant others can be a crucial source of support (Pritchard et al., 2020); socializing and educating family members about the rigors of nursing programs may facilitate their support for students. A variety of programs around the country have succeeded in increasing graduation rates among first-generation students, including pipeline programs that have successfully increased the diversity of candidates entering nursing. These programs include HRSA pipeline programs; HOSA-Future Health Professionals; and university-based programs such as the Niganawenimaanaanig program at Bemidji State University in Minnesota, created to support American Indian nursing students (HOSA, 2012; HRSA, 2017; Wilkie, 2020). Federal funding is available for these types of programs from sources that include HRSA's Health Careers Opportunity Program and Nursing Workforce Diversity Grant program. However, the need for such programs exceeds the available funding. Box 7-8 lists some of the ways in which nursing programs can support their students' success.

Data on Quality

One important tool for recruiting a more diverse student population is providing relevant data to prospective students so they can make informed decisions about where to study. These data could include NCLEX pass rates; however, these rates alone are insufficient to determine whether a school is likely to have the resources to support a student through to graduation. Data on student reten-

BOX 7-8
Examples of Supports for Nursing Students

Academic Supports

- Residential preparation programs held the summer before freshman year
- Booster programs held the summer after freshman year
- Personal education plans and student portfolios
- Supplemental instruction and study groups

Professional Development Supports

- Career shadowing
- Invited speaker series
- Resumé/interviewing workshop, mock interviews
- Attendance at a student research conference
- Mentored research projects
- Mentoring and sponsoring by professional nurses
- Service as peer mentor

SOURCE: Pritchard et al., 2020.

tion, graduation by demographic, full cost to attend, tuition, and other quality indicators can signal to both consumers and funders whether a nursing education program has the necessary infrastructure and support to retain students from diverse backgrounds. Pass rates can be reported by race, ethnicity, socioeconomic status, first-time college/university attendees, adult learners with children living at home, and status as an English as a second language (ESL) learner to help students choose a program that best suits their needs. It is also important for schools to provide on their websites demographic information about their current enrollees. As discussed above, NCSBN identified additional quality indicators for nursing education; as these indicators begin to be measured and reported, the data can help prospective students make more informed choices.

Educational Pathways and Options

As nursing education programs adapt their curricula and other learning experiences to better address SDOH and health equity, it will be important to consider the educational pathways students may follow, both in their initial preparation and as they progress in their careers. A key way of strengthening the nursing workforce will be to encourage nurses to pursue the next level of education and certification available to them and to improve access to these educational opportunities, especially for those from underrepresented communities (Jones et al., 2018; Phillips and Malone, 2014).

One way to improve access and encourage nurses to take the next step in their education is by offering expedited programs that allow them to complete their degree in less time. For example, there are articulation agreements, either among educational institutions or at the state or regional level, that align the content and requirements of programs. These types of agreements accelerate the RN-to-BSN and RN-to-MSN pathways and allow students to easily transfer credits between community colleges and universities (AACN, 2019b). There are also bridge programs available for LPNs who wish to pursue the ADN or BSN degree. Investments in articulation programs have been responsible in part for an increase in the number of employed nurses with a baccalaureate degree, from 49 percent in 2010 to 59 percent in 2019 (Campaign for Action, n.d.). Further progress in this area is needed, however, particularly for partnerships between baccalaureate nursing programs and academic institutions that serve underrepresented populations (e.g., tribal colleges, historically Black colleges and universities). A model of this type of partnership can be found in the New Mexico Nursing Education Consortium,[7] which coordinates prelicensure nursing curricula in 16 locations at state, tribal, and community colleges.

Nursing education can also be expedited through the use of a competency-based curriculum that allows students to progress by demonstrating the required

[7] See https://www.nmnec.org (accessed April 13, 2021).

competencies rather than meeting specific hour requirements (U.S. Department of Education, n.d.a). With this approach, which is currently used, for example, by Western Governors University, students can self-pace their education and potentially save time and money by learning the material quickly or tapping previous knowledge (WGU, 2020). This type of educational approach may be particularly useful for nontraditional students who are entering nursing with other experiences and education. For example, a person with a background as a nursing or medical assistant may find that he or she can quickly master some of the required material for a nursing degree, particularly at the beginning. Workers from other sectors may also be able to pivot to nursing. During the COVID-19 pandemic, a study identified health care jobs, such as nursing assistant, that out-of-work hospitality workers could quickly transition to pursue (Miller and Haley, 2020). While the study did not include jobs that required further education or certification, the shared skill sets that the authors identified include many skills that are central to nursing.

Another approach for increasing access to nursing education is to expand the use of distance learning opportunities. Distance learning gives students flexibility, and may be particularly beneficial for those from rural areas or other areas without a nursing school in the vicinity (NCSBN, 2020b). Rural areas face multiple challenges: rural populations have high rates of chronic disease and have difficulty accessing care because of provider shortages in these areas (see Chapter 2). Relative to their urban counterparts, rural nurses are less likely to hold a BSN (Merrell et al., 2020). Distance learning has been used for many years to reach rural populations, but there are challenges with respect to regulation and ensuring the quality of education (NCSBN, 2020a). Efforts have been made to assess and improve the quality of distance learning; Quality Matters, for example, is an organization that provides peer-reviewed evaluation of distance or hybrid programs using a set of quality standards.[8] While many nursing programs are adhering to these standards (Quality Matters, 2020), many are not, and the quality of distance learning remains uneven. The rapid rollout of distance learning during the COVID-19 pandemic has provided a unique opportunity to evaluate the effectiveness of different strategies for distance learning and to leverage this experience to expand and improve distance learning opportunities in the future.

STRENGTHENING AND DIVERSIFYING THE NURSING FACULTY

A system of nursing education that can prepare students from diverse backgrounds to address SDOH and health equity requires a diverse faculty (NACNEP, 2019; Thornton and Persaud, 2018). Unfortunately, the faculty currently teaching in nursing programs is overwhelmingly White and female: as of 2018, full-time faculty in nursing schools were about 93 percent female, and only 17.3 percent were from underrepresented groups, up from 11.5 percent in 2009 (AACN, 2020c).

---

[8] See https://www.qualitymatters.org (accessed April 13, 2021).

In addition to this lack of diversity, the number of faculty may be inadequate to prepare the next generation of nurses: not only were there 1,637 faculty vacancies in 2019 across 892 nursing schools, but the schools surveyed hoped to create 134 new faculty positions in that year (AACN, 2020c). These shortages contributed to decisions to turn away more than 80,000 qualified applicants, although other insufficiencies also played a part. The AACN report cites several key reasons for faculty shortages: increasing average age of faculty members and associated increasing retirement rates, high compensation in other settings that attracts current and potential nurse educators, and an insufficient pool of graduates from master's and doctoral programs (AACN, 2020c; Fang and Bednash, 2017). A 2020 NACNEP report calls the faculty shortage a "long-standing crisis threatening the supply, education, and training of registered nurses" and recommends federal efforts as well as a coordinated private–public response to address the shortage (NACNEP, 2020).

Finally, faculty must have the knowledge, skills, and competencies to prepare their students for the challenges of advancing health equity and fully understanding the implications of SDOH for their daily practice (NACNEP, 2019). If health equity and SDOH are to be integrated throughout the curriculum (as discussed earlier in this chapter), all faculty, including tenure-track faculty, clinical instructors, mentors, and preceptors, must have these competencies (Thornton and Persaud, 2018). To develop these competencies, nursing schools must commit resources and support to faculty development (Thornton and Persaud, 2018).

Diversifying the Faculty

As noted, diverse faculty are needed to broaden the perspectives and experiences to which nursing students are exposed and to serve as mentors and role models for diverse students (Phillips and Malone, 2014). Unfortunately, minority faculty members often face barriers similar to those faced by students, including an unwelcoming environment; feeling marginalized, underappreciated, and invisible; a lack of support; feelings of tokenism; and the inability to integrate into existing faculty structures (Beard and Julion, 2016; Hamilton and Haozous, 2017; Iheduru-Anderson, 2020; Kolade, 2016; Salvucci and Lawless, 2016; Whitfield-Harris and Lockhart, 2016). Faculty from underrepresented groups report feeling isolated, lacking in mentorship and collegial support, and burdened by having to represent the entire underrepresented community (Kolade, 2016; Whitfield-Harris et al., 2017). In addition, as discussed in Chapter 9, faculty from underrepresented racial and ethnic groups face a "diversity tax," in which they are asked to be part of efforts to improve diversity and inclusion to serve on committees; mentor underrepresented students; and participate in other activities that are uncompensated, unacknowledged, and unrewarded (Gewin, 2020). These demands on underrepresented faculty can lead to frustration, burnout, and a feeling that they have been given responsibility for institutional diversity (Gewin, 2020).

These experiences of minority faculty can result in high attrition and low satisfaction (Whitfield-Harris et al., 2017), and further research is needed on specific ways in which institutions can recruit and support a diverse faculty (Whitfield-Harris et al., 2017). Proposed approaches include cultivating an inclusive educational environment (Hamilton and Haozous, 2017), taking intentional action and holding open discourse to strengthen the institutional commitment to diversity (Beard and Julion, 2016), improving financial assistance and mentorship opportunities for faculty (Salvucci and Lawless, 2016), and conducting climate surveys to better understand the feelings and experiences of underrepresented faculty and using these data to improve the institutional culture (DeWitty and Murray, 2020). The challenges these faculty face and the opportunities to address these challenges highlight the importance of efforts by schools of nursing to recruit, support, and retain diverse faculty.

Faculty Development

Collectively, nursing school faculty need to be prepared to teach their students about the complex linkages among population health, SDOH, and health outcomes (NLN, 2019; Thornton and Persaud, 2018). To do so, as discussed above, nurse educators need to move beyond teaching abstract principles to integrating the core concepts and competencies related to these linkages into the entire learning experience across nursing education programs. They also need to create a truly inclusive and safe educational environment and prepare nurses to care for a diverse population, which, as discussed above, requires that they understand issues of racism and systems of marginalization and engage in critical self-reflection (O'Connor et al., 2019, Peek et al., 2020). Yet, many faculty in nursing schools lack the knowledge and experience needed to develop curricula and strategies for incorporating SDOH into all areas of nursing education (NACNEP, 2019; Valderama-Wallace and Apesoa-Varano, 2019).

Several approaches are available for preparing nursing school faculty to teach content related to SDOH and health equity. One approach, discussed above, is to actively recruit more diverse faculty who reflect the nation's population and provide different perspectives and role models for students (The Macy Foundation, 2020). Another approach is to encourage the development and dissemination of evidence-based methods for teaching nursing students how they can incorporate these core concepts into nursing practice. For example, educators involved in developing innovative models of classroom and experiential learning could focus on disseminating these models with the assistance of nursing associations and organizations, including through publication, continuing education programs, or faculty-to-faculty education and mentoring. Finally, institutions can provide in-depth and sustained learning opportunities for faculty, staff, and preceptors focused on how they can support their students in learning about SDOH and health equity both within and outside of the classroom (IOM, 2016b). While some funding sources are available for these types of efforts, including support from private foundations and HRSA grants for faculty development, the critical importance of this content to health outcomes argues for providing more such resources.

IMPLICATIONS OF COVID-19 FOR NURSING EDUCATION

It has been 100 years since a global event has had an impact on nursing education in the United States and around the world equal to that of the COVID-19 pandemic. Both World War I and the influenza pandemic of 1918 to 1920 led to transformations in nursing education, including standardization of training and professionalization of the field. The COVID-19 pandemic has already led to innovations that are likely to shape the future of nursing education. Faculty have adopted new teaching strategies, demonstrating creativity and adaptability, within a span of days or weeks, while such technologies as simulation-based education have quickly been adapted to replace in-person clinical hours (Jiménez-Rodríguez et al., 2020). In one example of a rapid pivot, educators at the University of Pennsylvania School of Nursing transitioned a community immersion course from in-person to virtual form when all in-person classes were canceled. While they faced challenges, the educators found that students were able to remain dedicated to their community partnerships and to think creatively about how to meet their learning objectives (Flores et al., 2020). These and similar innovations may ultimately guide the way to expanding and improving nursing education.

At the same time, however, the pandemic has highlighted challenges and inequities in nursing education. Simulated clinical experiences are practical only if a school and its students have access to computers with enough power to run the software, for example. While online learning has been in use for more than a decade, not all schools or faculty are prepared to deliver content in this way, nor are all students capable of accessing the necessary technology. Moreover, as practice settings have been emptied of non-COVID patients, programs have been facing multiple challenges in providing students with sufficient hours of instruction, training, and clinical practice. These challenges have underscored the limitations of traditional ways of educating nurses even as they have presented unique opportunities for innovation. To translate these short-term challenges into long-term improvements in nursing education will require

- evaluation of such practices as distance learning and virtual experiential learning to identify and disseminate best practices;
- a sense of urgency in the development of substantial changes, such as modifications of curriculum and the adoption of new technologies; and
- partnership with public- and private-sector organizations, associations, and researchers that can bring both resources and expertise to the tasks of strengthening nursing education.

CONCLUSIONS

Currently, most nursing schools tend to cover the topics of SDOH, health equity, and population health in isolated, stand-alone courses. This approach is insufficient for creating a foundational understanding of these critical issues and for preparing nurses to work in a wide variety of settings. This content needs to be integrated and sustained throughout nursing school curricula and paired with community-based experiential opportunities whereby students can apply their knowledge, build their skills, and reflect on their experiences.

Conclusion 7-1: A curriculum embedded in coursework and experiential learning that effectively prepares students to promote health equity, reduce health disparities, and improve the health and well-being of the population will build the capacity of the nursing workforce.

Preparing nursing students to address SDOH and improve health equity will require more than didactic learning and traditional clinical experiences. It will require that students engage actively in experiences that will expand and diversify their understanding of nursing practice, prepare them to care for diverse populations with empathy, and allow them to build the necessary skills and competencies for the nursing practice of tomorrow.

Conclusion 7-2: Increasing the number of nurses with PhD degrees who focus on the connections among social determinants of health, health disparities, health equity, and overall health and well-being will build the evidence base in this area. Building capacity in schools of nursing will require financial resources, including scholarship/loan repayment opportunities; adequate numbers of expert faculty available to mentor; and curriculum revisions to focus more attention on social determinants of health and health equity.

Having more nurses prepared at the PhD level will help build the knowledge base in the nursing profession for other nurses to translate (DNPs) and use in practice settings (LPNs, RNs, APRNs).

Conclusion 7-3: Learning experiences that develop nursing students' understanding of health equity, social determinants of health, and population health and prepare them to incorporate that understanding into their professional practice include opportunities to

- ***learn cultural humility and recognize one's own implicit biases;***
- ***gain experience with interprofessional collaboration and multisector partnerships to enable them to address social needs comprehensively and drive structural improvements;***

- ***develop such technical competencies as use of telehealth, digital health tools, and data analytics; and***
- ***gain substantive experience with delivering care in diverse community settings, such as public health departments, schools, libraries, workplaces, and neighborhood clinics.***

Building a diverse nursing workforce is a critical component of the effort to prepare nurses to address SDOH and health equity. While the nursing workforce has steadily grown more diverse, nursing schools need to continue and expand their efforts to recruit, support, and mentor diverse students.

> ***Conclusion 7-4: Successfully diversifying the nursing workforce will depend on holistic efforts to support and mentor/sponsor students and faculty from a wide range of backgrounds, including cultivating an inclusive environment; providing economic, social, professional, and academic supports; ensuring access to information on school quality; and minimizing inequities.***

REFERENCES

Aaberg, V. A. 2012. A path to greater inclusivity through understanding implicit attitudes toward disability. *Journal of Nursing Education* 51(9):505–510.

AAC&U (Association of American Colleges & Universities). 2019. *Majority of college students experience food insecurity, housing insecurity, or homelessness*. https://www.aacu.org/aacu-news/newsletter/majority-college-students-experience-food-insecurity-housing-insecurity-or (accessed March 29, 2021).

AACN (American Association of Colleges of Nursing). 2006. *The essentials of doctoral education for advanced nursing practice*. Washington, DC: American Association of Colleges of Nursing.

AACN. 2011. *The essentials of master's education in nursing*. https://www.aacnnursing.org/portals/42/publications/mastersessentials11.pdf (accessed July 6, 2021).

AACN. 2019a. *2018–2019 enrollment and graduations in baccalaureate and graduate programs in nursing*. Washington, DC: American Association of Colleges of Nursing.

AACN. 2019b. *Articulation agreements among nursing education programs*. https://www.aacnnursing.org/News-Information/Fact-Sheets/Articulation-Agreements (accessed January 25, 2021).

AACN. 2020a. *2019–2020 enrollment and graduations in baccalaureate and graduate programs in nursing*. https://www.aacnnursing.org/Store/product-info/productcd/IDSR_20ENROLLBACC (accessed January 8, 2021).

AACN. 2020b. *Essentials task force*. https://www.aacnnursing.org/About-AACN/AACN-Governance/Committees-and-Task-Forces/Essentials (accessed May 18, 2020).

AACN. 2020c. *Nursing faculty*. https://www.aacnnursing.org/news-information/fact-sheets/nursing-faculty-shortage (accessed March 9, 2021).

AACN. 2020c. *Curriculum improvement*. https://www.aacnnursing.org/Population-Health-Nursing/Curriculum-Improvement (accessed January 25, 2021).

AACN. 2020d. *Promising practices in holistic admissions review: Implementation in academic nursing*. https://www.aacnnursing.org/Portals/42/News/White-Papers/AACN-White-Paper-Promising-Practices-in-Holistic-Admissions-Review-December-2020.pdf (accessed January 25, 2021).

AACN. n.d. *Diversity & inclusion offerings*. https://www.aacnnursing.org/Diversity-Inclusion/Holistic-Admissions/Diversity-and-Inclusion-Offerings (accessed April 23, 2020).

AAPCHO (Association of Asian Pacific Community Health Organizations). 2009. *Pipeline programs to improve racial and ethnic diversity in the health professions*. https://www.aapcho.org/wp/wp-content/uploads/2012/11/PipelineToImproveDiversityInHealthProfessions.pdf (accessed June 2, 2021).

AARP. 2010. *Preparation and roles of nursing care providers in America*. http://championnursing.org/resources/preparation-and-roles-nursing-care-providers-america (accessed October 28, 2020).

Ackerman-Barger, K., D. Boatright, R. Gonzalez-Colaso, R. Orozco, and D. Latimore. 2020. Seeking inclusion excellence: Understanding racial microaggressions as experienced by underrepresented medical and nursing students. *Academic Medicine* 95(5):758–763.

Advisory Committee on Student Financial Assistance. 2013. *Federal Register* 78(152). https://fsapartners.ed.gov/sites/default/files/attachments/fregisters/FR080713AdvisoryCommitteeonStudentFinancialAssistance.pdf (accessed June 2, 2021).

Agner, J. 2020. Moving from cultural competence to cultural humility in occupational therapy: A paradigm shift. *American Journal of Occupational Therapy* 74(4):7404347010.

AHA (American Hospital Association). 2019. *Screening for social needs: Guiding care teams to engage patients*. https://www.aha.org/system/files/media/file/2019/09/screening-for-social-needs-tool-value-initiative-rev-9-26-2019.pdf (accessed November 11, 2020).

Aiken, L. H., D. Sloane, P. Griffiths, A. M. Rafferty, L. Bruyneel, M. McHugh, C. B. Maier, T. Moreno-Casbas, J. E. Ball, D. Ausserhofer, and W. Sermeus. 2017. Nursing skill mix in European hospitals: Cross-sectional study of the association with mortality, patient ratings, and quality of care. *BMJ Quality & Safety* 26(7):559–568.

Alleghany College of Maryland. 2020. *Nurse managed wellness clinic*. https://www.allegany.edu/health-clinics/nurse-managed-wellness-clinic (accessed June 2, 2021).

Allen, J. 2010. Improving cross-cultural care and antiracism in nursing education: A literature review. *Nurse Education Today* 30(4):314–320.

Arcaya, M. C., and J. F. Figueroa 2017. Emerging trends could exacerbate health inequities in the United States. *Health Affairs (Millwood)* 36(6):992–998.

Artinian, N. T., B. M. Drees, G. Glazer, K. Harris, L. S. Kaufman, N. Lopez, J. C. Danek, and J. Michaels. 2017. Holistic admissions in the health professions: Strategies for leaders. *College & University* 92(2):65–68.

Baker, C., A. H. Cary, and M. da Conceicao Bento. 2020. Global standards for professional nursing education: The time is now. *Journal of Professional Nursing* 37(1):86–92. doi: 10.1016/j.profnurs.2020.10.001.

Bandy, J. 2011. *What is service learning or community engagement?* Vanderbilt University Center for Teaching. https://cft.vanderbilt.edu/guides-sub-pages/teaching-through-community-engagement (accessed March 29, 2021).

Banister, G., H. M. Bowen-Brady, and M. E. Winfrey. 2014. Using career nurse mentors to support minority nursing students and facilitate their transition to practice. *Journal of Professional Nursing* 30(4):317–325.

Barton, A. J., T. A. Murray, and D. R. Spurlock, Jr. 2020. An open letter to members of the nursing education community. *Journal of Nursing Education* 59(4):183.

Batra, S., and J. Orban. 2020. *Social mission and accreditation standards*. Oral presentation at the National Center for Interprofessional Education and Practice NEXUS Summit 2020, October 15, 2020, Virtual.

Beard, K. V. 2014. How much diversity in nursing is enough? *American Journal of Nursing* 114(9):11.

Beard, K. V., and W. A. Julion. 2016. Does race still matter in nursing? The narratives of African-American nursing faculty members. *Nursing Outlook* 64:583–596. https://doi.org/10.1016/j.outlook.2016.06.005 PMID:27432213.

Bednash, G., E. T. Breslin, J. M. Kirschling, and R. J. Rosseter. 2014. PhD or DNP: Planning for doctoral nursing education. *Nursing Science Quarterly* 27(4):296–301.

Befus, D. R., T. Kumodzi, D. Schminkey, and A. S. Ivany. 2019. Advancing health equity and social justice in forensic nursing research, education, practice, and policy: Introducing structural violence and trauma-and violence-informed care. *Journal of Forensic Nursing* 15(4):199–205.

Bestsennyy, O., G. Gilbert, A. Harris, and J. Rost. 2020. *Telehealth: A quarter-trillion-dollar post-COVID-19 reality?* https://www.mckinsey.com/industries/healthcare-systems-and-services/our-insights/telehealth-a-quarter-trillion-dollar-post-covid-19-reality (accessed February 24, 2021).

Bjørk, I. T., K. Berntsen, G. Brynildsen, and M. Hestetun. 2014. Nursing students' perceptions of their clinical learning environment in placements outside traditional hospital settings. *Journal of Clinical Nursing* 23(19–20):2958–2967.

Blair, I. V., J. F. Steiner, and E. P. Havranek. 2011. Unconscious (implicit) bias and health disparities: Where do we go from here? *The Permanente Journal* 15(2):71–78. PMID: 21841929.

Breen, N., J. S. Jackson, F. Wood, D. Wong, and X. Zhang. 2019. Translational health disparities research in a data-rich world. *American Journal of Public Health* 109(S1):S41–S42.

Brennan, A. M. W., J. Barnsteiner, M. L. Siantz, V. T. Cotter, and J. Everett. 2012. Lesbian, gay, bisexual, transgendered, or intersexed content for nursing curricula. *Journal of Professional Nursing* 28(2):96–104.

Breslin, E. T., K. Nuri-Robins, J. Ash, and J. M. Kirschling. 2018. The changing face of academic nursing: Nurturing diversity, inclusivity, and equity. *Journal of Professional Nursing* 34(2):103–109.

Bresnick, J. 2017. Understanding the basics of clinical decision support systems. *Health IT Analytics*. https://healthitanalytics.com/features/understanding-the-basics-of-clinical-decision-support-systems (accessed November 11, 2020).

Brookings Institution. 2016. *Black-White disparity in student loan debt more than triples after graduation*. https://www.brookings.edu/research/black-white-disparity-in-student-loan-debt-more-than-triples-after-graduation (accessed November 11, 2020).

Broome, M. E., and J. Fairman. 2018. Changing the conversation about doctoral education in nursing. *Nursing Outlook* 66(2018):217–218.

Buhler-Wilkerson, K. 1993. Bringing care to the people: Lillian Wald's legacy to public health nursing. *American Journal of Public Health* 83(12):1778–1786.

Burnett, A., C. Moorley, J. Grant, M. Kahin, R. Sagoo, E. Rivers, L. Deravin, and P. Darbyshire. 2020. Dismantling racism in education: In 2020, the year of the nurse & midwife, "it's time." *Nurse Education Today* 93:104532. https://doi.org/10.1016/j.nedt.2020.104532.

Campaign for Action. 2019a. *New RN graduates by degree type, by gender*. https://campaignforaction.org/resource/new-rn-graduates-degree-type-gender (accessed May 13, 2020).

Campaign for Action. 2019b. *Nursing education and the path to population health improvement*. https://campaignforaction.org/wp-content/uploads/2019/03/NursingEducationPathtoHealthImprovement.pdf (accessed March 13, 2020).

Campaign for Action. 2020. *Campaign for Action dashboard*. https://campaignforaction.org/wp-content/uploads/2019/07/r2_CCNA-0029_2019-Dashboard-Indicator-Updates_1-29-20.pdf (accessed May 14, 2020).

Campaign for Action. n.d. *Transforming nursing education*. https://campaignforaction.org/issue/transforming-nursing-education (accessed May 14, 2020).

Campinha-Bacote, J. 2018. Cultural competemility: A paradigm shift in the cultural competence versus cultural humility debate—part I. *The Online Journal of Issues in Nursing* 24(1).

Castro-Sánchez, E., A. M. Russell, L. Dolman, and M. Wells. 2021. What place does nurse-led research have in the COVID-19 pandemic? *International Nursing Review* 1–5.

CCNE (Commission on Collegiate Nursing Education). 2018. *Standards for accreditation of baccalaureate and graduate nursing programs*. https://www.aacnnursing.org/Portals/42/CCNE/PDF/Standards-Final-2018.pdf (accessed September 29, 2020).

CDC (Centers for Disease Control and Prevention). 2018. *Health care provider/clinician apps*. https://www.cdc.gov/mobile/healthcareproviderapps.html (accessed November 11, 2020).

Center for Health Affairs. 2018. *LPNs crucial to nursing workforce diversity*. https://neohospitals.org/TheCenterForHealthAffairs/MediaCenter/NewsReleases/2018/August/Nursing-Workforce-Diversity (accessed May 14, 2020).

Cho, I., E. Kim, W. H. Choi, and N. Staggers. 2016. Comparing usability testing outcomes and functions of six electronic nursing record systems. *International Journal of Medical Informatics* 88:78–85.

Costello, M., A. Ballin, R. Diamond, and M. L. Gao. 2018. First generation college students and non-first generation college students: Perceptions of belonging. *Journal of Nursing Education and Practice* 8(12):59–65.

Devine, P. G., P. S. Forscher, A. J. Austin, and W. T. Cox. 2012. Long-term reduction in implicit race bias: A prejudice habit-breaking intervention. *Journal of Experimental Social Psychology* 48(6):1267–1278. https://doi.org/10.1016/j.jesp.2012.06.003.

DeWitty, V. P. 2018. What is holistic admissions review, and why does it matter? *Journal of Nursing Education* 57(4):195–196.

DeWitty, V. P., and T. A. Murray. 2020. Influence of climate and culture on minority faculty retention. *Journal of Nursing Education* 59(9):483–484.

DiAngelo, R. 2011. White fragility. *International Journal of Critical Pedagogy* 3(3):54–71.

DiAngelo, R. J. 2018. *White fragility: Why it's so hard for White people to talk about racism*. Boston, MA: Beacon Press.

Diefenbeck, C., B. Michalec, and R. Alexander. 2016. Lived experiences of racially and ethnically underrepresented minority BSN students: A case study specifically exploring issues related to recruitment and retention. *Nursing Education Perspectives* 37(1):41–44.

Duffy, M. T., M. A. Friesen, K. G. Speroni, D. Swengros, L. A. Shanks, P. A. Waiter, and M. J. Sheridan. 2014. BSN completion barriers, challenges, incentives, and strategies. *The Journal of Nursing Administration* 44(4):232–236.

Haffland, K. J., K. Hays, F. M. Ortiz, and B. A. Blanco. 2020. Incorporating an equity agenda into health professions education and training to build a more representative workforce. *Journal of Midwifery & Women's Health* 65(1):149–159.

El-Sayed, M., and J. El-Sayed. 2014. Achieving lifelong learning outcomes in professional degree programs. *International Journal of Process Education* 6(1):37–42.

Fairman, J. A., N. A. Giordano, K. McCauley, and A. Villaruel. 2020. Invitational summit: Re-envisioning research focused PHD programs of the future. *Journal of Professional Nursing* 37. doi: 10.1016/j.profnurs.2020.09.004.

Fang, D., and G. D. Bednash. 2017. Identifying barriers and facilitators to future nurse faculty careers for DNP students. *Journal of Professional Nursing* 33(1):56–67. doi: 10.1016/j.profnurs.2016.05.008.

FDA (U.S. Food and Drug Administration). 2020. *Digital health*. https://www.fda.gov/medical-devices/digital-health (accessed May 14, 2020).

Fee, E., and L. Bu. 2010. The origins of public health nursing: The Henry Street Visiting Nurse Service. *American Journal of Public Health* 100(7):1206–1207.

FitzGerald, C., and S. Hurst. 2017. Implicit bias in healthcare professionals: A systematic review. *BMC Medical Ethics* 18(1):19.

Flores, D. D., C. Bocage, S. Devlin, M. Miller, A. Savarino, and T. H. Lipman. 2020. When community immersion becomes distance learning: Lessons learned from a disrupted semester. *Pedagogy in Health Promotion*. Epub October 16, 2020. https://journals.sagepub.com/doi/pdf/10.1177/2373379920963596 (accessed November 11, 2020).

Forman, T. M., D. A. Armor, and A. S. Miller. 2020. A review of clinical informatics competencies in nursing to inform best practices in education and nurse faculty development. *Nursing Education Perspectives* 41(1):E3–E7.

Foronda, C., S. Liu, and E. B. Bauman. 2013. Evaluation of simulation in undergraduate nurse education: An integrative review. *Clinical Simulation in Nursing* 9(10):E409–E416.

Foronda, C., D. L. Baptiste, M. M. Reinholdt, and K. Ousman. 2016. Cultural humility: A concept analysis. *Journal of Transcultural Nursing* 27(3):210–217.

Foronda, C. L., D. L. Baptiste, T. Pfaff, R. Velez, M. Reinholdt, M. Sanchez, and K. W. Hudson. 2018. Cultural competency and cultural humility in simulation-based education: An integrative review. *Clinical Simulation in Nursing* 15:42–60.

Gaines, K. n.d. *Why nursing school accreditation matters*. https://nurse.org/education/nursing- school-accreditation (accessed April 30, 2020).

Gallagher, R. W., and J. R. Polanin. 2015. A meta-analysis of educational interventions designed to enhance cultural competence in professional nurses and nursing students. *Nurse Education Today* 35(2):333–340.

Gewin, V. 2020. The time tax put on scientists of colour. *Nature* 583:479–481.

Giddens, J. F. 2009. Changing paradigms and challenging assumptions: Redefining quality and NCLEX-RN pass rates. *Journal of Nursing Education* 48(3):123–124.

Giovenco, D. P., and T. E. Spillane. 2019. Improving efficiency in mobile data collection for place-based public health research. *American Journal of Public Health* 109(S2):S123–S125.

Glazer, G., A. Clark, and K. Bankston. 2016. Holistic admissions in nursing: We can do this. *Journal of Professional Nursing* 32(4).

Glazer, G., B. Tobias, and T. Mentzel. 2018. Increasing healthcare workforce diversity: Urban universities as catalysts for change. *Journal of Professional Nursing* 34(4):306–313.

Graham, C. L., S. M. Phillips, S. D. Newman, and T. W. Atz. 2016. Baccalaureate minority nursing students perceived barriers and facilitators to clinical education practices: An integrative review. *Nursing Education Perspectives* 37(3):130–137.

Greene, M. Z., M. K. FitzPatrick, J. Romano, L. H. Aiken, and T. S. Richmond. 2017. Clinical fellowship for an innovative, integrated BSN-PhD program: An academic and practice partnership. *Journal of Professional Nursing* 33(4):282–286.

Hamilton, N., and E. A. Haozous. 2017. Retention of faculty of color in academic nursing. *Nursing Outlook* 65(2):212–221. https:// doi.org/10.1016/j.outlook.2016.11.003. PMID: 28087139.

Hayden, J., R. Smiley, M. Alexander, S. Kardong-Edgren, and P. Jeffries. 2014. The NCSBN national simulation study: A longitudinal, randomized, controlled study replacing clinical hours with simulation in prelicensure nursing education. *Journal of Nursing Regulation* 5(2S):S1–S64.

Heath, S. 2019. Top considerations for SDOH screening, referral technologies. *Health IT Analytics*. https://patientengagementhit.com/news/top-considerations-for-sdoh-screening-referral-technologies (accessed April 21, 2021).

Hermer, J., A. Hirsch, B. Bekemeier, C. Nyirati, D. Wojnar, L. Wild, and G. Oneal. 2020. Integrating population health into nursing education: The process of gaining commitment from Washington's nursing deans and directors. *Journal of Professional Nursing* 36(2):6–12.

Higgins, L. W., J. A. Shovel, A. L. Bilderback, H. L. Lorenz, S. C. Martin, D. J. Rogers, and T. E. Minnier. 2017. Hospital nurses' work activity in a technology-rich environment: A triangulated quality improvement assessment. *Journal of Nursing Care Quality* 32(3):208–217.

Horn, C. 2020. *COVID-19 response: Virtual simulation keeps nursing students on track for graduation*. University of South Carolina. https://www.sc.edu/uofsc/posts/2020/04/covid_resilience_virtual_simulation_nursing.php#.X5S1e0JKjfY (accessed April 28, 2021).

HOSA (Future Health Professionals/Health Occupations Students of America). 2012. *About HOSA*. http://www.hosa.org/about (accessed March 30, 2020).

HRSA (Health Resources and Services Administration). 2017. *Health careers pipeline and diversity programs*. https://bhw.hrsa.gov/sites/default/files/bhw/health-workforce-analysis/program-highlights/diversity-and-pipeline-training-programs-2017.pdf (accessed April 30, 2020).

HRSA. 2019. *Strategic plan FY 2019–2022*. https://www.hrsa.gov/about/strategic-plan/index.html (accessed April 30, 2020).

HRSA. 2020. *2018 national sample survey of registered nurses*. https://data.hrsa.gov/DataDownload/NSSRN/GeneralPUF18/2018_NSSRN_Summary_Report-508.pdf (accessed April 30, 2020).

HRSA. 2021. *NHSC loan repayment program*. HRSA National Health Service Corps. https://nhsc.hrsa.gov/loan-repayment/nhsc-loan-repayment-program.html (accessed March 29, 2021).

Ibrahim, S. A., M. E. Charlson, and D. B. Neill. 2020. Big data analytics and the struggle for equity in health care: The promise and perils. *Health Equity* I(1):99–101.

Iheduru-Anderson, K. C. 2020. The White/Black hierarchy institutionalizes White supremacy in nursing and nursing leadership in the United States. *Journal of Professional Nursing*. Advance online publication. https://doi.org/10.1016/j.profnurs.2020.05.005.

Iheduru-Anderson, K. C., and M. M. Wahi. 2017. Prevention of lateral violence in nursing through education: The bullying awareness seminar. *The Journal of Nursing Education* 56(12):762–763.

IOM (Institute of Medicine). 2003. *Unequal treatment: Confronting racial and ethnic disparities in health care*. Washington, DC: The National Academies Press.

IOM. 2010. *Redesigning continuing education in the health professions*. Washington, DC: The National Academies Press.

IOM. 2011. *The future of nursing: Leading change, advancing health*. Washington, DC: The National Academies Press.

IOM. 2013. *Interprofessional education for collaboration: Learning how to improve health from interprofessional models across the continuum of education to practice: Workshop summary*. Washington, DC: The National Academies Press.

IOM. 2016a. *Assessing progress on the Institute of Medicine report* The Future of Nursing. Washington, DC: The National Academies Press.

IOM. 2016b. *A framework for educating health professionals to address the social determinants of health*. Washington, DC: The National Academies Press.

IPEC (Interprofessional Education Collaborative). 2016. *Core competencies for interprofessional collaborative practice: 2016 update*. Washington, DC: Interprofessional Education Collaborative. https://ipec.memberclicks.net/assets/2016-Update.pdf (accessed June 2, 2021).

Jamshidi, N., Z. Molazem, F. Sharif, C. Torabizadeh, and M. Najafi Kalyani. 2016. The challenges of nursing students in the clinical learning environment: A qualitative study. *Scientific World Journal* 2016:1846178.

Jiménez-Rodríguez, D., M. D. M. Torres Navarro, F. J. Plaza Del Pino, and O. Arrogante. 2020. Simulated nursing video consultations: An innovative proposal during COVID-19 confinement. *Clinical Simulation of Nursing* 48:29–37. doi: 10.1016/j.ecns.2020.08.004.

Johansson, P., D. E. Jones, C. C. Watkins, M. E. Haisfield-Wolfe, and F. Gaston-Johansson. 2011. Physicians' and nurses' experiences of the influence of race and ethnicity on the quality of healthcare provided to minority patients, and on their own professional careers. *Journal of National Black Nurses Association* 22(1):43–56.

Jones, C. B., M. Toles, G. J. Knafl, and A. S. Beeber. 2018. An untapped resource in the nursing workforce: Licensed practical nurses who transition to become registered nurses. *Nursing Outlook* 66(1):46–55.

Kaiser Permanente. 2019. *Kaiser Permanente launches social health network to address needs on a broad scale*. https://permanente.org/kaiser-permanente-launches-social-health-network-to-address-needs-on-a-broad-scale (accessed November 11, 2020).

Kamau-Small, S., B. Joyce, N. Bermingham, J. Roberts, and C. Robbins. 2015. The impact of the care equity project with community/public health nursing students. *Public Health Nursing* 32(2):169–176.

Katz, J. R., C. Barbosa-Leiker, and S. Benavides-Vaello. 2016. Measuring the success of a pipeline program to increase nursing workforce diversity. *Journal of Professional Nursing* 32(1):6–14.

Kleinman, A., and P. Benson. 2006. Anthropology in the clinic: The problem of cultural competency and how to fix it. *PLoS Medicine* 3(10).

Kolade, F. M. 2016. The lived experience of minority nursing faculty: A phenomenological study. *Journal of Professional Nursing* 32(2):107–114. https:// doi.org/10.1016/j.profnurs.2015.09.002.

Kononowicz, A. A., L. A. Woodham, S. Edelbring, N. Stathakarou, D. Davies, N. Saxena, L. Tudor Car, J. Carlstedt-Duke, J. Car, and N. Zary. 2019. Virtual patient simulations in health professions education: Systematic review and meta-analysis by the digital health education collaboration. *Journal of Medical Internet Research* 21(7):e14676. https://doi.org/10.2196/14676.

Koschmann, K. S., N. K. Jeffers, and O. Heidari. 2020. "I can't breathe": A call for antiracist nursing practice. *Nursing Outlook* 68(5):539–541. doi: 10.1016/j.outlook.2020.07.004.

Kumm, S., N. Godfrey, D. Martin, M. Tucci, M. Muenks, and T. Spaeth. 2014. Baccalaureate outcomes met by associate degree nursing programs. 2014. *Nurse Education* 39(5):216–220. doi: 10.1097/NNE.0000000000000060. PMID: 24978014.

Lake, E. T. 2020. How effective response to COVID-19 relies on nursing research. *Research in Nursing and Health* 43(3):213–214.

Larsen, R., L. Reif, and R. Frauendienst. 2012. Baccalaureate nursing students' intention to choose a public health career. *Public Health Nursing* 29:424–432. https://doi.org/10.1111/j.1525-1446.2012.01031.x.

Laternman, 2019 (May 2). Tuition or dinner? Nearly half of college students surveyed in a new report are going hungry. *The New York Times*. https://www.nytimes.com/2019/05/02/nyregion/hunger-college-food-insecurity.html (accessed March 29, 2021).

LCME (Liaison Committee on Medical Education). 2018. *Functions and structure of a medical school: Standards for accreditation of medical education programs leading to the MD degree*. http://lcme.org/wp-content/uploads/filebase/standards/2019-20_Functions-and-Structure_2018-09-26.docx (accessed November 16, 2020).

Levine, S., C. Varcoe, and A. J. Browne. 2020. "We went as a team closer to the truth": Impacts of interprofessional education on trauma-and violence-informed care for staff in primary care settings. *Journal of Interprofessional Care* 35(1):46–54.

Lewis and Clark Community College. n.d. *Lewis and Clark mobile health unit*. https://www.lc.edu/Mobile_Clinics (accessed February 21, 2021).

Lim, F., M. Johnson, and M. Eliason. 2015. A national survey of faculty knowledge, experience, and readiness for teaching lesbian, gay, bisexual, and transgender health in baccalaureate nursing programs. *Nursing Education Perspectives* 36:144–152.

Linden, M. A., and S. J. Redpath. 2011. A comparative study of nursing attitudes towards young male survivors of brain injury: A questionnaire survey. *International Journal of Nursing Studies* 48(1):62–69.

Loftin, C., S. D. Newman, B. P. Dumas, G. Gilden, and M. L. Bond. 2012. Perceived barriers to success for minority nursing students: An integrative review. *International Scholarly Research Network Nursing* 2012:806543.

Love, R., and J. M. Carrington. 2020. Introducing telehealth skills into the doctor of nursing practice curriculum. *Journal of the American Association of Nurse Practitioners*. Epub ahead of print. doi: 10.1097/JXX.0000000000000505.

Mann, K., J. Gordon, and A. MacLeod. 2009. Reflection and reflective practice in health professions education: A systematic review. *Advances in Health Sciences Education Theory and Practice* 14(4):595–621.

Marion-Martins, A. D., and D. L. M. Pinho. 2020. Interprofessional simulation effects for healthcare students: A systematic review and meta-analysis. *Nurse Education Today* 94:104568.

Marken, P. A., C. Zimmerman, C. Kennedy, R. Schremmer, and K. Smith. 2010. Human simulators and standardized patients to teach difficult conversations to interprofessional health care teams. *American Journal of Pharmaceutical Education* 74(7):120.

Massachusetts Department of Higher Education Nursing Initiative. 2016. *Massachusetts nursing of the future nursing core competencies*. https://www.mass.edu/nahi/documents/NOFRN Competencies_updated_March2016.pdf (accessed January 12, 2021).

McCue, P. L. 2017. The pre-collegiate pipeline to diversify the nursing workforce. *Open Access Dissertations*. Paper 575.

McMenamin, P. 2015. *Diversity among registered nurses: Slow but steady progress*. ANA Community blog. https://community.ana.org/blogs/peter-mcmenamin/2015/08/21/rn-diversity-note?ssopc=1 (accessed June 2, 2021).

Menzel, N., L. H. Willson, and J. Doolen. 2014. Effectiveness of a poverty simulation in Second Life®: Changing nursing student attitudes toward poor people. *International Journal of Nursing Education Scholarship* (11)11. doi: 10.1515/ijnes-2013-0076.

Merrell, M., J. Probst, E. Crouch, D. Abshire, S. McKinney, and E. Haynes. 2020. A national survey of RN-to-BSN programs: Are they reaching rural students? *Journal of Nursing Education* 59(10):557–565.

Metzger, M., and J. Taggart. 2020. A longitudinal mixed methods study describing 4th year baccalaureate nursing students' perceptions of inclusive pedagogical strategies. *Journal of Professional Nursing* 36(4):229–235.

Metzger, M., T. Dowling, J. Guinn, and D. T. Wilson. 2020. Inclusivity in baccalaureate nursing education: A scoping study. *Journal of Professional Nursing* 36(1):5–14.

Miller, S., and P. Haley. 2020. *Transitioning from hospitality to health care occupations*. Federal Reserve Bank of Atlanta. https://www.frbatlanta.org/cweo/workforce-currents/2020/08/28/transitioning-from-hospitality-to-health-care-occupations (accessed February 24, 2021).

Minority Nurse. 2013. *Mentors to the max*. https://minoritynurse.com/mentors-to-the-max (accessed November 11, 2020).

Morton, J. L., F. M. Weierbach, R. Sutter, K. Livsey, E. Goehner, J. Liesveld, and M. K. Goldschmidt. 2019. New education models for preparing pre-licensure students for community-based practice. *Journal of Professional Nursing* 35(6):491–498.

Mosher, D. K., J. N. Hook, L. E. Captari, D. E. Davis, C. DeBlaere, and J. Owen. 2017. Cultural humility: A therapeutic framework for engaging diverse clients. *Practice Innovations* 2(4):221.

Murray, T. A., D. C. Pole, E. M. Ciarlo, and S. Holmes. 2016. A nursing workforce diversity project: Strategies for recruitment, retention, graduation, and NCLEX-RN success. *Nursing Education Perspectives* 37(3):138–143. PMID: 27405194.

NACNEP (National Advisory Council on Nurse Education and Practice). 2016. *Preparing nurses for new roles in population health management*. https://www.hrsa.gov/sites/default/files/hrsa/advisory-committees/nursing/reports/2016-fourteenthreport.pdf (accessed May 15, 2020).

NACNEP. 2019. *Integration of social determinants of health in nursing education, practice, and research*. https://www.hrsa.gov/sites/default/files/hrsa/advisory-committees/nursing/reports/nacnep-2019-sixteenthreport.pdf (accessed March 29, 2021).

NACNEP. 2020. *Preparing nurse faculty, and addressing the shortage of nurse faculty and clinical preceptors*. https://www.hrsa.gov/sites/default/files/hrsa/advisory-committees/nursing/reports/nacnep-17report-2021.pdf (accessed March 29, 2021).

NASEM (National Academies of Sciences, Engineering, and Medicine). 2016a. *Big data and analytics for infectious disease research, operations, and policy: Proceedings of a workshop*. Washington, DC: The National Academies Press

NASEM. 2016b. *Developing a national STEM workforce strategy: A workshop summary*. Washington, DC: The National Academies Press.

NASEM. 2017. *Communities in action: Pathways to health equity*. Washington, DC: The National Academies Press.

NASEM. 2018a. *Exploring a business case for high-value continuing professional development: Proceedings of a workshop*. Washington, DC: The National Academies Press.

NASEM. 2018b. *How people learn II: Learners, contexts, and cultures*. Washington, DC: The National Academies Press.

NASEM. 2018c. *Improving health professional education and practice through technology: Proceedings of a workshop*. Washington, DC: The National Academies Press.

NASEM. 2019. *Integrating social care into the delivery of health care: Moving upstream to improve the nation's health*. Washington, DC: The National Academies Press.

NCDHHS (North Carolina Department of Health and Human Services). 2020. *North Carolina health atlas*. https://schs.dph.ncdhhs.gov/data/hsa (accessed November 11, 2020).

NCSBN (National Council of State Boards of Nursing). 2019. *NCLEX-RN examination*. https://www.ncsbn.org/2019_RN_TestPlan-English.pdf (accessed May 1, 2020).

NCSBN. 2020a. *Number of candidates taking NCLEX examination and percent passing, by type of candidate*. https://www.ncsbn.org/Table_of_Pass_Rates_2019_Q4.pdf (accessed May 1, 2020).

NCSBN. 2020b. *Distance education*. https://www.ncsbn.org/6662.htm (accessed November 11, 2020).

NEJM (*New England Journal of Medicine*) Catalyst. 2018. *Healthcare big data and the promise of value-based care*. https://catalyst.nejm.org/doi/full/10.1056/CAT.18.0290 (accessed November 11, 2020).

New York State. n.d. *Leading the way to college affordability*. https://www.ny.gov/programs/tuition-free-degree-program-excelsior-scholarship (accessed May 15, 2020).

NLN (National League for Nursing). 2013. *Interprofessional education and healthcare simulation symposium*. http://www.nln.org/docs/default-source/professional-development-programs/white-paper-symposium-ipe-in-healthcare-simulation-2013-(pdf).pdf?sfvrsn=0 (accessed February 24, 2021).

NLN. 2015a. *A vision for the changing faculty role: Preparing students for the technological world of health care*. A diving Document from the National League for Nursing NLN Board of Governors. http://www.nln.org/docs/default-source/about/nln-vision-series-%28position-statements%29/nlnvision_8.pdf?sfvrsn=4 (accessed January 25, 2021).

NLN. 2015b. *Interprofessional collaboration in education and practice*. http://www.nln.org/docs/default-source/default-document-library/ipe-ipp-vision.pdf?sfvrsn=14 (accessed January 25, 2021).

NLN. 2016. *Accreditation standards for nursing education programs*. http://www.nln.org/docs/default-source/accreditation-services/cnea-standards-final-february-201613f2bf5c78366c709642ff00005f0421.pdf?sfvrsn=12 (accessed January 10, 2020).

NLN. 2019. *A vision for integration of the social determinants of health into nursing education curricula*. http://www.nln.org/docs/default-source/default-document-library/social-determinants-of-health.pdf?sfvrsn=2 (accessed January 10, 2020).

NONPF (National Organization of Nurse Practitioner Faculties). 2018. *NONPF supports telehealth in nurse practitioner education 2018*. https://cdn.ymaws.com/www.nonpf.org/resource/resmgr/2018_Slate/Telehealth_Paper_2018.pdf (accessed January 18, 2020).

NYSIM (City University of New York Grossman School of Medicine). 2017. *NYSIM Center*. http://nysimcenter.org (accessed May 18, 2020).

O'Connor, M. R., W. E. Barrington, D. T. Buchanan, D. Bustillos, M. Eagen-Torkko, A. Kalkbrenner, and A. B. de Castro. 2019. Short-term outcomes of a diversity, equity, and inclusion institute for nursing faculty. *Journal of Nursing Education* 58(11):633–640.

O'Lynn, C. 2017. Rethinking indicators of academic quality in nursing programs. *Journal of Nursing Education* 56(4):195–196.

Peek, M. E., M. B. Vela, and M. H. Chin. 2020. Practical lessons for teaching about race and racism: Successfully leading free, frank, and fearless discussions. *Academic Medicine* 95(12S):S139–S144.

Periyakoil, V. S. 2019. Building a culturally competent workforce to care for diverse older adults: Scope of the problem and potential solutions. *Journal of the American Geriatrics Society* 67(2):S423–S432.

Phillips, J. M., and B. Malone 2014. Increasing racial/ethnic diversity in nursing to reduce health disparities and achieve Health Equity. *Public Health Reports* 129(Suppl 2):45–50.

Phillips, K. E., A. Roberto, S. Salmon, and V. Smalley. 2020. Nursing student interprofessional simulation increases empathy and improves attitudes on poverty. *Journal of Community Health Nursing* 37(1):19–25.

Poore, J. A., D. L. Cullen, and G. L. Schaar. 2014. Simulation-based interprofessional education guided by Kolb's experiential learning theory. *Clinical Simulation in Nursing* 10(5):e241–e247.

Porter, K., G. Jackson, R. Clark, M. Waller, and A. G. Stanfill. 2020. Applying social determinants of health to nursing education using a concept-based approach. *Journal of Nursing Education* 59(5):293–296.

Pritchard, T. J., J. D. Perazzo, J. A. Holt, B. P. Fishback, M. McLaughlin, K. D. Bankston, and G. Glazer. 2016. Evaluation of a summer bridge: Critical component of the Leadership 2.0 Program. *Journal of Nursing Education* 55(4):196–202.

Pritchard, T. J., G. Glazer, K. D. Bankston, and K. McGinnis. 2020. Leadership 2.0: Nursing's next generation: Lessons learned on increasing nursing student diversity. *The Online Journal of Issues in Nursing* 25(2).

Purnell, T. S., J. K. Marshall, I. Olorundare, R. W. Stewart, S. Sisson, B. Gibbs, and L. A. Cooper. 2018. Provider perceptions of the organization's cultural competence climate and their skills and behaviors targeting patient-centered care for socially at-risk populations. *Journal of Health Care for the Poor and Underserved* 29(1):481–496.

Quality Matters. 2020. *QM-Certified Programs*. https://www.qualitymatters.org/qm-membership/faqs/qm-certified-programs (accessed November 11, 2020).

Richmond, T. S., and M. Foman. 2019. Firearm violence: A global priority for nursing science. *Journal of Nursing Scholarship* 51:229–240. https://doi.org/10.1111/jnu.12421.

RINIMC (Rhode Island Nurses Institute Middle College Charter High School). n.d. *RINIMC Charter High School*. https://rinimc.org/rinimc-charter-high-school (accessed March 29, 2021).

Rosa, W. E., M. T. Ojemeni, V. Karanja, G. Cadet, A. Charles, C. McMahon, and S. Davis. 2019. Education equity in nursing: A cornerstone of sustainable development goal attainment. *Public Health Nursing* 36(4):447–448.

Rutledge, C. M., K. Kott, P. A. Schweickert, R. Poston, C. Fowler, and T. S. Haney. 2017. Telehealth and eHealth in nurse practitioner training: Current perspectives. *Advances in Medical Education and Practice* 8:399–409. https://doi.org/10.2147/AMEP.S116071.

RWJF (Robert Wood Johnson Foundation). 2020. *Future of nursing scholars: PhD nurse profiles*. http://futureofnursingscholars.org/phd-nurse-profiles (accessed November 11, 2020).

RWJF. 2021. *Future of nursing scholars*. http://futureofnursingscholars.org (accessed June 2, 2021).

Sabin, J. A., F. P. Rivara, and A. G. Greenwald. 2008. Physician implicit attitudes and stereotypes about race and quality of medical care. *Medical Care* 46(7):678–685.

Sabio, C., and N. Petges. 2020. Understanding the barriers to BSN education among ADN students: A qualitative study. *Teaching and Learning in Nursing* 15(1):45–52.

Salvucci, C., and C. A. Lawless. 2016. Nursing faculty diversity: Barriers and perceptions on recruitment, hiring, and retention. *Journal of Cultural Diversity* 23(2):65–75. PMID: 27439233.

Sanner, S., D. E. E. Baldwin, K. A. Cannella, and J. Charles. 2010. The impact of cultural diversity forum on students' openness to diversity. *Journal of Cultural Diversity* 17(2).

Scheel, L. S., M. D. Peters, and A. C. M. Møbjerg. 2017. Reflection in the training of nurses in clinical practice settings: A scoping review protocol. *JBI Database of Systematic Reviews and Implementation Reports* 15(12):2871–2880.

Schmidt, S., M. George, and J. Bussey-Jones. 2016. Welcome to the neighborhood: Service-learning to understand social determinants of health and promote local advocacy. *Diversity Equality Health Care* 13(6):389–390.

Schroeder, C., and R. DiAngelo. 2010. Addressing whiteness in nursing education: The sociopolitical climate project at the University of Washington School of Nursing. *Advances in Nursing Science* 33(3):244–255. doi: 10.1097/ANS.0b013e3181eb41cf. PMID: 20693833.

Schroeder, K., B. Garcia, R. S. Phillips, and T. H. Lipman. 2019. Addressing social determinants of health through community engagement: An undergraduate nursing course. *Journal of Nursing Education* 58(7):423–426.

Sharma, M., A. D. Pinto, and A. K. Kumagai. 2018. Teaching the social determinants of health: A path to equity or a road to nowhere? *Academic Medicine* 93(1):25–30.

Shiffrin, R. M. 2016. Drawing causal inference from big data. *Proceedings of the National Academy of Sciences* 113(27):7308–7309.

Shin, S., J. H. Park, and J. H. Kim. 2015. Effectiveness of patient simulation in nursing education: Meta-analysis. *Nurse Education Today* 35(1):176–182. doi: 10.1016/j.nedt.2014.09.009.

Siegel, J., D. L. Coleman, and T. James. 2018. Integrating social determinants of health into graduate medical education: A call for action. *Academic Medicine* 93(2):159–162.

Spector, N., J. Silvestre, M. Alexander, B. Martin, J. Hooper, A. Squires, and M. Ojemeni. 2020. NCSBN regulatory guidelines and evidence-based quality indicators for nursing education programs. *Journal of Nursing Regulation* 11(2S):S1–S64.

Spetz, J. 2018. Projections of progress toward the 80% bachelor of science in nursing recommendation and strategies to accelerate change. *Nursing Outlook* 66(4):394–400.

Squires, A., C. Kovner, F. Faridaben, and D. Chyun. 2013. Assessing nursing student intent for PhD study. *Nurse Education Today* 34(11):1405–1410.

SSIH (Society for Simulation in Healthcare). n.d. *About simulation*. https://www.ssih.org/About-SSH/About-Simulation (accessed January 12, 2021).

Storfjell, J., B. Winslow, and J. Saunders. 2017. *Catalysts for change: Harnessing the power of nurses to build population health in the 21st century*. Princeton, NJ: Robert Wood Johnson Foundation.

Strauss, V. 2020. *Housing and food insecurity affecting many college students, new data says*. https://www.washingtonpost.com/education/2020/02/20/housing-food-insecurity-affecting-many-college-students-new-data-says (accessed January 12, 2021).

Sukhera, J., M. Wodzinski, M. Rehman, and C. M. Gonzalez. 2019. The implicit association test in health professions education: A meta-narrative review. *Perspectives in Medical Education* 8(5):267–275.

Sullivan, L. W. 2004. *Missing persons: Minorities in the health professions. A report of the Sullivan Commission on Diversity in the Healthcare Workforce*. The Sullivan Commission. https://campaignforaction.org/wp-content/uploads/2016/04/SullivanReport-Diversity-in-Healthcare-Workforce1.pdf (accessed March 29, 2021).

Szanton, S. L., J. W. Wolff, B. Leff, R. J. Thorpe, E. K. Tanner, C. Boyd, Q. Xue, J. Guralnik, D. Bishai, and L. N. Gitlin.2014. CAPABLE trial: A randomized controlled trial of nurse, occupational therapist and handyman to reduce disability among older adults: Rationale and design. *Contemporary Clinical Trials* 38(1):102–112. https://doi.org/10.1016/j.cct.2014.03.005.

Taylor, H., C. Loftin, and H. Reyes. 2014. First-time NCLEX-RN pass rate: Measure of program quality or something else? *Journal of Nursing Education* 53(6):336–341.

The Macy Foundation. 2020. *Addressing harmful bias and eliminating discrimination in health professions learning environments*. Conference recommendations February 24–27, 2020. Atlanta, GA: Josiah Macy Jr. Foundation.

The Poverty Simulation. n.d. *The Poverty Simulation*. http://www.povertysimulation.net/about (accessed May 14, 2020).

ThinkTank, n.d. *The cost of poverty experience*. https://thinktank-inc.org/cope (accessed November 11, 2020).

Thornton, M., and S. Persaud. 2018. Preparing today's nurses: Social determinants of health and nursing education. *The Online Journal of Issues in Nursing* 23(3).

Tilden, V. P., K. S. Cox, J. E. Moore, and M. D. Naylor. 2018. Strategic partnerships to address adverse social determinants of health: Redefining health care. *Nursing Outlook* 66(3):233–236.

Topaz, M., and L. Pruinelli. 2017. Big data and nursing: Implications for the future. *Studies in Health Technology and Informatics* 232:165–171.

Turk, M. T., and A. M. Colbert. 2018. Using simulation to help beginning nursing students learn about the experience of poverty: A descriptive study. *Nurse Education Today* 71:174–179. Epub September 29, 2018. doi: 10.1016/j.nedt.2018.09.035. PMID: 30292059.

Tyczkowski, B. L., and J. Reilly. 2017. DNP-prepared nurse leaders: Part of the solution to the growing faculty shortage. *The Journal of Nursing Administration* 47(7–8):359–360.

UND (University of North Dakota). 2020. *RAIN: No excuses orientation*. https://cnpd.und.edu/rain/no-excuses.html (accessed November 11, 2020).

U.S. Department of Education. n.d.a. *Competency-based learning or personalized learning*. https://www.ed.gov/oii-news/competency-based-learning-or-personalized-learning (accessed November 11, 2020).

U.S. Department of Education. n.d.b. *Public service loan forgiveness*. https://studentaid.gov/manage-loans/forgiveness-cancellation/public-service (accessed September 2, 2020).

Valderama-Wallace, C. P., and E. C. Apesoa-Varano. 2019. "Social justice is a dream": Tensions and contradictions in nursing education. *Public Health Nursing* 36(5):735–743.

Velasquez, D., and A. Mehrotra. 2020. Ensuring the growth of telehealth during COVID-19 does not exacerbate disparities in care. *Health Affairs Blog*. doi: 10.1377/hblog20200505.591306.

Villarruel, A. M., and M. E. Broome. 2020. Beyond the naming: Institutional racism in nursing. *Nursing Outlook* 68(4):375–376.

von Wendt, C. E. A., and L. Niemi-Murola. 2018. Simulation in interprofessional clinical education. *Simulation in Healthcare* 13(2):131–138.

Waite, R., and D. Nardi. 2019. Nursing colonialism in America: Implications for nursing leadership. *Journal of Professional Nursing* 35(1):18–25. doi: 10.1016/j.profnurs.2017.12.

Walker, K., M. Arbour, and J. Waryold. 2016. Educational strategies to help students provide respectful sexual and reproductive health care for lesbian, gay, bisexual, and transgender persons. *Journal of Midwifery and Women's Health* 61(6):737–743.

Wallace, J., K. Decosimo, and M. Simon. 2019. Applying data analytics to address social determinants of health in practice. *North Carolina Medical Journal* 80:244–248.

WGU (Western Governors University). 2020. *Competency-based education*. https://www.wgu.edu/about/competency-based-education.html (accessed November 11, 2020).

Whitfield-Harris, L., and J. S. Lockhart. 2016. The workplace environment for African American faculty employed in predominantly White institutions. *The Association of Black Nursing Faculty Journal* 27(2):28–38. PMID: 27263232.

Whitfield-Harris, L., J. S. Lockhart, R. Zoucha, and R. Alexander. 2017. The lived experience of Black nurse faculty in predominantly White schools of nursing. *Journal of Transcultural Nursing* 28(6):608–615.

WHO (World Health Organization). Regional Office for the Eastern Mediterranean. 2015. *The growing need for home health care for the elderly: Home health care for the elderly as an integral part of primary health care services*. https://apps.who.int/iris/handle/10665/326801 (accessed March 29, 2021).

Wilkie, M. L. 2020. Empowered by cultural identity and catalyzed by resilience: A path to support American Indian nursing student success. *Creative Nursing* 26(1):43–47.

Williams, S. D., K. Hansen, M. Smithey, J. Burnley, M. Koplitz, K. Koyama, and A. Bakos. 2014. Using social determinants of health to link health workforce diversity, care quality and access, and health disparities to achieve health equity in nursing. *Public Health Reports* 129(1):32–36.

Wilson, A. H., S. Sanner, and L. E. McAllister. 2010. An evaluation study of a mentoring program to increase the diversity of the nursing workforce. *Journal of Cultural Diversity* 17(4).

Wise, P. H. 2012. Emerging technologies and their impact on disability. *The Future of Children* 169–191.

Yale School of Nursing. 2020. *Simulation technology redirects nursing curriculum during COVID-19*. https://nursing.yale.edu/news/simulation-technology-redirects-nursing-curriculum-during-covid-19 (accessed January 12, 2021).

Yen, P. Y., and S. Bakken. 2012. Review of health information technology usability study methodologies. *Journal of the American Medical Informatics Association* 19(3):413–422.

Yoder, C. M., and M. S. Pesch. 2020. An academic–fire department partnership to address social determinants of health. *Journal of Nursing Education* 59(1):34–37.

Zandee, G., D. Bossenbroek, M. Friesen, K. Blech, and R. Engbers. 2010. Effectiveness of community health worker/nursing student teams as a strategy for public health nursing education. *Public Health Nursing* 27(3):277–284.

8[1]

Nurses in Disaster Preparedness and Public Health Emergency Response

By failing to prepare, you are preparing to fail.

—Benjamin Franklin, writer, philosopher, politician

In the past decade, 2.6 billion people around the world have been affected by earthquakes, floods, hurricanes, and other natural disasters. Nurses have been and continue to be pivotal in safeguarding the public during and after these disasters, as well as public health emergencies—most recently, the COVID-19 pandemic. They educate and protect people, engage with and build trust with the community, help people prepare and respond, and foster resilience to help communities fully recover. But fundamental reform is needed in nursing education, practice, research, and policy across both health care and public health settings to ensure that all nurses—from front-line professionals to researchers—have the baseline knowledge, skills, abilities, and autonomy they need to protect populations at greatest risk and improve the readiness, safety, and support of the nursing workforce.

The increasing frequency of natural and environmental disasters, along with public health emergencies such as the COVID-19 pandemic, highlights the critical importance of having a national nursing workforce prepared with the knowledge, skills, and abilities to respond. COVID-19 has revealed deep chasms within a fragmented U.S. health care system that have resulted in significant excess

[1] This chapter was commissioned by the Committee on the Future of Nursing 2020–2030 (Veenema, 2020).

mortality and morbidity, glaring health inequities, and an inability to contain a rapidly escalating pandemic. Most severely affected by these systemic flaws are individuals and communities of color that suffer disproportionately from the compound disadvantages of racism, poverty, workplace hazards, limited health care access, and preexisting health conditions that reflect the role of social determinants of health (SDOH) and inequities in access to health and health care that are a primary focus of this report. As natural disasters and public health emergencies continue to threaten population health in the decades ahead, articulation of the roles and responsibilities of nurses in disaster preparedness and public health emergency response will be critical to the nation's capacity to plan for and respond to such events.

As described in the conceptual model framework developed by the committee to guide this study (see Figure 1-1 in Chapter 1), strengthening nurses' capacity to aid in disaster preparedness and public health emergency response is one of the key ways to enhance nursing's role in addressing SDOH and improving health and health care equity. This chapter explores the contribution of nurses during the COVID-19 pandemic and across sentinel historical events and describes the impact of natural disasters and public health emergencies on SDOH and health and health care equity. It also illuminates the multiple and systemic challenges encountered by nurses in these past events, and identifies bold and essential changes needed in nursing education, practice, and policy across health care and public health systems and organizations to strengthen and protect the nursing profession during and after such events. Only when equipped with the salient knowledge, skills, and abilities can nurses be fully effective in helping to protect the well-being of underserved populations, striving for health equity, and advocating for themselves and other health care workers.

ROLES OF NURSES DURING NATURAL DISASTERS AND PUBLIC HEALTH EMERGENCIES

The ability to care for and protect the nation's most vulnerable citizens depends substantially on the preparedness of the nursing workforce. The myriad factors related to national nurse education and training—licensure and certification, scope of practice, mobilization and deployment, safety and protection, crisis leadership, and health care and public health systems support—together define nursing's capacity and capabilities in disaster response. The nursing workforce available to participate in U.S. disaster and public health emergency response includes all licensed nurses (licensed practical/vocational nurses [LPN/LVNs] and registered nurses [RNs]), civilian and uniformed services nurses at the federal and state levels, nurses who have recently retired, and those who volunteer (e.g., National Disaster Medical System, Medical Reserve Corps, National Voluntary Organizations Active in Disasters, and American Red Cross [ARC]). Each of these entities plays a critical role in the nation's ability to respond to and recover from disasters and large-scale public health emergencies such as the COVID-19 pandemic.[2]

Nurses' General Roles in Disasters

Across a broad spectrum of clinical and community settings and through all phases of a disaster event (see Figure 8-1), nurses, working with physicians and other members of the health care team, play a central role in response. Before, during, and after disasters, nurses provide education, community engagement, and health promotion and implement interventions to safeguard the public health. They provide first aid, advanced clinical care, and lifesaving medications; assess and triage victims; allocate scarce resources; and monitor ongoing physical and mental health needs. Nurses also assist with organizational logistics by developing operational response protocols and security measures and performing statistical analysis of individual- and community-level data.

Beyond these contributions, nurses activate organizational emergency operations plans, participate in incident command systems, oversee the use of personal protective equipment (PPE), and provide crisis leadership and communications, often at risk to their own health. In the community, they open and manage shelters; organize blood drives; and provide outreach to underserved populations, including by addressing social needs. Nurses also assist with care for the frail elderly (Heagele and Pacqiao, 2018; Kleier et al., 2018), assist with childbirth to ensure that women have healthy babies during a disaster (Badakhsh et al., 2010; de Mendoza et al., 2012; Role of the nurse, 2012), and work to reunite families separated during response activities. Disasters place unprecedented demands on health care systems and often test nurses' knowledge, skills, abilities, and personal commitment as health care professionals.

Nurses' Roles in Pandemics and Other Infectious Disease Outbreaks

Nurses' roles in pandemics and other infectious disease outbreaks are multifaceted and may include

- supporting and advising in epidemic surveillance and detection, such as contact tracing;
- working in point-of-distribution clinics to screen, test, and distribute vaccines and other medical countermeasures;
- employing prevention and response interventions;
- providing direct hospital-based treatment for impacted individuals;
- educating patients and the public to decrease risk for infection;

[2] For the sake of brevity, the term "disaster" is used throughout the remainder of this chapter to refer to both natural disasters and public health emergencies.

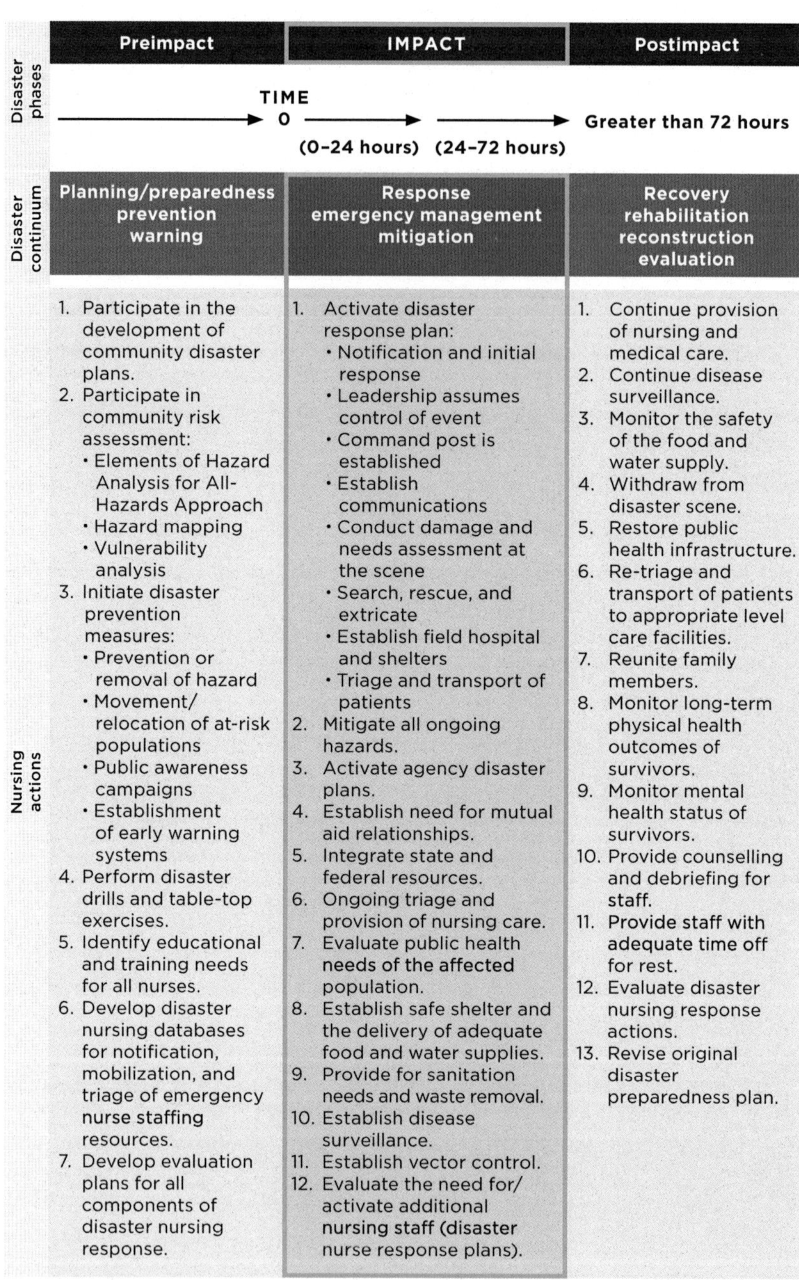

Disaster phases	Preimpact	IMPACT	Postimpact
	TIME 0 →	→ (0–24 hours) → (24–72 hours)	→ Greater than 72 hours
Disaster continuum	Planning/preparedness prevention warning	Response emergency management mitigation	Recovery rehabilitation reconstruction evaluation
Nursing actions	1. Participate in the development of community disaster plans. 2. Participate in community risk assessment: • Elements of Hazard Analysis for All-Hazards Approach • Hazard mapping • Vulnerability analysis 3. Initiate disaster prevention measures: • Prevention or removal of hazard • Movement/relocation of at-risk populations • Public awareness campaigns • Establishment of early warning systems 4. Perform disaster drills and table-top exercises. 5. Identify educational and training needs for all nurses. 6. Develop disaster nursing databases for notification, mobilization, and triage of emergency nurse staffing resources. 7. Develop evaluation plans for all components of disaster nursing response.	1. Activate disaster response plan: • Notification and initial response • Leadership assumes control of event • Command post is established • Establish communications • Conduct damage and needs assessment at the scene • Search, rescue, and extricate • Establish field hospital and shelters • Triage and transport of patients 2. Mitigate all ongoing hazards. 3. Activate agency disaster plans. 4. Establish need for mutual aid relationships. 5. Integrate state and federal resources. 6. Ongoing triage and provision of nursing care. 7. Evaluate public health needs of the affected population. 8. Establish safe shelter and the delivery of adequate food and water supplies. 9. Provide for sanitation needs and waste removal. 10. Establish disease surveillance. 11. Establish vector control. 12. Evaluate the need for/activate additional nursing staff (disaster nurse response plans).	1. Continue provision of nursing and medical care. 2. Continue disease surveillance. 3. Monitor the safety of the food and water supply. 4. Withdraw from disaster scene. 5. Restore public health infrastructure. 6. Re-triage and transport of patients to appropriate level care facilities. 7. Reunite family members. 8. Monitor long-term physical health outcomes of survivors. 9. Monitor mental health status of survivors. 10. Provide counselling and debriefing for staff. 11. Provide staff with adequate time off for rest. 12. Evaluate disaster nursing response actions. 13. Revise original disaster preparedness plan.

FIGURE 8-1 Disaster nursing timeline.
SOURCE: Veenema, 2018.

- providing health systems and community-based leadership; and
- counseling and supporting community members to assuage fear and anxiety (Veenema et al., 2020).

Public health nurses have helped coordinate and implement disaster plans (Jakeway et al., 2008), and it was a school nurse working in Queens, New York, in 2009 who first observed and then notified the Centers for Disease Control and Prevention (CDC) about the H1N1 outbreak (Molyneux, 2009).

Infectious disease outbreaks have been occurring more frequently and at a higher intensity over the past few decades (Fauci and Morens, 2012; Lam et al., 2018). Both the health care system and individual front-line health care workers must be adequately prepared to respond to such events (Imai et al., 2008; Lam et al., 2018; Siu, 2010). Preparedness at the system level includes understanding the capacity of a hospital or health care system in advance of a potential public health emergency, including workforce capacity and capabilities and access to PPE, medical supplies, medical gases, and ventilators. It also requires having an action plan that includes the essential elements of managing the challenges such an event may impose on the institution (Siu, 2010; Toner et al., 2020; WHO, 2018). However, the preparedness of the U.S. health care system to manage a pediatric surge during a pandemic has been recognized as lacking (Anthony et al., 2017). Preparedness for front-line workers includes clinical skills and knowledge for providing care for patients and protecting the public from becoming ill (Lam et al., 2018; Ruderman et al., 2006; Shih et al., 2007).

Response plans and nurses' willingness to respond will vary based on the amount of information available about the pathogen and its transmission, the severity of the disease, and the public's attitude toward the outbreak (Chung et al., 2005; Lam and Hung, 2013; Lam et al., 2018; Shih et al., 2007). When certain aspects of the disease are uncertain or the information is inconsistent, nurses become less confident and more anxious about performing their duties during an outbreak (Lam et al., 2018; Shih et al., 2007). The more severe the disease outbreak, the more likely it is that nurses will be prone to greater anxiety and fear of infection (Koh et al., 2012; O'Boyle et al., 2006). Even if this fear does not stop them from working during the outbreak, they are more likely to have a negative attitude and decreased morale when caring for infected patients. Nurse attitudes can also be strongly impacted by the mass media and news outlets (Lam et al., 2018; Shih et al., 2009). During disease outbreaks, the media will focus on the number of deaths and the severity of the disease, making it challenging for nurses to maintain a positive attitude when working with patients. Perceptions of the disease created in the media can also cause panic in the general public, which directly affects front-line nurses both in health systems and in the community (Lam and Hung, 2013; O'Boyle et al., 2006; Shih et al., 2007, 2009).

The disaster nursing timeline (see Figure 8-1) and many state, local, and organizational response plans are based on the single occurrence of an acute event. It is important to note that infectious disease outbreaks are slow-moving disasters with multiple waves that create unique challenges for health system response. There is much to be learned from the events of 2020 and the devastating sequence of events that unfolded during the COVID-19 response.

Nurses' Roles in the COVID-19 Pandemic

In December 2019, the novel coronavirus known as the severe acute respiratory syndrome coronavirus 2 (SARS-CoV-2) was first detected in China. By March 2020, the World Health Organization (WHO) had declared the COVID-19 outbreak a pandemic, which was to become the worst public health emergency in more than 100 years, with more than 120 million cases detected worldwide and 30.5 million cases confirmed in the United States as of April 1, 2021.[3] Nurses have performed a variety of roles during the COVID-19 pandemic, while health care organizations and hospitals have had to treat innumerable patients across the United States for COVID-related illness alongside other complex and serious conditions (Veenema et al., 2020).

Roles and responsibilities for nurses shifted rapidly to accommodate patient surges and the sudden unanticipated demand for health care services. Nurses were required to take on multiple new roles (e.g., non–critical care nurses asked to care for patients critically ill with COVID-19), provide end-of-life care, and serve as a means of vital communications between hospitalized patients and their families (Veenema et al., 2020). These shifts may have lowered the skill mix in intensive care units (ICUs) below required standards, with potential risks to patients' safety and quality of care (Bambi et al., 2020). As of April 1, 2021, 552,957 people in the United States had died from COVID-19,[4] including an estimated 551 nurses.[5] Evidence gathered from nurses throughout the pandemic reveals the multiple challenges they have encountered during the pandemic response. Nurses have reported inadequate supplies of PPE, insufficient knowledge and skills for responding to the pandemic, a lack of authority for decision making related to workflow redesign and allocation of scarce resources, staffing shortages, and a basic lack of trust between front-line nurses and nurse executives and hospital administrators (ANA, 2020a,b; Mason and Friese, 2020; Veenema et al., 2020).

Nurses have experienced significant psychological and moral distress during the pandemic (Altman, 2020; Labrague and De Los Santos, 2020; Pappa et al., 2020; Shechter et al., 2020). Results of a survey conducted by the American Nurses Association (ANA, 2020a) reveal that 87 percent of nurses were afraid

[3] See https://gisanddata.maps.arcgis.com/apps/opsdashboard/index.html#/bda7594740fd40299423467b48e9ecf6 (accessed April 1, 2021).

[4] See https://gisanddata.maps.arcgis.com/apps/opsdashboard/index.html#/bda7594740fd40299423467b48e9ecf6 (accessed April 1, 2021).

[5] See https://www.theguardian.com/us-news/ng-interactive/2020/dec/22/lost-on-the-frontline-our-findings-to-date (accessed March 18, 2021).

to go to work, 36 percent had cared for an infectious patient without having adequate PPE, and only 11 percent felt well prepared to care for a patient with COVID-19. A follow-up survey conducted by ANA (2020c) revealed that intermittent shortages of PPE for nurses persisted 7 months into the pandemic, particularly for those working in smaller rural hospitals, home care, and palliative care. Nurses were asked to extend and reuse N95 masks long after CDC's recommended guidelines, leading ANA to request that the Defense Production Act (DPA) be invoked to produce N95 masks (Lasek, 2020). In particular, nurses working in long-term care facilities, home care, palliative care, and small rural hospitals were particularly vulnerable as caregivers in environments with high risk and high mortality (ANA, 2020c).

The mental health burden of the pandemic on nurses has been profound (see Chapter 10). Nurses of Asian/Pacific Islander (API) descent have experienced discrimination from patients who have refused care from them or made disparaging remarks about their ethnic origins. The Asian Pacific Policy and Planning Council released a report on August 27, 2020, detailing 2,583 incidents of discrimination against APIs in the United States from March 19 to August 5, 2020 (*Attacks against AAPI community*, 2020). The psychological and mental health implications for nurses of API descent represent one of the many challenges nurses have faced during the pandemic.

Nurses' Response to Human-Caused Disasters

In addition to natural disasters and public health emergencies, the United States is currently experiencing significant increases in gun-related violence, civil unrest against systemic racism, and social upheaval associated with growing political polarization (see Box 8-1). Active shooters in hospitals, school shootings, and random acts of foreign and domestic terrorism have forced a widening aperture for national preparedness, and nurses are involved in responding to the care needs of victims of these events (Lavin et al., 2017).

DISASTERS' IMPACT ON POPULATION HEALTH

A disaster is defined as "a serious disruption of the functioning of a community or a society at any scale due to hazardous events interacting with conditions of exposure, vulnerability and capacity, leading to one or more of the following: human, material, economic and environmental losses and impacts" (UNISDR, 2017). More than 2.6 billion people globally have been affected by natural disasters, such as earthquakes, tsunamis, and heat waves, in the past decade, and these disasters have led to massive injuries, mental health issues, and illnesses that can overwhelm local health care resources and prevent them from delivering comprehensive and definitive medical care (WHO, 2020). During 2019 alone, the United States experienced 14 separate billion-dollar disasters, including inland floods, severe storms,

BOX 8-1
Pulse Nightclub Shooting

What would become one of the worst mass shootings in U.S. history occurred on June 12, 2016, in Orlando, Florida. Around 2:00 AM, a gunman opened fire at a popular gay nightclub, Pulse Orlando, killing 50 people and injuring another 53 (Shapiro, 2016). Fortunately, the Orlando Regional Medical Center (ORMC), the only Level 1 trauma center in the region, was just a few blocks away. Within a few hours, the hospital had treated 44 of the shooting victims, 36 of whom had arrived within the first 36 minutes of the hospital's response (Willis and Philp, 2017). Just a few months prior to the Pulse Nightclub shooting, there had been a community-wide exercise in disaster response that involved responding to an active shooter. More than 500 volunteers, 50 agencies, and 15 hospitals across central Florida had participated. Staff from ORMC stated that participation in such mass-casualty drills was one of the reasons they were prepared to respond to the Pulse Nightclub tragedy (Willis and Philp, 2017). These drills included practicing roles within the Hospital Incident Command System, which the nurse leaders were able to execute during the event. By understanding what is expected of them and feeling confident in their previously assigned roles, they were able to provide quality, timely care to the victims while managing the large influx of patients that arrived with no emergency medical services notice or triage.

two hurricanes, and a major wildfire event (Smith, 2020). Disaster planning for emergency preparedness is, then, imperative. In the near future, such factors as climate change and climate change–related events, including global warming and sea-level rise; the depletion of resources and associated societal factors; and the growth of "megacities" and populations shifts (IFRC, 2019; UN, 2016) are likely to converge to increase the risk of future disasters (IPCC, 2012, 2014; Watts et al., 2018). Human-caused disasters, such as school and other mass shootings and random acts of terrorism, create additional hazards for human health.

Health Inequities in Disasters

While disasters impact populations, research has shown that those impacts are not equally distributed. Disasters often amplify the inequities already present in society and harm high-risk and highly vulnerable communities far more than others (Davis et al., 2010). Although every person who is exposed to a disaster is impacted in some form, the disproportionate impact on high-risk and highly vulnerable populations, including the elderly, individuals with disabilities, the immunosuppressed, the underserved, and those living in poverty, is unequivocal (Maltz, 2019; UNISDR, 1982). Severe and morbid obesity, the complex causes of which are rooted in SDOH, also creates increased vulnerability to disasters.

In fact, the intersection of SDOH, severe or morbid obesity, and disaster vulnerability is postulated to create "triple jeopardy" for these individuals (Gray, 2017).

Health and health care disparities, such as lack of access to primary care and specialty providers, the presence of comorbid conditions, and lack of health insurance, together with poverty, not only put people at increased risk for injury or death during disasters but also are often exacerbated during a disaster. For example, more than 4,600 excess deaths are believed to have resulted from Hurricane Katrina because of interruptions in medical care and basic utilities, which especially impacted those with chronic conditions who required medical equipment powered by electricity (Kishore et al., 2018). This number was much higher than the number of people who died as a direct result of the hurricane and indicates how quickly chronic conditions can revert to acute medical emergencies, greatly increasing the mortality of those most underserved.

Studies show that although the majority of Americans are considered unprepared for the occurrence of a disaster, those of lower socioeconomic status (SES) and lower educational attainment are generally less prepared than their wealthier and more educated counterparts in part because of the costs associated with preparedness actions, such as obtaining insurance and taking measures to prepare for earthquakes (SAMHSA, 2017). In a national household survey, for example, 65 percent of respondents said they had no disaster plans or had plans that were inadequate (Petkova et al., 2016). And according to national survey data from the Federal Emergency Management Agency (FEMA), fewer than half of Americans are familiar with local hazards, less than 40 percent have created a household emergency plan, and only about half (52 percent) have disaster supplies at home (FEMA, 2014).

When communities are warned about impending disasters, research shows that those of lower SES may be less likely to respond because of the cost and resources associated with evacuation (Thiede and Brown, 2013). When a disaster strikes, a range of impacts continue to affect those of lower SES compared with those of higher SES more severely, including homelessness, physical injuries, and financial effects. Families of lower SES are more likely to experience greater impacts from disasters, including damage to their homes from strong winds, floods, or earthquakes because of their homes' lower construction quality and increased likelihood of being located in flood-prone areas; lack of insurance coverage; insufficient savings; and lack of understanding of the governmental systems that provide aid to victims (Hallegatte et al., 2016). They may not know how to access aid and may feel uncomfortable working with these systems, especially if they are undocumented immigrants in fear of being deported. Families may even be unable to reach assistance centers because of a lack of transportation and child care or the inability to miss work. Those of lower SES are more vulnerable to homelessness after a disaster and experience extreme difficulty in obtaining housing loans to help them rebuild their damaged homes (SAMHSA, 2017). This plethora of hardships experienced by people of lower SES and people of color during and after a disaster also leads to an increased likelihood of experiencing depression and posttraumatic stress.

Relationship to Race and Ethnicity

Health inequities seen in natural disasters and infectious disease outbreaks are often directly related to race and ethnicity. The COVID-19 pandemic has had a disproportionate effect on Black, Hispanic, and American Indian populations, who have experienced greater levels of suffering and death. Long-standing racial and ethnic inequities in access to health care services prior to the pandemic have translated into disparities in access to COVID-19 testing and treatment (Duke Margolis Center for Health Policy, 2020; Poteat et al., 2020). Zoning laws and low income levels have disadvantaged some racial and ethnic groups and contributed to living conditions that have made it difficult for individuals to socially distance (Davenport et al., 2020). The added burdens of chronic disease and persistent underfunding of American Indian health systems have resulted in the nation's Indigenous population being at high risk of poor outcomes from the disease (AMA, 2020). COVID-19-related unemployment and economic devastation have impacted all communities, with Black and Hispanic workers experiencing the highest rates of COVID-19 infection (BLS, 2020). Box 8-2 describes how one county in Texas became a COVID-19 "hotspot."

BOX 8-2
COVID-19 in Hidalgo County, Texas

Hidalgo County, Texas, in the Rio Grande Valley on the U.S.–Mexico border became a coronavirus hotspot, with 15,153 confirmed cases and 456 deaths as of July 25, 2020.[a] Hidalgo County has a high prevalence of diabetes and obesity, along with poverty and poor access to health care, exacerbating the life-threatening side effects of the coronavirus (Killough et al., 2020; Najmabadi and Gutierrez, 2020). Furthermore, 92 percent of the Hidalgo Country residents are Hispanic, a population that has been disproportionately affected by the pandemic because of their essential worker status (Erdman, 2020).

After a broad reopening in May 2020, Texas saw a surge in cases across the state. Hospitals were referred to as "war zones" (Brooks and O'Brien, 2020; Killough et al., 2020). More than 1,200 medical personnel were sent to the region, including U.S. Navy and Army nurses and physicians, to provide desperately needed relief to the overworked hospital staff. The county suffered the deaths of five nurses from COVID-19 (Hernandez, 2020), as they were responsible for more critically ill patients and were constantly working overtime with no end in sight as their patient load continued to grow.

[a] See https://www.hidalgocounty.us/coronavirusupdates (accessed April 5, 2021).

Nurses' Roles in Addressing Disparities

In the future, nurses could play a role in helping to address these disparities before, during, and after a disaster. Community resilience, which "refers to community capabilities that buffer it from or support effective responses to disasters," is of growing importance in disaster preparedness, particularly in underresourced areas (Wells et al., 2013, p. 1172). This concept engages the community in disaster planning, such as creating "community emergency response teams" and helping families compile their own disaster preparedness kits (Wells et al., 2013). When adequate in number, public health and school nurses can help with these community engagement activities and advance preparedness in at-risk populations, such as low-income families and the homebound elderly (Spurlock et al., 2019). Some disasters may not call on nurses to use technical clinical practice skills, but rather their skills in networking, communications, creation of partnerships, resource identification, and assessment, as well as their understanding of SDOH that result in increased vulnerabilities to a disaster event. Disasters often limit or eliminate access to transportation; access to care, food, and shelter; and employment. By understanding how these factors affect a person's health and well-being and related potential resources, nurses can help build community resilience (Heagele, 2017). Additionally, nurses can play a role in advocating for a health equity approach in preparation for future pandemics that addresses historical and current structural as well as systemic racial prejudice and discrimination that result in health disparities.

Equitable access to and distribution of tests, treatments, contact tracing, and vaccines especially for underserved populations, is instrumental to the success of the response to COVID-19 as well as future pandemics. Nurses' capacity to advance health equity in the United States includes supporting fair, equitable, and transparent allocation of vaccine during the nation's COVID-19 vaccine campaign and future infectious disease emergencies. Nurses' awareness of the relationship between the historical experience of individuals and communities and how SDOH impact trust in the health care system and vaccine hesitancy is a precursor to the critically important work of framing community health education and messaging to counter misinformation. With this understanding, nurses can be trusted sources of health information and work actively to educate their communities, particularly in the areas of preventing disease spread and dispelling vaccine-related misinformation. Nurses should be able and willing to participate in all of these activities during an ongoing pandemic (Martin, 2011).

NURSES' ROLE IN SHELTERING DURING DISASTERS

During disasters, nurses staff shelters that house people displaced by these events. Shelters are critical in disaster response, providing temporary housing for those displaced by such events as earthquakes and hurricanes (see Box 8-3).

During Hurricanes Gustav and Ike in 2008, more than 3,700 patients were treated by nurses in shelters for acute and chronic illnesses (Noe et al., 2013). After Hurricane Katrina in 2006, nearly 1,400 evacuation shelters were opened to accommodate 500,000 evacuees from the Gulf region (Jenkins et al., 2009). People who receive care in shelters, including children, the elderly, and those with chronic medical conditions, are often economically disadvantaged and highly vulnerable to a disaster's health impacts (Laditka et al., 2008; Springer and Casey-Lockyer, 2016). For example, one study of evacuees living in Red Cross shelters after Hurricane Katrina found that nearly half lacked health insurance, 55 percent had a preexisting chronic disease, and 48 percent lacked access to medication (Greenough et al., 2008). Nurses can help ensure that such evacuees receive appropriate care, including for physical and mental illnesses, and help prevent unnecessary deaths that may result from disruptions in health care services.

After a disaster, people must often spend extended periods in shelters until they can find alternative housing, greatly affecting their social, mental, and physical well-being. For example, studies have found that disaster victims are at increased risk for posttraumatic stress disorder, and the close proximity to others in which they must live in shelters, combined with poor infection control, greatly

BOX 8-3
Lessons Learned from Nurses' Role in Evacuation During Hurricane Sandy

On October 28, 2012, Hurricane Sandy made landfall in Atlantic City, New Jersey. The storm eventually claimed nearly 150 lives and caused billions of dollars of damage along the U.S. East Coast. Hospitals across New York City, including the New York University Langone Medical Center (NYULMC), began preparing for Hurricane Sandy in the week before landfall. Nurses assisted with storm preparations and the evacuation of patients from NYULMC, including helping to triage, move, and discharge patients; printing medical records; ensuring sufficient staffing; communicating with patients and their families; and identifying other hospitals that could take patients. Many had worked during Hurricane Irene the year before and expected a similar outcome, but instead had to adapt rapidly to "an unplanned evacuation that ended in hospital closure" (VanDevanter et al., 2017, p. 637).

Many nurses felt unprepared to help evacuate the entire hospital, had little clarity on what role they were to play during the disaster, and had "limited knowledge of hospital disaster policies and procedures" (VanDevanter et al., 2017, p. 638). The lessons learned from nurses' response to this disaster highlight the importance of education and training for nurses in disaster response, including in scenarios of short- and long-term power outages. Event management, triage, and evacuation are critical skills for nurses.

increases the potential for infectious disease outbreaks in these settings. The health needs of those residing in shelters long-term are often much greater than the needs of those who suffer acute injuries, such as traumas (e.g., penetrating wounds, bone fractures), from the disaster itself. For example, a review of more than 30,000 people treated in shelters after Hurricane Katrina found that most of the care provided was "primary care or preventive in nature, with only 3.8 percent of all patients requiring referral to a hospital or emergency department" (Jenkins et al., 2009, p. 105). An assessment conducted after Hurricanes Gustav and Ike identified similar postdisaster health care needs within shelters (Noe et al., 2013).

Historically, nurses have delivered care to shelter populations, perhaps most familiarly in working with ARC. For example, ARC nurses at a shelter housing Hurricane Katrina evacuees set up hand sanitizing stations to help prevent infectious disease outbreaks. ARC nurses have worked to understand the functional, physical, and mental health needs of displaced persons; ensure that shelters are safe environments; and "maximiz[e] the effectiveness of nurses and other licensed care providers in disaster shelters" (Springer and Casey-Lockyer, 2016).

NURSES' PREPAREDNESS FOR DISASTER RESPONSE

Critical lessons learned during the response to prior infectious disease outbreaks, such as the 2003 severe acute respiratory syndrome (SARS) coronavirus outbreak, the 2009 H1N1 influenza pandemic, and the Ebola virus outbreak in West Africa, were not applied to workforce planning for future infectious disease outbreaks such as COVID-19 (Hick et al., 2020). These prior public health emergencies illuminated glaring gaps in emergency preparedness and workforce development and the harmful effects on nurses, and multiple calls to improve nurse readiness for pandemic response have been issued (Catrambone and Vlasich, 2017; Corless et al., 2018; Veenema et al., 2016a).

Basic knowledge about health system emergency preparedness is generally lacking among nurses, including school nurses, who, as discussed above, are expected to play key roles during public health emergencies (Baack and Alfred, 2013; Labrague et al., 2018; Rebmann et al., 2012; Usher et al., 2015). For example, in a survey of more than 5,000 nurses across the Spectrum Health system, 78 percent of respondents said they had little or no familiarity with emergency preparedness and disaster response (ASPR, 2019). Similarly, studies evaluating curricular content in U.S. schools of nursing (Charney et al., 2019; Veenema et al., 2019) and globally (Grochtdreis et al., 2016) disclose a notable absence of health care emergency preparedness content and little evidence that the few students who receive instruction in this context achieve competency in these skills. Furthermore, the willingness of individual nurses and other health care providers to respond to disasters is variable, and research suggests that many feel unequipped to respond (Connor, 2014; Veenema et al., 2008) or to keep themselves safe (Subbotina and Agrawal, 2018).

This educational gap is striking given that studies have shown that the more knowledgeable nurses are about infectious disease manifestation, transmission, and protection, the more confident and successful they will be when working during an outbreak (Liu and Liehr, 2009; Shih et al., 2009). Moreover, nurses who have previous experience working with an infectious disease outbreak are more confident and better prepared during a subsequent outbreak (Koh et al., 2012; Lam and Hung, 2013; Liu and Liehr, 2009), more knowledgeable about infection control and prevention measures, and more skilled in treating those with such infectious diseases. Nurses with a strong sense of their professional value—those who believe their role as a nurse is not just a job but a responsibility to serve and protect the public—are more likely to work during an infectious disease outbreak (Koh et al., 2012). Their outlook often causes them to struggle in balancing their duty as a nurse to provide care with their personal safety and health during an outbreak (Chung et al., 2005).

Gaps in education and training are evident in nursing leadership as well (Knebel et al., 2012; Langan et al., 2017; Veenema et al., 2016b, 2017). Nurse leadership, an important component of nurses' roles (see Chapter 9), is essential in any organization experiencing a disaster (Samuel et al., 2018). Thus, greater effort to develop and evaluate training programs for nurse leaders is warranted. Such programs can cultivate communication, business, and leadership competencies, and these nurse leaders, in turn, can improve health care's response, outcomes for patients, staff well-being, and the financial stability of hospitals (Shuman and Costa, 2020). Results of the April 2020 ANA survey indicated gaps in crisis leadership resulting in a lack of trust between nursing and hospital leadership and front-line nursing staff.

Areas in which action needs to be taken to advance national nurse readiness for responding to disasters, including pandemics, are detailed below. First, however, it is critical to identify and understand the gaps in the U.S. health care system both within and outside of the nursing workforce that have contributed to an ongoing lack of disaster readiness (Veenema et al., 2020). A range of factors that influence nursing workforce development and nurses' safety and support during disasters extend across the governmental, system (e.g., large regional health systems), and organizational (e.g., individual hospitals, clinics, and other types of health care settings) levels. Aggressive actions taken now to transform nursing education, practice, and policy across health care and public health systems and organizations can improve the readiness, safety, and support of the national nursing workforce for COVID-19 as well as future disasters. The factors reviewed below that affect nurse preparedness include government strategies, research funding, education and accreditation, responsibilities of hospitals and health care organizations, and the role of professional nursing organizations. The interactions among nurses, health care institutions, and government have been identified as crucial to an effective pandemic response (Lam et al., 2018).

Government Strategies

The federal government has wide-ranging responsibilities for disaster preparedness and response across various agencies. The Office of the Assistant Secretary for Preparedness and Response (ASPR) within the U.S. Department of Health and Human Services (HHS) "leads the nation's medical and public health preparedness for, response to, and recovery from disasters and public health emergencies" (HHS, 2019). ASPR's many roles during these events include coordinating the HHS Emergency Support Functions, overseeing the National Disaster Medical System, supporting the Hospital Preparedness Program, and maintaining and distributing the Strategic National Stockpile.[6] ASPR's strategies for identifying risks and informing preparedness and response efforts also include the National Biodefense Strategy and the National Health Security Strategy. Federal response strategies and frameworks beyond those of ASPR include FEMA's National Response Framework and CDC's Public Health Emergency Preparedness and Response Capabilities.

Concern has been expressed that the above federal strategies may not accurately reflect and incorporate the capacity of the nursing workforce to respond to disasters. Veenema and colleagues (2016a) identify the need for a systematic review of national policies and planning documents addressing disasters to ensure that they elevate, prioritize, and address the practice of disaster nursing in federal, state, and local emergency management operations. For instance, the 2017–2022 Health Care Preparedness and Response Capabilities provides a framework for health care coalition capabilities, including health care and medical readiness, health care and medical response coordination, continuity of health care service delivery, and medical surge (ASPR, 2016). Noteworthy, however, is that many of the capabilities outlined in this framework depend on a trained nursing workforce.

Ensuring that nurses are educationally prepared and available will be instrumental to success in mass vaccination and other disaster-related efforts. In terms of local government decisions, for example, school nurses are responsible for safe reentry of children to K–12 education during disasters. Lessons learned from the reopening of schools in other jurisdictions and other countries, as well as CDC guidance, can inform the incorporation of such practices as pandemic public health interventions into schools. The roles and responsibilities expected of nurses within existing local, state, and federal preparedness and response strategies need to be clarified to equip nurses with the knowledge, skills, and abilities needed to execute those roles safely and to build and maintain them across the nursing workforce. Additionally, nursing expertise that draws on both clinical and public health nursing knowledge can actively inform policy makers

---

[6] See https://www.phe.gov/about/aspr/Pages/default.aspx (accessed June 4, 2021).

from the local to the federal levels to ensure nurses' robust preparation for and response to disasters.

Research Funding

Scientific evidence is foundational to the delivery of safe, high-quality nursing care to individuals and communities affected by a disaster, yet data suggest that this evidence base is underdeveloped (Veenema et al., 2020). Research gaps have been identified (Stangeland, 2010), and priorities related to disaster nursing have been articulated (Ranse et al., 2014). A 2016 consensus report articulates specific recommendations for advancing research on disaster nursing, including the articulation of a research agenda based on a needs assessment to document gaps in the literature, nursing knowledge and skills, and available resources; expansion of research methods to include interventional studies and use both quantitative and qualitative designs; and an effort to increase the number of PhD-prepared nurse scientists serving as principal investigators on disaster research projects (Veenema et al., 2016a).

However, funding for this work has been insufficient. Support for public health emergency preparedness and response (PHEPR) research in general has repeatedly stopped and restarted, resulting in an evidence base comprising one-off studies. There has been little funding for academic public health emergency programs since 2015, with the exception of CDC's Center for Preparedness and Response's Broad Agency Announcement for Public Health Emergency Preparedness and Response Applied Research, and no funding for academic disaster nursing. Overall funding for disaster research has declined since 2009 (NASEM, 2020). A report recently released by the National Academies (NASEM, 2020) concludes,

A report recently released by the National Academies concludes the public health emergency preparedness and response (PHEPR) response field is currently "relying on fragmented and largely uncoordinated efforts," (NASEM, 2020, p. 7) often with no clear linkage to overall system goals. Collectively, these deficiencies have contributed to a field based on long-standing practice not evidence-based practices (NASEM, 2020). To address these deficiencies, the PHEPR field needs a coordinated intergovernmental, multidisciplinary effort with defined objectives to prioritize and align research efforts and investments in a research infrastructure to strengthen the capacity to conduct research before, during, and following public health emergencies (NASEM, 2020).

Education and Accreditation

In 2017, the Centers for Medicare & Medicaid Services (CMS) enacted the Emergency Preparedness Rule, which established requirements for planning, preparing, and training for emergencies (CMS, 2016, 2019). The rule was intended to advance health care preparedness, but it did not address the preparedness of the nursing workforce. The rule was designed to promote preparedness at the health care organization level, allowing the organization flexibility in testing and training for staff, including nurses. Accreditors are required to ensure that the criteria for the rule are met, but they do not evaluate the level of knowledge among staff or require additional training or workforce development. Gaps in nursing's emergency preparedness within these organizations can occur even if they have met the CMS emergency preparedness criteria.

Maintaining adequate and safe staffing levels during a disaster needs to be a key consideration in the development of a workforce emergency strategy. The Joint Commission has a vested interest in nursing workforce issues, viewing nursing as part of its mission to support high-quality and safe care for the public. The Joint Commission has produced recommendations designed to increase the professionalism of nursing and diversify the nursing workforce, and it has implemented measures to improve the safety and quality of nursing care practices. While The Joint Commission does not specifically require reporting of nurse-to-patient ratios, it does have some related metrics around patient outcomes (The Joint Commission, 2020). The lack of metrics that specifically measure whether facilities have the plans, procedures, and human resources needed to surge the workforce during a disaster leaves them vulnerable to staffing shortages and increases the likelihood that they will need to turn to a crisis standards of care staffing model.

Fundamental and seismic change also is required in nursing education if the profession is to keep pace with the increasing numbers of natural disasters and public health emergencies. The major threats to global human health (climate change, air pollution, influenza, emerging infectious diseases, vaccine hesitancy) (WHO, 2019) receive minimal coverage in most nursing school curricula. COVID-19 represents a harbinger of public health emergencies to come, highlighting the vital role of disaster response education and training for nurses. Yet, repeatedly, empirical evidence shows that nurses are ill prepared to respond to these events (Charney et al., 2019; Labrague et al., 2018; Veenema, 2018). Overall, the preparedness of the nursing workforce is a factor in prelicensure education and lifelong learning inclusive of training (e.g., regular drills and exercises). Nursing preparedness requires that all organizations employing nurses, from schools of nursing to hospitals to other health-related organizations, engage in this agenda. To equip nurses to respond to future disaster events, schools of nursing need to produce nurses capable of providing culturally meaningful care, using data to drive health decisions, and addressing SDOH to optimize population health outcomes (Duke Margolis Center for Health Policy, 2020). And as noted earlier, PhD-prepared nurse scientists are essential to conduct disaster research and educate a cadre of future nurse researchers and educators to sustain and advance the field. Nursing curricula need to be updated to reflect the realities of these increasing threats to human health.

The American Association of Colleges of Nursing (AACN) establishes the standards for curriculum for academic nursing programs through a series of *Essentials* documents that are currently being revised and are targeted to be released in early 2021 (see Chapter 7 for more detailed information). Population health competencies that specifically address disaster response are included in the revised *Essentials*, and their addition has the potential to drive transformational change across academic programs. Greater emphasis on disaster and public health emergency response competencies and skills should have beneficial effects for nurses during disasters, including greater resilience, increased practical and theoretical knowledge, a broader view of the "clinical and organizational big picture," and reduced psychological impact in case of sudden reassignment to a different clinical setting (Bambi et al., 2020). While all schools need to increase content in general disaster preparedness, it is also worth considering incorporating additional hazard-specific content to build capacity for nurses to respond to the kinds of emergencies that are most likely in the geographic area where they will live and practice. Schools of nursing can expand their use of educational technology, including telenursing and virtual simulations to increase interprofessional disaster training opportunities in partnership with community disaster response agencies.

The Commission on Collegiate Nursing Education (CCNE) Standards and Professional Nursing Guidelines Standards for Accreditation of Baccalaureate and Graduate Nursing Programs are applied at accreditation site visits to schools of nursing (AACN, 2011) to confirm that academic programs align with *Essentials*. CCNE evaluators' confirmation of the adoption of the new *Essentials* standards on incorporating disaster response content into education and training programs could produce evidence of graduates' related clinical competence (Veenema et al., 2020).

Disasters, including such events as the COVID-19 pandemic, interrupt academic progression and student mastery of clinical competencies and can delay graduations. Schools of nursing and state boards of nursing would be well served to establish options for supporting clinical rotations in the health care setting, such as expanding the role of virtual or simulated learning and alternative, non-traditional sites for clinical placements. Working with clinical and community partners, schools of nursing would benefit from establishing back-up plans to ensure that academic programs continue during public health emergencies. A particular emphasis on addressing health care equity in the face of disaster would be of prime importance.

Responsibilities of Hospitals and Health Care Organizations

The COVID-19 pandemic has revealed profound problems with the financing and delivery of American health care, presenting both challenges and opportunities for nursing, and has exposed systemic vulnerabilities that afflict the well-being and resilience of nurses and other health professionals. Hospitals and other organizations employing nurses, nurse leaders, physicians, and others have a responsibility to create a safe working environment for nurses, ensuring adequate staffing levels, access to appropriate levels of PPE, and physical and mental health support services for protracted disaster events. Hospital administrators and nursing and medical executives need to be held accountable for having policies in place to ensure a safe working environment for nurses during disaster response. Hospital disaster plans need to accommodate changes in clinical duties and nurse staffing to meet demand, and identify alternative nurse staffing resources to aid in the response. Long-term care facilities, home care agencies, and community health clinics need to include the same accommodations.

Nurse executives in various health and health care organizations across communities can work together to plan for circumstances that may require surging nurses across settings to meet emerging health care needs. Nurses well educated in addressing SDOH would be of particular value in contributing to the development and implementation of preparedness and response strategies that meet the needs of diverse high-risk, high-vulnerability populations. Stockpiling and procurement of adequate supplies (e.g., testing supplies, PPE, medical gases) are critical for keeping nurses safe at work. Health system leaders, mandated to have emergency management response plans in place, can ensure that all disaster and pandemic response plans address training content, including issues of health equity and communication with and protection of their workforce.

The Role of Professional Nursing Organizations

Professional nursing organizations have an important role in ensuring that their members and the profession at large have the expertise and support to respond to unanticipated events that threaten the health of the public. These organizations have advocated for the support and protection of nurses during past disasters and continue to do so today. The Tri-Council for Nursing (Tri-Council) is an alliance of five nursing organizations focused on leadership for education, practice, and research. Working with specialty nursing organizations, such as the Emergency Nurses Association and the Council of Public Health Nursing Organizations, the Tri-Council could advocate for a broad and forward-thinking national plan to advance disaster nursing and PHEPR. A special emphasis should be the care of individuals, families, and communities that are disproportionally affected by disasters. Nursing organizations uniting around the COVID-19 response can use this experience to establish a foundation for preparing the profession to meet future disaster-related challenges.

CONCLUSIONS

COVID-19, while historic, is but one example of the significant burden imposed by disasters and public health emergencies on the health of populations, health care professionals, and nurses in particular. The pandemic has created multiple challenges, particularly for managing its effects across diverse and highly vulnerable populations, and exacerbated existing health inequities. Future natural disasters and infectious disease outbreaks will present similar, if not greater challenges for the nursing profession. Bold, anticipatory action is needed to advance nurse readiness for these events.

Conclusion 8-1: The nation's nurses are not currently prepared for disaster and public health emergency response.

Conclusion 8-2: A bold and expansive effort, executed across multiple platforms, will be needed to fully support nurses in becoming prepared for disaster and public health emergency response. It is essential to convene experts who can develop a national strategic plan articulating the existing deficiencies in this regard and action steps to address them, and, most important, establishing where responsibility will lie for ensuring that those action steps are taken.

Conclusion 8-3: Rapid action is needed across nursing education, practice, policy, and research to address the gaps in nursing's disaster preparedness and improve its capacity as a profession to advocate for population health and health equity during such events.

REFERENCES

AACN (American Association of Colleges of Nursing). 2011. *The essentials of master's education in nursing*. https://www.aacnnursing.org/Portals/42/Publications/MastersEssentials11.pdf (accessed July 15, 2020).

Altman, M. 2020 (April 8). Facing moral distress during the COVID-19 crisis. *American Association of Critical Care Nurses Blog*. https://www.aacn.org/blog/facing-moral-distress-during-the-covid-19-crisis (accessed March 31, 2021).

AMA (American Medical Association). 2020. *Why COVID-19 is decimating some Native American communities*. https://www.ama-assn.org/delivering-care/population-care/why-covid-19-decimating-some-native-american-communities (accessed March 18, 2021).

ANA (American Nurses Association). 2020a. *COVID-19 survey: March 20–April 10*. https://www.nursingworld.org/practice-policy/work-environment/health-safety/disaster-preparedness/coronavirus/what-you-need-to-know/covid-19-survey-results (accessed April 5, 2021).

ANA. 2020b. *ANA survey of 14K nurses finds access to PPE remains a top concern*. https://www.nursingworld.org/news/news-releases/2020/ana-survey-of-14k-nurses-finds-access-to-ppe-remains-a-top-concern (accessed October 9, 2020).

ANA. 2020c. *Update on nurses and PPE: Survey reveals alarming conditions*. https://www.nursingworld.org/~4a558d/globalassets/covid19/ana-ppe-survey-one-pager---final.pdf (accessed April 5, 2021).

Anthony, C., T. J. Thomas, B. M. Berg, R. V. Burke, and J. S. Upperman. 2017. Factors associated with preparedness of the US healthcare system to respond to a pediatric surge during an infectious disease pandemic: Is our nation prepared? *American Journal of Disaster Medicine* 12(4):203–226.

ASPR (Office of the Assistant Secretary for Preparedness and Response). 2016. *2017–2022 health care preparedness and response capabilities*. https://www.phe.gov/Preparedness/planning/hpp/reports/Documents/2017-2022-healthcare-pr-capablities.pdf (accessed July 26, 2020).

ASPR. 2019. *TRACIE emergency preparedness information modules for nurses in acute care settings*. https://files.asprtracie.hhs.gov/documents/aspr-tracie-emergency-preparedness-information-modules-for-nurses-and-economic-framework.pdf (accessed June 6, 2021).

Attacks against AAPI community continue to rise during pandemic over 2,500 racist incidents reported since March. 2020. Press Release. Stop AAPI Hate, Asian Pacific Policy & Planning Council, Chinese for Affirmative Action, and San Francisco State University Asian American Studies. http://www.asianpacificpolicyandplanningcouncil.org/wp-content/uploads/PRESS_RELEASE_National-Report_August27_2020.pdf (accessed March 31, 2021).

Baack, S., and D. Alfred. 2013. Nurses' preparedness and perceived competence in managing disasters. *Journal of Nursing Scholarship* 45(3):281–287. doi: 10.1111/jnu.12029.

Badakhsh, R., E. Harville, and B. Banerjee. 2010. The childbearing experience during a natural disaster. *Journal of Obstetric, Gynecologic, & Neonatal Nursing* 39(4):489–497.

Bambi, S., P. Iozzo, and A. Lucchini. 2020. New issues in nursing management during the COVID-19 pandemic in Italy. *American Journal of Critical Care* 29(4):e92–e93. doi: 10.4037/ajcc2020937.

BLS (U.S. Bureau of Labor Statistics). 2020. *Occupational employment and wages, registered nurses*. U.S. Department of Labor. https://www.bls.gov/oes/current/oes291141.htm (accessed July 24, 2021).

Brooks, B., and B. O'Brien. 2020 (July 22). *Texas county stores bodies in trucks as state sets one-day record for COVID-19 deaths*. Thomson Reuters. https://www.reuters.com/article/us-health-coronavirus-usa/texas-county-stores-bodies-in-trucks-as-state-sets-one-day-record-for-covid-19-deaths-idUSKCN24N2F2 (accessed March 31, 2021).

Catrambone, C. D., and C. Vlasich. 2016. *Global Advisory Panel on the Future of Nursing & Midwifery (GAPFON): Recommendations, strategies, and outcomes*. Sigma Repository. https://sigma.nursingrepository.org/handle/10755/623881 (accessed March 31, 2021).

Charney, R. L., R. P. Lavin, A. Bender, J. C. Langan, R. S. Zimmerman, and T. G. Veenema. 2019. Ready to respond: A survey of interdisciplinary health-care students and administrators on disaster management competencies. Online ahead of print, September 30, 2019. *Disaster Medicine and Public Health Preparedness* Sep 30:1–8. doi :10.1017/dmp.2019.96.

Chung, B. P. M., T. K. S. Wong, E. S. B. Suen, and J. W. Y. Chung. 2005. SARS: Caring for patients in Hong Kong. *Journal of Clinical Nursing* 14(4):510–517. doi: 10.1111/j.1365-2702.2004. 01072.x.

CMS (Centers for Medicare & Medicaid Services). 2016. Emergency preparedness requirements for Medicare and Medicaid participating providers and suppliers final rule. *Federal Register* 81(180). https://www.federalregister.gov/documents/2016/09/16/2016-21404/medicare-and-medicaid-programs-emergency-preparedness-requirements-for-medicare-and-medicaid (accessed July 26, 2020).

CMS. 2019. *Emergency preparedness rule*. https://www.cms.gov/Medicare/Provider-Enrollment-and-Certification/SurveyCertEmergPrep/Emergency-Prep-Rule (accessed July 26, 2020).

Connor, S. B. 2014. When and why health care personnel respond to a disaster: The state of the science. *Prehospital and Disaster Medicine* 29(3):270–274. doi: 10.1017/S1049023X14000387.

Corless, I. B., D. Nardi, J. A. Milstead, E. Larson, K. M. Nokes, S. Orsega, A. Kurth, K. Kirksey, and W. Woith. 2018. Expanding nursing's role in responding to global pandemics 5/14/2018. *Nursing Outlook* 66(4):412–415.

Davenport, C., A. Gregg, and C. Timberg. 2020 (March 22). Working from home reveals another fault line in America's racial and educational divide. *The Washington Post*. https://www.washingtonpost.com/business/2020/03/22/working-home-reveals-another-fault-line-americas-racial-educational-divide (accessed March 31, 2021).

Davis, J. R., S. Wilson, A. Brock-Martin, S. Glover, and E. R. Svendsen. 2010. The impact of disasters on populations with health and health care disparities. *Disaster Medicine and Public Health Preparedness* 4(1):30.

de Mendoza, V. B., J. Savage, E. Harville, and G. P. Giarratano. 2012. Prenatal care, social support, and health-promoting behaviors of immigrant Latina women in a disaster recovery environment. *Journal of Obstetric, Gynecologic & Neonatal Nursing* 41:S133.

Duke Margolis Center for Health Policy. 2020. *Response and reform: Reflections on COVID-19.* 2019–2020 Duke Margolis Scholars. https://healthpolicy.duke.edu/sites/default/files/2020-11/Respond%20and%20Reform%20Reflections%20on%20COVID19.pdf (accessed March 31, 2021).

Ebola nurses labour in the spirit of Nightingale [Editorial]. 2014. *The Spectator*, p. A.12.

Erdman, S. L. 2020. *Hispanics a disproportionate risk from COVID-19 over work, living conditions, health experts say.* CNN Health. https://www.cnn.com/2020/06/10/health/hispanics-disparity-coronavirus/index.html (accessed March 31, 2021).

Fauci, A. S., and D. M. Morens. 2012. The perpetual challenge of infectious diseases. *New England Journal of Medicine* 366:454–461. doi: 10.1056/NEJMra1108296.

FEMA (Federal Emergency Management Agency). 2014. Preparedness in America: Research insights to increase individual, organizational, and community action. https://www.ready.gov/sites/default/files/2020-08/Preparedness_in_America_August_2014.pdf (accessed March 31, 2021).

Gray, L. 2017. Social determinants of health, disaster vulnerability, severe and morbid obesity in adults: Triple jeopardy? *International Journal of Environmental Research and Public Health* 14(12):1452.

Greenough, P. G., M. D. Lappi, E. B. Hsu, S. Fink, Y. H. Hsieh, A. Vu, C. Heaton, and T. D. Kirsch. 2008. Burden of disease and health status among Hurricane Katrina-displaced persons in shelters: A population-based cluster sample. *Annals of Emergency Medicine* 51(4):426–432. doi: 10.1016/j.annemergmed.2007.04.004.

Grochtdreis, T., N. de Jong, N., Harenberg, S. Görres, and P. Schröder-Bäck. 2016. Nurses' roles, knowledge and experience in national disaster preparedness and emergency response: A literature review. *South Eastern European Journal of Public Health*. doi: 10.4119/seejph-1847.

Hallegatte, S., A. Vogt-Schilb, M. Bangalore, and J. Rozenberg. 2016. *Unbreakable: Building the resilience of the poor in the face of natural disasters*. Washington, DC: World Bank Publications.

Heagele, T. 2017. Disaster-related community resilience: A concept analysis and a call to action for nurses. *Public Health Nursing* 34(3):295–302.

Heagele, T., and D. Pacqiao. 2018. Disaster vulnerability of elderly and medically frail populations. *Health Emergency and Disaster Nursing* 2016-0009. doi: 10.24298/hedn.2016-0009.

Hernandez, S. 2020. *Hidalgo County get 1,274 new COVID-19 cases, nurses die, doctors isolated.* KVEO-TV. https://www.valleycentral.com/news/local-news/hidalgo-county-get-1274-new-covid-19-cases-nurses-die-doctors-isolated (accessed March 31, 2021).

HHS (U.S. Department of Health and Human Services). 2019. *Saving lives and protecting Americans from 21st century health security threats*. Office of the Assistant Secretary for Preparedness and Response. https://www.phe.gov/about/aspr/Pages/default.aspx (accessed July 22, 2020).

Hick, J. L., D. Hanfling, M. K. Wynia, and A. T. Pavia. 2020 (March 5). *Duty to plan: Health care, crisis standards for care and coronavirus-SARS-CoV-2*. National Academy of Medicine. https://nam.edu/duty-to-plan-health-care-crisis-standards-of-care-and-novel-coronavirus-sars-cov-2 (accessed July 21, 2020).

IFRC (International Federation of the Red Cross). 2019. *World disaster report 2018*. International Federation of Red Cross and Red Crescent Societies. https://www.ifrc.org/en/publications-and-reports/world-disasters-report (accessed March 31, 2021).

Imai, T., K. Takahashi, M. Todoroki, H. Kunishima, T. Hoshuyama, R. Ide, and D. Koh. 2008. Perception in relation to a potential influenza pandemic among healthcare workers in Japan: Implications for preparedness. *Journal of Occupational Health* 50(1):13–23. doi: 10.1539/joh.50.13.

IPCC (Intergovernmental Panel on Climate Change). 2012. *Managing the risks of extreme events and disasters to advance climate change adaptation: A special report of Working Groups I and II of the Intergovernmental Panel on Climate Change*. Cambridge, UK: Cambridge University Press.

IPCC. 2014. *Climate change 2014: Impacts, adaptation, and vulnerability: Contribution of Working Group II to the Fifth Assessment Report of the Intergovernmental Panel on Climate Change*. Geneva, Switzerland: Intergovernmental Panel on Climate Change.

Jakeway, C. C., G. LaRosa, A. Cary, and S. Schoenfisch. 2008. The role of public health nurses in emergency preparedness and response: A position paper of the association of state and territorial directors of nursing. *Public Health Nursing* 25(4):353–361.

Jenkins, J. L., M. McCarthy, G. Kelen, L. M. Sauer, and T. Kirsch. 2009. Changes needed in the care for sheltered persons: A multistate analysis from Hurricane Katrina. *American Journal of Disaster Medicine* 42:101–106. doi: 10.5055/ajdm.2009.0015.

Killough, A., E. Lavandera, and K. Jones. 2020 (July 22). *Texas COVID-19 hot spot is facing a "tsunami" of patients, overwhelming hospitals*. CNN. https://www.cnn.com/2020/07/22/us/hidalgo-county-south-texas-covid-19/index.html (accessed March 31, 2021).

Kishore, N., D. Marqués, A. Mahmud, M. V. Kiang, I. Rodriguez, A. Fuller, P. Ebner, C. Sorensen, F. Racy, J. Lemery, L. Maas, J. Leaning, R. A. Irizarry, S. Balsari, and C. O. Buckee. 2018. Mortality in Puerto Rico after Hurricane Maria. *New England Journal of Medicine* 379(2):162–170. doi: 10.1056/NEJMsa1803972.

Kleier, J. A., D. Krause, and T. Ogilby. 2018. Hurricane preparedness among elderly residents in South Florida. *Public Health Nursing* 35(1):3–9.

Knebel, A. R., L. Toomey, and M. Libby. 2012. Nursing leadership in disaster preparedness and response. *Annual Review of Nursing Research* 30(1):21–45. doi: 10.1891/0739-6686.30.21.

Koh, Y., D. Hegney, and V. Drury. 2012. Nurses' perceptions of risk from emerging respiratory infectious diseases: A Singapore study. *International Journal of Nursing Practice* 18(2):195–204. doi: 10. 1111/j.1440-172X.2012.02018.x.

Labrague, L. J., and J. A. A. De Los Santos. 2020. COVID-19 anxiety among front-line nurses: Predictive role of organisational support, personal resilience and social support. *Journal of Nursing Management* 28(7):1653–1661. doi: 10.1111/jonm.13121.

Labrague, L. J., K. Hammad, D. S. Gloe, D. M. McEnroe-Petitte, D. C. Fronda, A. A. Obeidat, M. C. Leocadio, A. R. Cayaban, and E. C. Mirafuentes. 2018. Disaster preparedness among nurses: A systematic review of literature. *International Nursing Review* 65(1):41–53. doi: 10.1111/inr/12369.

Laditka, S. B., J. N. Laditka, S. Xirasagar, C. B. Cornman, C. B., Davis, and J. V. Richter. 2008. Providing shelter to nursing home evacuees in disasters: Lessons from Hurricane Katrina. *American Journal of Public Health* 98(7):1288–1293. doi: 10.2105/AJPH.2006.107748.

Lam, K. K., and S. Y. M. Hung. 2013. Perceptions of emergency nurses during the human swine influenza outbreak: A qualitative study. *International Emergency Nursing* 21(4):240–246. doi: 10.1016/ j.ienj.2012.08.008.

Lam, S. K. K., E. W. Y. Kwong, M. S. Y. Hung, S. M. C. Pang, and V. C. L. Chiang. 2018. Nurses' preparedness for infectious disease outbreaks: A literature review and narrative synthesis of qualitative evidence. *Journal of Clinical Nursing* 27(7–8):e1244–e1255. doi: 10.1111/jocn.14210.

Langan, J. C., R. Lavin, K. A. Wolgast, and T. G. Veenema. 2017. Education for developing and sustaining a health care workforce for disaster readiness. *Nursing Administration Quarterly* 41(2):118–127.

Lasek, A. 2020 (September 4). *Nurses ask feds to invoke Defense Production Act for N95 masks; Survey finds "unacceptable" reuse levels*. McKnight's Long-Term Care News. https://www.mcknights.com/news/clinical-news/nurses-ask-feds-to-invoke-defense-production-act-for-n95-masks-survey-finds-unacceptable-reuse-levels (accessed March 31, 2021).

Lavin, R. P., T. G. Veenema, W. J. Calvert, S. R. Grigsby, and J. Cobbina. 2017. Nurse leaders' response to civil unrest in the urban core. *Nursing Administration Quarterly* 41(2):164–169.

Liu, H., and P. Liehr. 2009. Instructive messages from Chinese nurses' stories of caring for SARS patients. *Journal of Clinical Nursing* 18(20):2880–2887. doi: 10.1111/j.1365-2702.2009.02857.x.

Maltz, M. 2019. Caught in the eye of the storm: The disproportionate impact of natural disasters on the elderly population in the United States. *Elder Law Journal* 27:157.

Martin, S. D. 2011. Nurses' ability and willingness to work during pandemic flu. *Journal of Nursing Management* 19(1):98–108.

Mason, D., and C. Friese. 2020 (March 19). Protecting health care workers against COVID-19: And being prepared for future pandemics. *JAMA Health Forum*. https://jamanetwork.com/channels/health-forum/fullarticle/2763478#top (accessed March 31, 2021).

Molyneux, J. 2009. AJN speaks with Mary Pappas, school nurse who alerted CDC to swine flu outbreak. *Off the charts: Blog of the American Journal of Nursing*. https://ajnoffthecharts.com/mary-pappas-school-nurse-just-carrying-on-despite-swine-flu-outbreak (accessed March 31, 2021).

Najmabadi, S., and M. Gutierrez, Jr. 2020 (July 2). "How many more are coming?" What it's like inside hospitals as coronavirus grips Texas' Rio Grande Valley. *Texas Tribune*. https://www.texastribune.org/2020/07/02/texas-coronavirus-hospital-rio-grande-valley (accessed March 31, 2021).

NASEM (National Academies of Sciences, Engineering, and Medicine). 2020. *Evidence-based practice for public health emergency preparedness and response*. Washington, DC: The National Academies Press.

Noe, R. S., A. H. Schnall, A. F. Wolkin, M. N. Podgornik, A. D. Wood, J. Spears, and S. A. R. Stanley. 2013. Disaster-related injuries and illnesses treated by American Red Cross Health Services during Hurricanes Gustav and Ike. *South Medicine Journal* 106(1):102–108. doi: 10.1097/SMJ.0b013e31827c9e1f.

O'Boyle, C., C. Robertson, and M. Secor-Turner. 2006. Nurses' beliefs about public health emergencies: Fear of abandonment. *American Journal of Infection Control* 34(6):351–357. doi: 10.1016/j.ajic.2006.01.012.

Pappa, S., V. Ntella, T. Giannakas, V. G. Giannakoulis, E. Papoutsi, and P. Katsaounou. 2020. Prevalence of depression, anxiety, and insomnia among healthcare workers during the COVID-19 pandemic: A systematic review and meta-analysis. *Brain, Behavior, and Immunity* 88:901–907.

Petkova, E., J. Schlegelmilch, J. Sury, T. Chandler, C. Herrera, S. Bhaskar, E. Sehnert, S. Martinez, S. Marx, and I. Redlener. 2016. *The American preparedness project: Where the US public stands in 2015*. National Center for Disaster Preparedness at Columbia University's Earth Institute, Research Brief 2016. https://academiccommons.columbia.edu/doi/10.7916/D84Q7TZN (accessed April 5, 2021).

Poteat, T., G. Millett, L. E. Nelson, and C. Beyrer. 2020. Understanding COVID-19 risks and vulnerabilities among Black communities in America: The lethal force of syndemics. *Annals of Epidemiology* 47:1–3.

Ranse, J., A. Hutton, B. Jeeawody, and R. Wilson. 2014. What are the research needs for the field of disaster nursing? An international Delphi study. *Prehospital and Disaster Medicine* 29(5):448.

Rebmann, T., M. B. Elliott, D. Reddick, and Z. D. Swick. 2012. US school/academic institution disaster and pandemic preparedness and seasonal influenza vaccination among school nurses. *American Journal of Infection Control* 40(7):584–589.

Ruderman, C., C. S. Tracy, C. M. Bensimon, M. Bernstein, L. Hawryluck, R. Z. Shaul, and R. E. Upshur. 2006. On pandemics and the duty to care: Whose duty? Who cares? *BMC Medical Ethics* 7(1):5. doi: 10.1186/1472-6939-7-5.

SAMHSA (Substance Abuse and Mental Health Services Administration). 2017. Greater impact: How disasters affect people of low socioeconomic status. *Disaster Technical Assistance Center Supplemental Research Bulletin*. https://www.samhsa.gov/sites/default/files/dtac/srb-low-ses_2.pdf (accessed March 31, 2021).

Samuel, P., M. T. Quinn Griffin, M. White, and J. Fitzpatrick. 2018. Crisis leadership efficacy of nurse practitioners. *Journal for Nurse Practitioners* 11(9). doi:10.1016/j.nurpra.2015.06.010.

Shapiro, J. 2016. What to know about the Pulse Nightclub shooting in Orlando. *Time*. https://time.com/4365260/orlando-shooting-pulse-nightclub-what-know (accessed March 31, 2021).

Shechter, A., F. Diaz, N. Moise, D. E. Anstey, S. Ye, S., Agarwal, J. Birk, D. Brodie, D. Cannone, B. Chang, J. Claassen, T. Cornelius, L. Derby, M. Dong, R. Givens, B. Hochman, S. Homma, I. Kronish, S. Lee, W. Manzano, L. Mayer, C. McMurry, V. Moitre, P. Pham, L. Rabbani, R.

Rivera, A. Schwartz, J. Schwartz, P. Shapiro, K. Shaw, A. Sullivan, C. Vose, L. Wasson, D. Edmondson, and M. Abdalla. 2020. Psychological distress, coping behaviors, and preferences for support among New York healthcare workers during the COVID-19 pandemic. *General Hospital Psychiatry* 66:1–8.

Shih, F. J., M. L. Gau, C. C. Kao, C. Y. Yang, Y. S. Lin, Y. C. Liao, and S. J. Sheu. 2007. Dying and caring on the edge: Taiwan's surviving nurses' reflections on taking care of patients with severe acute respiratory syndrome. *Applied Nursing Research* 20(4):171–180. doi: 10.1016/j.apnr.2006.08.007.

Shih, F. J., S. Turale, Y. S. Lin, M. L. Gau, C. C. Kao, C. Y. Yang, Y. C. and Liao. 2009. Surviving a life-threatening crisis: Taiwan's nurse leaders' reflections and difficulties fighting the SARS epidemic. *Journal of Clinical Nursing* 1824:3391–3400. doi: 10.1111/j.1365- 2702.2008.02521.x.

Shuman, C. J., and D. K. Costa. 2020. Stepping in, stepping up, and stepping out: Competencies for intensive care unit nursing leaders during disasters, emergencies, and outbreaks. *American Journal of Critical Care* 29(5):403–406.

Siu, J. Y. M. 2010. Another nightmare after SARS: Knowledge perceptions of and overcoming strategies for H1N1 influenza among chronic renal disease patients in Hong Kong. *Qualitative Health Research* 20(7):893–904. doi: 10.1177/1049732310367501.

Smith, A. B. 2020. *2010-2019: A landmark decade of billion-dollar weather and climate disasters*. National Oceanic and Atmosphere Administration. https://www.climate.gov/news-features/blogs/beyond-data/2010-2019-landmark-decade-us-billion-dollar-weather-and-climate (accessed March 31, 2021).

Springer, J., and M. Casey-Lockyer. 2016. Evolution of a nursing model for identifying client needs in a disaster shelter: A case study with the American Red Cross. *Nursing Clinics of North America* 51(4):647–662. doi: 10.1016/j.cnur.2016.07.009.

Spurlock, W. R., K. Rose, T. G.Veenema, S. K. Sinha, D. Gray-Miceli, S. Hitchman, N. Foster, L. Slepski-Nash, and E. T. Miller. 2019. American Academy of Nursing on policy position statement: Disaster preparedness for older adults. *Nursing Outlook* 67(1):118–121.

Stangeland, P. A. 2010. Disaster nursing: A retrospective review. *Critical Care Nursing Clinics of North America* 22(4):421–436. doi: 10.1016/j.ccell.2010.09.003.

Subbotina, K., and N. Agrawal. 2018. Natural disasters and health risks of first responders. In *Asia-Pacific security challenges*. Cham, Switzerland: Springer. Pp. 85–122.

The Joint Commission. 2020. *Health care staffing services*. https://www.jointcommission.org/measurement/measures/health-care-staffing-services (accessed July 26, 2020).

The role of the nurse in emergency preparedness. 2012. *Journal of Obstetrical Gynecology Neonatal Nursing* 41(2):322–324. PMID: 22376141.

Thiede, B. C., and D. L. Brown. 2013. Hurricane Katrina: Who stayed and why? *Population Research Policy Review* 32(6):803–824. doi: 10.1007/s11113-013-9302-9.

Toner, E., R. Waldhorn, T. G. Veenema, A. Adalja, D. Meyer, E. Martin, L. Sauer, M. Watson, L. D. Biddison, A. Cicerno, and T. Inglesby. 2020. *National action plan for expanding and adapting the healthcare system for the duration of the COVID-19 pandemic*. Baltimore, MD: Johns Hopkins Bloomberg School of Public Health, Center for Health Security.

UN (United Nations), Department of Economic and Social Affairs, Population Division. 2016. *The world's cities in 2016—data booklet* (ST/ESA/SER.A/392).

UNISDR (United Nations International Strategy for Disaster Reduction). 1982. *Disasters and the disabled*. https://www.undrr.org/publication/disasters-and-disabled (accessed March 31, 2021).

UNISDR. 2017. *Terminology*. https://www.undrr.org/terminology/disaster (accessed July 24, 2021).

Usher, K., M. L. Redman-MacLaren, J. Mills, C. West, E. Casella, E. Hapsari, S. Bonita, R. Rosaldo, A. Liswar, and Y. Zang. 2015. Strengthening and preparing: Enhancing nursing research for disaster management. *Nurse UNISEducation in Practice* 15(1):68–74. doi: 10.1016/j.nepr.2014.03.006.

VanDevanter, B., V. H. Raveis, C. T. Kovner, M. McCollum, and R. Keller. 2017. Challenges and resources for nurses participating in a Hurricane Sandy hospital evacuation. *Journal of Nursing Scholarship* 49(6):635–643. doi: 10.1111/jnu.12329.

Veenema, T. G. (ed.). 2018. (4th Edition). *Disaster nursing and emergency preparedness for chemical, biological, and radiological terrorism and other hazards*. New York: Springer Publishing Company.

Veenema, T. G. 2020. *The role of nurses in disaster preparedness and response*. Chapter commissioned by the Committee on the Future of Nursing 2020–2030. Washington, DC: National Academies of Sciences, Engineering, and Medicine.

Veenema, T. G., B. Walden, N. Feinstein, and J. P. Williams. 2008. Factors affecting hospital-based nurses' willingness to respond to a radiation emergency. *Disaster Medicine and Public Health Preparedness* 2(4):224–229.

Veenema, T. G., A. Griffin, A. R. Gable, L. MacIntyre, N. Simons, M. Couig, J. Walsh, Jr., R. Proffitt Lavin, A. Dobalian, and E. Larson. 2016a. Nurses as leaders in disaster preparedness and response—A call to action. *Journal of Nursing Scholarship* 48(2):187–200. doi: 10.1111/jnu.12198.

Veenema, T. G., S. L. Losinski, S. M. Newton, and S. Seal. 2016b. Exploration and development of standardized nursing leadership competencies during disasters. *Health Emergencies and Disaster Nursing* 4(1):1–13.

Veenema, T. G., K. Deruggiero, S. L. Losinski, and D. Barnett. 2017. Hospital administration and nursing leadership in disasters: An exploratory study using concept mapping. *Nursing Administration Quarterly* 41(2):151–163.

Veenema, T. G., R. P. Lavin, S. Schneider-Firestone, M. P. Couig, J. Langan, K. Qureshi, D. Scerpella, and L. Sasnett. 2019. National assessment of nursing schools and nurse educators readiness for radiation emergencies and nuclear events. *Disaster Medicine and Public Health Preparedness* 13(5–6):936–945.

Veenema, T. G., D. Meyer, S. Bell, M. Couig, C. Friese, R. Lavin, J. Stanley, E. Martin, M. Montegue, E. Toner, M. Schoch-Spana, A. Cicero, T. Ingelsby, L. Sauer, M. Watson, L. D. Biddison, A. Cicerno, and T. Inglesby. 2020. *Recommendations for improving national nurse preparedness for pandemic response: Early lessons from COVID-19*. Baltimore, MD: Johns Hopkins Bloomberg School of Public Health, Center for Health Security.

Watts, N., M. Amann, S. Ayeb-Karlsson, K. Belesova, T. Bouley, M. Boykoff, P. Byass, W. Cai, D. Campbell-Lendrum, J. Chambers, P. Cox, M. Daly, N. Dasandi, M. Davies, M. Depledge, A. Depoux, P. Dominguez-Salas, P. Drummond, P. Ekins, A. Flahault, H. Frumkin, L. Georgeson, M Ghanei, D. Grace, H. Graham, R. Grojsman, A. Haines, I. Hamilton, S. Hartinger, A. Johnson, I. Kelman, G. Kiesewetter, D. Kniveton, L. Liang, M. Lott, R. Lower, G. Mace, M. Sewe, M. Maslin, S. Mikhaylov, J. Milner, A. Latifi, M. Moradi-Lakeh, K. Morrissey, K. Murray, T. Neville, M. Nilsson, T. Oreszczyn, F. Owfi, D. Pencheon, S. Pye, M. Rabbaniha, E. Robinson, J. Rocklöv, S. Schütte, J. Shumake-Guillemot, R. Steinbach, M. Tabatabaei, N. Wheeler, P. Wilkinson, P. Gong, H. Montgomer, and A. Costello. 2018. The Lancet Countdown on health and climate change: From 25 years of inaction to a global transformation for public health. *Lancet* 391(10120):581–630.

Wells, K. B., J. Tang, E. Lizaola, F. Jones, A. Brown, A. Stayton, A., M. Williams, A. Chandra, D. Eisenman, S. Fogleman, and A. Ploug. 2013. Applying community engagement to disaster planning: Developing the vision and design for the Los Angeles County Community Disaster Resilience Initiative. *American Journal of Public Health* 103(7):1172–1180. doi: 10.2105/ajph.2013.301407.

WHO (World Health Organization). 2018. *Essential steps for developing or updating a national pandemic influenza preparedness plan* (No. WHO/WHE/IHM/GIP/2018.1). Geneva, Switzerland: World Health Organization.

WHO. 2019. *Ten threats to global health in 2019*. https://www.who.int/news-room/spotlight/ten-threats-to-global-health-in-2019 (accessed March 31, 2021).

WHO. 2020. *Essential emergency and surgical care*. https://www.who.int/surgery/challenges/esc_disasters_emergencies/en (accessed March 31, 2021).

Willis, J., and L. Philp. 2017. Orlando health nurse leaders reflect on the pulse tragedy. *Nurse Leader* 15(5):319–322. doi: 10.1016/j.mnl.2017.07.007.

9

Nurses Leading Change

Minister to the world in a way that can change it.
Minister radically in a real, active, practical,
and get your hands dirty way.

—Chimamanda Ngozi Adichie, author

As demonstrated by the COVID-19 pandemic, nurses at every level and across all settings are positioned to lead. Nurses can lead teams, promote community health, advocate for systems change and health policy, foster the redesign of nursing education, and advance efforts to achieve health equity. Even so, educational institutions and health systems can better prepare and empower new and practicing nurses, including licensed practical nurses, registered nurses, advanced practice registered nurses, and those with doctoral degrees to develop and grow in leadership roles. To this end, it will be necessary to place more intentional focus on providing models and opportunities for the emergence of more diverse nurse leaders who can reflect the people and families they care for and can mentor and serve as role models for underrepresented students.

Creating a future in which opportunities to optimize health are more equitable will require disrupting the deeply entrenched prevailing paradigms of health care, which in turn will require enlightened, diverse, courageous, and competent leadership. The seminal Institute of Medicine report *Crossing the Quality Chasm: A New Health System for the 21st Century* (IOM, 2001) calls for broad and sweeping transformation of the health care system in order to improve the quality of care. It identifies six aims for improvement that define quality health care: to provide care that is safe, effective, patient-centered, timely, efficient, and equitable (IOM, 2001). The Institute for Healthcare Improvement (IHI) has found that progress on health equity has lagged behind that on the other five aims, calling it "the forgotten aim" of health care (Feely, 2016). The *Crossing the Quality Chasm* report emphasizes the importance of leadership in achieving the six aims, noting that leaders have a wide variety of roles and responsibilities that include

> creating and articulating the organization's vision and goals, listening to the needs and aspirations of those working on the front lines, providing direction, creating incentives for change, aligning and integrating improvement efforts, and creating a supportive environment and a culture of continuous improvement that encourages and enables success. (IOM, 2001, p. 137)

It must be emphasized that having this type of leadership only at the top of an organization or initiative is not enough. Rather, leadership is needed at multiple levels to "provide clear strategic and sustained direction and a coherent set of values and incentives to guide group and individual actions" (IOM, 2001, p. 137) and to ensure that health equity is a strategic priority at every level (Feely, 2016).

This chapter focuses on how nurse leaders can, and do, address social determinants of health (SDOH) and health equity in all settings and all nursing roles. It begins by articulating how nurses are well suited to lead in such efforts, and then outlines the committee's vision for nursing leadership specific to these challenges in the future. Next is a discussion of the competencies that will enhance nurses' ability to lead effective change. Finally, the chapter explores ways to help achieve the committee's vision for nursing leadership through training and leadership development specific to advancing an agenda of greater health equity.

NURSES LEADING IN HEALTH EQUITY

Nurses have a rich history of both advocacy and the provision of holistic care that includes meeting social needs of individuals and focusing on SDOH. As presented in this report, there are numerous examples illustrating how nurses are already working effectively as leaders on equity issues across a variety of settings. If nurses are to build on this rich tradition, it will not be enough for them to see themselves as leaders; the organizations that employ them will have to provide them with ample opportunities, resources, and mentorship to fully realize their leadership potential. This is the case even for nurses who are self-employed, who can benefit from opportunities provided by the external systems around them.

Nursing's Focus on Social Determinants

Nurses have always been key to the health and well-being of individuals and communities, but a new generation of nurse leaders is now needed—one that recognizes the importance of SDOH and diversity and is able to use and build on the increasing evidence base supporting the link between SDOH and health status. Today's nurses are called on to lead in the development of effective strategies for improving the nation's health (Lathrop, 2013; Ogbolu et al., 2018) with due attention to the needs of the most underserved individuals, neighborhoods, and communities and the crucial importance of advancing health equity.

Leadership can be defined as a process of social influence that maximizes the efforts of others toward achievement of a goal (Kruse, 2013). Leaders set direction, build an inspiring vision, press for change, and create new ways of thinking and doing. Nurses as a professional group manifest many of the characteristics of strong leadership—including courage, humility, caring, compassion, intelligence, empathy, awareness, and accountability—that are essential to leading the way on health equity (Shapiro et al., 2006). In addition to their deep understanding of how health intersects with SDOH (Olshansky, 2017), they have a holistic view of people across systems and settings, they are active listeners, they establish therapeutic relationships, and they practice person-centered care. Increasingly, nurses are serving as innovators and codesigners of health care in their roles in the public health and health care systems (Jouppila and Tianen, 2020), and by continuing to learn and apply improvement and innovation skills, will be able to help create new care models for the decade ahead. Given the wide range of settings and roles in which nurses at all levels serve (see Chapter 1), their leadership in this regard can have broad and far-reaching impacts on equity in health and health care.

THE COMMITTEE'S VISION FOR NURSING LEADERSHIP

Implementing change to address SDOH and advance health equity will require the contributions of nurses in all roles and all settings, and recognition that no one nurse can successfully implement change without the collaboration of others. Clinical nurses manage the nursing care of patients and coordinate care, making decisions and communicating with families and other health care professionals. These nurses can influence clinical practice environments and local organizational culture, as well as organizational processes and policies, often working with members of other health care disciplines. Public health and school nurses and other community-based nurses engage with the community to identify and address individual- and community-level needs, often working with professionals from other disciplines and sectors. Some nurses serve on boards, manage organizations, direct programs, and have direct responsibility for developing policies and practices. Nurses leading community organizations often lead team members and partner with community members and organizations in other sectors. Nurses serving on health care boards can exert leadership influence on the organization's policies and structures while not leading day-to-day organizational operations. Still other nurses work with but outside the health care system, advocating for and working toward public- and private-sector policies and structures that can have positive impacts on health and well-being. These nurses (e.g., a public health nurse advocating for more equitable transportation policy) may lead individuals and organizations as part of a multidisciplinary, multisector coalition. And nurses with formal leadership roles, such as nurse managers, chief executive officers (CEOs), and deans, can use their positions to establish organizational cultures and implement practices that advance health equity. In addition to collaboration among members of the nursing profession and across other disciplines and sectors, the creation of enduring change requires the involvement of individuals and community members. Rather than a more hierarchal system of leadership, collaborative leadership assumes that everyone involved has unique contributions to make and that constructive dialogue and joint resources are needed to achieve ongoing goals (Eckert et al., 2014).

Each of the various leadership roles described above involves different skills and responsibilities, as shown in the framework for nurse leadership in Table 9-1. It is important to note that an individual nurse may lead in multiple areas of this framework and can lead in both formal and informal capacities. While some nursing positions (e.g., CEO, dean, nurse manager) entail more explicit leadership responsibilities, all nurses can lead according to their own interests, capacities, and opportunities. For example, a staff nurse who has no official leadership position in the workplace can lead others by modeling behaviors that promote a culture of diversity, equity, and inclusion, and can also lead beyond health care through involvement in political advocacy. As noted earlier, fulfillment of this potential will require support, encouragement, mentorship, and advancement opportunities, with nurses operating to the full scope of their education, training, and expertise.

The subsections below detail the leadership roles nurses can play at the four levels shown in Table 9-1: leading self, leading others, leading health care, and leading beyond health care. Nurses engaging in each of these leadership levels are important to advancing health equity. Together, the various roles at these four levels constitute the committee's vision for nursing leadership.

Leading Self

Before nurses can lead others, they need to be able to lead themselves. To address SDOH, nurses need to understand and acknowledge how social determinants affect them personally, and to be aware of implicit biases that may influence the decisions they make and the outcomes of the people and communities they serve. They must understand and manage their own emotional responses, invest in their own physical and mental health, serve as role models for others, and continue their personal and professional development. Nurses can lead at this level by advocating for themselves and others in the workplace, functioning as effective team players, and developing coping and self-care skills (NASEM, 2020).

Part of leading oneself is seeing oneself as a leader and viewing leadership as an integral part of one's role. One barrier to effective leadership is that not all nurses see themselves in this way or have the bandwidth to take on or un-

TABLE 9-1 A Framework for Nurse Leadership

Leadership Role	Nurses Leading Self	Nurses Leading Others	Nurses Leading Health Care	Nurses Leading Beyond Health Care
Engage the community	Get to know the community and its unique strengths and needs	Facilitate opportunities to become involved in the community	Assess community needs and engage with the community and other partners to address them	Lead and work with community, state, and national coalitions to address structural and systemic barriers
Represent and communicate the nursing perspective	Provide the nursing perspective with other health professionals, patients, and communities	Lead and serve on staff work groups, serve as a union representative, participate in interprofessional collaboration	Lead and participate in multisectoral collaborations, serve in professional associations and organizations	Serve on boards and expert panels, pursue political office and appointed political positions, hold C-suite positions
Advocate	Advocate for self (e.g., report workplace hazards and bullying, speak up for self)	Advocate for others, help other nurses be healthy and well, advocate for patient and community needs	Advocate for organizational policies and structures that support nurses and promote equity	Advocate for legislative and regulatory changes at the community, state, and national levels
Improve equity	Practice nursing with compassion and cultural humility, understand and address own bias	Set a culture of equity, diversity, and inclusion among staff	Lead with a health equity lens; implement policies and systems that promote equity and address racism, discrimination, and bias in the organization	Work to dismantle structural racism and discrimination
Improve health care	Provide quality health care	Encourage innovation and quality improvement efforts in the workplace	Implement programs and lead/translate research and evidence to improve quality of care, address structural barriers, and reach underserved populations	Pursue policies and systems at the state and federal levels that ensure access to quality care for all

SOURCE: CCL, 2010.

derstand what leadership entails (Dyess et al., 2016; Sherman, 2019). Given the right environment and support, however, nurses can overcome these barriers. (See Chapter 7 for further discussion of implicit bias and Chapter 10 for further discussion of self-care.)

Leading Others

In the pursuit of health equity, nurses have the opportunity to lead others, including other nurses, students, health care professionals, staff, community members, and partners. Leading others may occur in a wide range of contexts, including working with clinical nurse managers, community organization leaders, nurses engaging in policy development, and educators and research teams. Leading and managing effective teams requires building and maintaining trusting relationships among team members, communicating effectively, and supporting each team member. In this role, nurses can leverage and actively promote diversity within their teams and create an atmosphere of equity, inclusion, innovation, support, and growth. As team leaders, they can use their position to motivate and empower others to work to identify and address social in addition to health care needs, take action on health equity, and provide the tools and resources needed to do so.

One example of nurses leading others in pursuit of health equity is Cultivando Juntos, a community wellness program aimed at helping farmworkers live longer, healthier lives (Berger, 2019). Two nursing students designed the program, which has expanded to include a biostatistician, a postdoctoral fellow, and undergraduate nursing students. The team meets with local Hispanic farmworkers to discuss their health and well-being and to conduct demonstrations on cooking healthy food. Baseline and longitudinal data are collected across the program to track progress on outcomes that include HgbA1c and lipid levels and body mass index (Berger, 2019). This program is an example of nurses leading others by bringing multiple sectors together to engage with a community in order to address the community's needs.

Nurses Leading Health Care

Nurses lead in numerous ways within health care, both in health care organizations and beyond their organizational boundaries. Within an organization, nurses can assess the organization's readiness to address issues of equity and recommend related improvement. For example, a staff nurse on an inpatient unit can advocate for incorporating an assessment tool that can systematically collect data on SDOH within the electronic health record. Or a nursing director within a health care organization can engage other leaders, as well as members of the community, in initiating a healthy foods program within the hospital and connecting with related community-based agencies. Nurses can also identify and disseminate best and evidence-based practices to ensure equitable health care services within departments and across patient populations, improving and sustaining a supportive culture of care for both staff and those they serve, and advocate for policy changes that address population health and SDOH at the organizational and public policy levels. Nurses leading at higher levels within health care, such as nurse CEOs, chief nursing officers (CNOs), and chief operating officers, can work collaboratively with their organization to set direction and develop a vision and strategies for advancing organization-wide goals that include the drive for greater health equity through engagement with SDOH to meaningfully impact communities served by the health system. Successful organizational leaders can span boundaries between disciplines and sectors in an inclusive way to create meaningful, respectful, and sustainable partnerships to address issues of health equity. For example, public health nurse leaders can bring together representatives of the community served along with leaders from other sectors, including health care, transportation, housing, and food security, to address community needs (see the section below on leading multisector partnerships).

Nurses also have the capacity to lead in health care more broadly. For example, a nurse can seek to influence SDOH by working with a specialty organization such as the National Black Nurses Association, which focuses on the professional development of Black nurses and the delivery of culturally competent care, or serve as a leader for the Council of Public Health Nursing Organizations (CPHNO) or the National Rural Health Association. Many nurses also serve on boards of health care organizations, where they can provide their unique perspective on health-related issues facing individuals, families, and communities (Harper and Benson, 2019). And nurses can serve as leaders in a variety of interprofessional contexts within health care; an example is a nurse researcher leading a multiorganizational research team. In each of these contexts and roles, nurses can share nursing's perspective and expertise while collaborating with others to address health disparities, SDOH, and health equity.

Leading Beyond Health Care

Nurses have myriad opportunities to lead entirely outside the traditional boundaries of health care, in both the public and private sectors. In the public sector, they can lead through positions in local, state, and national government organizations, such as departments of human services, public health, and education. Nurses can be appointed to senior government positions or stand for election to political office, positions in which they can use their expertise and voice to advocate for policy change in the areas of SDOH and health equity. Applying her expertise, U.S. House of Representatives member Lauren Underwood, a registered nurse, discussed the disproportionate health and economic impacts of COVID-19 on communities of color, particularly Black Americans, in a Committee on Education and Labor virtual hearing in June 2020, calling these disparities "the pandemic inside this pandemic."[1] She also sponsored a number of bills to eliminate disparities, such as H.R. 6142,[2] focused on maternal health outcomes among minority populations.

A number of other nurses serve in state legislatures, the U.S. Congress, state and federal executive branch positions, and national and state commissions and committees. Nurse leaders also can bring nursing perspective and expertise to private organizations. For example, Microsoft employs a CNO, and AARP has been served by several nurse CEOs. Nurses can facilitate and convene multisector partnerships, leading efforts to disseminate and implement interventions aimed at improving population health, and can engage communities and partners through local, regional, and national networks. Just as nurses serve as board members within health care, they can also serve on boards for programs or organizations that are outside of health care but have impact on health. The Nurses on Boards Coalition works to create opportunities for nurses to participate in a wide range of boards outside of health care, from boards of local schools or places of worship to those of Fortune 500 companies and large international corporations (Harper and Benson, 2019). In the next 10 years, nurse leaders in these types of positions can become drivers for change within their communities by advocating for social change and health equity, and bringing nursing's perspective to organizational and public policy-making discussions.

LEADERSHIP COMPETENCIES FOR ADVANCING HEALTH EQUITY

While nurses' specific leadership roles vary depending on the focus of their work, the setting in which they work, and the people whom they lead, there are certain skills and competencies on which all nurse leaders need to draw as they work to advance health equity by creating a vision and culture of equity, putting the necessary structures and supports in place, and working both within and across boundaries to achieve the vision of health for all. The committee identified eight skills and competencies that are essential for nurse leadership in nearly every setting, which are described in turn below:

- visioning for health equity,
- leading multisector partnerships,
- leading change,
- innovating and improving,
- teaming across boundaries,

[1] The full committee hearing is available at https://edlabor.house.gov/hearings/inequities-exposed-how-covid-19-widened-racial-inequities-in-education-health-and-the-workforce- (accessed April 8, 2021).

[2] See https://www.congress.gov/bill/116th-congress/house-bill/6142?q=%7B%22search%22%3A%5B%22Black+Maternal+Health+Momnibus+Act%22%5D%7D&s=1&r=1 (accessed April 8, 2021).

- creating a culture of equity,
- creating systems and structures for equity, and
- mentoring and sponsoring.

Visioning for Health Equity

In all types of work, a leader is responsible for articulating a vision, setting direction and goals, and developing clear expectations for individuals and teams. Nurse leaders are no exception, whether the vision they create is for providing quality patient care in a clinic, meeting the needs of a community, setting the direction and goals for an organization or company, or redesigning the nation's health care system. In the context of this report, nurse leaders at all levels and in all settings can work collectively with others to develop and communicate a clear and compelling vision for a future state of greater health equity. The creation of a vision for greater health equity can be squarely rooted in existing data demonstrating profound differences in care quality and health outcomes among people of color compared with their White counterparts (Betancourt et al., 2017).

The most effective visions are a shared product (Boyatzis et al., 2015). Nurse leaders can articulate ideas for a vision, and develop a shared vision by working collaboratively with others. Fully understanding the needs, hopes, and aspirations of a community or population is critical to achieving an effective shared vision (Kouzes and Posner, 2009). To this end, nurse leaders can engage in dialogue with community members, whether that community consists of patients in a clinical setting; a subpopulation such as juveniles in the justice system; or residents of a neighborhood, city, or state. Regardless of the specific target community, this engagement requires a nurse leader to apply such skills as listening, acknowledging, and collaborating in order to create trusted relationships that are needed to build community-centric, community-informed solutions to complex health and social needs. Additionally, data collection and analysis to identify, assess, and prioritize opportunities for advancing health equity is essential (Wesson et al., 2019).

Nurses can work with communities to identify and address their needs in a number of ways, including collecting and analyzing data, leading community meetings, presenting at city council meetings, and working to implement and evaluate strategies for eliminating health disparities. One established mechanism in which nurse leaders can engage is community health needs assessments, which are a statutory requirement for nonprofit hospitals (see Chapter 4 for a fuller description). Ensuring that these needs assessments explicitly target health disparities and prioritize SDOH and that they are conducted with input from members of the community on which they focus are examples of the considerations nurses can advance while helping to align community needs with culturally sensitive and relevant resources. Nurse leaders in both health care systems and public health (the entities involved in developing these needs assessments) can use these data to develop nurse-led and other innovative solutions for meeting the identified needs (Swider et al., 2017).

Leading Multisector Partnerships

Strategic partnerships involving a broad range of stakeholders are essential to address factors that perpetuate structural inequities in health and health care (NASEM, 2017). In the Framework for Achieving Health Equity of IHI, developing partnerships with community organizations is identified as one of the framework's fundamental elements (Laderman and Whittington, 2016). Nurses are skilled in working on and leading clinical teams. However, the role of the interprofessional health team is evolving beyond individual clinical encounters and extending beyond the walls of health care systems into the communities where people live (NASEM, 2019a; Pittman, 2019). Multisector models involving innovative interprofessional collaboration among, for example, police, emergency services, the legal system, housing, and public works and the health care system are showing promise and demonstrating positive health outcomes for underserved populations (Hardin and Mason, 2020).

The ability to develop and lead multisector partnerships is critical to achieving health equity for a number of reasons (NASEM, 2017). First, community needs are complex and wide-ranging, and necessarily involve actors from multiple sectors (e.g., employment services, education transportation, health). Collaboration across sectors is essential to break down existing silos that are counterproductive to improving health and health care (NAM, 2017). Second, collaboration among partners introduces "more expertise and knowledge than what resides in any one stakeholder group" (Wakefield, 2018), and multisector partnerships can leverage unique skills and resources from multiple stakeholders (e.g., faith leaders, philanthropists, researchers). Third, working with community partners can help nurses reach underserved populations, including the homeless, recent immigrants, and non-English-speaking families. Fourth, multisector partnerships increase a community's capacity to make sustainable changes by bringing energy, expertise, and perspectives from multiple arenas. Fifth, multisector partnerships can simultaneously address upstream, midstream, and downstream SDOH and ensure alignment of efforts across these levels. Finally, bringing people together from multiple sectors can facilitate and encourage creative approaches; the intersections across boundaries are "where the promise of innovation lies" (Pittman, 2019, p. 27). As Johansson (2004, p. 2) puts it, "When you step into an intersection of fields, disciplines, or cultures, you can combine existing concepts into a large number of extraordinary new ideas."

It is important for multisector partnerships to be formal, structured, and collaborative relationships (Siegel et al., 2018) in which partners have mutual respect for one another, and time and attention are devoted to maintaining those relationships (Chandra et al., 2016). Trust among partners is also essential for a collaborative relationship, and once established, can serve as a foundation for future collaborations (Wakefield, 2018). Nurses leading and engaged in multisector partnerships can help ensure that collaborative efforts are based on an understanding that health is a value shared among all partners (Erickson et al., 2017; Mason et al., 2019; Realized Worth, 2018).

Nurses need to be able to build partnerships that include a focus on integrating clinical and nonclinical services and ensuring access to health and human services. Collaborative multisector efforts are common in the work of public health nurse leaders, and their experience and expertise can inform new approaches. Nurses currently have limited opportunities to learn from such efforts working in traditional health care systems. There is a need to start providing nurses with substantial exposure to experiences that involve developing and maintaining effective cross-sector partnerships, rather than what is often quite limited observational experience in public health and other social services settings.

While nurses have long worked at the intersection of individuals, families, other health professionals, social workers, educators, and others to improve health, more nurses will increasingly need to apply and expand this skill set to participating in or leading community-engaged multisector partnerships. The *Crossing the Quality Chasm* report (IOM, 2001) calls for health care leaders to invest in their nursing workforce to enable nurses to achieve their full potential as individuals, team members, and leaders. Going forward, then, there is an expanding need to build and engage teams that reach beyond health care to include other sectors. Just as working in health care teams represented a "fundamental shift" in perspective in 2001 (IOM, 2001, p. 139), so, too, working across health and social sectors for the benefit of individuals and communities will require a fundamental shift in perspective, resources, and academic preparation.

Leading Change

Reducing disparities and achieving health equity will require nurse leaders to be skilled in leading change. To be effective, these efforts will need to be anchored in the theoretical constructs of change management and occur at multiple levels, within clinical practice, organizations, communities, populations, health authorities, and nations (Browne et al., 2018). Evidence suggests that health care leaders are knowledgeable about disparities and what can be done to eliminate them, but that a number of barriers to successful change exist (Betancourt et al., 2017). These barriers, including a lack of leadership buy-in, competing organizational priorities, existing culture, and ineffective execution, can be addressed through effective change management (Betancourt et al., 2017). Effective change management requires that individuals learn and apply new behaviors and skills, as well as lead and collaborate with others in driving change within and outside of the organizations where they work. Empirically based interventions to drive change that can reduce health disparities include developing a vision for change (as discussed above), aligning executive support, engaging a coalition of committed stakeholders, setting expectations, establishing clear goals and a plan for change, anchoring change in the existing culture, measuring progress, iterating as needed, and communicating status reports and results (Betancourt et al., 2017). Nurses at all levels can exert substantial influence on SDOH by using their experience and knowledge to engage in such change management efforts.

Innovating and Improving

Changing the prevailing health care paradigm to address SDOH and advance health equity will require innovation. The U.S. Department of Commerce's Advisory Committee on Measuring Innovation in the 21st Century Economy defines innovation as the "design, invention, development, and/or implementation of new or altered products, services, processes, systems, organizational structures, or business models for the purpose of creating new value" (ESA, 2007). For the complex work of eliminating disparities and impacting SDOH, knowledge and skill in innovation will be an important competency for nurses. Nurse leaders can facilitate the creation of innovative approaches by challenging the status quo, breaking down traditional barriers to change, teaching and encouraging team members to solve problems using design thinking, identifying best practices, and facilitating the translation and adoption of new ideas.

Virtually all nurses have opportunities to innovate by developing new ideas for improving health and translating these ideas into practice and policy. Over the past several years, nurse-designed and nurse-led innovations addressing SDOH among underserved populations have increasingly appeared in the literature. As described in Chapter 4, for example, nurses in the Netherlands developed and implemented Buurtzorg, an innovative nurse-led, nurse-run organization of self-managed teams that provide home care to individuals in their neighborhoods (Monsen and de Blok, 2013). Similarly, the SOAR (Supporting Older Adults at Risk) program reimagined how to prepare and support frail older adults in the transition back to their homes following a hospital admission. The program addresses issues of transportation, nutrition, and medication access (IHI, 2018).

Yet, while some nurses are already leading efforts focused on health equity in their work settings and communities, this focus is not consistent across the profession. It is a leader's responsibility to create an environment that allows for innovation (IOM, 2000). Leaders can provide a forum for continual innovation in and testing of strategies for improving population health and health equity, and ensure that their organization is flexible and able to adapt to those changes (IOM, 2001). For example, leaders of front-line health teams can encourage team members to share their own observations and ideas for improving patient health and facilitate the transfer of new ideas across professional boundaries (IOM, 2001). Likewise, nurse leaders working in the community or in multisector partnerships can encourage communication and collaboration without regard for traditional boundaries and recognize that innovative ideas can surface from an array of individuals across sectors, such as those working in aging-related services or Medicaid managed care organizations.

Nurses have a rich tradition of working creatively to solve problems and improve the quality of care in clinical settings (Thomas et al., 2016), and these experiences and skills can apply to efforts designed to address SDOH. These types of initiatives require systematic, continuous, data-driven, and rigorous processes of assessment, innovation, implementation, evaluation, and diffusion or translation of the evidence or best practices into tangible strategies or policies for improving population health. For example, IHI's Model for Improvement for quality improvement initiatives uses a Plan-Do-Study-Act (PDSA) cycle that involves planning exactly how the intervention will be implemented; implementing it; studying whether and how it is being conducted; and then acting to either adapt it, adopt it as a standard practice, collect more data, or abandon it (IHI, 2020). This model has been used with great success in the clinical setting. Transforming Care at the Bedside (TCAB), was one such model using the PDSA cycle. A partnership between the Robert Wood Johnson Foundation and IHI, TCAB created learning collaboratives at the front lines of care on medical-surgical units that engaged nurses and other front-line staff in generating and testing ideas that led to processes and practices that improved the efficiency, safety, and satisfaction of care.[3] This process has the potential to be equally successful in addressing SDOH and health equity (IHI, 2020).

Teaming Across Boundaries

As nurses work within and across organizations to address SDOH and advance health equity, they will need the skills to develop, engage, and lead cross-boundary teams. Cross-boundary teaming is a strategy for driving innovation that engages diverse stakeholders and subject-matter experts to expand the range of views and ideas on which teams can draw (Edmondson and Harvey, 2018). In cross-boundary teams, individuals work across knowledge boundaries. Teams are diverse in expertise, knowledge, and educational background, characterized by deep-level differences or what Edmondson and Harvey call "knowledge diversity" (p. 3480).

Addressing SDOH and advancing health equity will require a cross-boundary team approach that includes not only people from different disciplines and sectors but also individuals and organizations from within the community. Regardless of the composition of the team, the cross-boundary team leader will need to support each team member, balance the use of resources, facilitate communication, and ensure the team's effectiveness. A leader's job is to "optimize the performance of teams that provide various services in pursuit of a shared set of aims" (IOM, 2001). Evidence suggests that high-performing team members listen to one an-

[3] See http://www.ihi.org/Engage/Initiatives/Completed/TCAB/Pages/default.aspx for more information about TCAB (accessed April 8, 2021).

other and show sensitivity to feelings and needs (Duhigg, 2016). To support the team and optimize its performance, a nurse leader will need to work to help its members achieve their full potential, both individually and collectively. This investment may include providing support and time for self-care, providing access to and time for ongoing professional development, and supporting individuals as they seek higher levels of education and responsibility. Facilitating nurses' well-being and self-care is one particularly important way in which nurse leaders can support and optimize cross-boundary teams (see Chapter 10 on the importance of facilitating nurse well-being).

Creating a Culture of Equity

Nurse leaders in many positions of authority, including academic leaders (DeWitty and Murray, 2020), journal editors (Villarruel and Broome, 2020), educators (Graham et al., 2016), and managers (ANA, 2018), can act to call out and dismantle racism. To advance equity in society, nursing needs first to work to create a culture of equity within the profession itself. Nursing has a history of racism that continues to impact the experiences of nursing faculty, nurses in practice, communities, and patients (DeWitty and Murray, 2020; Iheduru-Anderson, 2020a; Villarruel and Broome, 2020; Waite and Nardi, 2019; Whitfield-Harris et al., 2017). The nursing profession's substantive and sustained attention is required to address and eliminate racism in nursing and in broader organizations where nurses work. Waite and Nardi (2019, p. 20) call on nurse leaders to "urge their colleagues and students to characterize, name, contest, and transform the norms, traditions, structures, and establishments that preserve White supremacy through continued effects of American colonialism." Over the past few years, the nursing literature, including statements issued by national nursing organizations, has reflected increased attention to these issues.

Nurse leaders must acknowledge existing disparities and facilitate open, honest, and respectful discussions about factors that drive disparities (Oruche, and Zapolski, 2020; Purtzer and Thomas, 2019) and the challenges staff face as they engage in this work within organizations and with communities. It will be essential for these discussions to include opportunities for and support of the expression of patient and community perspectives (NASEM, 2017). Specific strategies for promoting equity and inclusion include (1) creating safe spaces to engender trust and open communication; (2) reassessing recruitment and advancement processes; (3) examining and redesigning equity policies, procedures, and practices; (4) requiring a diverse pool of applicants for applicant selection; (5) moving from mentorship to sponsorship, which focuses on protégé advancement; (6) creating an infrastructure to monitor and track progress with development programs; and (7) dismantling racism, including applying an equity lens to all practices (Fitzsimmons and Peters-Lewis, 2021). Nurse leaders need to set an example of inclusion and confront negative and toxic cultural norms in nursing, such as bullying and in-fighting (Kaiser, 2017). Nurse leaders need to be knowledgeable about and able to lead others in cultural humility and culturally competent practices, which are critical for reducing health disparities and improving access to high-quality health care (Powell, 2016).

In a recent analysis of six models of cultural competence, Botelho and Lima (2020) argue that existing approaches to the delivery of culturally appropriate care may assist with cultural respect, but tend to oversimplify patients' cultural experiences and overlook the complexities associated with power dynamics (Botelho and Lima, 2020). They propose the practices of not only cultural humility but also relational ethics[4] to facilitate cross-cultural work. To practice cultural humility, clinicians relinquish their role as experts in a culturally diverse world where power imbalances exist and embrace an attitude characterized by constant questioning, openness, self-awareness, absence of ego, and self-reflection and -critique, willingly interacting with diverse individuals. Practicing with cultural humility can foster mutual empowerment, respect, partnerships, optimal care, and lifelong learning (Foronda et al., 2016, p. 213). (See Chapter 7 for further discussion of cultural humility.)

Creating Systems and Structures for Equity

Nurse leaders at all levels and in all settings can help create systems and structures that promote equity and do not unintentionally exacerbate inequalities through unintended incentives. For example, working midstream (see Chapter 2), a nurse leader who oversees a home visiting program can educate around the concept of equitable care and establish expectations of nurses that encourage the provision of equitable care, including meeting social needs, rather than orienting nursing's interventions to the volume of visits they make (IOM, 2001). A nurse leader who manages an organization can develop organization-wide policies that put equity at the forefront of the staff's work, and ensure that the provision of services does not exacerbate existing inequalities. Upstream, a nurse leader can influence government policy by advocating for policies that improve equity, such as a city transportation policy that prioritizes traditionally underserved rather than higher-income neighborhoods, or by highlighting exposure to noise pollution and associated health impacts related to building low-income housing near railroad tracks.

The goal of health equity is more likely to be achieved when it becomes deeply ingrained in official systems and structures and becomes inherent in a cultural shift that includes inner reflections on bias and structural racism (Chin, 2020), rather than being pursued through one-off initiatives or well-intentioned

[4] Relational ethics is defined in health care as actions that take place within relationships and consider the existence of the other (i.e., patient, nurse) (Bergum and Dossetor, 2005). Core tenets include mutual respect, engagement, embodied knowledge, environment, and uncertainty; the most important tenet is mutual respect (Pollard, 2015).

efforts that are not formalized. Systems and structures are never neutral—they either entrench or dismantle existing health inequities. Nurse leaders have a responsibility to advocate for and build systems that promote equitable health for all.

Mentoring and Sponsoring

The transformation toward a health system that is more equitable and just will require explicit preparation of and support for future nurse leaders in multiple settings (AACN, 2016). A key strategy for achieving this goal is mentorship and sponsorship of the next generation of nurses and nurse leaders. Mentoring is critical across the trajectory of nurses' professional lives, particularly as they take on new and increasingly complex leadership roles (Vitale, 2018). Given the overarching need for nurse leaders with expertise and commitment to achieving equity in health and health care, and given the need for more nurses with expertise in such priority areas as care for the aging, maternal mortality, mental and behavioral health, rural health, and public health (see Chapter 3), mentoring is critical to building and supporting the next generation of nurses.

Mentoring is associated with positive benefits, including professional development, greater skills, a better fit with one's choice of specialty, and greater life–work balance (Disch, 2018). In mentoring new nurses in the application of concepts related to health equity or in needed specialty areas as identified above, nurses with experience can encourage collaboration among nurses of different ages and at different professional development stages. In general, a lack of support and mentoring by senior nurses has negative impacts on well-being and workforce turnover (IOM, 2011), and mentoring is therefore a critical part of building capacity in the profession and of mitigating the loss of knowledge and experience that results when retiring nurses leave the profession.

A particularly critical role for nurse leaders is mentoring nurses from traditionally underrepresented communities to build a more diverse nursing workforce and increase the number of nurses from underrepresented groups in leadership positions (Phillips and Malone, 2014). Mentoring is a critical component of recruiting, supporting, and advancing nurses of color through the ranks of leadership (DeWitty and Murray, 2020; Iheduru-Anderson, 2020b; Whitfield-Harris et al., 2017). As discussed in Chapter 3, diversity in the nursing workforce—and in nursing leadership in particular—is essential to achieving health equity. There are relatively few nurses of color in leadership positions, particularly in more senior executive positions (Phillips and Malone, 2014; Schmieding, 2000). A 2019 National Academies report on increasing the number of professionals of color in science, technology, engineering, and mathematics found that structured mentorship programs in minority-serving institutions[5]

[5] Institutions serving people of color are commonly defined in two distinct categories: historically Black colleges and universities and tribal colleges and universities (NASEM, 2019).

can improve leadership diversity in nursing and the health care field generally (NASEM, 2019b). One such effort is being led by the Center to Champion Nursing in America (CCNA) in its convenings of mentor training programs with historically Black colleges and universities (HBCUs). CCNA will continue to convene mentoring programs in Hispanic- and American Indian–serving nursing schools as well (CCNA, 2020).

Serving as a sponsor becomes even more critical than mentoring when a more active role is required to help nurses rise in leadership ranks (Williams and Dawson, 2021). The expectations of a sponsor include being a staunch advocate for career advancement for the protégé, including making assignments and connecting the protégé to key decision makers while keeping her or him protected from negative influences. Sponsors take advantage of the organizations and people in their sphere to present their protégés in the most positive light, with the goal of career advancement. This more active approach has been shown to be especially helpful in helping nurses of color rise in the leadership ranks (Beckwith et al., 2016).

ACHIEVING THE COMMITTEE'S VISION OF NURSE LEADERSHIP

As previously noted, many nurse leaders are currently focused on incorporating equity into their work. To achieve the committee's vision, however, a significant investment in broader and deeper development of nurse leadership will be needed. New and established nurse leaders—at all levels and in all settings—are needed to lead change that results in meeting social needs, eliminating health disparities, addressing SDOH, and ultimately achieving equity in health and health care, with the aim of improved health for all individuals and communities. Nurse leaders need to both develop and expand the leadership competencies described in this chapter, and implement strategies targeted to achieving diversity among nurse leaders. Nurse leadership competencies and knowledge can be developed through approaches that encompass education, fellowships, and nursing organizations, as discussed below.

Increasing Diversity in Nurse Leadership

Diverse leaders can serve as particularly important role models, provide guidance and mentoring for other nurses, influence the allocation of resources, and shape policies aimed at eliminating inequities (Phillips and Malone, 2014). The prior *The Future of Nursing* report identifies the need for a renewed focus on diversity in nursing, calling for the development of novel education models that promote respect for diversity along a number of dimensions, such as race, ethnicity, geography, background, and personal experiences (IOM, 2011). Even when nurse leaders hold similar positions, salary disparities are seen among racial and ethnic groups. Among nurse leaders with the highest salaries (ranging from clinical staff to C-suite executives), only 11 percent are Black, compared with 27 percent who are Asian American, 25 percent who are Hispanic, and 21 percent who are White. Not only are few Black nurses in positions of leadership at all, but even fewer advance to careers as nurse executives (Iheduru-Anderson, 2020a; Jeffries et al., 2018).

Understanding and addressing the reasons for the diversity gap in nursing leadership is essential. The existing literature identifies racism as a significant factor (Iheduru-Anderson, 2020a). Nursing's roots in the United States have been shaped within the context of colonialism, a history that has influenced the makeup of the profession's leaders (Waite and Nardi, 2019). As discussed earlier, acknowledging and addressing how racism has been internalized and how it has manifested within the field, including in the advancement of nurses of color, is key (Brathwaite, 2018; Waite and Nardi, 2019). Other barriers include stereotyping; a lack of career development opportunities (Carroll, 2020); a lack of mentorship (Ihederu-Anderson, 2020b); inadequate support systems; isolation; the perception of being overlooked for positions in contrast to White counterparts (Kolade, 2016); and the cultural taxation or diversity tax (Gewin, 2020), characterized by the role assigned to the ethnic representative of a group involving the expectation that this individual will provide unofficial diversity consultation.[6]

Numerous innovative programs aimed at cultivating diversity in nursing leadership have been developed and implemented. A number of these programs target nurses early in the trajectory of development (in prebaccalaureate or baccalaureate programs), while others are aimed at later stages of professional growth. Examples of programs focused on early leadership training include EMBRACE (Engaging Multiple communities of BSN [bachelor of science in nursing] students in Research and Academic Curricular Experiences), which was developed to provide comprehensive experiences in research and leadership for undergraduate students of color who are underrepresented in nursing, and the Duke University School of Nursing's Making a Difference program (Carter et al., 2015; Stacciarini and McDaniel, 2019). Likewise, the University of North Dakota has a program called Recruitment & Retention of American Indians into Nursing (RAIN), which provides academic support and assistance to American Indian nursing students, from prenursing programs through doctoral education (UND, 2020). (See Chapter 7 for further discussion of recruiting and supporting underrepresented students.) To fully support the goal of diversity in nurse leadership, such programs will need to be evaluated and scaled.

Nursing Education, Fellowships, and Certificates

While nursing school curricula often include some information about public health, SDOH, and health equity, they do not always prepare students to engage

[6] Cultural taxation refers to the phenomenon whereby faculty who are individuals of color are asked routinely to take on extra, uncompensated work to address a lack of diversity in their institutions.

fully with and serve as leaders on these issues. Nursing education traditionally has emphasized the development of clinical skills over leadership and management skills (Joseph and Huber, 2015). As discussed in Chapter 7, the American Association of Colleges of Nursing's (AACN's) *Essentials*[7] provides an outline for the necessary curriculum content and expected competencies for graduates of baccalaureate, master's, and doctor of nursing practice (DNP) programs. Introducing the concept of health equity in school is a necessary first step in professional role development and leadership, but nurses also need to take every opportunity to supplement their preparation through continuing education.

A number of fellowships support education in leadership skills with a focus on health equity and community health.[8] Nearly all of these fellowships are interdisciplinary, bringing together professionals from multiple sectors, including health care, business, community organizing, education, and the law. These types of fellowships present opportunities for nurses to grow their leadership skills, to collaborate and innovate with professionals from multiple disciplines and sectors, and to develop and implement projects within their areas of interest that relate directly to achieving health equity. In addition to equity-specific fellowships, a wide variety of fellowships available for nurses are focused on general leadership skills that can be transferred to any area and any setting, including addressing SDOH and pursuing health equity.

One fellowship specifically for nurses and focused on equity is the Environmental Health Nurse Fellowship, which trains nurses to work with communities to address environmental health threats. In 2019, the Alliance of Nurses for Healthy Environments (ANHE) launched this fellowship to focus on environmental health equity and justice and on the disproportionate impact of environmental conditions on underserved groups. The 30 fellows, all of whom are nurses, work with mentors to help communities identify environmental needs and build support for community-driven solutions (ANHE, 2019).

The Global Nursing Leadership Institute[9] (GNLI) fellowship, sponsored by the International Council of Nurses and supported by the Burdett Trust for Nursing, is available to nurses worldwide. This fellowship is focused on policy leadership, with a special emphasis on strengthening political and policy understanding and influence. Its framework includes in-depth work on the United Na-

---

[7] The February 2021 final draft (AACN, 2021) is available at https://www.aacnnursing.org/Portals/42/AcademicNursing/pdf/Essentials-Final-Draft-2-18-21.pdf?ver=hNeCl7OjgamIA9sHgDi_Yw%3d%3d×tamp=1613742420447 (accessed April 8, 2021).

[8] See, for example, the Atlantic Fellows for Health Equity at The George Washington University Health Workforce Institute, the Diversity and Health Equity Fellowship of the American Hospital Association, and the Robert Wood Johnson Foundation's Health Policy Fellows and Culture of Health Leaders programs.

[9] See https://www.icn.ch/what-we-do/projects/global-nursing-leadership-institutetm-gnli (accessed April 8, 2021).

tions' Sustainable Development Goals, which reflect multiple SDOH. The focus of 2020 was on health disparities in the context of the COVID-19 pandemic.

Many certificate programs in the United States can help nurses develop leadership skills that can be leveraged to lead work in equity in health and health care. Examples include the Health Equity Certificate at the University of Pittsburgh School of Public Health[10] and the Graduate Certificate in Health Equity at the Vanderbilt University Medical Center.[11]

The Role of Nursing Organizations

Most professional nursing organizations recognize and specifically call out leadership as an essential competency for nurses in all settings (NAHN, 2020; NCEMNA, 2020; NLN, 2005; Quad Council, 2018). These organizations offer leadership courses, resources, and support, most pertaining to leadership in general rather than leadership on health equity, for current and aspiring nurse leaders. Nursing organizations also have undertaken specific initiatives to develop and support nurse leaders that include content related to equity in health and health care. Examples include the following: (1) the American Public Health Association Public Health Nursing Section, with the vision of advancing social justice and equity to achieve population health for all[12]; (2) the Future of Nursing: Campaign for Action, with the vision of working toward an America in which everyone can live a healthier life, supported by nurses as essential partners in providing care and promoting health equity and well-being[13]; (3) the Black Coalition Against COVID-19,[14] an interprofessional multisector coalition, co-led by the National Black Nurses Association, focused on urgently mobilizing and coordinating all available community assets in a collaborative effort with the government of Washington, DC; and (4) the National Coalition of Ethnic Minority Nurse Associations (NCEMNA), which stands as a unified force advocating for equity and justice in nursing and health care for ethnic minority populations.[15] In addition, professional associations offer nurses an opportunity to build leadership competencies by leading within the association. While some nursing associations are small and others large, each can offer nurses an opportunity to meet other nurses, join boards and workgroups, and help guide the association's direction, especially toward the goals germane to this report.

Nursing associations that are organized around a racial or ethnic identity may offer a particularly good opportunity for underrepresented nurses to hone their

---

[10] See https://catalog.upp.pitt.edu/preview_program.php?catoid=73&poid=23709&returnto=6375 (accessed April 8, 2021).

[11] See https://www.vumc.org/healthequity/graduate-certificate-health-equity (accessed April 8, 2021).

[12] See https://www.apha.org/apha-communities/member-sections/public-health-nursing (accessed June 7, 2021).

[13] See https://campaignforaction.org/about (accessed June 7, 2021).

[14] See https://blackcoalitionagainstcovid.org (accessed June 7, 2021).

[15] See https://ncemna.org/about (accessed June 7, 2021).

leadership skills. The NCEMNA is an umbrella organization of five national ethnic nurse associations: the Asian American/Pacific Islander Nurses Association, the National Alaska Native American Indian Nurses Association, the National Association of Hispanic Nurses (NAHN), the National Black Nurses Association, and the Philippine Nurses Association of America. One of the five strategic goals of the NCEMNA is to "promote ethnic minority nurse leadership in areas of health policy, practice, education and research" through the implementation of leadership development and mentorship programs (NCEMNA, 2020).

CONCLUSIONS

All nurses have the capability to lead and engage in meaningful roles in addressing SDOH and health equity, with their specific roles and functions depending on individual interests, capacities, and opportunities.

> ***Conclusion 9-1: Nurse leaders at every level and across all settings can strengthen the profession's long-standing focus on social determinants of health and health equity to meet the needs of underserved individuals, neighborhoods, and communities and to prioritize the elimination of health inequities.***

Given that social determinants that affect health exist largely outside of the health care system (e.g., poverty, literacy, housing, transportation, and food security), addressing SDOH and eliminating health disparities will require collaboration and partnership among a broad group of stakeholders. Public health nurses have a long history of working collaboratively to meet social needs and address SDOH, and their experiences can be used as models for other nurses seeking to work collaboratively across sectors.

> ***Conclusion 9-2: Achieving health equity will require multisector collaboration, and nurse leaders can participate in and lead these efforts.***

> ***Conclusion 9-3: Many community and public health nurse leaders have expertise and experience in leading cross-sector partnerships to meet social needs and address social determinants of health, and their expertise can be leveraged to inform the broader nursing profession in both practice and education.***

Racism and discrimination are deeply entrenched in U.S. society and its institutions, and the nursing profession is no exception. Nurse leaders have an important role to play in acknowledging the history of racism within the profession and in moving forward to dismantle structural racism and mitigate the effects of discrimination and implicit bias on health. Role modeling listening, engagement, and inclusivity within and outside of nursing will be necessary to foster trust and achieve needed change. A critical part of these efforts will be building a more diverse nursing workforce and supporting these nurses in their pursuit of and success in leadership roles.

Conclusion 9-4: Nurse leaders have a responsibility to address structural racism, cultural racism, and discrimination based on identity (e.g., sexual orientation, gender), place (e.g., rural, urban), and circumstances (e.g., disability, mental health condition) within the nursing profession and to help build structures and systems at the societal level that address these issues to promote health equity.

Conclusion 9-5: A critical role for nurse leaders is mentoring and sponsoring nurses from traditionally underrepresented communities in order to build a more diverse nursing workforce and increase the number of underrepresented nurses in leadership positions.

REFERENCES

AACN (American Association of Colleges of Nursing). 2016. *Advancing healthcare transformation: A new era for academic nursing*. https://www.aacnnursing.org/Portals/42/Publications/AACN-New-Era-Report.pdf (accessed April 8, 2021).

AACN. 2021. The essentials: Core competencies for professional nursing education: Final draft. https://www.aacnnursing.org/Portals/42/AcademicNursing/pdf/Essentials-Final-Draft-2-18-21.pdf?ver=hNeCl7OjgamIA9sHgDi_Yw%3d%3d×tamp=1613742420447 (accessed April 16, 2021).

ANA (American Nurses Association). 2018. *The nurse's role in addressing discrimination: Protecting and promoting inclusive strategies in practice settings, policy, and advocacy*. Position Statement. https://www.nursingworld.org/~4ab207/globalassets/practiceandpolicy/nursing-excellence/ana-position-statements/social-causes-and-health-care/the-nurses-role-in-addressing-discrimination.pdf (accessed April 8, 2021).

ANHE (Alliance of Nurses for Healthy Environments). 2019. *ANHE environmental health nurse fellowship: 2019–2020 cohort*. https://envirn.org/anhe-fellowship (accessed April 8, 2021).

Beckwith, A. L., D. R. Carter, and T. Peters. 2016. The underrepresentation of African American women in executive leadership: What's getting in the way? *Journal of Business Studies Quarterly* 7(4):115–134.

Berger, M. W. 2019 (October 23). Cultivando Juntos takes shape in Kennett Square. *Penn Today*. https://penntoday.upenn.edu/news/cultivando-juntos-takes-shape-kennett-square (accessed April 8, 2021).

Bergum, V., and J. B. Dossetor. 2005. *Relational ethics: The full meaning of respect*. Hagerstown, MD: University Publishing Group.

Betancourt, J. R., A. Tan-McGrory, K. S. Kenst, T. H. Phan, and L. Lopez. 2017. Organizational change management for health equity: Perspectives from the disparities leadership program. *Health Affairs (Millwood)* 36(6):1095–1101.

Botelho, M. J., and C. A. Lima. 2020. From cultural competence to cultural respect: A critical review of six models. *Journal of Nursing Education* 59(6):311–318. doi: 10.3928/01484834-20200520-03.

Boyatzis, R. E., K. Rochford, and S. N. Taylor. 2015. The role of the positive emotional attractor in vision and shared vision: Toward effective leadership, relationships, and engagement. *Frontiers in Psychology* 6:670.

Brathwaite, B. 2018. Black, Asian and minority ethnic female nurses: Colonialism, power and racism. *British Journal of Nursing* 27(5):254–258.

Browne, A. J., C. Varcoe, M. Ford-Gilboe, C. Nadine Wathen, V. Smye, B. E. Jackson, B. Wallace, B. Pauly, C. P. Herbert, J. G. Lavoie, S. T. Wong, and A. Blanchet Garneau. 2018. Disruption as opportunity: Impacts of an organizational health equity intervention in primary care clinics. *International Journal for Equity in Health* 17(1):154.

Carroll, D. 2020. *Diversity: Lack of African American presence in nursing leadership. DNP qualifying manuscripts*. 45. https://repository.usfca.edu/dnp_qualifying/45 (accessed April 15, 2021).

Carter, B. M., D. L. Powell, A. L. Derouin, and J. Cusatis. 2015. Beginning with the end in mind: Cultivating minority nurse leaders. *Journal of Professional Nursing* 31(2):95–103.

CCL (Center for Creative Leadership). 2010. *Executive nurse fellows program, outcome and competency chart*. Princeton, NJ: Robert Wood Johnson Foundation.

CCNA (Center to Champion Nursing in America). 2020. *Mentoring for better health*. Campaign for Action. https://campaignforaction.org/resource/mentoring-for-better-health (accessed June 7, 2021).

Chandra, A., C. E. Miller, J. D. Acosta, S. Weilant, M. Trujillo, and A. Plough. 2016. Drivers of health as a shared value: Mindset, expectations, sense of community, and civic engagement. *Health Affairs* 35(11):1959–1963.

Chin, M. 2020. Advancing health equity in patient safety: A reckoning, challenge, and opportunity. *BMJ Quality and Safety*. Epub ahead of print. doi: 10.1136/bmjqs-2020-012599.

DeWitty, V. P., and T. A. Murray. 2020. Influence of climate and culture on minority faculty retention. *Journal of Nursing Ethics* 59(9):483–484.

Disch, J. 2018. Rethinking mentoring. *Critical Care Medicine* 46(3):437–441.

Duhigg, D. 2016 (February 25). What Google learned from its quest to build the perfect team. *The New York Times Magazine*. https://www.nytimes.com/2016/02/28/magazine/what-google-learned-from-its-quest-to-build-the-perfect-team.html (accessed April 8. 2021).

Dyess, S. M., R. O. Sherman, B. Pratt, and L. Chiang-Hanisko. 2016. Growing nurse leaders: Their perspectives on nursing leadership and today's practice environment. *Online Journal for Issues in Nursing* 21(1). http://ojin.nursingworld.org/MainMenuCategories/ANAMarketplace/ANAPeriodicals/OJIN/TableofContents/Vol-21-2016/No1-Jan-2016/Articles-Previous-Topics/Growing-Nurse-Leaders.html (accessed April 9, 2021).

Eckert, R., M. West, D. Altman, K. Steward, and B. Pasmore. 2014. *Delivering a collective leadership strategy for health care*. Greensboro, NC: Center for Creative Leadership and Kings Fund.

Edmondson, A. C., and J.-F. Harvey. 2018. Cross-boundary teaming for innovation: Integrating research on teams and knowledge in organizations. *Human Resource Management Review* 28(4):347–360.

Erickson, J., B. Milstein, L. Schafer, K. E. Pritchard, C. Levitz, C. Miller, and A. Cheadle. 2017. *Progress along the pathway for transforming regional health: A pulse check on multi-sector partnerships*. ReThink Health and the Center for Community Health and Evaluation. https://www.rethinkhealth.org/wp-content/uploads/2017/03/2016-Pulse-Check-Narrative-Final.pdf (accessed April 8, 2021).

ESA (Economics and Statistics Administration, U.S. Department of Commerce). 2007. Innovation measurement. *Federal Register* 72(71):18627. https://www.govinfo.gov/content/pkg/FR-2007-04-13/pdf/07-1827.pdf (accessed April 8, 2021).

Feely, D. 2016 (August 11). Equity: The forgotten aim? *Institute for Healthcare Improvement Blog*. http://www.ihi.org/communities/blogs/equity-the-forgotten-aim (accessed April 8, 2021).

Fitzsimmons, M. J., and A. Peters-Lewis. 2021, March 1. Creating more diverse C-suites: From intention to outcomes. *Voice of Nursing Leadership*. American Organization for Nursing Leadership. https://www.aonl.org/news/voice/mar-2021/creating-more-diverse-csuite-from-intention (accessed April 8, 2021).

Foronda, C., D. L. Baptiste, M. M. Reinholdt, and K. Ousman. 2016. Cultural humility: A concept analysis. *Journal of Transcultural Nursing* 27(3):210–217.

Gewin, V. 2020. The time tax put on scientists of colour. *Nature* 583(7816):479–481.

Graham, C. L., S. M. Phillips, S. D. Newman, and T. W. Atz. 2016. Baccalaureate minority nursing students perceived barriers and facilitators to clinical education practices: An integrative review. *Nursing Education Perspective* 37(3):130–137.

Hardin, L., and D. J. Mason. 2020. Lessons from complex care in a COVID-19 world. *JAMA Health Forum* 1(7):e200908.

Harper, K. J., and L. S. Benson. 2019. The importance and impact of nurses serving on boards. *Nursing Economics* 37(4):209–212.

Iheduru-Anderson, K. C. 2020a. The white/black hierarchy institutionalizes White supremacy in nursing and nursing leadership in the United States. *Journal of Professional Nursing*. Epub ahead of print. doi: 10.1016/j.profnurs.2020.05.005.

Iheduru-Anderson, K. 2020b. Barriers to career advancement in the nursing profession: Perceptions of Black nurses in the United States. *Nursing Forum* 55(4):664–677.

IHI (Institute for Healthcare Improvement). 2018 (October 23). How "flipped" discharge can help your largest patient population. *Institute for Healthcare Improvement Blog*. http://www.ihi.org/communities/blogs/how-flipped-discharge-can-help-your-largest-patient-population (accessed April 8, 2021).

IHI. 2020. *Science of improvement: How to improve*. http://www.ihi.org/resources/Pages/HowtoImprove/ScienceofImprovementHowtoImprove.aspx (accessed April 8, 2021).

IOM (Institute of Medicine). 2000. *Exploring innovation and quality improvement in health care micro-systems: A cross-case analysis*. Washington, DC: National Academy Press.

IOM. 2001. *Crossing the quality chasm: A new health system for the 21st century*. Washington, DC: National Academy Press.

IOM. 2011. *The future of nursing: Leading change, advancing health*. Washington, DC: The National Academies Press.

Jefferies, K., L. Goldberg, M. Aston, and G. Tomblin Murphy. 2018. Understanding the invisibility of black nurse leaders using a black feminist poststructuralist framework. *Journal of Clinical Nursing* 27(15–16):3225–3234.

Johansson, F. 2004. *The Medici effect: Breakthrough insights at the intersection of ideas, concepts & cultures*. Boston, MA: Harvard Business School Press.

Joseph, M. L., and D. L. Huber. 2015. Clinical leadership development and education for nurses: Prospects and opportunities. *Journal of Healthcare Leadership* 7:55–64.

Jouppila, T., and T. Tiainen. 2020. Nurses' participation in the design of an intensive care unit: The use of virtual mock-ups. *Health Environments Research & Design Journal*. doi: 10.1177/1937586720935407.

Kaiser, J. A. 2017. The relationship between leadership style and nurse-to-nurse incivility: Turning the lens inward. *Journal of Nursing Management* 25(2):110–118.

Kolade, F. M. 2016. The lived experience of minority nursing faculty: A phenomenological study. *Journal of Professional Nursing* 32(2):107–114.

Kouzes, J. M., and B. Z. Posner. 2009. To lead, create a shared vision. *Harvard Business Review* 87(1):20–21.

Kruse, K. 2013 (April 9). What is leadership? *Forbes*. https://www.forbes.com/sites/kevinkruse/2013/04/09/what-is-leadership/?sh=98657e85b90c (accessed April 8, 2021).

Laderman, M., and J. Whittington. 2016. A framework for improving health equity. *Healthcare Executive* 31(3):82–85.

Lathrop, B. 2013. Nursing leadership in addressing the social determinants of health. *Policy, Politics, & Nursing Practice* 14(1):41–47.

Mason, D. J., G. R. Martsolf, J. Sloan, A. Villarruel, and C. Sullivan. 2019. Making health a shared value: Lessons from nurse-designed models of care. *Nursing Outlook* 67(3):213–222.

Monsen, K. A., and J. de Blok. 2013. Buurtzorg: Nurse-led community care. *Creative Nursing* 19(3):122–127.

NAHN (National Association of Hispanic Nurses). 2020. *About NAHN*. https://nahnnet.org/about (accessed April 8, 2021).

NAM (National Academy of Medicine). 2017. *Vital directions for health and health care*. Discussion Paper Series. https://nam.edu/initiatives/vital-directions-for-health-and-health-care/vital-directions-for-health-health-care-discussion-papers (accessed April 8, 2021).

NASEM (National Academies of Sciences, Engineering, and Medicine). 2017. *Communities in action: Pathways to health equity*. Washington, DC: The National Academies Press.

NASEM. 2019a. *Integrating social care into the delivery of health care: Moving upstream to improve the nation's health*. Washington, DC: The National Academies Press.

NASEM. 2019b. *Minority serving institutions: America's underutilized resource for strengthening the STEM workforce*. Washington, DC: The National Academies Press.

NASEM. 2020. *Educating health professionals to address the social determinants of mental health: Proceedings of a workshop*. Washington, DC: The National Academies Press.

NCEMNA (National Coalition of Ethnic Minority Nurse Associations). 2020. *History*. https://ncemna.org/history (accessed April 8, 2021).

NLN (National League for Nursing). 2005. *NLN core competencies for academic nurse educators*. http://www.nln.org/professional-development-programs/competencies-for-nursing-education/nurse-educator-core-competency (accessed April 8, 2021).

Ogbolu, Y., D. A. Scrandis, and G. Fitzpatrick. 2018. Barriers and facilitators of care for diverse patients: Nurse leader perspectives and nurse manager implications. *Journal of Nursing Management* 26(1):3–10.

Olshansky, E. F. 2017. Social determinants of health: The role of nursing. *American Journal of Nursing* 117(12):11.

Oruche, U. M., and T. C. B. Zapolski. 2020. The role of nurses in eliminating health disparities and achieving health equity. *Journal of Psychosocial Nursing and Mental Health Services* 58(12):2–4.

Phillips, J. M., and B. Malone. 2014. Increasing racial/ethnic diversity in nursing to reduce health disparities and achieve health equity. *Public Health Reports* 129(Suppl 2):45–50.

Pittman, P. 2019. *Activating nursing to address unmet needs in the 21st century*. Princeton, NJ: Robert Wood Johnson Foundation.

Pollard, C. 2015. What is the right thing to do: Use of a relational ethic framework to guide clinical decision-making. *International Journal of Caring Sciences* 8(2):362–368.

Powell, D. L. 2016. Social determinants of health: Cultural competence is not enough. *Creative Nursing* 22(1):5–10.

Purtzer, M. A., and J. J. Thomas. 2019. Intentionality in reducing health disparities: Caring as connection. *Public Health Nursing (Boston, Mass.)* 36(3):276–283.

Quad Council (Quad Council Coalition Competency Review Task Force). 2018. *Community/public health nursing [C/PHN] competencies*. https://www.cphno.org/wp-content/uploads/2020/08/QCC-C-PHN-COMPETENCIES-Approved_2018.05.04_Final-002.pdf (accessed April 8, 2021).

Realized Worth. 2018. *Multi-sector partnerships—The key to a brighter future?* https://www.realizedworth.com/2018/07/07/multi-sector-partnerships-the-key-to-a-brighter-future (accessed April 8, 2021).

Schmieding, N. J. 2000. Minority nurses in leadership positions: A call for action. *Nursing Outlook* 48(3):120–127.

Shapiro, M. L., J. Miller, and K. White. 2006. Community transformation through culturally competent nursing leadership: Application of theory of culture care diversity and universality and tri-dimensional leader effectiveness model. *Journal of Transcultural Nursing* 17(2):113–118.

Sherman, R. O. 2019. A new generation of nurse leaders. *Nurse Leader* 17(4):276–277.

Siegel, B., J. Erickson, B. Milstein, and K. E. Pritchard. 2018. Multisector partnerships need further development to fulfill aspirations for transforming regional health and well-being. *Health Affairs* 37(1):30–37.

Stacciarini, J. R., and A. M. McDaniel. 2019. Embrace: Developing an inclusive leadership program with and for undergraduate nursing students. *Journal of Professional Nursing* 35(1):26–31.

Swider, S. M., P. F. Levin, and V. Reising. 2017. Evidence of public health nursing effectiveness: A realist review. *Public Health Nursing* 34(4):324–334.

Thomas, T. W., P. C. Seifert, and J. C. Joyner. 2016. Registered nurses leading innovative changes. *Online Journal of Issues in Nursing* 21(3):3.

UND (University of North Dakota). 2020. *Recruitment & retention of American Indians into nursing*. https://cnpd.und.edu/rain (accessed April 8, 2021).

Villarruel, A. M., and M. E. Broome. 2020. Beyond the naming: Institutional racism in nursing. *Nursing Outlook* 68(4):375–376.

Vitale, T. R. 2018. Nurse leader mentorship. *Nursing Management* 49(2):8–10.

Waite, R., and D. Nardi. 2019. Nursing colonialism in America: Implications for nursing leadership. *Journal of Professional Nursing* 35(1):18–25. doi: 10.1016/j.profnurs.2017.12.013. PMID: 30709460.

Wakefield, M. 2018. The next era of regulation: Partnerships for change. *Journal of Nursing Regulation* 9(1):4–10.

Wesson, D. E., C. R. Lucey, and L. A. Cooper. 2019. Building trust in health systems to eliminate health disparities. *Journal of the American Medical Association* 322(2):111–112.

Whitfield-Harris, L., J. S. Lockhart, R. Zoucha, and R. Alexander. 2017. The lived experience of black nurse faculty in predominantly white schools of nursing. *Journal of Transcultural Nursing* 28(6):608–615.

Williams, E., and M. Dawson. 2021, March. Cultivating diversity in nursing leadership: Role of the sponsors. *Voice of Nursing Leadership*. American Hospital Association. https://www.aonl.org/news/voice-of-nursing-leadership (accessed June 7, 2021).

10

Supporting the Health and Professional Well-Being of Nurses

I believe that everything affecting our society affects nurses and that eventually will hemorrhage over to the nursing profession.

—Denetra Hampton, RN, documentary filmmaker of *Racism: The African American Nursing Experience Short Film*

Nurses' health and well-being are affected by the demands of their workplace, and in turn, their well-being affects their work and the people they care for. As it has in so many other areas, COVID-19 has imposed new challenges for the well-being of nurses. But it also has offered opportunities to give nurses' well-being the attention it deserves and to address the systems, structures, and policies that create workplace hazards and stresses that lead to burnout, fatigue, and poor physical and mental health. This issue will take on even greater urgency over the coming years as nurses are asked to assume a more prominent role in advancing health equity. For nurses to address the many social determinants that influence health—from housing, to violence, to poor air quality—they must first feel healthy, well, and supported themselves. Policy makers, employers of nurses, nursing schools, nurse leaders, professional associations, and nurses themselves all have a role in ensuring the well-being of the nursing workforce.

Nurses are committed to meeting the diverse and often complex needs of people with competence and compassion. While nursing is viewed as a "calling" by many nurses, it is a demanding profession. During the course of their work, nurses encounter physical, mental, emotional, and ethical challenges. Depending on the role and setting of the nurse's work, these may include incurring the risk of infection and physical or verbal assault, meeting physical demands, managing and supporting the needs of multiple patients with complex needs, having emotional conversations with patients and families, and confronting challenging social and ethical issues. Nurses, particularly those who work in communities and public health settings, may also face the stress of encountering health inequities laid bare, such as hazardous housing and food insecurity. Nurses' health and well-being are affected by these stresses and demands of their work, and in turn, their well-being affects their work, including increasing the risk of medical errors and compromising patient safety and care (Melnyk et al., 2018). As shown in the framework introduced in Chapter 1 (see Figure 1-1), well-being is one of five key areas with the potential to enhance nurses' ability to address social determinants of health (SDOH) and advance health and health care equity.

With the emergence of COVID-19, the day-to-day demands of nursing have been illuminated and exacerbated. Nurses are coping with unrealistic workloads; insufficient resources and protective equipment; risk of infection; stigma directed at health care workers; and the mental, emotional, and moral burdens of caring for patients with a new and unpredictable disease (Shechter et al., 2020; Squires et al., 2020). Nurses are accustomed to setting aside their own needs and fears to care for people and take on the burdens and stresses of families and communities (Epstein and Delgado, 2010). However, if nurses are not supported in maintaining their physical, emotional, and mental well-being and integrity, their ability to serve and support patients, families, and communities will be compromised (e.g., McClelland et al., 2018).

In this chapter, the committee briefly describes the impact of nurse well-being, then presents a framework for well-being in the context of the health care professions. The chapter examines aspects of nurses' physical, mental, social, and moral[1] well-being and health, and concludes with a review of approaches for addressing nurses' health and well-being in various areas.

THE FAR-REACHING IMPACT OF NURSE WELL-BEING

Nurse well-being—or the lack thereof—has impacts on nurses, patients, health care organizations, and society (NASEM, 2019a). Well-being affects individual nurses in terms of physical and mental health, joy and meaning in their work, professional satisfaction, and engagement with their job. Nurses' well-being affects patients and their perceptions of the quality of care they receive

[1] Moral well-being is defined by Thompson (2018) as "the highest attainable development of innate capacities that enable humans to flourish as embodied, individuated but necessarily interdependent social organisms by managing the adaptive challenges of vulnerability, constraint, connection, and cooperation in an uncertain, risky environment."

(e.g., McClelland et al., 2018; Melnyk et al., 2018; Ross et al., 2017; Salyers et al., 2017), and it also affects the health care system, impacting turnover rates and the costs of hiring and training new nurses (Jones and Gates, 2007; Lewin Group, 2009; Li and Jones, 2013). With more than 1 million nurses projected to retire between 2020 and 2030 (Buerhaus et al., 2017), retaining established nurses and supporting new nurses is vital to the growth and sustainability of the workforce. The costs associated with nurse turnover are high. According to the most recent annual *National Health Care Retention and RN Staffing Report*, the average cost of turnover for a hospital-based registered nurse (RN) is $44,400. Consequently, nurse turnover costs the average hospital $3.6–$6.1 million per year (NSI Nursing Solutions, 2020). Ensuring nurse well-being is not just good for nurses, then; it is essential for the health and safety of patients, the functioning of health systems, and the financial health of health care organizations.

A FRAMEWORK FOR WELL-BEING

Well-being is an inherently complex concept, encompassing an individual's appraisal of physical, social, and psychological resources needed to meet a psychological, physical, or social challenge (Dodge at al., 2012). The 2019 National Academies report *Taking Action Against Clinician Burnout* (NASEM, 2019a) adopts an existing definition of well-being:

> an integrative concept that characterizes quality of life with respect to an individual's health and work-related environmental, organizational, and psychosocial factors. Well-being is the experience of positive perceptions and the presence of constructive conditions at work and beyond that enables workers to thrive and achieve their full potential. (Chari et al., 2018, p. 590)

Professional well-being is associated with individuals' job satisfaction, including being able to find meaning and fulfillment in work, feeling engaged, and having a high-quality work experience (Danna and Griffin, 1999; Doble and Santha, 2008; NASEM, 2019a). Well-being is often classified into *objective* well-being, or the satisfaction of physical needs, such as food, clothing, and shelter, and *subjective* well-being, or the emotional and psychological support needed to flourish (NASEM, 2019b; Prilleltensky, 2012). For the purposes of this report, the committee has chosen to examine well-being using a broad lens, encompassing many aspects of a nurse's physical, mental, social, and moral well-being.

Taking Action Against Clinician Burnout (NASEM, 2019a) uses a visual framework to describe clinician burnout and professional well-being (see Figure 10-1). While focused primarily on addressing burnout, this framework demonstrates how the physical, social, and legal environments at different

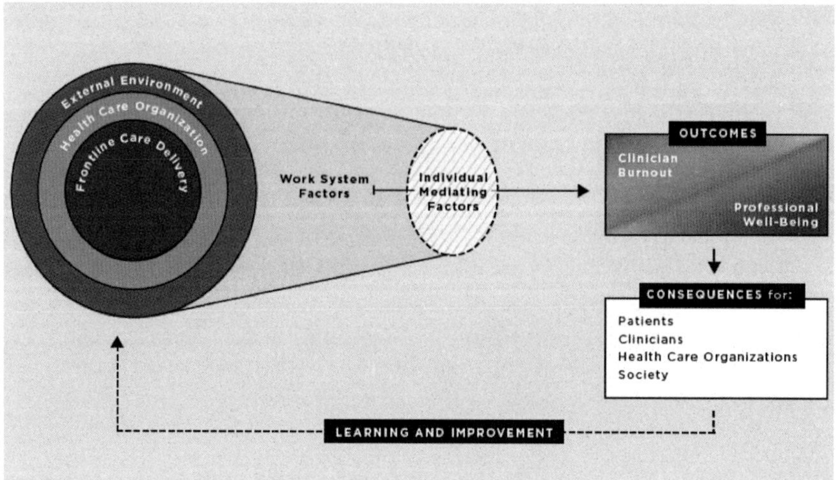

FIGURE 10-1 Systems model of burnout and well-being.
SOURCE: NASEM, 2019a.

levels work together to impact clinician well-being. The first level, "external environment," represents the health care industry, laws, regulations, standards, and societal values. The second level, "health care organization," encompasses the leadership and management, governance, and policies and structures of the organization. The third level, "frontline care delivery," represents the actions of and interactions among team members, local organizational conditions, technologies in the workplace, the physical environment, and work activities. Together, these three levels shape and constrain the day-to-day work environment of clinicians, called "work system factors." These work system factors include both job demands, such as workload and administrative burden, and job resources, such as organizational culture, teamwork, and professional relationships. These factors are mediated by individual factors, such as personality, coping strategies, resilience, and social support, and ultimately impact the health and well-being of clinicians.

While this framework was designed with the clinical environment in mind, it can be applied to nurses working in other environments, including communities, schools, and non–health care organizations. The specific work factors will vary from setting to setting—for example, some nurses will contend with electronic health records (see Box 10-1), while others will not—but the general schema holds true for most nurses in most settings.

BOX 10-1
Technological Factors Impacting Nurses' Well-Being

There is increasing evidence that the growing use of electronic health records (EHRs) and other technologies in the workplace is burdening health care workers and adding to their stressful and demanding work environment. Research has indicated that nurses spend a great deal of time charting in and reviewing EHRs, and that this can deplete their time, negatively impact their morale (Berwick et al., 2017), and take time away from their ethical and professional commitments to spend more time with patients and families (ANA, 2015). Many reports have considered the burden imposed by clinical documentation and other clerical tasks (Arndt et al., 2017; Baumann et al., 2018; Shanafelt et al., 2016; Sinsky et al., 2016; Tai-Seale et al., 2017). Accordingly, there have been many demands for a significant redesign of clinical documentation (Haas et al., 2019; Ommaya et al., 2018; Sinsky and Linzer, 2020).

Another technological source of workplace stress is clinical alarms, which notify nurses that a patient is in distress. One study conducted over a period of 12 days found an average of 350 clinical alarms per patient per day in an intensive care unit (Yue et al., 2016). In a review of the research, Yue and colleagues (2016) found that alarm-related adverse events, including patient deaths due to failures to monitor alarm devices, are common in clinical practice. Factors associated with alarm-related adverse events include alarm fatigue, missed alarms, and inappropriate parameter settings.

THE STATE OF NURSES' HEALTH AND WELL-BEING

This section provides a brief overview of nurses' health and well-being in the following areas: physical, occupational, mental and behavioral, moral, and social. It should be noted that both within and across these categories, some issues are interrelated and may exacerbate or reinforce others. For example, it has been demonstrated that chronic stress can create biological conditions that lead to obesity (Yau and Potenza, 2013). In addition, obesity has been associated with high-demand, low-control work environments and with working long hours (Schulte et al., 2007). These conditions—stress, high-demand and low-control work environments, and long hours—are common in nursing work environments, which may place nurses at risk of obesity. Obesity, in turn, has been associated with higher risk of occupational injury (Jordan et al., 2015; Nowrouzi et al., 2016; Schulte et al., 2007), for which nurses are already at high risk. It should be noted as well that most of the evidence cited in this chapter relates to nurses in clinical settings. While there is some limited research on other settings, including home visiting (Mathiews and Salmond, 2013), rural communities (Terry et al.,

2015), prisons (Walsh and Freshwater, 2009), and schools (Jameson and Bowen, 2018), the vast majority of research on nurses' well-being focuses on their work in clinical care, pointing to a need for more research on nurse well-being in all settings, including public and community health.

Physical Health

The physical health of American nurses is often worse than that of the general population, especially with regard to nutrition, sleep, and physical activity (Gould et al., 2019). Box 10-2 shows a snapshot of the physical health of nurses.

Occupational Safety and Health

There is a high prevalence of occupational injuries to health care workers, especially among nurses (OSHA, n.d.). Nurses may be exposed to a number of hazards in the workplace, including infectious agents; needle sticks; slips and falls; and injuries due to standing, bending, and lifting patients (Dressner and Kissinger, 2018). While nursing involves inherent risks due to proximity to infectious agents and other hazards and the physical demands of the work, these risks may be exacerbated by workplaces that are understaffed and underresourced. Nurse staffing levels have been associated with occupational injuries (Hughes, 2008), including musculoskeletal injuries and disorders. In addition, as described in Chapter 8, the COVID-19 pandemic has revealed the extent to which nurses' jobs put them at risk of physical harm due to lack of adequate personal protective equipment (PPE) and severe staffing shortages. Nurses of color may be particularly at risk of COVID-19-related harms. As of September 2020, nurses of color made up half of the estimated 213 total RN deaths from COVID-19; nurses of Filipino descent accounted for 31.5 percent of those total deaths (Akhtar, 2020). The Centers for Disease Control and Prevention (CDC) reviewed data from March to May 2020 in 13 states (n = 438) and found that greater than 50 percent of the health care workers hospitalized because of COVID-19 were Black; 36.3 percent of the hospitalized health care workers were working in nurse functions that included nurse and certified nursing assistant (CNA) (Kambhampati et al., 2020).

Patient safety is a frequent topic in discussion of improving care and is also a measure of nurses' quality of care (AHRQ, 2019; Vaismoradi et al., 2020). Patient safety, staff safety, and equity have become a highlighted area of need, declining as health care workers face the challenge of the short- and long-term effects of structural racism, inequities, and bias. These challenges include caring for patients who are often the most underrepresented in the community, who lack adequate access to health care, and who tend to work in low-wage jobs and to have increased exposure to illness among the general public. Chin (2020) discusses the necessity of aligning health care organizations' approaches and intentionality toward patient safety and equity. One of the ways health care organizations and leadership can be more intentional is by stratifying data with patient and clinician

BOX 10-2
A Snapshot of the Physical Health of American Nurses

Obesity/Overweight[a,b]

- The average body mass index for nurses is 27.94, which falls into the overweight category.
- Roughly half (52 percent) of nurses say that they have adequate access to healthy food choices while at work.
- Only 11 percent of nurses report a daily intake of at least two servings of fruits and two and a half servings of vegetables.
- Fewer than half (47 percent) of nurses report not engaging in regular muscle-strengthening exercise, 46 percent in vigorous cardio exercise, and 20 percent in light or moderate exercise.
- Just over one-third (37 percent) of nurses say they have adequate access to employer-based exercise facilities and programs.
- Only 44 percent of nurses rate their health as good, 25 percent as very good, and 5 percent as excellent.

Sleep[a]

- Just 60 percent of nurses report getting 7 or more hours of sleep. The National Sleep Foundation recommends 7 to 9 hours of sleep for individuals aged 18–64.

Consequences of Shift Work and Long Hours[c,d]

- Long-term insomnia is reported by 32 percent of night workers and 26 percent of rotating shift workers.
- Compared with the morning/day shift, there is an 18 percent increase in injury risk during the afternoon/evening shift and a 34 percent increase during the night shift.
- There is a 40 percent increase in the risk for cardiovascular disease among shift workers.
- The majority (79 percent) of newly licensed nurses work 12-hour shifts, a near majority work the night shift (44 percent), and more than half (61 percent) work overtime (mandatory or voluntary) weekly.
- Nurses working weekly overtime are associated with a 32 percent increase in the risk of a needle stick, while those working night shift are associated with a 16 percent increase in the risk of a sprain or strain injury.

Smoking[e,f]

- Around 7 percent of registered nurses (RNs) smoke tobacco, while almost 25 percent of licensed practical nurses do so.
- From 2003 to 2010–2011, the prevalence of smoking among RNs declined by 36 percent.
- Smoke-free policies among 689 schools of nursing increased from 36 percent in 2015 to 91 percent in 2017.

---

[a] ANA Enterprise, 2020.
[b] Carpenter et al., 2020.
[c] Trinkoff et al., 2008.
[d] Stimpfel et al., 2015.
[e] Sarna et al., 2014.
[f] Sarna et al., 2019.

input, and nurses are a critical component of this process. As mentioned in Chapter 8, leaders and organizations will have to support an actual culture of equity throughout, and will require intentional change.

Mental and Behavioral Health

Mental health is defined as "a state of well-being in which every individual realizes his or her own potential, can cope with the normal stresses of life, can work productively and fruitfully, and is able to make a contribution to his or her community" (WHO, 2004). Mental health issues, including stress, burnout, and depression, are common among nurses (Adriaenssens et al., 2015; Da Silva et al., 2016; Gómez-Urquiza et al., 2016, 2017; Mark and Smith, 2012; McVicar, 2003). Whereas the exact prevalence of posttraumatic stress disorder (PTSD)[2] among nurses is unclear (see Schuster and Dwyer, 2020), intensive care unit nurses are particularly exposed to repeated trauma and stress and often experience PTSD, anxiety, depression, and burnout (Mealer et al., 2017).

These mental health issues have effects on multiple levels. They adversely impact individual nurses' quality of life and enjoyment of work (Tarcan et al., 2017); they increase absenteeism and staff turnover (Burlison et al., 2016; Davey et al., 2009; Lavoie-Tremblay et al., 2008; Oyama et al., 2015); and they impact nurses' ability to provide quality and safe care, resulting in such consequences as general and medication administration errors, poor relationships with patients and coworkers, and lower patient satisfaction (Gärtner et al., 2010). In addition, nurses with mental health concerns may be stigmatized and discriminated against by RN licensing boards. A recent study by Halter and colleagues (2019) found that of 30 boards that asked questions about mental illness, 22 asked questions not compliant with the Americans with Disabilities Act (ADA).

Studies have found that caring for patients on the front lines of the COVID-19 pandemic can increase stress, depression, anxiety, and PTSD for nurses (Kang et al., 2020; Lai et al., 2020). Early research results suggest that the pandemic has placed nurses at high risk of mental health sequelae, particularly anxiety, depression, and peritraumatic dissociation (Azoulay et al., 2020). Box 10-3 describes how addressing the COVID-19 crisis has impacted nurses' health and well-being.

Burnout

Burnout is an increasingly prevalent problem among clinicians, including nurses, and it has significant consequences for patients, organizations, teams,

[2] The American Psychiatric Association defines PTSD as "a psychiatric disorder that may occur in people who have experienced or witnessed a traumatic event such as a natural disaster, a serious accident, a terrorist act, war/combat, or rape or who have been threatened with death, sexual violence or serious injury" (see https://www.psychiatry.org/patients-families/ptsd/what-is-ptsd [accessed April 13, 2021]).

BOX 10-3
COVID-19 and Nurses' Health and Well-Being

Nurses can struggle with determining how to uphold their professional ethical values in the context of competing obligations to patients, their own families, and their health. Many clinicians already faced anxiety, burnout, depression, stress, and risk of suicide prior to the pandemic, but the COVID-19 crisis has presented an even greater hardship that can exacerbate existing levels of burnout and mental health stressors (Squires et al., 2020; Ulrich et al., 2020). Sources of stress identified in a recent qualitative study of nurses caring for COVID-19 patients between May and July 2020 included personal experiences of social isolation, witnessing large numbers of deaths, increased patient acuity, caring for families, the uncertainty of how to care for patients, and severe staffing shortages and organizational issues (Squires et al., 2020). Nurses may experience varying degrees of moral suffering that result in moral residue and fatigue as they respond to complex and often unsolvable ethical trade-offs in caring for patients with COVID-19 (Rosa et al., 2020). Adding to these stressors, nurses are acting as de facto social intermediaries for patients who are isolated from their families. For example, nurses are using technology to help patients stay connected with their families when visitors are not permitted (Shapiro, 2020). COVID-19 is also highlighting the challenges that nurses and nurse leaders have in reporting staff safety issues and equity issues (Rangchari and Woods, 2020).

The disproportionate impact of COVID-19 on people of color (see Chapter 2) has highlighted the need for nurses to focus on caring for the underserved and addressing social and structural barriers to health. Nurses at the front lines see firsthand the consequences of social and economic injustice when the people most negatively affected by the disease are people of color, immigrants, and other vulnerable groups who are providing essential services often without needed protections, who lack basic access to health services, and who live in overcrowded communities. Absent interventions, as COVID-19 rates ebb and peak around the United States, the impact on nurses is likely to be long-lasting (Nelson and Lee-Winn, 2020).

and nurses themselves. Burnout syndrome is characterized by three components: emotional exhaustion, depersonalization (e.g., cynicism, apathy), and a low sense of personal accomplishment at work (Maslach and Jackson, 1981). Estimated rates of burnout among U.S. nurses have ranged between 35 and 45 percent (Aiken et al., 2002; Moss et al., 2016), although many studies focus only on the emotional exhaustion component of burnout, painting an incomplete picture (NASEM, 2019a). The consequences of burnout can include poor patient outcomes, high turnover rates, increased costs, and clinician illness and suicide (NASEM, 2019a). Factors including high workloads, staff shortages, extended shifts (Stimpfel et al., 2012), and the burden of documentation (see Box 10-1) can all contribute to nurse burnout. Another known contributor to burnout is a mismatch between the skills and preparation of workers and the jobs that they are expected to perform (Maslach, 2017).

Nurses in all roles and settings can experience burnout. Nursing students may experience academic and emotional burnout before they even enter the workforce (Ríos-Risquez et al., 2018). A shift toward preventive care and care management based in primary care or patient-centered medical homes means there is a growing demand on nurses to take on more complex patients and associated tasks, increasing burnout among nurses in primary care (Duhoux et al., 2017). Nurses in other settings that entail prolonged contact with patients such as critical care, oncology, and psychiatric nursing experience burnout as well (Cañadas-De la Fuente et al., 2017; Jackson et al., 2018). While data are lacking on burnout among nurse practitioners, some evidence shows they can experience burnout comparable to that experienced by nurses and physicians (Hoff et al., 2019). Nurses who work in long-term care settings face particular occupational stressors, such as physical or verbal abuse from residents with dementia, frequent physical transfers of residents, exposure to death and declining health among residents, and caring for individuals with very different care needs (Woodward et al., 2016).

Compassion Fatigue

Compassion fatigue, considered distinct from burnout, is defined as "a health care practitioner's diminished capacity to care as a consequence of repeated exposure to the suffering of patients, and from the knowledge of their patients' traumatic experiences" (Cavanagh et al., 2020, p. 640). Compassion fatigue occurs when a nurse's ability to empathize with people is reduced as a result of repeated exposure to others' suffering (Peters, 2018). Research suggests a number of factors that can lead to compassion fatigue, some of which are organizational and some of which are individual. Organizational factors include chronic and intense patient contact, prolonged stress, a lack of support, high workload, hours per shift, and time constraints that hinder quality care (Peters, 2018). Individual factors include a personal history of trauma, a lack of awareness about compassion fatigue, an inability to maintain professional boundaries (e.g., taking on extra shifts), and a lack of self-care (Peters, 2018).

Suicide

Nurses, like physicians, are at higher risk than the general population for suicide (Davidson et al., 2020a; NASEM, 2019a). Longitudinal data from 2005 through 2016 showed that nurses committed suicide at a higher rate relative to the general population. Both female and male nurses were at greater risk of suicide (female incident rate ratio [IRR] = 1.395, 95% confidence interval [CI] 1.323–1.470, $p < .001$; male IRR = 1.205, 95% CI 1.083, 1.338, $p < .001$) (Davidson et al., 2020a). Despite this increased risk, relatively little attention has been paid to understanding and preventing nurse suicide (Davidson et al., 2018a).

Behavioral Health

Estimates indicate that nurses have the same rate of substance use disorders (SUDs) as the general population (Strobbe and Crowley, 2017; Worley, 2017), with approximately 10 percent of the nursing population having an SUD (Worley, 2017). In addition to the general risk factors that are associated with SUD, including genetic predisposition, history of trauma or abuse, early age at first use of a substance, and comorbid mental health disorders, nurses may also have unique risk factors that include access to controlled substances, workplace stress, and lack of education about SUDs (Worley, 2017). Nursing students are also at risk of SUDs (ANA, 2015; Strobbe and Crowley, 2017).

Moral Well-Being

Nurses in all roles and settings are confronted with ethical challenges that have the potential to cause moral suffering (ANA, 2015), including moral distress or moral injury (Rushton, 2018). When nurses are unable to convert their moral choices into action because of internal or external constraints, moral distress ensues and threatens their integrity (Ulrich and Grady, 2018). Moral distress also arises to varying degrees in response to moral uncertainty, moral conflicts or dilemmas involving competing ethical values or commitments, or tensions resulting from not being able to share moral concerns with others (Morley et al., 2019). Moral distress, the most well-researched form of moral suffering, occurs in response to moral adversity that threatens or violates an individual's professional values and integrity, and is associated with myriad negative consequences (Burston and Tuckett, 2013; Epstein and Delgado, 2010; Morley et al., 2019; Rushton et al., 2016). Nurses can experience moral distress when they feel inadequately supported, when health care resources are inappropriately used, and when there is disagreement between the patient's care plan and the patient's family's wishes (Burston and Tuckett, 2013; Epstein et al., 2019). For example, nurses may experience moral distress when asked to provide life support care that is not in the best interest of the patient (Kasman, 2004). Moral injury, a more extreme form of moral suffering, occurs when there is "a betrayal of what's right, by someone who holds legitimate authority … in a high stakes situation" (Shay, 2014, p. 182). It involves a violation of one's moral code by witnessing, participating in, or precipitating a variety of moral harms. While the roots of the concept began in the military, nurses and other clinicians increasingly are exploring its application in health care.

Nurses can suffer from moral distress when they lack the resources or capacity to help their patients (Kelly and Porr, 2018) or are unable to take the ethically appropriate action because of constraints or moral adversities (Ulrich et al., 2020). Nurses working in communities or with people with complex health needs and social risks, such as SUDs and psychological and behavioral disorders, and those working in high-intensity settings or palliative care can experience moral distress due to the complex moral and ethical issues they confront (Englander et al., 2018; SAMHSA, 2000; Welker-Hood, 2014; Wolf et al., 2019). Nurses who work in clinical care often lose contact with patients when they leave the clinical setting (Wolf et al., 2016), which makes it difficult to help these patients with their nonclinical needs, such as food, safe housing, and a support network. This can leave nurses feeling that their efforts are futile without societal commitment to systemic reforms.

Addressing issues of health equity can involve confronting sexism, racism, ableism, xenophobia, and trauma, which can be uncomfortable and challenging for all involved (Munnangi et al., 2018). In addition, the historical roots of trauma are often "invisible" (Comas-Díaz et al., 2019; Helms et al., 2012), with individuals of color suffering from race-based stress (Comas-Díaz et al., 2019). Moreover, nurses may not feel empowered to raise their concerns about these inequities because of fear of retaliation or compromised relationships (Ulrich et al., 2019). When the claims or voices of nurses and other clinicians are discounted, their stress is heightened (Hurst, 2008).

In the context of COVID-19 (see Box 10-3), evidence is emerging that nurses have experienced moral distress as they have addressed the stark ethical tensions (Morley et al., 2019; Ulrich et al., 2020) created by the pandemic, facing a gap between "what they can do and what they believe they should do" (Pearce, 2020; Rosa et al., 2020). This situation led the American Nurses Association (ANA) to develop guidance to help nurses understand their ethical obligations during a pandemic, particularly with respect to preserving their integrity and well-being (ANA, 2020a,b). Upholding the ethical mandate of nurses to provide respectful, equitable care for all persons and the responsibility to address issues of social justice can be especially challenging during a pandemic (ANA, 2015; ANA and AAN, 2020). Moral injury has become a focus of inquiry both prior to and during the pandemic (Dean et al., 2020; Kopacz et al., 2019; Maguen and Price, 2020; Rushton et al., 2021), and early data suggest that it is emerging as a factor associated with the difficult ethical trade-offs experienced by clinicians in the context of the pandemic (Hines et al., 2020; Williams et al., 2020) and in response to the deaths of Black individuals at the hands of police (Barbot, 2020). The practice setting and ethical climate of the health care organization are postulated as factors that influence the prevalence of moral distress (Rathert et al., 2016; Sauerland et al., 2014). More research is needed to understand the relevance of moral injury among health care professionals and to study its relationship to various measures of well-being and moral resilience (Rushton, 2018).

Social Health and Well-Being

The nature of nursing work means that nurses are constantly interacting with other people, including individuals, families, communities, physicians and other providers, administrators, staff, and other nurses. While these social interactions are essential to the work of caring for individuals and communities, they can also be a source of stress and adversely impact nurse well-being. This section explores three types of negative social interactions: bullying and incivility, workplace violence, and racism and discrimination.

Bullying and Incivility

Bullying and incivility among nurses is a major problem in nursing practice and can result in mental health issues, burnout, and nurses leaving positions or the profession entirely (Spence Laschinger et al., 2012; Weaver, 2013). There is an expected culture within nursing in which young or new nurses will encounter bullying, gossip and belittling, intimidation, hostility, exclusion, and hazing from other staff nurses, supervisors, and managers (Caristo and Clements, 2019; Echevarria, 2013; Meissner; 1986). A survey of more than 10,000 RNs and nursing students found that half of respondents had experienced bullying in the workplace (ANA, n.d.). While the terms "bullying" and "incivility" are often used interchangeably,[3] bullying is distinguished by its repetitive nature and is perpetrated by a person in a position of power (Rutherford et al., 2018). ANA defines bullying as "repeated, unwanted, harmful actions intended to humiliate, offend, and cause distress in the recipient," and incivility as "one or more rude, discourteous, or disrespectful actions that may or may not have a negative intent behind them" (ANA, n.d.).

Psychological safety, the perception that it is safe to take risks within the team, is one important factor in creating healthy, civil, integrity-preserving workplaces (Edmonson, 1999, 2018; Edmondson and Lei, 2014). Low levels of psychological safety in the culture of some health care organizations can undermine nurses' ability to contribute fully and to thrive in the workplace (Edmonson, 2002; Moore and McAuliffe, 2010, 2012; Newman et al., 2017; Ünal and Seren, 2016). Nurses—particularly those who work in clinical settings—work in teams where hierarchy, power imbalances, and interpersonal aggression can occur (Nembhard and Edmonson, 2006). Maslach and Leitner (2017) suggest that improving civility among the interprofessional team may be a leverage point for reducing burnout. However, there is limited research on the relationship between workplace hierarchies and bullying behaviors among nurses and between nurses and other health care providers (Wech et al., 2020).

---

[3] The term "lateral violence" is also used interchangeably with "bullying" and "incivility" (Pfeifer and Vessey, 2017).

Workplace Violence

In the United States, health care workers experience the highest level of assault of all occupations, and among health care workers, nurses and patient care assistants experience the highest rates of violence (Groenewold et al., 2018; OSHA, 2015). Aggression and assault can result in long-term effects on nurses that include posttraumatic stress and lower levels of productivity (Gates et al., 2011). Nurses endure both emotional and physical abuse from patients (Gabrovec, 2017; Gates et al., 2011). An ANA health risk assessment of nurses during 2013–2016 indicated that 25 percent of nurses had experienced violence at the hands of patients or their family members (ANA, 2017). However, incidents of assault are substantially underreported by as much as 50 percent because of a lack of workplace reporting policies, a lack of confidence in the reporting system, and fear of retaliation (OSHA, 2015).

A 2018 survey of more than 8,000 critical care nurses found that 80 percent of respondents had experienced verbal abuse at least once during the past year, nearly half physical abuse and discrimination, and 40 percent reported sexual harassment (Ulrich et al., 2019). Patients and family members were reported as the most frequent source of abuse (73 percent and 64 percent, respectively), followed by physicians (41 percent) and other nurses (34 percent). Fewer than half of nurses reported that their organization had zero tolerance policies for verbal abuse, while 62 percent reported such policies for physical abuse. These data paint a picture of work environments that are hostile to the psychological safety and well-being of nurses (Ulrich et al., 2019).

While much of the research on workplace violence focuses on hospital settings, nurses working in other settings are also at risk of violence and aggression. Home visiting nurses, who often work alone in dynamic environments characterized by potentially high-risk situations, are at risk of verbal and physical assault while in the community or people's homes (Mathiews and Salmond, 2013). The incidence of workplace violence in home nursing is likely underreported because of factors including the perception that violence is part of the job and the moral conflict nurses face between duty to their patients and duty to report an incident of violence (Mathiews and Salmond, 2013). While many organizations are attempting to respond to these challenges, education and training alone are likely insufficient to address the root factors that contribute to them (Geoffrion et al., 2020).

Racism and Discrimination

As discussed in Chapter 2, racism can significantly impact the physical and mental health of individuals. Health can be affected by structural racism (policies and systems), cultural racism (stereotypes, beliefs, and implicit biases), and discrimination (being treated differently based on race) (Williams et al., 2019). Microaggressions, which are brief and commonplace daily indignities, are also correlated with poor health (Cruz et al., 2019; Nadal et al., 2016; Ong and Burrow, 2017; Sue et al., 2007). Nurses may encounter racism, discrimination, and microaggressions from a number of sources, including employers, educators, managers, colleagues, and patients. Nurses and other clinicians of color can experience hardship, burnout, and the increased emotional labor and burden of an already emotionally demanding job while dealing with the personal negative consequences of racism from patients (Cottingham et al., 2018; Paul-Emile et al., 2016). Accommodating patients' preferences regarding the race, gender, or religion of their providers has been common practice in the United States, often in a context of little guidance on how to approach these situations (Paul-Emile, 2012). This practice can have adverse effects on clinicians, especially when they are rejected by patients or subject to abuse because of their race. However, nurses' experiences of racism are not limited to these types of discrete events but are part of the larger system of structural racism in the United States (Waite and Nardi, 2019).

Black nurses in particular have long reported encountering racism in the workplace (Bennett et al., 2019; Wojciechowski, 2020). Internationally educated nurses (IENs)—those who completed a nursing education program in a country outside that of their employer and who have migrated to the United States (see also Chapter 3)—also contend with racism and discrimination (Ghazal et al., 2020). As described in Chapter 8, in the wake of COVID-19, which was first discovered in China, Asian nurses have reported verbal and physical attacks, and some patients have refused their care (AHA, 2020a). Discrimination against Asian American and Pacific Islander (AAPI) nurses is not a new phenomenon, having existed since at least the mid-19th century. However, Stop AAPI Hate, a national coalition focused on tracking and addressing anti-Asian discrimination during the COVID-19 pandemic, reported 3,795 hate incidents between March 2020 and February 2021.[4] These experiences may lead to increased anxiety, fear for personal safety, and poor physical health (AHA, 2020a).

Lesbian, gay, bisexual, transgender, and queer/questioning (LGBTQ) nurses have also reported discrimination and harassment based on sexual orientation or gender identity and expression (Eliason et al., 2011, 2017). In a recent qualitative study of 277 LGBTQ+[5] health care professionals, Eliason and colleagues (2017) found that these health care workers faced both work-related stress and hostility from coworkers and patients. Reported consequences included lack of promotions, tenure denials, and negative comments and gossip (Eliason et al., 2017). Avery-Desmarais and colleagues (2020) examined problematic substance use (PSU) and its relationship with stress among a convenience sample of 394

[4] See https://secureservercdn.net/104.238.69.231/a1w.90d.myftpupload.com/wp-content/uploads/2021/03/210312-Stop-AAPI-Hate-National-Report-.pdf?fbclid=IwAR3jLV0DTBnIy_NK3322T4fWDjZhJaY9A6w05elGLG83bJZ47SVckBrPwKQ (accessed April 13, 2021).

[5] Lesbian, gay, bisexual, transgender, queer, and other sexual/gender minorities.

lesbian, gay, and bisexual nurses. They found that the incidence of PSU was higher among this group than among either the general population of nurses or the general lesbian, gay, and bisexual population.

Nurses with disabilities[6] can experience discrimination in the workplace (Neal-Boylan et al., 2015), in nursing school (Neal-Boylan and Smith, 2016), and by nursing boards, as mentioned previously (Halter et al., 2019), and encounter negative stereotypes about their ability to do their job or provide effective care (Neal-Boylan et al., 2012). Nursing students with learning disabilities can encounter difficulties in nursing programs (Northway et al., 2015), including negative perceptions that conflate the need for accommodations for disabilities with a student's capability as a nurse and professional (Marks and McCulloh, 2016). Nurses in the workforce may be reluctant to disclose a disability or mental illness (Hernandez et al., 2016; Peterson, 2017; Rauch, 2019) or to request a need for accommodations, which could increase the risk of injury to the health care team and potentially patients (Davidson et al., 2016). There has been a call for both health care organizations and nursing schools to see beyond disability as a disqualifier for nursing practice, and instead value professionals with disabilities who can offer unique and different perspectives (Marks and Ailey, 2014; Marks and McCulloh, 2016). New research on disabilities in the general population can increase awareness and depth of understanding, and more research on the health and experience of nurses themselves will build effective strategies for nurses with disabilities to achieve success (Davidson et al., 2016).

APPROACHES TO IMPROVING WELL-BEING

As shown in Figure 10-1, nurse well-being is impacted by the external environment, organizational structure and policies, and the conditions of day-to-day work. These three factors are mediated by individual factors, including personality, resilience, and social support. Together, these structural and individual factors can either strengthen or diminish nurse well-being. The responsibility for addressing nurse well-being lies with both nurses themselves and the systems, organizations, and structures that support them. Some barriers to well-being can be addressed only at the organizational and external environmental levels. For example, the burden of technology on nurses must be lifted by federal regulators, insurance companies, technology companies, and the like. However, individual nurses also have an important role to play in promoting their own well-being.

[6] The definition of disabilities is based on the 1990 ADA and the 2008 ADA Amendments Act, in which a disability is defined as a physical or mental impairment or limitation that significantly affects a person in major life activities that include but are not limited to "caring for oneself, performing manual tasks, seeing, hearing, eating, sleeping, walking, standing, lifting, bending, speaking, breathing, learning, reading, concentrating, thinking, communicating, and working" (American Disabilities Act, Title 42, Chapter 126, § 12111; https://www.ada.gov/pubs/adastatute08.htm#12102 [accessed April 13, 2021]).

There is emerging evidence that despite the constraints imposed by the system, some nurses are able to remain healthy and whole and grow in response to adversity (Cui et al., 2021; Itzhaki et al., 2015; Okoli et al., 2021; Traudt et al., 2016). Nurses need the skills and tools that enable them to exercise their autonomy, agency, and competence within these systems. Further investigation is needed to understand the individual and system characteristics that create the conditions for nurses to thrive in the midst of complexity, uncertainty, and unpredictability.

This section first examines individual-level approaches to well-being and then turns to a review of approaches at the systems level. The committee notes that although there exists no menu of ready-to-implement, evidence-based interventions for improving nurse well-being (NASEM, 2019a), a great number of efforts currently being pursued can offer inspiration and opportunities for evaluation, replication, and scalability. However, as noted by Melnyk and colleagues (2020) in a recent systematic review of interventions focused on improving physicians' and nurses' physical and mental well-being, more randomized controlled trials (RCTs) are needed to examine the efficacy of such interventions as many of the available studies have weaknesses in their methodologies.

Individual-Level Interventions

While health care organizations must create the workplace conditions for well-being and integrity to thrive, nurses are also responsible for identifying their own needs and investing in their well-being (Ross et al., 2017). This responsibility arises from their inherent human dignity and their professional ethical mandate to invest in their own integrity and well-being so they can execute the responsibilities of their nursing role (ANA, 2015). Provision 5 of the ANA Code of Ethics states that nurses should "eat a healthy diet, exercise, get sufficient rest, maintain family and personal relationships, engage in adequate leisure and recreational activities, and attend to spiritual or religious needs" (ANA, 2015, p. 35).

Although nurses are often knowledgeable about the importance of these issues, that knowledge does not always translate into action (Ross et al., 2017). Ross and colleagues (2017) identify a number of intrinsic and extrinsic factors that affect nurses' participation in health-promoting behaviors. Intrinsic factors include personal characteristics and beliefs, perceived benefits and barriers, self-efficacy, gender and age, fatigue, depression, and anxiety. Extrinsic factors include norms, social support, role modeling, financial and time constraints, and institutional support. Shift work and work schedules, as well as competing demands outside of work, such as caring for adult or child dependents, are additional barriers to participation (Ross et al., 2017).

Below, the committee examines interventions and initiatives directed at improving individual nurses' health and well-being in a number of areas. Many such initiatives address multiple areas of well-being and use multiple approaches. For example, the Healthy Nurse, Healthy Nation (HNHN) Grand Challenge, an effort of ANA and its partners, seeks to transform the health of 4 million RNs through a focus on physical activity, nutrition, rest, quality of life, and safety (ANA Enterprise, 2018). Organizations that participate in HNHN have developed a number of individual-focused initiatives, such as offering onsite fitness opportunities, walking programs, increased access to healthy food, mindfulness resources, and dedicated rooms for nurses to reset and relax (ANA Enterprise, 2018, 2019; Jarrín et al., 2017). Other well-being initiatives are focused on a specific behavior or health characteristic, but one that may have consequences for multiple areas of well-being. For example, poor sleep patterns are associated with poor physical and mental health, an increased risk of obesity, and an increased risk of accidents both in and outside of the workplace (IOM, 2006).

The initiatives and ideas described below are designed to improve the health of nurses by addressing a wide variety of targets:

- physical activity, diet, and sleep;
- substance use;
- resilience;
- mental health;
- ethical competence;
- incivility, bullying, and workplace violence; and
- racism, prejudice, and discrimination.

Physical Activity, Diet, and Sleep

A recent systematic review of workplace interventions to address obesity in nurses found limited evidence of successful interventions. The authors recommend that interventions be tailored to the unique aspects of nurses' working lives (Kelly and Wills, 2018) and that interventions not be universal but targeted toward those who are obese. In their systematic review, Melnyk and colleagues (2020) found that visual triggers, pedometers, and health coaching can increase participation in physical activity. The Nurses Living Fit program was effective in reducing nurses' body mass index (BMI) over a 12-week intervention period; however, the effects of the program on BMI were not sustained (Speroni et al., 2014).

A recent scoping review of studies looked at interventions targeted at nurses who work shifts and aimed at improving sleep patterns or managing fatigue (Querstret et al., 2020). In these studies, most of which were conducted in Italy, Taiwan, and the United States interventions fell into three primary categories: napping, working different shift patterns, and exposure to light or light attenuation. With regard to napping interventions, the authors found mixed results. For studies that measured performance at work as an outcome, there was improvement on some measures (e.g., information processing improving after a 30-minute nap). Studies that examined shift patterns (e.g., rotating shift patterns, fixed night versus day shifts, 8-hour versus 12-hour rotating shifts) found that shift patterns including night shifts were associated with poorer sleep quality and increased fatigue. Results of light exposure studies were similarly mixed. Four studies found that self-reported energy levels increased with exposure to bright light. Another study, however, found no effect of an intervention involving light visors on fatigue or sleep. The scoping review found no studies conducted on samples involving nurse midwives. Querstret and colleagues (2020) conclude that the literature is inconsistent regarding how to intervene to improve sleep and reduce fatigue for nurses who work shifts, and that the interventions and measures used in these studies were disparate in nature.

Substance Use

A recent position statement from the Emergency Nurses Association and the International Nurses Society on Addictions called for four primary actions to address nurses with SUDs (Strobbe and Crowley, 2017): providing education to nurses and other employees, adopting alternative-to-discipline (ATD) approaches, considering drug diversion in the context of personal use as a symptom and not a criminal offense, and ensuring that nurses and nursing students are aware of the risks associated with SUDs and have a way to report concerns safely. The two primary approaches to treating nurses with SUDs have been either a disciplinary approach or an ATD program (Monroe et al., 2013; NCSBN, 2011; Russell, 2020). Monroe and colleagues (2013) conclude that ATD programs have a greater impact than disciplinary programs on protecting the health and safety of the public, as they identify and enroll more nurses and in turn remove more nurses with SUDs from direct patient care. These programs have been adopted by many state boards of nursing (Russell, 2020). In an analysis of 27 state board of nursing programs, Russell (2020) found a lack of consistency among them and suggests that more research is needed to identify the essential components of such programs. Common components identified in at least half of the programs included an alcohol/drug abstinence requirement, use of mood-altering medications for psychiatric/medical conditions, an Alcoholics Anonymous or Narcotics Anonymous program, and restricted hours or shifts (Russell, 2020).

In a retrospective study of 7,737 nurses participating in SUD programs between 2007 and 2015, Smiley and Reneau (2020) found that bimonthly random drug tests, a minimum of 3 years in a program, and daily check-ins were associated with successful program completion. They also found that structured group meetings were helpful. The best results were for those nurses who stayed in a program at least 5 years and were tested twice per month. The authors recommend that an expert panel review these results and develop formal guidelines for such programs, and that boards of nursing test these guidelines in their ATD programs. In addition, health care organizations and employers have a responsibility to detect early patterns of drug diversion[7] proactively before they become severe. To this end, organizations are using such technologies as automated dispensing cabinets, advanced analytics, and machine learning.[8]

Resilience

Training focused on building individual resilience is often offered to prepare nurses for the fatigue, stress, workload, and burnout they may face (Taylor, 2019). Resilience refers to "the capacity of dynamic systems to withstand or recover from significant disturbances" (Masten, 2007, p. 923). Humans are thought to have an innate resilience potential that evolves over time and fluctuates depending on the context; the interplay of individual factors; social, community, environmental, and societal conditions; and moral/ethical values and commitments (Rushton, 2018; Szanton et al., 2010). Resilience includes "the ability to face adverse situations, remain focused, and continue to be optimistic for the future," and it is described as a "vital characteristic" for nurses in the complex health care system. Resilience is associated with reduced symptoms of burnout, improved mental health, and reduced turnover (Rushton et al., 2015).

Taylor (2019) suggests offering resilience interventions at the primary, secondary, and tertiary levels. At the primary level, such interventions would focus on building self-awareness, coping skills, and communications skills. At the secondary level, they might include screening for burnout and providing the associated resources and supports nurses will need. Finally, at the tertiary level, interventions would target nurses whose resilience threshold had been breached and support their healing and return to work. Understanding and addressing resilience among nurses holds promise for attenuating the effects of workplace demands that exceed personal resources (Yu et al., 2019). A nurse suicide task force led by ANA[9] has been refocused on resilience and is making resources available that can address mental health, particularly during the response to the COVID-19 pandemic (Davidson et al., 2020a).

However, focusing only on individual resilience is insufficient to create workplaces designed to preserve integrity and well-being (Taylor, 2019). Every system, including the human system, has limits beyond which it cannot recover and can become permanently degraded. The challenge is to better understand how to recognize the symptoms of those thresholds and to develop strategies that

---

[7] Drug diversion is "the deflection of prescription drugs from medical sources into the illegal market" (see https://www.cms.gov/Medicare-Medicaid-Coordination/Fraud-Prevention/Medicaid-Integrity-Education/Downloads/infograph-Do-You-Know-About-Drug-Diversion-%5BApril-2016%5D.pdf [accessed April 13, 2021]).

[8] See https://www.fiercehealthcare.com/hospitals/industry-voices-as-covid-19-flare-ups-continue-healthcare-organizations-must-double-down (accessed April 13, 2021).

[9] See https://www.nursingworld.org/get-involved/share-your-expertise/pro-issues-panel/moral-resilience-panel (accessed April 16, 2021).

support human systems, teams, and organizations in adapting healthfully to the adversities they inevitably encounter by modifying those characteristics that are amenable to intervention (Moss et al., 2016). In addition to improving the resilience of individuals, organizations can seek to identify and ameliorate the negative conditions that systematically undermine health and well-being (Gregory et al., 2018). Barratt (2018) suggests that efforts to improve individual resilience focus on building the resilience of teams and organizations to give individuals the support and resources they need. Resilience is discussed further in the section on system-level approaches later in this chapter.

Mental Health

Promising approaches for fostering nurses' mental health and well-being include the development of skills in mindfulness and cognitive-behavioral therapy/skills-building interventions. Mindfulness skills are aimed at building awareness of one's reactions and being able to choose how to respond in the moment. The development of new neuropathways to calm a reactive nervous system is not aimed at tolerating intolerable situations, but at restoring stability so individuals can choose the responses that best reflect their values and commitments. Mindfulness interventions, including mindfulness-based stress reduction and mindfulness-based cognitive therapy, are increasingly being used to treat anxiety and depression (Hofmann and Gomez, 2017), and may be particularly effective in fostering self-compassion (Wasson et al., 2020). Recent reviews of RCTs have found that mindfulness-based interventions are effective in treating a range of clinical symptoms and disorders, including anxiety, depression, psychological and emotional distress, and general "quality of life" concerns (Hofmann and Gomez, 2017).

One evidence-based skills-building intervention based on cognitive-behavioral therapy that integrates mindfulness—MINDBODYSTRONG—(adapted from the COPE cognitive-behavioral skills-building intervention) is delivered by a nurse to new nurse residents. MINDBODYSTRONG comprises eight weekly sessions focused on caring for the mind, caring for the body, and building skills (Sampson et al., 2020). Evidence from an RCT supports MINDBODYSTRONG's efficacy in improving mental health, healthy lifestyle beliefs, healthy lifestyle behaviors, and job satisfaction (Sampson et al., 2019), sustaining its positive impacts over time (Sampson et al., 2020).

In a recent systematic review, Melnyk and colleagues (2020) found that interventions involving mindfulness and those using cognitive-behavioral therapy were effective in addressing stress, anxiety, and depression in clinicians (Melnyk et al., 2020). Deep breathing and gratitude interventions also showed promise. These findings are consistent with those of other reviews (e.g., Lomas et al., 2018). The programs reviewed by Melnyk and colleagues (2020) typically included eight weekly 1- to 2.5-hour sessions plus about 9 hours of mindfulness practice at home; however, the authors conclude that these programs were potentially too time-intensive for clinicians to accommodate within their schedules. They also note that many hospitals do not have mindfulness trainers available to implement these programs.

Given the challenges of implementing time-intensive interventions highlighted by Melnyk and colleagues (2020), there is also promising evidence that brief mindfulness interventions may have positive impacts on compassion, although Hofmann and Gomez (2017) observe that it is unclear whether brief interventions can have the same kind of impact on anxiety and depression as that of the longer interventions. Box 10-4 describes promising interventions that use mobile technologies to support mindfulness and other well-being skills.

Another promising approach to early screening and treatment is the Healer Evaluation Assessment and Referral (HEAR) program, first piloted with nurses in 2016 (Davidson et al., 2018b, 2020b). This program, a collaboration between the University of California, San Diego, and the American Foundation for Suicide Prevention, includes a set of educational presentations focused on burnout, depression, and suicide, as well as an encrypted and confidential web-based assessment tool designed to identify and refer individuals at risk for depression and suicide. The pilot assessment showed it to be an effective screening tool (Davidson et al., 2018b). Three years after the pilot, 527 nurses have been screened, with 9 percent of those screened expressing thoughts of taking their own life; 176 nurses have received treatment, and 98 have accepted referrals for treatment.

Ethical Competence

Organizations are investing in programs aimed at building mindfulness, ethical competence, and resilience through experiential and discovery learning, simulation, and communities of practice (Brown and Ryan, 2003; Grossman et al., 2004; Rushton et al., 2021; Shapiro et al., 2005; Singleton et al., 2014). These programs, coupled with programs aimed at cultivating nurses' competencies to address ethical concerns through systematic processes that engage the voice of the front line and provide nurses with skills for constructively and confidently raising their concerns, are important leverage points for creating workplaces where moral resilience is fostered and ethical practice is routine (Grace et al., 2014; Hamric and Epstein, 2017; Robinson et al., 2014; Rushton et al., 2021; Trotochaud et al., 2018; Wocial et al., 2010). These resources also need to be aligned with system changes that remove the impediments to nurses' well-being and integrity and build moral community (Hamric and Wocial, 2016; Liaschenko and Peter, 2016; Traudt et al., 2016). Adopting systematic methods for building a culture that fosters ethical practice and integrity by investing in structural elements and processes in health care organizations will be essential to amplify interventions aimed at building individual capacities (Nelson et al., 2014; Pavlish

BOX 10-4
Mobile Technology and Mental Health Interventions

Mobile technology and mHealth has become a growing field of innovation, study, and research (Park, 2016), and has the potential to help nurses and other clinicians maintain their well-being. mHealth is a combination of eHealth or telehealth service delivery, health care tracking, mobile computing, medical sensor, and communication technologies (Istepanian et al., 2004). mHealth has many advantages, it allows users to access services in most places, at any time, and bypasses traditional barriers created by infrastructure, such as roads and transportation (WHO, 2011).

There has been a steady increase in the use of smartphones and the emergence of several mental health–focused apps (Donker et al., 2013). Systematic reviews have shown that these apps, including those focused on mindfulness and meditation (Huberty et al., 2019) and on behavior change (Han and Lee, 2018; Lyzwinski et al., 2019), hold promise for reducing symptoms of mental illness and managing symptoms of other chronic illness. However, research in this area is growing, and studies have found that many apps lack clinical evidence or meaningful input from users (Subhi et al., 2015), or have been studied with small sample sizes (Goodwin et al., 2016; Rathbone and Prescott, 2017; Wang et al., 2018; Wood et al., 2017). Other challenges include limited adoption of new app-based health interventions because of age or access to traditional health care services (Alsswey and Al-Samarraie, 2020; Subhi et al., 2015). The near ubiquity and adoption of information technology and data systems in health care and the steady growth of younger nurses entering the workforce means that nurses, especially during periods of public health emergencies and crises, provide an optimal pool of potential users for evidence-based mental health apps.

In the coming years and with higher mobile usage in place (Alexopoulos et al., 2020), additional research will support the determination of best practices for helping nurses maintain their mental health or access mental health resources through the use of mobile technology. In the meantime, several resources have been launched with a focus on health care workers. A mental health partner initiative between the University of North Carolina at Chapel Hill and Cooper University Health Care created an app called Heroes Health, launched in July 2020 that is aimed at first responders and health care workers. The app allows them to answer weekly questions that assess their mental health, and users are connected to resources based on their answers (Heroes Health, 2020). An additional feature to which a health care organization can subscribe allows its employees to give feedback through an aggregate dashboard. Brigham and Women's Hospital in Boston released an app for emergency providers called "Rose" that collects data from users through a journal feature and questionnaires. The app's built in AI platform then uses these data to identify trends in stress and burnout, allowing the organization to find warning patterns or triggers that mark adverse mental health symptoms in staff (Drees, 2020; Landi, 2020). Artificial intelligence technology in the app is equipped to read key words and phrases and detect signs of mental health problems, including trauma (Miliard, 2020).

et al., 2020). These efforts are synergistic with those aimed at building psychological safety (Nelson et al., 2014) and models of just culture for safe, quality care.

Incivility, Bullying, and Workplace Violence

In its 2015 position statement (ANA, 2015), ANA articulated the responsibilities of both individual nurses and employers in ending workplace bullying, incivility, and workplace violence. With regard to bullying, Rutherford and colleagues (2019) conducted an integrative review of studies of interventions addressing the bullying of prelicensure nursing students and nursing professionals, finding that those interventions fell into three main categories: education, nurses as leaders, and policy changes. The authors conclude that educational interventions are important to reducing or eliminating bullying behavior and may be of the most benefit to students. These types of interventions range from journaling to teaching nurses how to address being a target of bullying or incivility.

One intervention, described by Aebersold and Schoville (2020), used role play simulations with debriefing sessions and an educational component with senior-level undergraduate nursing students. Preliminary qualitative evidence from this intervention indicated that simulation can be an effective strategy for addressing incivility and bullying in the workplace, although this was a small pilot study with a convenience sample of nursing students. Pfeiffer and Vessey (2017) conducted an integrative review of bullying and lateral violence (BLV) among nurses in Magnet® accredited health care organizations.[10] The authors found that a variety of terms were used to describe BLV, making it difficult to synthesize and compare findings across studies. Although Magnet accreditation standards promote a model of collegiality and teamwork, BLV remains prevalent and exists in both Magnet and non-Magnet organizations. Pfeiffer and Vessey (2017) call for more studies examining the prevalence of BLV in these accredited organizations and also more research aimed at better understanding factors within organizations and interventions that can effectively reduce the occurrence of BLV. In sum, the level of evidence for the effectiveness of bullying interventions among nurses is limited and there is a need for rigorous, well-designed RCTs to build this evidence base; multiple, stratified interventions may be needed (Rutherford et al., 2019).

As mentioned previously, workplace violence is also a concern for nurses, particularly those who work in emergency department settings (Gillespie et al., 2014a,b). Interventions that have been developed to address workplace violence include a hybrid educational intervention with online and classroom components (Gillespie et al., 2014a) and a multicomponent intervention that includes environmental changes, education, training, and changes in policies and procedures

[10] These are health care organizations that are accredited through the American Nurses Credentialing Center. This model is considered to be the gold standard for nursing (Pfeiffer and Vessey, 2017).

(Gillespie et al., 2014b), although these are not strictly focused on nurses. The hybrid educational intervention showed promise with a small sample of employees from a pediatric emergency department, with the research team concluding that to achieve significant learning and retention, the hybrid model is preferred. The multicomponent intervention was promising, but only two of six sites reported significant decreases in violent events. The authors also note that emergency department workers did not report most of the violent events that occurred because of such factors as time constraints and fear of being blamed (Gillespie et al., 2014b). There is a need for more research to examine how to ameliorate workplace violence among health care workers, and for replication and rigorous RCTs of promising interventions.

Racism, Prejudice, and Discrimination

As discussed in Chapter 4, there has been a shift in patient care settings away from cultural competency toward cultural humility, and toward a focus on a lifelong approach to learning about diversity and the role of individual bias and systemic power in health care interactions. Specific approaches to weaving cultural humility concepts into nursing and interprofessional education are discussed in Chapter 7. In addition, as noted in Chapter 7, research on the efficacy of interventions designed to reduce implicit bias has found that many of these interventions are ineffective, and some may even increase implicit biases (FitzGerald et al., 2019). Chapter 7 describes an evidence-based intervention, the prejudice habit-breaking intervention (Cox and Devine, 2019; Devine et al., 2012), that has been tested in RCTs and is aimed at overcoming bias through conscious self-regulation or breaking the bias "habit." Reducing prejudice and discrimination may also be possible through simple and brief interventions, such as 10-minute nonconfrontational conversations, although more research is needed to test such interventions with racial outgroups (Williams and Cooper, 2019).

Another concept that can be considered in relationship to well-being is that of "wellness as fairness" (Prilleltensky, 2012). As described in earlier chapters of this report, nurses are being called on to dismantle racism and to advance the social mission of making health better and fairer. Similarly, in the public health field, it is acknowledged that a focus on both individual personal transformation and structural change is needed to detect, confront, and prevent racism (Margaret and Came, 2019). Margaret and Came (2019, p. 317) note that White public health practitioners can become allies in antiracism work by addressing the following three interdependent and overlapping areas: "(1) understanding and addressing power; (2) skills for working across difference; and (3) building and sustaining relationships." Rigorous, well-designed studies are needed to test these and other promising approaches with nurse educators, nursing students, and practicing nurses.

Systems-Level Approaches

The responsibility for nurse well-being is shared between individual nurses and those who shape the environment in which they practice. Individual nurses' dedication to their own well-being is enhanced by the support of the system, its leaders, and a culture in which well-being is prioritized. The 2019 National Academies report on clinician burnout makes clear that while interventions focused on individuals have their place, these strategies alone are insufficient to address the systemic contributions to the factors that erode clinician well-being (NASEM, 2019a). The evidence demonstrates that integrated, systematic, organization-focused interventions are more effective at reducing burnout and improving well-being. A systems approach focuses on the structure, organization, and culture of workplaces (Dzau et al., 2018; Shanafelt and Noseworthy, 2017; Shanafelt et al., 2017), and considers the complex interplay of factors that impact well-being and other outcomes (NASEM, 2019a; Plsek and Greenhalgh, 2001; Rouse, 2008).

An integrated and systematic approach requires the involvement of a broad range of stakeholders, including nurse leaders, educational institutions, health care organizations and other employers of nurses, policy makers, and professional associations. Some stakeholders will have the capacity to make sweeping changes to policies and work environments, while others will focus more on facilitating individual and team well-being. Because the factors that contribute to burnout and poor well-being are multiple, varied, complex, and context-dependent, efforts on all levels and in all areas are welcome and necessary. The National Academy of Medicine's (NAM's) Clinician Well-Being Knowledge Hub has detailed, illustrative case studies from the Virginia Mason Kirkland Medical Center, and The Ohio State University's Colleges of Medicine and Nursing, Emergency Medicine Residency Program, and Wexner Medical Center.[11]

Stakeholder actions could include restructuring systems and implementing initiatives to prevent burnout, reduce administrative burden, enable technological solutions to support the provision of care, reduce the stigma and barriers that prevent health professionals from seeking support, and increase investment in research on clinician well-being (NASEM, 2019a). All stakeholders can consider the role technology can play in improving well-being (see Box 10-4). Well-being initiatives will vary considerably based on the setting and role of nurses; for example, nurses who are working directly with patients during a pandemic disease outbreak will have different needs and wants from those of nurses who are leading community efforts to change housing policies. This section describes how different stakeholders—nurse leaders, educational institutions, employers, policy makers, and nursing associations and organizations—can continue working toward improving nurse well-being, and provides several examples of action in these areas.

[11] See https://nam.edu/clinicianwellbeing/case-studies (accessed April 13, 2021).

Nurse Leaders

Nurse leaders have the potential to dramatically impact nurse well-being by shaping the day-to-day work life of nurses, setting the culture and tone of the workplace, developing and enforcing policies, and serving as exemplars of well-being (Ross et al., 2017). The leadership style and effectiveness of nurse leaders have been associated with outcomes including the health of the work environment, patient outcomes and mortality, job satisfaction, work engagement, burnout, and retention (Bamford et al., 2013; Boamah et al., 2018; Cummings et al., 2010a,b; Rushton and Pappas, 2020; Spence Laschinger and Fida, 2014; Spence Laschinger et al., 2012; Wei et al., 2018). Nurse leaders have a responsibility to create a safe work environment with a culture of inclusivity and respect, and to implement and enforce strong policies to protect nurses. In particular, nurse leaders must be skilled in recognizing signals of toxicity and strategically responding to them (Rutherford et al., 2019). This responsibility is not limited to acute care or hospital settings; nurses on all fronts and at every point in the workforce pipeline deserve support from their leaders.

The specific ways in which leaders can impact nurse well-being depend on their role and scope of authority and responsibility. Nurse executives with influence over organizational policies can advocate for adequate pay and benefits, and address staffing and scheduling issues to prevent nurses from being overworked. Nurse leaders who manage teams can support well-being by addressing workplace safety and incivility and bullying, and by creating a culture in which all nurses feel supported and respected (Spence Laschinger et al., 2009). For example, leaders could implement a "see something, say something" program in which nurses are encouraged to report any unsafe workplace conditions, including violence and bullying.

Nurse leaders can also use their position to serve as educators and role models for their staff (NASEM, 2019a; Ross et al., 2017). They might do so by, for example, investing in programs aimed at developing resilience skills, teaching skills based on cognitive-behavioral therapy, creating norms of self-care within the work day, and setting firm work–life boundaries for self and staff. The effects of stress and trauma related to the COVID-19 pandemic will impact the workforce at both the individual and staffing levels for years to come, and leaders will need vigilance and a long-term strategy to build the health of the teams providing care.

For example, Menschner and Maul (2016) report that some community-based health care organizations and health care networks are fostering a healthy life–work balance by encouraging employees to leave work mobile phones in the office after their shifts and ensuring that they do not work beyond their designated 40 hours. Nurse leaders can also serve as role models by examining their own health promotion behaviors and maintaining their own health and well-being (Ross et al., 2017). And they can be advocates for making environmental changes in the workplace, such as by holding standing or walking meetings, advocating for healthy work schedules, or implementing programs to help nurses cope with the stresses of work.

Leadership can be particularly important during times of transition and challenge. For example, during the early days of the COVID-19 pandemic,[12] health centers with level-headed, disciplined, and unified leadership were able to quickly implement plans, limit confusion, and prepare staff for the changes ahead (Canton and Company, 2020). Rosa and colleagues (2020) outline steps for nurse leaders to take to promote health system resilience during the COVID-19 pandemic. These include specific local and organizational recommendations aimed at mitigating burnout and moral suffering and building a culture of well-being. The transition associated with integrating SDOH and health equity further into nursing practice will not be as swift or as bleak as the transition to COVID-19 care, but it will similarly require strong leadership and steady hands to guide the way and advocate for nurse well-being amid the changes (Rosa et al., 2020). Nurse leaders will be essential in helping to shift the priorities and workflow of nurses and to supporting nurses through this transition (AHA, 2020b).

Educational Institutions

The foundation for nurse well-being starts long before nurses enter the workplace. While more data are available on the poor well-being of medical students, research suggests that nursing students are similarly stressed out, exhausted, and disengaged (Michalec et al., 2013; Rudman and Gustavsson, 2012). While evidence on burnout and poor well-being among nursing students is quite limited (NASEM, 2019a), there is an emerging body of evidence on the important role of resilience (see also the earlier discussion of resilience in the section on individual-level interventions). Resilience of prelicensure nursing students has a significant inverse relationship with academic intention to leave (Van Hoek et al., 2019) and moral distress (Krautscheid et al., 2020). Strategies to support resilience include positive reframing (Amsrud et al., 2019; Mathad et al., 2017; Stacey et al., 2020; Thomas and Revell, 2016), reflection (He et al., 2018), and mindfulness (Stacey et al., 2020). Integration points for resilience within the clinical and didactic components of curricula are needed for sustainable impact on nursing student behavior (Cleary et al., 2018). In a recent systematic review of resilience among health care professions, Huey and Palaganas (2020) outline individual, organizational, and environmental factors that impact student resilience and promising interventions. Further work is needed to understand the relationship among factors that support well-being

[12] The American Hospital Association developed a workforce checklist for use by leaders to consider how they can support their workforce during the pandemic. See https://www.aha.org/system/files/media/file/2020/07/aha-covid19-pathways-workforce.pdf (accessed April 13, 2021).

and resilience among nursing students in all programs of study (Stephens, 2013; Thomas and Revell, 2016).

Nursing educational institutions have a responsibility to ensure students' well-being, and to impart to them the skills and resources necessary for well-being throughout their nursing career. Consistent with the recommendations of the National Academies report focused on addressing burnout (NASEM, 2019a), educational institutions, like health care organizations, can invest in interventions that build individual resilience and well-being while dismantling the impediments within the system itself. This process begins with executive leadership and faculty commitment to a learning culture in which systems, processes, incentives, rewards, and resources are aligned to amplify rather than degrade well-being. One way to accelerate change is through investment in a leadership position assigned the role of championing individual and system alignment of well-being activities. Routine assessment of well-being and factors known to undermine it is then conducted annually, with leadership accountable for remediating modifiable factors and expanding efforts to deepen culture change. These strategies, recommended in the National Academies report (NASEM, 2019a), require attention to supporting faculty, staff, and students in contributing to a culture of well-being as a strategic priority.

As part of the effort to make well-being an institutional priority, conscious attention is needed to creating a culture in which well-being and integrity are not an afterthought but are integrated throughout the curriculum in visible and meaningful ways. Specific inclusion of content that links nursing students' well-being to the profession's Code of Ethics reinforces that self-stewardship is an ethical imperative rather than an optional activity (ANA, 2015). Including program outcomes focused on well-being and ethical competence is a tangible way to elevate the importance of developing and sustaining well-being as a foundational skill for the nursing profession, as explicitly reflected in the American Association of Colleges of Nursing's *Essentials*[13] for nursing education. Faculty, like students, require expanded resources that enable them to embody their commitment to well-being and serve as role models and coaches for students (Feeg et al., 2021; Robichaux, 2012). Statewide, regional, and national initiatives to build capacity among faculty and students in these foundational areas are vital.

There are a variety of concrete ways in which nursing schools can facilitate student well-being (see Box 10-5)—for example, by ensuring that the workload is reasonable, providing easy-to-access support and mentoring for students, setting a culture and an example of well-being, and teaching self-care and mindfulness skills, such as reflective practice, journaling, or various forms of artistic expression (Song and Lindquist, 2015). These skills can be integrated throughout the curriculum with reinforcement at regular intervals. For these interventions to be

---

[13] See https://www.aacnnursing.org/Education-Resources/AACN-Essentials (accessed April 13, 2021).

BOX 10-5
Examples of Nursing Schools' Well-Being Initiatives

The Compassionate Care Initiative (CCI) (Bauer-Wu and Fontaine, 2015) is an integrated, multifaceted program within the University of Virginia School of Nursing. CCI serves students, faculty, and staff and promotes well-being through such initiatives as coursework, resilience activities, workshops, retreats, and meditation and yoga classes. CCI incorporates four central concepts: resilience, mindfulness, interprofessional collaboration, and a healthy work environment. The initiative conducts research on compassion, resilience, and self-care, and also has an Ambassador program in which student-clinicians, faculty, and community members implement changes in their workplaces and meet monthly to share successes and challenges.

The Ohio State University College of Nursing has a 5-year strategic plan focused on student, trainee, and faculty well-being, with outcomes monitored on an annual basis (Cappelucci et al., 2019). LIVE WELL is a core tenet of this plan aimed at producing nurses, leaders, researchers, and health professionals who Lead, Innovate, Vision, and Execute, and are Wellness-focused, Evidence-based, Lifelong Learners, and Lights for the World. The College has a LIVE WELL curriculum that promotes healthy lifestyles for students, faculty, and staff through seminars, events, and wellness activities.

effective, it will be necessary for nursing education organizations to carefully assess the impact of recruitment narratives and organizational norms that conflate perfectionism with excellence, establish patterns of unhealthy competition, or reinforce systemic racism or social injustice. Such an assessment requires scrutinizing grading and pedagogical practices, encouraging a diversity of learning styles, and eliminating norms of chronic overwork as the standard to be achieved. Attention is needed to how faculty norms and behaviors impact the adoption of those norms by students. For example, students who witness exhausted and overworked faculty who do not demonstrate investment in their own health and well-being experience dissonance when those same faculty urge them to adopt healthy habits and well-being practices.

Nursing students' well-being can also be enhanced by advancing opportunities for interdisciplinary education and interventions aimed at fostering professionalism and interprofessional practice to support well-being (IOM, 2014). Currently, core competencies for both interprofessional[14] and single-discipline[15] education lack robust requirements for developing capacities that enable well-be-

---

[14] See https://www.aacom.org/docs/default-source/insideome/ccrpt05-10-11.pdf?sfvrsn=77937f97_2 (accessed April 13, 2021).

[15] See https://www.aacnnursing.org/Education-Resources/AACN-Essentials (accessed April 13, 2021).

ing and integrity. Often when included, such content is elective or optional. However, there are signs of progress, animated by concerns about the detrimental effects of the learning environment and recommendations to redress them (Larsen et al., 2018). Interprofessional initiatives, such as the NAM's Action Collaborative on Clinician Well-Being and Resilience,[16] represent a coordinated method for learning with and from colleagues (IOM, 2014).

Employers

Organizations that employ nurses—including hospitals, nursing homes, schools, prisons, community organizations, and others—play a major role in shaping the conditions that promote nurse well-being or the lack thereof. In the framework for burnout and well-being shown earlier in Figure 10-1, there are a number of areas in which employers can make an impact.

First, an organization's leadership, governance, and management can make monitoring and improving nurse well-being a priority and be accountable for making the organizational changes necessary to dismantle the impediments to achieving that priority. This includes alignment of budgeting with desired outcomes of improved well-being in the nursing workforce. Nurses are also well equipped to take on roles as chief wellness officers in health care systems (Kishore et al., 2018).

Second, an organization can shape the environment, culture, and policies that affect nurses. An organization can redesign the work system so that nurses have adequate resources (e.g., staffing, scheduling, workload, job control, physical environment), and design systems that encourage and facilitate interprofessional collaboration, communication, and professionalism (NASEM, 2019c). For example, a health care organization can ensure that nurses not only have sufficient PPE, but also "psychological PPE" (see Box 10-6).

Third, employers can help support individual nurses in bolstering personal capabilities that may modify the effects of work systems on well-being; for example, employers can offer education, resources, and training in mindfulness, resilience, and healthy habits.

As discussed previously, for individual approaches to be effective, they must be coupled with redesign of organizational processes, structures, and policies to animate sustainable culture shifts that make interventions feasible and normative (Rushton and Sharma, 2018; Stanulewicz et al., 2020). For example, if an organization encourages nurses to use meditation to decompress during shifts but organizational culture frowns on nurses taking breaks, the initiative is likely to have limited impact. End users of these initiatives (front-line nurses) can be engaged proactively in designing a diversity of resources that they perceive to be valuable in fostering their well-being rather than having such resources

[16] See https://nam.edu/initiatives/clinician-resilience-and-well-being (accessed April 13, 2021).

imposed on them (Richards, 2020). The Wikiwisdom™ Forum: Wisdom from Nurses (Richards, 2020) is one such effort, sponsored by New Voice Strategies, the Johns Hopkins University School of Nursing, and the *American Journal of Nursing* to facilitate online conversations with front-line nurses who are battling the COVID-19 pandemic.

For organizations employing nurses who are dispersed in a community (e.g., public health nurses, school nurses) rather than concentrated in a clinical setting, monitoring and communicating with them about well-being may be even more critical. Nurses in community settings and in clinical settings face different risks; nurses working in the community may deal with, for example, isolation or violence in a patient's home or neighborhood, and have less opportunity for breaks (Mathiews and Salmond, 2013; Terry et al., 2015). The dispersed nature

BOX 10-6
Psychological Personal Protective Equipment (PPE)

Just as health care organizations provide PPE, schedule adequate staff, and ensure safety in the workplace, they are also responsible for providing "psychological PPE" to their employees (IHI, 2020). The Institute for Healthcare Improvement (IHI) describes psychological PPE as "individual and system-level actions owned by unit and team leaders that provide protection and support for staff's mental health that can be deployed both before providing care and after a shift has ended." These guidelines (see the figure below) were created specifically for health care staff working during the COVID-19 pandemic, but they may be adaptable for use in other contexts and settings as well (IHI, 2020).

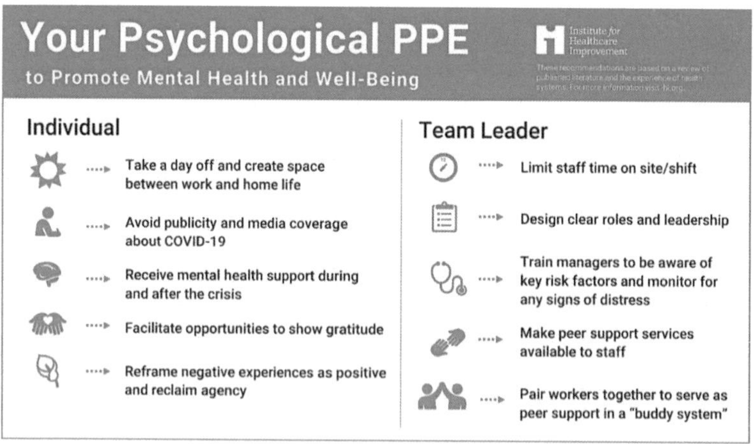

SOURCE: IHI, 2020.

of community nurses means that employers have less opportunity to observe their well-being and less control over the work environment. More research is needed on improving the well-being of nonclinical nurses; in the interim, given the lack of evidence, employers need to think creatively and communicate with nurses about their needs.

There are a variety of existing organizational initiatives to improve nurse well-being through changes to the work environment, as described below. The previously discussed Magnet Recognition program of the American Nurses Credentialing Center (ANCC) is an organizational model designed to improve the work environment for nurses in a hospital setting. The model is focused on improving those components of a nurse's work environment that can be adjusted, such as sufficient staffing, leadership, clinical autonomy, interdisciplinary collaboration, and shared governance. The committee notes that these components match many of the work system factors that contribute to burnout (NASEM, 2019a). As of 2019, about 10 percent of U.S. hospitals had achieved Magnet designation (ANCC, 2019). Another ANCC initiative, the Pathway to Excellence program, recognizes health care organizations that demonstrate a culture in which a work environment that engages and empowers its workers is fostered. Meeting the 12 standards focused on workplace excellence is associated with promising data suggesting improved patient care, decreased emotional exhaustion, and higher job satisfaction (Jarrín et al., 2017).

Programs such as Schwartz Center Rounds offer interprofessional opportunities to explore the psychological, spiritual, and moral aspects of clinical work in a facilitated format. The creation of well-being and a feeling of psychological safety among teams is enabled by a culture of safety, norms of professional responsibility to speak up, leadership, support from peers and leaders, familiarity with team members, and inclusiveness (O'Donovan and McAuliffe, 2020). Evidence suggests that such programs foster communication, teamwork and support (Lown and Manning, 2010), and psychological well-being (Maben et al., 2018). Further research is needed to support the design, implementation, and evaluation of interventions aimed at building psychological safety within health care teams (O'Donovan and McAuliffe, 2020).

The American Association of Critical-Care Nurses (AACN) has developed a set of standards for establishing and sustaining healthy work environment (HWE) standards. Initially released in 2005 and revised in 2016, the HWE standards have been widely adopted nationally and in several other countries. The six essential standards are "skilled communication, true collaboration, effective decision making, appropriate staffing, meaningful recognition, and authentic leadership" (AACN, 2016, p. 10). Outcomes for organizations improve when they actively implement these standards (AACN, 2016). A survey of more than 8,000 acute and critical care nurses (Ulrich et al., 2019) demonstrated that units that intentionally address work environment issues scored better on every indicator of HWE standards, including collaboration, leadership, staffing, intent to leave, and decision making. Notably, these elements were consistently more highly rated at the unit level than at the health care organization level, suggesting that there may be opportunities to intervene at the unit/team level to leverage changes in practice and culture. AACN has also developed the AACN Healthy Work Environment Assessment tool, designed to assist organizations in monitoring their progress in implementing the standards (Connor et al., 2018).

Meaningful recognition of the value each person brings to the organization is one key element of AACN's HWE standards. Such recognition ought to be systematic, consistent, and meaningful to those it intends to acknowledge. Programs such as the Daisy Award[17] give patients, families, and colleagues opportunities to publicly recognize the contributions of individual nurses (Barnes et al., 2016). Recognition by the people served reinforces the meaning of nurses' work by acknowledging their behaviors and their impact on others (Lefton, 2012). It can also help mitigate the unintended negative consequences of the "hero" narrative by connecting the contribution nurses make to patient outcomes explicitly, visibly, and meaningfully (Stokes-Parish et al., 2020).

Health care organizations can also learn from other sectors in using such well-being frameworks as PERMA (Positive Emotion, Engagement, Relationships, Meaning, Achievement). PERMA has been proposed as a model for institutional leadership and culture change to overcome the tendency in many health care organizations to look to quick fixes and partial solutions to stem the tide of burnout and degraded well-being among clinicians (Slavin et al., 2012). The committee points out that all of these existing programs focus on the acute care setting. In the future, programs that recognize and incentivize health care organizations to distinguish their cultures as enabling the well-being of nurses have the potential to be expanded beyond acute care organizations to other settings where nurses work. Adopting standards and programs such as those described above offers organizations a roadmap for aligning efforts to produce meaningful and sustainable change.

Policy Makers

There have been sweeping changes in the structure and regulatory environment of U.S. health care in recent years, and some of these changes have impacted the well-being of clinicians (NASEM, 2019a). One frequently cited example is the growing administrative burden placed on clinicians, such as the documentation requirements associated with electronic health records (see Box 10-1). Efforts to reduce this burden at the federal level include the Centers for Medicare & Medicaid's (CMS's) Patients over Paperwork initiative, an attempt to simplify Medicare documentation requirements, and a U.S. Department of Health and Human Services (HHS) draft Strategy on Reducing Regulatory and

---

[17] See https://www.daisyfoundation.org/daisy-award (accessed April 13, 2021).

Administrative Burden Relating to the Use of Health IT and EHR (ONC, 2020). Policy makers can work together with nurses, other clinicians, workplaces, and patients to develop policies that meet the needs of health care while promoting the well-being of nurses.

During the COVID-19 pandemic, CMS and other regulators and payers have made changes to policies to lift or lessen administrative and technological burdens on clinicians, including nurses. There have been calls to make many of these changes permanent to transform health care, with the goal of achieving the Quadruple Aim outcomes of better care for individuals, better health for the population, lower costs, and better experience for clinicians (Bodenheimer and Sinsky, 2014; Sinsky and Linzer, 2020). For instance, in a recent commentary, Sinsky and Linzer (2020) call for a reconsideration of the pre-COVID-19 status quo and recommend that certain policy and practice changes related to COVID-19 remain in place (e.g., permitting verbal orders, allowing clinicians to provide telehealth services from their homes). As noted in Chapter 4, the Triple Aim is focused primarily on optimizing the health system's performance (see Bodenheimer and Sinsky, 2014). The "fourth aim," addressing clinicians' well-being and improving their work life, also targets improving the quality of patient-centered care, and these two need to be in balance so one or the other is not compromised (Bodenheimer and Sinsky, 2014).

Nursing Associations and Organizations

Nursing associations and organizations, individually and collectively, have a pivotal role in supporting nurse well-being. Professional organizations such as ANA, AACN, and others have leveraged their organizational infrastructure to curate resources; offer programs; and interpret and disseminate reports, research, and best practices. In May 2020, the American Nurses Foundation, the philanthropic arm of ANA, launched a national well-being initiative[18] for nurses to address the increased stress on nurses due to the COVID-19 pandemic. This initiative is a collaboration among ANA, AACN, the Emergency Nurses Association (the ENA), and the American Psychiatric Nurses Association (APNA), and includes peer-to-peer conversations; hotlines; cognitive processing techniques; and other preventive approaches, such as apps for stress reduction. The National Black Nurses Association (NBNA) has an NBNA Affirmations webpage in which nurses can submit their favorite quotes or positive affirmations,[19] and also has a Twitter campaign called #NBNAResilient. The National Association of Hispanic

[18] For more information, see https://www.nursingworld.org/news/news-releases/2020/american-nurses-foundation-launches-national-well-being-initiative-for-nurses (accessed April 13, 2021).

[19] See https://www.nbna.org/affirmations (accessed April 13, 2021).

Nurses (NAHN) conducts educational programming that includes webinars focused on stress and compassion fatigue.[20]

Nursing organizations are poised to be the collective voice of their members on critically important issues including nurse well-being by naming the problem and advocating for solutions. They have a vital role in shaping the narrative about the challenges nurses face to avoid reinforcing a victim perspective by offering an evidence-informed array of solutions that can be customized for the unique needs of members within their organizations. They have represented various nursing specialties in such interprofessional initiatives as the NAM's Action Collaborative to bring the voice of nurses to the table. Professional organizations also provide systems of support, build community and connection among their members, and inspire engagement in addressing the systemic impediments to nurse well-being. Professional organizations have a pivotal role in educating their communities about the factors that degrade their well-being, such as burnout, and in disseminating resources to address them (Cochran et al., 2020).

CONCLUSIONS

To care responsibly for people—especially as they practice in more settings with more diverse people with complex needs—nurses need to feel healthy, well, and supported. The systems that educate and employ nurses have a duty to fully support them as they take on new roles to advance health equity. While nurses have experienced roadblocks to well-being before—from burnout, to compassion fatigue, to injuries and infection—COVID-19 has intensified their stress and left them feeling unprotected and unsupported.

Conclusion 10-1: All environments in which nurses work affect the health and well-being of the nursing workforce. Ultimately, the health and well-being of nurses influence the quality, safety, and cost of the care they provide, as well as organizations and systems of care. The COVID-19 crisis has highlighted the shortcomings of historical efforts to address nurses' health and well-being.

Nurse well-being is impacted by physical, mental, moral, and social factors originating in a range of sources from the individual to the system level. Improving the well-being of nurses will therefore require multilevel and multifaceted approaches that address their physical, mental, moral, and social health and create safe, supportive, and ethically grounded environments. Occupational health hazards, workplace violence, stress and mental health issues, moral suffering, compassion fatigue, burnout, and bullying and incivility all need to be addressed

[20] See http://www.nahnnet.org/NAHN/Events/Webinars/NAHN/Content/Webinars.aspx?hkey=5c3658d1-a2e6-4ea2-8b4f-da0f622bf2dc (accessed April 13, 2021).

through reform aimed at changing workplace policies and culture to support the well-being of nurses and ensure their capacity and ability to provide quality care for people, families, and communities.

> ***Conclusion 10-2: The lack of sufficient data and evidence about the negative impacts of burnout, fatigue, and stressful work environments on nurses' health and well-being hinders understanding of the severity of these issues and limits the ability to address them appropriately. Many programs and initiatives seek to improve nurses' health and well-being; however, the translation of effective evidence-based interventions into practice, further research, and rigorous studies are needed to understand the impact of these programs and initiatives and their relationship to system factors.***

> ***Conclusion 10-3: Structural racism, cultural racism, and discrimination exist within nursing as in other professions. Nurses of color experience discrimination and bias within the workplace and educational systems, compounded by the lack of diversity among the nursing workforce and faculty. Nurses, educators, and health care leaders have a responsibility to address structural racism, cultural racism, and discrimination within the nursing profession across educational and practice settings, and to build structures and systems that promote inclusivity and health equity.***

As the future of nursing demands that nurses increasingly address social needs and SDOH, attention to nurse well-being will be critical. Addressing social needs and SDOH requires in turn cognitive, emotional, and moral work that is not currently supported; that is, time and payment for this work are largely not available. If nurses and other clinicians are expected to fulfill their professional mandates for social justice, including addressing complex social needs and SDOH, and to spend the time and cognitive effort to address both health and social issues, system-wide changes will be needed to provide space and support for that shift. More well-designed, methodologically sound research studies are needed to develop additional knowledge in this area.

> ***Conclusion 10-4: Coordinated and collaborative action at the individual and systems levels, encompassing individual nurses, educators, employers, health systems, professional organizations, and government agencies, is needed to promote nurses' health and well-being.***

Ensuring nurse well-being necessitates an investment in individual strategies within a systems approach that addresses the structures and policies responsible for the workplace hazards and stresses that lead to poor health. This investment is analogous to that needed to address SDOH in the society at large. It is not sufficient to ask people or nurses simply to make better choices when the structures and systems that surround them are designed to promote poor health and inequity. Approaches to supporting nurse well-being must not be simply short-term, discrete initiatives; they must be embedded systematically into every aspect of nursing, from education to retirement, and in every practice setting. COVID-19 has served as an inflection point for giving nurses' well-being the attention it deserves and for restructuring systems, organizations, and policies to promote their physical, mental, moral, and social health.

REFERENCES

AACN (American Association of Critical-Care Nurses). 2016. *AACN standards for establishing and sustaining healthy work environments*. https://www.aacn.org/WD/HWE/Docs/HWEStandards.pdf (accessed December 15, 2020).

Adriaenssens, J., V. De Gucht, and S. Maes. 2015. Determinants and prevalence of burnout in emergency nurses: A systematic review of 25 years of research. *International Journal of Nursing Studies* 52(2):649–661.

Aebersold, M., and R. Schoville. 2020. How to prevent the next generation of nurses from "eating their young." *Clinical Simulation in Nursing* 38:27–34.

AHA (American Hospital Association). 2020a. *COVID-19: Acknowledging and addressing racism and xenophobia*. https://www.aha.org/system/files/media/file/2020/05/COVID-19_Xenophobia_Resource.pdf (accessed April 9, 2021).

AHA. 2020b. Workforce. *COVID-19 pathways to recovery: Considerations and resources to guide hospitals and health systems*. https://www.aha.org/system/files/media/file/2020/07/aha-covid19-pathways-workforce.pdf (accessed October 6, 2020).

AHRQ (Agency for Healthcare Research and Quality). 2019. *Nursing and patient safety*. Patient Safety Network. https://psnet.ahrq.gov/primer/nursing-and-patient-safety (accessed April 9, 2021).

Aiken, L. H., S. P. Clarke, D. M. Sloane, J. Sochalski, and J. H. Silber. 2002. Hospital nurse staffing and patient mortality, nurse burnout, and job dissatisfaction. *Journal of the American Medical Association* 288(16):1987–1993.

Akhtar, A. 2020 (September 29). Filipinos make up 4% of nurses in the US, but 31.5% of nurse deaths from COVID-19. *Business Insider*. https://www.businessinsider.com/filipinos-make-up-disproportionate-covid-19-nurse-deaths-2020-9 (accessed October 9, 2020).

Alexopoulos, A. R., J. G. Hudson, and O. Otenigbagbe. 2020. The use of digital applications and COVID-19. *Community Mental Health Journal* 56(7):1202–1203.

Alsswey, A., and H. Al-Samarraie. 2020. Elderly users' acceptance of mHealth user interface (UI) design-based culture: The moderator role of age. *Journal on Multimodal User Interfaces* 14(1):49–59. doi: 10.1007/s12193-019-00307-w.

Amsrud, K. E., A. Lyberg, and E. Severinsson. 2019. Development of resilience in nursing students: A systematic qualitative review and thematic synthesis. *Nurse Education Practice* 41:102621.

ANA (American Nurses Association). 2015. *Code of ethics*. Silver Spring, MD: American Nurses Association.

ANA. 2017. *Executive summary: American Nurses Association health risk appraisal*. https://www.nursingworld.org/~4aeeeb/globalassets/practiceandpolicy/work-environment/health--safety/ana-healthriskappraisalsummary_2013-2016.pdf (accessed May 14, 2020).

ANA. 2020a. *Crisis standard of care: COVID-19 pandemic*. https://www.nursingworld.org/~496044/globalassets/practiceandpolicy/work-environment/health--safety/coronavirus/crisis-standards-of-care.pdf (accessed October 15, 2020).

ANA. 2020b. *Provision 5: Self-care and COVID-19*. https://www.nursingworld.org/~4a1fea/globalassets/covid19/provision-5_-self-care--covid19-final.pdf (accessed October 15, 2020).

ANA. n.d. *Violence, incivility, & bullying*. https://www.nursingworld.org/practice-policy/work-environment/violence-incivility-bullying (accessed April 9, 2021).

ANA and AAN (American Academy of Nursing). 2020. *The American Academy of Nursing and the American Nurses Association call for social justice to address racism and health equity in communities of color (News Release)*. https://www.nursingworld.org/news/news-releases/2020/the-american-academy-of-nursing-and-the-american-nurses-association-call-for-social-justice-to-address-racism-and-health-equity-in-communities-of-color (accessed October 15, 2020).

ANA Enterprise. 2018. Healthy nurse, health nation: Year one highlights 2017–2018. *American Nurse Today* 13(11):1–12. https://www.nursingworld.org/~4ab632/globalassets/docs/ana/practice/hnhn17-18highlights.pdf (accessed April 9, 2021).

ANA Enterprise. 2019. Healthy nurse healthy nation: Year two highlights 2018-2019. *American Nurse Today* 14(9):1–12. https://www.healthynursehealthynation.org/globalassets/all-images-view-with-media/about/2019-hnhn_highlights.pdf (accessed April 9, 2021).

ANA Enterprise. 2020. *Year Three Highlights 2019–2020*. https://www.healthynursehealthynation.org/globalassets/all-images-view-with-media/about/2020-hnhn_sup-8.pdf (accessed January 8, 2021).

ANCC (American Nurses Credentialing Center). 2019. *Find a Magnet organization*. https://www.nursingworld.org/organizational-programs/magnet/find-a-magnet-organization (accessed April 19, 2021).

Arndt, B. G., J. W. Beasley, M. D. Watkinson, J. L. Temte, W. J. Tuan, C. A. Sinsky, and V. J. Gilchrist. 2017. Tethered to the EHR: Primary care physician workload assessment using EHR event log data and time-motion observations. *Annals of Family Medicine* 15(5):419–426.

Avery-Desmarais, S., K. A. Sethares, C. Stover, A. Batchelder, and M. K. McCurry. 2020. Substance use and minority stress in a population of lesbian, gay and bisexual nurses. *Substance Use & Misuse* 55(12):1958–1967.

Azoulay. E., A. Cariou, F. Bruneel, A. Demoule, A. Kouatchet, D. Reuter, V. Souppart, A. Combes, K. Klouche, L. Argaud, F. Barbier, M. Jourdain, J. Reignier, L. Papazian, B. Guidet, G. Geri, M. Resche-Rigon, O. Guisset, V. Labbe, B. Megarbane, G. Van Der Meersch, C. Guitton, D. Friedman, F. Pochard, M. Darmon, and N. Kentish-Barnes. 2020. Symptoms of anxiety, depression, and peritraumatic dissociation in critical care clinicians managing patients with COVID-19. A cross-sectional study. *American Journal of Respiratory and Critical Care Medicine* 202:1388–1398.

Bamford, M., C. A. Wong, and H. Spence Laschinger. 2013. The influence of authentic leadership and areas of work life on work engagement of registered nurses. *Journal of Nursing Management* 21(3):529–540.

Barbot, O. 2020. George Floyd and our collective moral injury. *American Journal of Public Health* 110(9):1253–1253.

Barnes, B., M. Barnes, and C. D. Sweeney. 2016. Supporting recognition of clinical nurses with the Daisy award. *Journal of Nursing Administration* 46(4):164–166.

Barratt, C. 2018. Developing resilience: The role of nurses, healthcare teams and organisations. *Nursing Standard* 33(7):43–49.

Bauer-Wu, S., and D. Fontaine. 2015. Prioritizing clinician wellbeing: The University of Virginia's compassionate care initiative. *Global Advances in Health and Medicine* 4(5):16–22. doi: 10.7453/gahmj.2015.042.

Baumann, L. A., J. Baker, and A. G. Elshaug. 2018. The impact of electronic health record systems on clinical documentation times: A systematic review. *Health Policy* 122(8):827–836.

Bennett, C., E. K. Hamilton, and H. Rochani. 2019. Exploring race in nursing: Teaching nursing students about racial inequality using the historical lens. *Online Journal of Issues in Nursing* 24(2).

Berwick, D. M., S. Loehrer, and C. Gunther-Murphy. 2017. Breaking the rules for better care. *Journal of the American Medical Association* 317(21):2161–2162.

Boamah, S. A., H. K. Spence Laschinger, C. Wong, and S. Clarke. 2018. Effect of transformational leadership on job satisfaction and patient safety outcomes. *Nursing Outlook* 66(2):180–189.

Bodenheimer, T., and C. Sinsky 2014. From triple to quadruple aim: Care of the patient requires care of the provider. *Annals of Family Medicine* 12(6):573–576.

Brown, K. W., and R. M. Ryan. 2003. The benefits of being present: Mindfulness and its role in psychological well-being. *Journal of Personality and Social Psychology* 84(4):822–848.

Buerhaus, P., D. Auerbach, L. Skinner, and D. Staigner. 2017. State of the registered nurse workforce as a new era of health reform emerges. *Nursing Economic$* 35(5):229–237.

Burlison, J. D., R. R. Quillivan, S. D. Scott, S. Johnson, and J. M. Hoffman. 2016. The effects of the second victim phenomenon on work-related outcomes: Connecting self-reported caregiver distress to turnover intentions and absenteeism. *Journal of Patient Safety* 17(3):195–199. doi: 10.1097/PTS.0000000000000301.

Burston, A. S., and A. G. Tuckett. 2013. Moral distress in nursing: Contributing factors, outcomes and interventions. *Nursing Ethics* 20(3):312–324.

Cañadas-De la Fuente, G. A., J. Gómez-Urquiza, E. Ortega-Campos, G. Cañadas, L. Albendín-García, and E. De la Fuente-Solana. 2017. Prevalence of burnout syndrome in oncology nursing: A meta-analytic study. *Psychooncology* 27(5):1426–1433.

Canton and Company. 2020. *Finding the "next normal": FQHC resilience during the COVID-19 pandemic*. https://cantoncompany.com/2020/04/22/finding-the-next-normal-fqhc-resilience-during-the-covid-19-pandemic (accessed April 19, 2021).

Cappelucci, K., M. Zindel, H. C. Knight, N. Busis, and C. Alexander. 2019. Clinician well-being at The Ohio State University: A case study. *NAM Perspectives*. Discussion Paper. Washington, DC: National Academy of Medicine. doi: 10.31478/201908b.

Caristo, J. M., and P. T. Clements. 2019. Let's stop "eating our young": Zero-tolerance policies for bullying in nursing. *Nursing2020 Critical Care* 14(4):45–48.

Carpenter, H., T. Mulvey, and L. Gould. 2020. *Examining and improving nurse wellness: Healthy nurse, healthy nation*. Norwood, MA: Infusion Nurses Society. https://indd.adobe.com/view/8b585881-bb8c-42a3-ad05-7b0dc1773874 (accessed June 8, 2021).

Cavanagh, N., G. Cockett, C. Heinrich, L. Doig, K. Fiest, J. R. Guichon, S. Page, I. Mitchell, and C. J. Doig. 2020. Compassion fatigue in healthcare providers: A systematic review and meta-analysis. *Nursing Ethics* 27(3):639–665.

Chari, R., C-C. Chang, S. Sauter, E. Petrun Sayers, J. Cerully, P. Schulte, A. Schill, and L. Uscher-Pines. 2018. Expanding the paradigm of occupational safety and health: A new framework for worker well-being. *Journal of Occupational Environmental Medicine* 60(7):589–593.

Chin, M. 2020. Advancing health equity in patient safety: A reckoning, challenge, and opportunity. *BMJ Quality and Safety*. Epub ahead of print. doi: 10.1136/bmjqs-2020-012599.

Cleary, M., D. Visentin, S. West, V. Lopez, and R. Kornhaber. 2018. Promoting emotional intelligence and resilience in undergraduate nursing students: An integrative review. *Nurse Education Today* 68:112–120.

Cochran, K. L., K. Doo, A. Squires, T. Shah, S. Rinne, and M. Mealer. 2020. Addressing burnout syndrome from a critical care specialty organization perspective. *AACN Advanced Critical Care* 31(2):158–166.

Comas-Díaz, L., G. M. Hall, and H. A. Neville. 2019. Racial trauma: Theory, research, and healing: Introduction to the special issue. *American Psychologist* 74(1):1–5.

Connor, J. A., S. I. Ziniel, C. Porter, D. Doherty, M. Moonan, P. Dwyer, L. Wood, and P. A. Hickey. 2018. Interprofessional use and validation of the AACN healthy work environment assessment tool. *American Journal of Critical Care* 27(5):363–371.

Cottingham, M. D., A. H. Johnson, and R. J. Erickson. 2018. I can never be too comfortable: Race, gender, and emotion at the hospital bedside. *Qualitative Health Research* 28(1):145–158.

Cox, W. T. L., and P. G. Devine. 2019. The prejudice habit-breaking intervention: An empowerment-based confrontation approach. In *Confronting prejudice and discrimination,* edited by R. K. Mallett and M. J. Monteith. New York: Elsevier. Pp. 249–274.

Cruz, D., C. Mastropaolo, and Y. Rodriguez. 2019. Perceived microaggressions in health care: A measurement study. *PLoS One* 14:e0211620.

Cui, P. P., P. P. Wang, K. Wang, Z. Ping, P. Wang, and C. Chen. 2021. Post-traumatic growth and influencing factors among frontline nurses fighting against COVID-19. *Occupational and Environmental Medicine* 78(2):129–135

Cummings, G. G., T. MacGregor, M. Davey, H. Lee, C. Wong, E. Lo, M. Muise, and E. Stafford. 2010a. Leadership styles and outcome patterns for the nursing workforce and work environment: A systematic review. *International Journal of Nursing Studies* 47(3):363–385.

Cummings, G. G., W. Midodzi, C. Wong, and C. Estabrooks. 2010b. The contribution of hospital nursing leadership styles to 30-day patient mortality. *Nursing Research* 59(5):331–339.

da Silva, A. T., C. de Souza Lopes, E. Susser, and P. Rossie Menezes. 2016. Work-related depression in primary care teams in Brazil. *American Journal of Public Health* 106(11):1990–1997.

Danna, K., and R. Griffin. 1999. Health and well-being in the workplace: A review and synthesis of the literature. *Journal of Management* 25(3):357–384.

Davey, M. M., G. Cummings, C. V. Newburn-Cook, and E. A. Lo. 2009. Predictors of nurse absenteeism in hospitals: A systematic review. *Journal of Nursing Management* 17(3):312–330.

Davidson, P. M., C. H. Rushton, J. Dotzenrod, C. A. Godack, D. Baker, and M. N. Nolan. 2016. Just and realistic expectations for persons with disabilities practicing nursing. *AMA Journal of Ethics* 18(10):1034–1040.

Davidson, J. E., J. Mendis, A. R. Stuck, G. DeMichele, and S. Zisook. 2018a. *Nurse suicide: Breaking the silence. NAM Perspectives.* Discussion Paper. Washington, DC: National Academy of Medicine. doi: 10.31478/201801a.

Davidson, J., Zisook, S., Kirby, B., DeMichele, G., and W. Norcross. 2018b. Suicide prevention: A Healer education and referral program for nurses. *Journal of Nursing Administration* 48(2):85–892.

Davidson, J. E., J. Proudfoot, K. Lee, G. Terterian, and S. Zisook. 2020a. A longitudinal analysis of nurse suicide in the United States (2005-2016) with recommendations for action. *Worldviews on Evidence Based Nursing* 17(1):6–15.

Davidson, J. E., R. Accardi, C. Sanchez, S. Zisook, and L. A. Hoffman. 2020b. Sustainability and outcomes of a suicide prevention program for nurses. *Worldviews on Evidence-Based Nursing* 17(24):24–31.

Dean, W., B. Jacobs, and R. A. Manfredi. 2020. Moral injury: The invisible epidemic in COVID health care workers. *Annals of Emergency Medicine* 76(4):385–386.

Devine, P. G., P. S. Forscher, A. J. Austin, and W. T. L. Cox. 2012. Long-term reduction in implicit race bias: A prejudice habit-breaking intervention. *Journal of Experimental Social Psychology* 48(6):1267–1278. doi: 10.1016/j.jesp.2012.06.003.

Doble, S. E., and J. C. Santha. 2008. Occupational well-being: Rethinking occupational therapy outcomes. *Canadian Journal of Occupational Therapy* 75(3):184–190.

Dodge, R., A. Daly, J. Huyton, and L. Sanders. 2012. The challenge of defining wellbeing. *International Journal of Wellbeing* 2(3):222–235. doi: 10.5502/ijw.v2i3.4.

Donker, T., K. Petrie, J. Proudfoot, J. Clarke, M-R. Birch, and H. Christensen. 2013. Smartphones for smarter delivery of mental health programs: A systematic review. *Journal of Medical Internet Research* 15(11):e247. doi: 10.2196/jmir.2791.

Drees, J. 2020. Johns Hopkins digital health startup selected for pilot to help clinicians prevent COVID-19 burnout. *Beckers Hospital Review.* https://www.beckershospitalreview.com/digital-transformation/johns-hopkins-digital-health-startup-selected-for-pilot-to-help-clinicians-prevent-covid-19-burnout.html (accessed April 9, 2021).

Dressner, M. A., and S. P. Kissinger. 2018. Occupational injuries and illnesses among registered nurses. *Monthly Labor Review.* Bureau of Labor Statistics. doi: 10.21916/mlr.2018.27.

Duhoux, A., M. Menear, M. Charron, M. Lavoie-Tremblay, and M. Alderson. 2017. Interventions to promote or improve the mental health of primary care nurses: A systematic review. *Journal of Nursing Management* 25(8):597–607.

Dzau, V. J., D. G. Kirch, and T. J. Nasca. 2018. To care is human—Collectively confronting the clinician-burnout crisis. *New England Journal of Medicine* 378(4):312–314.

Echevarria, I. M. 2013. Change your appetite: Stop "eating the young" and start mentoring. *Nursing2020 Critical Care* 8(3):20–24.

Edmondson, A. 1999. Psychological safety and learning behavior in work teams. *Administrative Science Quarterly* 44(2):350–383.

Edmondson, A. 2002. The local and variegated nature of learning in organizations: A group-level perspective. *Organization Science* 13(2):128–146.

Edmondson, A. C. 2018. *The fearless organization: Creating psychological safety in the workplace for learning, innovation, and growth*. Hoboken, NJ: John Wiley & Sons.

Edmondson, A. C., and Z. Lei. 2014. Psychological safety: The history, renaissance, and future of an interpersonal construct. *Annual Review of Organizational Psychology and Organizational Behavior* 1(1):23–43.

Eliason, M. J., J. DeJoseph, S. Dibble, S. Deevey, and P. Chin. 2011. Lesbian, gay, bisexual, transgender, and queer/questioning nurses' experiences in the workplace. *Journal of Professional Nursing* 27(4):237–244.

Eliason, M. J., C. Streed, and M. Henne. 2017. Coping with stress as an LGBTQ+ health care professional. *Journal of Homosexuality* 65(5):561–578.

Englander, H., D. Collins, S. P. Perry, M. Rabinowitz, E. Phoutrides, and C. Nicolaidis. 2018. We've learned it's a medical illness, not a moral choice: Qualitative study of the effects of a multicomponent addiction intervention on hospital providers' attitudes and experiences. *Journal of Hospital Medicine* 13(11):752–758. doi: 10.12788/jhm.2993.

Epstein, E. G., and S. Delgado. 2010. Understanding and addressing moral distress. *Online Journal of Issues in Nursing* 15(3):1.

Epstein, E. G., P. B. Whitehead, C. Prompahakul, L. R. Thacker, and A. B. Hamric. 2019. Enhancing understanding of moral distress: The measure of moral distress for health care professionals. *The American Journal of Bioethics* 10(2):113–124.

Feeg, V. D., D. J. Mancino, C. H. Rushton, K. J. Waligora Mendez, and J. Baierlein. 2021. Ethical dilemmas for nursing students and faculty: In their own voices. *Nursing Education Perspective* 42(1):29–35.

FitzGerald, C., A. Martin, D. Berner, and S. Hurst. 2019. Interventions designed to reduce implicit prejudices and implicit stereotypes in real world contexts: A systematic review. *BMC Psychology* 7(1):29.

Gabrovec, B. 2017. Prevalence of violence toward community nurses: A questionnaire survey. *Workplace Health & Safety* 65(11):527–532.

Gärtner, F. R., K. Nieuwenhuijsen, F. J. van Dijk, and J. K. Sluiter. 2010. The impact of common mental disorders on the work functioning of nurses and allied health professionals: A systematic review. *International Journal of Nursing Studies* 47(8):1047–1061.

Gates, D. M., G. Gillespie, and P. Succop. 2011. Violence against nurses and its impact on stress and productivity. *Nursing Economics* 29(2):59–66, quiz 67.

Geoffrion, S., D. J. Hills, H. M. Ross, J. Pich, A. T. Hill, T. K. Dalsbo, S. Riahi, B. Martinez-Jarreta, and S. Guay. 2020. Education and training for preventing and minimizing workplace aggression directed toward healthcare workers. *The Cochrane Database of Systematic Reviews*. doi: 10.1002/14651858.CD011860.pub2.

Ghazal, L. V., C. Ma, M. Djukic, and A. Squires. 2020. Transition-to-U.S. practice experiences of internationally educated nurses: An integrative review. *Western Journal of Nursing Research* 42(5):373–392.

Gillespie, G. L., S. L. Farra, and D. M. Gates. 2014a. A workplace violence educational program: A repeated measures study. *Nurse Education in Practice* 14(5):468–472.

Gillespie, G. L., D. M. Gates, T. Kowalenko, S. Bresler, and P. Succop. 2014b. Implementation of a comprehensive intervention to reduce physical assaults and threats in the emergency department. *Journal of Emergency Nursing* 40(6):586–591.

Gómez-Urquiza, J. L., A. B. Aneas-López, E. I. Fuente-Solana, L. Albendín-García, L. Díaz-Rodríguez, and G. A. Fuente. 2016. Prevalence, risk factors, and levels of burnout among oncology nurses: A systematic review. *Oncology Nursing Forum* 43(3):e104–e120.

Gómez-Urquiza, J. L., E. I. De la Fuente-Solana, L. Albendín-García, C. Vargas-Pecino, E. M. Ortega-Campos, and G. A. Cañadas-De la Fuente. 2017. Prevalence of burnout syndrome in emergency nurses: A meta-analysis. *Critical Care Nurse* 37(5):e1–e9.

Goodwin, J., J. Cummins, L. Behan, and S. M. O'Brien. 2016. Development of a mental health smartphone app: Perspectives of mental health service users. *Journal of Mental Health* 25(5):434–440.

Gould, L., H. Carpenter, D. R. Farmer, D. Holland, and Dawson, J. M. 2019. Healthy nurse, healthy nation™ (HNHN): Background and first year results. *Applied Nursing Research* 49:64–69.

Grace, S. M., J. Rich, W. Chin, and H. P. Rodriguez. 2014. Flexible implementation and integration of new team members to support patient-centered care. *Healthcare* 2(2):145–151.

Gregory, S. T., T. Menser, and B. T. Gregory. 2018. An organizational intervention to reduce physician burnout. *Journal of Healthcare Management* 63(5):338–352.

Groenewold, M. R., R. Sarmiento, K. Vanoli, W. Raudabaugh, S. Nowlin, and A. Gomaa. 2018. Workplace violence injury in 106 US hospitals participating in the Occupational Health Safety Network (OHSN), 2012–2015. *American Journal of Industrial Medicine* 61(2):157–166.

Grossman, P., L. Niemann, S. Schmidt, and H. Walach. 2004. Mindfulness-based stress reduction and health benefits: A meta-analysis. *Journal of Psychosomatic Research* 57(1):35-43.

Haas, D. A., J. D. Halmaka, and M. Suk. 2019 (January 10). 3 ways to make electronic health records less time-consuming for physicians. *Harvard Business Review*. https://hbr.org/2019/01/3-ways-to-make-electronic-health-records-less-time-consuming-for-physicians (accessed April 9, 2021).

Halter, M. J., D. G. Rolin, M. Adamaszek, M. C. Ladenheim, and B. Frese Hutchens. 2019. State nursing licensure questions about mental illness and compliance with the Americans with Disabilities Act. *Journal of Psychosocial Nursing and Mental Health Services* 57(8):17–22.

Hamric, A. B., and E. G. Epstein. 2017. A health system-wide moral distress consultation service: Development and evaluation. *Hospital Ethics Committee Forum* 29(2):127–143.

Hamric, A. B., and L. D. Wocial. 2016. Institutional ethics resources: Creating moral spaces. *Hastings Center Report* 46(S1):S22–S27.

Han, M., and E. Lee. 2018. Effectiveness of mobile health application use to improve health behavior changes: A systematic review of randomized controlled trials. *Healthcare Informatics Research* 24(3):207–226. doi: 10.4258/hir.2018.24.3.207.

He, W., A. J. Holton, and G. Farkas. 2018. Impact of partially flipped instruction on immediate and subsequent course performance in a large undergraduate chemistry course. *Computers & Education* 125:120–131.

Helms, J. E., G. Nicolas, and C. E. Green. 2012. Racism and ethnoviolence as trauma: Enhancing professional and research training. *Traumatology* 18(1):65–74.

Hernandez, S. H. A., B. J. Morgan, and M. B. Parshall. 2016. Resilience, stress, stigma, and barriers to mental healthcare in U.S. Air Force nursing personnel. *Nursing Research* 65(6):481–486.

Heroes Health. 2020. *A collaboration between UNC Chapel Hill and many others*. https://heroeshealth.unc.edu (accessed April 9, 2021).

Hines, S. E., K. H. Chin, A. R. Levine, and E. M. Wickwire. 2020. Initiation of a survey of healthcare worker distress and moral injury at the onset of the COVID-19 surge. *American Journal of Industrial Medicine* 63(9):830–833.

Hoff, T., S. Carabetta, and G. E. Collinson. 2019. Satisfaction, burnout, and turnover among nurse practitioners and physician assistants: A review of the empirical literature. *Medical Care Research and Review* 76(1):3–31. doi: 10.1177/1077558717730157.

Hofmann, S. G., and A. F. Gómez. 2017. Mindfulness-based interventions for anxiety and depression. *Psychiatric Clinics of North America* 40(4):739–749. doi: 10.1016/j.psc.2017.08.008.

Huberty, J., J. Green, C. Glissmann, L. Larkey, M. Puzia, and C. Lee. 2019. Efficacy of the mindfulness meditation mobile app "Calm" to reduce stress among college students: Randomized controlled trial. *JMIR mHealth and uHealth* 7(6):e14273. doi: 10.2196/14273.

Huey, C. W. T., and J. C. Palaganas. 2020. What are the factors affecting resilience in health professionals? A synthesis of systematic reviews. *The Medical Teacher* 42(5):550–560.

Hughes, R. (ed.). 2008. *Patient safety and quality: An Evidence-Based Handbook for Nurses* (Vol. 3). Rockville, MD: Agency for Healthcare Research and Quality.

Hurst, S. A. 2008. Vulnerability in research and health care: Describing the elephant in the room? *Bioethics* 22(4):191–202.

IHI (Institute for Healthcare Improvement). 2020. *Psychological PPE: Promote health care workforce mental health and well-being*. http://www.ihi.org/resources/Pages/Tools/psychological-PPE-promote-health-care-workforce-mental-health-and-well-being.aspx (accessed April 9, 2021).

IOM (Institute of Medicine). 2006. *Sleep disorders and sleep deprivation: An unmet public health problem*. Washington, DC: The National Academies Press.

IOM. 2014. *Establishing transdisciplinary professionalism for improving health outcomes: Workshop summary*. Washington, DC: The National Academies Press.

Istepanian, R. S. H., E. Jovanov, and Y. T. Zhang. 2004. Guest editorial introduction to the special section on M-Health: Beyond seamless mobility and global wireless health-care connectivity. *IEEE Transactions on Information Technology in Biomedicine* 8(4):405–414. doi: 10.1109/TITB.2004.840019.

Itzhaki, M., A. Peles-Bortz, H. Kostistky, D. Barnoy, V. Filshtinsky, and I. Bluvstein. 2015. Exposure of mental health nurses to violence associated with job stress, life satisfaction, staff resilience, and post-traumatic growth. *International Journal of Mental Health Nursing* 24(5):403–412.

Jackson, J., V. Vandall-Walker, B. Vanderspank-Wright, P. Wishart, and S. Moore. 2018. Burnout and resilience in critical care nurses: A grounded theory of managing exposure. *Intensive and Critical Care Nursing* 48:28–35.

Jameson, B. E., and F. Bowen. 2018. Use of the worklife and levels of burnout surveys to assess the school nurse work environment. *Journal of School Nursing* 36(4):272–282. doi: 1059840518813697.

Jarrín, O. F., Y. Kang, and L. H. Aiken. 2017. Pathway to better patient care and nurse workforce outcomes in home care. *Nursing Outlook* 65(6):671–678.

Jones, C., and M. Gates. 2007. The costs and benefits of nurse turnover: A business case for nurse retention. *Online Journal of Issues in Nursing* 12(3).

Jordan, G., B. Nowrouzi-Kia, B. Gohar, and B. Nowrouzi. 2015. Obesity as a possible risk factor for lost-time injury in registered nurses: A literature review. *Safety and Health at Work* 6(1):1–8.

Kambhampati, A. K., A. C. O'Halloran, M. Whitaker, S. Magill, N. Chea, S. Chai, P. Kirley, R. Herlihy, B. Kawasaki, J. Meek, K. Yousey-Hindes, E. Anderson, K. Openo, M. Monroe, P. Ryan, S. Kim, L. Reeg, K. Como-Sabetti, R. Danila, S. Shrum Davis, S. Tores, G. Barney, N. Spina, N. Bennett, C. Felsen, L. Billing, J. Shiltz, M. Sutton, N. West, W. Schaffner, H. Keipp Talbot, R. Chatelain, M. Hill, L. Brammer, A. Fry, A. Hall, J. Wortham, S. Garg, L. Kim, and COVID-NET Surveillance Team. 2020. COVID-19-associated hospitalizations among health care personnel—COVID-NET, 13 states, March 1–May 31, 2020. *Morbidity and Mortality Weekly Report* 69(43):1576–1583. doi: 10.15585/mmwr.mm6943e3.

Kang, L., S. Ma, M. Chen, J. Yang, Y. Wang, R. Li, L. Yao, H. Bai, Z. Cai, B. Xiang Yang, S. Hu, K. Zhang, G. Wang, C. Ma, and Z. Liu. 2020. Impact on mental health and perceptions of psychological care among medical and nursing staff in Wuhan during the 2019 novel coronavirus disease outbreak: A cross-sectional study. *Brain, Behavior, and Immunity* 87:11–17.

Kasman, D. L. 2004. When is medical treatment futile? A guide for students, residents, and physicians. *Journal of General Internal Medicine* 19(10):1053–1056.

Kelly, P., and C. Porr. 2018. Ethical nursing care versus cost containment: Considerations to enhance RN practice. *Online Journal of Issues in Nursing* 23(1).

Kelly, M., and J. Wills. 2018. Systematic review: What works to address obesity in nurses? *Occupational Medicine* 68(4):228–238. doi: 10.1093/occmed/kqy038. PMID: 29579241.

Kishore, S., J. Ripp, T. Shanafelt, B. Melnyk, D. Rodgers, T. Brigham, N. Busis, D. Charney, P. Cipriano, L. Minor, P. Rothman, J. Spisso, D. G. Kirch, T. Nasca, and V. Dzau. 2018 (October 26). Making the case for the chief wellness officer in America's health systems: A call to action. *Health Affairs Blog*. doi: 10.1377/hblog20181025.308059.

Kopacz, M., D. Ames, and H. Koenig. 2019. It's time to talk about physician burnout and moral injury. *Lancet Psychiatry* 6(11):e28. doi: 10.1016/S2215-0366(19)30385-2.

Krautscheid, L., L. Mood, S. M. McLennon, T. C. Mossman, M. Wagner, and J. Wode. 2020. Examining relationships between resilience protective factors and moral distress among nursing students. *Nursing Education Perspectives* 41(1):43–45.

Lai, J., S. Ma, Y. Wang, Z. Cai, J. Hu, N. Wei, J. Wu, H. Du, T. Chen, R. Li, H. Tan, L. Kang, L. Yao, M. Huang, H. Wang, G. Wang, Z. Liu, and S. Hu. 2020. Factors associated with mental health outcomes among health care workers exposed to coronavirus disease 2019. *JAMA Network Open* 3(3):e203976.

Landi, H. 2020. Brigham and Women's taps mental health startup to use AI to track providers' stress. *Fierce Healthcare*. https://www.fiercehealthcare.com/tech/brigham-and-women-s-teams-up-mental-health-startup-to-track-providers-stress-during-covid-19 (accessed April 19, 2021).

Larsen, R., J. Ashley, T. Ellens, R. Frauendienst, K. Jorgensen-Royce, and M. Zelenak. 2018. Development of a new graduate public health nurse residency program using the core competencies of public health nursing. *Public Health Nursing* 35(6):606–612.

Lavoie-Tremblay, M., D. Wright, N. Desforges, C. Gélinas, C. Marchionni, and U. Drevniok. 2008. Creating a healthy workplace for new-generation nurses. *Journal of Nursing Scholarship* 40(3):290–297.

Lefton, C. 2012. Strengthening the workforce through meaningful recognition. *Nursing Economics* 30(6):331–338, 355.

Lewin Group. 2009. *Wisdom at work: Retaining experienced RNs and their knowledge—Case studies of top performing organizations*. https://www.rwjf.org/en/library/research/2009/03/wisdom-at-work.html (accessed April 9, 2021).

Li, Y., and C. B. Jones 2013. A literature review of nursing turnover costs. *Journal of Nursing Management* 21(3):405–418.

Liaschenko, J., and E. Peter. 2016. Fostering nurses' moral agency and moral identity: The importance of moral community. *Hastings Center Report* 46(1):S18–S21.

Lomas, T., J. Medina, I. Ivtzan, S. Rupprecht, and F. J. Eiroa Orosa. 2018. Mindfulness-based interventions in the workplace: An inclusive systematic review and meta-analysis of their impact upon wellbeing. *Journal of Positive Psychology* 14:1–16.

Lown, B. A., and C. F. Manning. 2010. The Schwartz Center rounds: Evaluation of an interdisciplinary approach to enhancing patient-centered communication, teamwork, and provider support. *Academic Medicine* 85(6):1073–1081.

Lyzwinski, L. N., L. Caffery, M. Bambling, and S. Edirippulige. 2019. The mindfulness app trial for weight, weight-related behaviors, and stress in university students: Randomized controlled trial. *JMIR Mhealth and Uhealth* 7(4):e12210. doi: 10.2196/12210.

Maben, J., C. Taylor, J. Dawson, M. Leamy, I. McCarthy, E. Reynolds, S. Ross, C. Shuldham, L. Bennett, and C. Foot. 2018. Health services and delivery research. In *A realist informed mixed-methods evaluation of Schwartz Center Rounds® in England*. Southampton, UK: NIHR Journals Library.

Maguen, S., and M. A. Price. 2020. Moral injury in the wake of coronavirus: Attending to the psychological impact of the pandemic. *Psychological Trauma: Theory, Research, Practice, and Policy* 12(S1):S131–S132.

Margaret, J., and H. Came. 2019. Organizing—What do white people need to know to be effective antiracism allies within public health? In *Racism: Science and tools for the public health professional*, edited by C. L. Ford, D. M. Griffith, M. A. Bruce, and K. L. Gilbert. Washington, DC: APHA Press. Pp. 315–326.

Mark, G., and A. P. Smith 2012. Occupational stress, job characteristics, coping, and the mental health of nurses. *British Journal of Health Psychology* 17(3):505–521.

Marks, B., and S. Ailey. 2014. White paper on inclusion of students with disabilities in nursing educational programs for the California Committee on Employment of People with Disabilities (CCEPD). *California Committee on the Employment of People with Disabilities*. doi: 10.13140/RG.2.1.4741.9606.

Marks, B., and K. McCulloh. 2016. Success for students and nurses with disabilities: A call to action for nurse educators. *Nurse Educator* 41(1):9–12.

Maslach, C. 2017. Finding solutions to the problem of burnout. *Consulting Psychology Journal: Practice and Research* 69(2):143–152.

Maslach, C., and S. E. Jackson. 1981. The measurement of experienced burnout. *Journal of Organizational Behavior* 2(2):99–113.

Maslach, C., and M. P. Leiter. 2017. Understanding burnout: New models. In *The handbook of stress and health: A guide to research and practice*, edited by C. L. Cooper and J. C. Quick. Hoboken, NJ: Wiley Blackwell. Pp. 36–56.

Masten, A. 2007. Resilience in developing systems: Progress and promise as the fourth wave rises. *Development and Psychopathology* 19(3):921–930.

Mathad, M. D., B. Pradhan, and S. K. Rajesh. 2017. Correlates and predictors of resilience among baccalaureate nursing students. *Journal of Clinical and Diagnostic Research* 11(2):jc05–jc08.

Mathiews, A., and S. Salmond. 2013. Opening the door to improve visiting nurse safety: An initiative to collect and analyze protection practices and policies. *Home Healthcare Now* 31(6):319–321.

McClelland, L. E., A. S. Gabriel, and M. J. DePuccio. 2018. Compassion practices, nurse well-being, and ambulatory patient experience rating. *Medical Care* 56(1):4–10. doi: 10.1097/MLR.0000000000000834.

McVicar, A. 2003. Workplace stress in nursing: A literature review. *Journal of Advanced Nursing* 44(6):633–642.

Mealer, M., J. Jones, and P. Meek. 2017. Factors affecting resilience and development of posttraumatic stress disorder in critical care nurses. *American Journal of Critical Care* 26(3):184–192.

Meissner, J. E. 1986. Nurses: Are we eating our young? *Nursing* 16(3):51–53.

Melnyk, B. M., L. Orsolini, A. Tan, C. Arslanian-Engoren, G. D'Eramo Melkus, J. Dunbar-Jacob, V. Hill Rice, A. Millan, S. Dunbar, L. Braun, J. Wilbur, D. Chyun, K. Gawlik, and L. Lewis. 2018. A national study links nurses' physical and mental health to medical errors and perceived worksite wellness. *Journal of Occupational and Environmental Medicine* 60(2):126–131.

Melnyk, B. M., S. A. Kelly, J. Stephens, K. Dhakal, C. McGovern, S. Tucker, J. Hoying, K. McRae, S. Ault, E. Spurlock, and S. B. Bird. 2020. Interventions to improve mental health, well-being, physical health, and lifestyle behaviors in physicians and nurses: A systematic review. *American Journal of Health Promotion* 34(8):929–941.

Menschner, C., and A. Maul 2016. *Strategies for encouraging staff wellness in trauma-informed organizations*. Center for Health Care Strategies. https://www.chcs.org/media/ATC-Staff-Wellness-121316_FINAL.pdf (accessed April 9, 2021).

Michalec, B., C. Diefenbeck, and M. Mahoney. 2013. The calm before the storm? Burnout and compassion fatigue among undergraduate nursing students. *Nurse Education Today* 33(4):314–320.

Miliard, M. 2020 (August 17). Brigham and Women's pilots new program to support provider mental health. *Healthcare IT News*. https://www.healthcareitnews.com/news/brigham-and-womens-pilots-new-program-support-provider-mental-health (accessed April 9, 2021).

Monroe, T. B., H. Kenaga, M. S. Dietrich, M. A. Carter, and R. L. Cowan. 2013. The prevalence of employed nurses identified or enrolled in substance use monitoring programs. *Nursing Research* 62(1):10–15.

Moore, L., and E. McAuliffe. 2010. Is inadequate response to whistleblowing perpetuating a culture of silence in hospitals? *Clinical Governance* 15(3).

Moore, L., and E. McAuliffe. 2012. To report or not to report? Why some nurses are reluctant to whistle blow. *Clinical Governance* 17(4).

Morley, G., J. Ives, C. Bradbury-Jones, and F. Irvine. 2019. What is "moral distress"? A narrative synthesis of the literature. *Nursing Ethics* 26(3):646–662. doi: 10.1177/0969733017724354.

Moss, M., V. Good, D. Gozal, R. Kleinpell, and C. Sessler. 2016. A Critical Care Societies Collaborative statement: Burnout syndrome in critical care health-care professionals. A call for action. *American Journal of Respirator and Critical Care Medicine* 194(1):106–113.

Munnangi, S., L. Dupiton, A. Boutin, and G. Angus. 2018. Burnout, perceived stress, and job satisfaction among trauma nurses at a Level I safety-net trauma center. *Journal of Trauma Nursing* 25(1):4–13. doi: 10.1097/JTN.0000000000000335.

Nadal, K. L., C. N. Whitman, L. S. Davis, T. Erazo, and K. C. Davidoff. 2016. Microaggressions toward lesbian, gay, bisexual, transgender, queer, and genderqueer people: A review of the literature. *Journal of Sex Research* 53(4–5):488–508.

NASEM (National Academies of Sciences, Engineering, and Medicine). 2019a. *Taking action against clinician burnout: A systems approach to professional well-being*. Washington, DC: The National Academies Press.

NASEM. 2019b. *Strengthening the military family readiness system for a changing American society*. Washington, DC: The National Academies Press.

NASEM. 2019c. *A design thinking, systems approach to well-being within education and practice: Proceedings of a workshop*. Washington, DC: The National Academies Press.

NCSBN (National Council of State Boards of Nursing). 2011. *Substance use disorder in nursing: A resource manual and guidelines for alternative and disciplinary monitoring programs*. https://www.ncsbn.org/SUDN_11.pdf (accessed April 9, 2021).

Neal-Boylan, L., and D. Smith. 2016. Nursing students with physical disabilities: Dispelling myths and correcting misconceptions. *Nurse Educator* 41(1):13–18.

Neal-Boylan, L., A. Hopkins, R. Skeete, S. B. Hartmann, L. I. Iezzoni, and M. Nunez-Smith. 2012. The career trajectories of health care professionals practicing with permanent disabilities. *Academic Medicine* 87(2):172–178.

Neal-Boylan, L., B. Marks, and K. J. McCulloh. 2015. Supporting nurses and nursing students with disabilities. *American Journal of Nursing* 115(10):11.

Nelson, S. M., and A. E. Lee-Winn. 2020. The mental turmoil of hospital nurses in the COVID-19 pandemic. *Psychological Trauma: Theory, Research, Practice, and Policy* 12(S1):S126–S127.

Nelson, W. A., E. Taylor, and T. Walsh. 2014. Building an ethical organizational culture. *Health Care Management (Frederick)* 33(2):158–164.

Nembhard, I. M., and A. C. Edmondson. 2006. Making it safe: The effects of leader inclusiveness and professional status on psychological safety and improvement efforts in health care teams. *Journal of Organizational Behavior* 27(7):941–966.

Newman, A., R. Donohue, and N. Eva. 2017. Psychological safety: A systematic review of the literature. *Human Resource Management Review* 27.

Northway, R., M. Parker, N. James, L. Davies, K. Johnson, and S. Wilson. 2015. Research teaching in learning disability nursing: Exploring the views of student and registered learning disability nurses. *Nurse Education Today* 35(12):1155–1160. https://nsinursingsolutions.com/Documents/Library/NSI_National_Health_Care_Retention_Report.pdf (accessed October 9, 2020).

Nowrouzi, B., E. Giddens, B. Gohar, S. Schoenenberger, M. Bautista, and J. Casole. 2016. The quality of work life of registered nurses in Canada and the United States: A comprehensive literature review. *International Journal of Occupational and Environmental Health* 22(4):1–18.

NSI Nursing Solutions. 2020. *2020 NSI national health care retention & RN staffing report*. https://www.nsinursingsolutions.com/Documents/Library/NSI_National_Health_Care_Retention_Report.pdf (accessed April 9, 2021).

O'Donovan, R., and E. McAuliffe. 2020. Exploring psychological safety in healthcare teams to inform the development of interventions: Combining observational, survey and interview data. *BMC Health Services Research* 20(1):810.

Okoli, C. T. C., S. Seng, A. Lykins, and J. T. Higgins. 2021. Correlates of post-traumatic growth among nursing professionals: A cross-sectional analysis. *Journal of Nursing Management* 29(2):307–316.

Ommaya, A. K., P. F. Cipriano, D. B. Hoyt, K. A. Horvath, P. Tang, H. L. Paz, M. S. DeFrancesco, S. T. Hingle, S. Butler and C. A. Sinsky. 2018. *Care-centered clinical documentation in the digital environment: Solutions to alleviate burnout. NAM Perspectives*. Discussion Paper. Washington, DC: National Academy of Medicine. doi: 10.31478/201801c.

ONC (Office of the National Coordinator for Health Information Technology). 2020. *Strategy on reducing regulatory and administrative burden relating to the use of health IT and EHRs: Final Report*. https://www.healthit.gov/sites/default/files/page/2020-02/BurdenReport_0.pdf (accessed April 9, 2021).

Ong, A. D., and A. L. Burrow. 2017. Microaggressions and daily experience: Depicting life as it is lived. *Perspectives on Psychological Science* 12(1):173–175.

OSHA (Occupational Safety and Health Administration). 2015. *Workplace violence in healthcare*. https://www.osha.gov/sites/default/files/OSHA3826.pdf (accessed April 9, 2021).

OSHA. n.d. *Healthcare overview*. https://www.osha.gov/healthcare (accessed April 9, 2021).

Oyama, Y., Y. Yonekura, and H. Fukahori. 2015. Nurse health-related quality of life: Associations with patient and ward characteristics in Japanese general acute care wards. *Journal of Nursing Management* 23(6):775–783.

Park, Y-T. 2016. Emerging new era of mobile health technologies. *Healthcare Informatics Research* 22(4):253–254. doi: 10.4258/hir.2016.22.4.253.

Paul-Emile, K. 2012. Patient racial preferences and the medical culture of accommodation. *UCLA Law Review* 60:462.

Paul-Emile, K., A. K. Smith, B. Lo, and A. Fernández. 2016. Dealing with racist patients. *New England Journal of Medicine* 374(8):708–711.

Pavlish, C. L., J. Henriksen, K. Brown-Saltzman, E. M. Robinson, U. S. Warda, C. Farra, B. Chen, and P. Jakel. 2020. A team-based early action protocol to address ethical concerns in the intensive care unit. *American Journal of Critical Care* 29(1):49–61.

Pearce, K. 2020. In fight against COVID-19, nurses face high-stakes decisions, moral distress. *Johns Hopkins University HUB*. https://hub.jhu.edu/2020/04/06/COVID-nursing-cynda-rushton-qa (accessed April 9, 2021).

Peters, E. 2018. Compassion fatigue in nursing: A concept analysis. *Nursing Forum* 53(4):466–480.

Peterson, A. L. 2017. Experiencing stigma as a nurse with mental illness. *Journal of Psychiatric and Mental Health Nursing* 24(5):314–321.

Pfeifer, L. E., and J. A. Vessey. 2017. An integrative review of bullying and lateral violence among nurses in Magnet® organizations. *Policy, Politics, and Nursing Practice* 18(3):113–124.

Plsek, P. E., and T. Greenhalgh. 2001. The challenge of complexity in health care. *British Medical Journal* 323(7313):625–628.

Prilleltensky, I. 2012. Wellness as fairness. *American Journal of Community Psychology* 49(1–2):1–21.

Querstret, D., K. O'Brien, D. J. Skene, and J. Maben. 2020. Improving fatigue risk management in health care: A scoping review of sleep-related/fatigue management interventions for nurses and midwives. *International Journal of Nursing Studies* 106. https://doi.org/10.1016/j.ijnurstu.2020.103745.

Rangachari, P., and J. L. Woods. 2020. Preserving organizational resilience, patient safety, and staff retention during COVID-19 requires a holistic consideration of the psychological safety of healthcare workers. *International Journal of Environmental Research and Public Health* 17(12):4267.

Rathbone, A. L., and J. Prescott. 2017. The use of mobile apps and SMS messaging as physical and mental health interventions: Systematic review. *Journal of Medical Internet Research* 19(8):e295.

Rathert, C., J. Mittler, and L. McClelland. 2016. Caring health care work environments and patient-centered care. In *The evolving healthcare landscape: How employees, organizations, and institutions are adapting and innovating*, edited by A. Avgar and T. Vogus. Champaign, IL: Labor and Employment Relations Association.

Rauch, S. 2019. Medicalizing the disclosure of mental health: Transnational perspectives of ethical workplace policy among healthcare workers. *World Medical and Health Policy* 11(4):424–439.

Richards, C. 2020. Wisdom from nurses. *Wikiwisdom Forum*. New Voice Strategies, John Hopkins School of Nursing, and *American Journal of Nursing*. https://static1.squarespace.com/static/5c237f83f2e6b174633d77df/t/5f5bddf47d362d682dfeb547/1599856128213/WikiWisdom-Nurses.pdf (accessed April 9, 2021).

Ríos-Risquez, M. I., M. García-Izquierdo, E. de Los Ángeles Sabuco-Tebar, C. Carrillo-Garcia, and C. Solano-Ruiz. 2018. Connections between academic burnout, resilience, and psychological well-being in nursing students: A longitudinal study. *Journal of Advanced Nursing* 74(12):2777–2784.

Robichaux, C. 2012. Developing ethical skills: From sensitivity to action. *Critical Care Nurse* 32(2):65–72.

Robinson, E. M., S. M. Lee, A. Zollfrank, M. Jurchak, D. Frost, and P. Grace. 2014. Enhancing moral agency: Clinical ethics residency for nurses. *Hastings Center Report* 44(5):12–20.

Rosa, W. E, A. E. Schlak, and C. Rushton. 2020. A blueprint for leadership during COVID-19: Minimizing burnout and moral distress among the nursing workforce. *Nursing Management* 51(8):28–34. doi: 10.1097/01.NUMA.0000688940.29231.6f.

Ross, A., M. Bevans, A. T. Brooks, S. Gibbons, and G. R. Wallen. 2017. Nurses and health-promoting behaviors: Knowledge may not translate into self-care. *Association of Perioperative Registered Nurses* 105(3):267–275.

Rouse, W. 2008. Health care as a complex adaptive system: Implications for design and management. *Bridge: Linking Engineering and Society* 38(1):17–25. Washington, DC: National Academy of Engineering.

Rudman, A., and J. P. Gustavsson. 2012. Burnout during nursing education predicts lower occupational preparedness and future clinical performance: A longitudinal study. *International Journal of Nursing Studies* 49(8):988–1001.

Rushton, C. H. 2006. Defining and addressing moral distress: Tools for critical care nursing leaders. *AACN Advanced Critical Care* 17(2):161–168. https://pubmed.ncbi.nlm.nih.gov/16767017 (accessed April 9, 2021).

Rushton, C. H. 2018. *Moral resilience: Transforming moral suffering in healthcare*. New York: Oxford University Press.

Rushton, C., and S. Pappas. 2020. System recommendations to address burnout and support clinician well-being: Implications for critical care nurses. *AACN Advanced Critical Care* 31(2):141–145.

Rushton C. H., and M. Sharma. 2018. Designing sustainable systems for ethical practice. In *Moral resilience: Transforming moral suffering in healthcare*, edited by C. H. Rushton. New York: Oxford University Press. Pp. 206–242.

Rushton, C. H., J. Batcheller, K. Schroeder, and P. Donohue. 2015. Burnout and resilience among nurses practicing in high-intensity settings. *American Journal of Critical Care* 24(5):412–420.

Rushton, C. H., M. Caldwell, and M. Kurtz. 2016. Moral distress: A catalyst in building moral resilience. *American Journal of Nursing* 116(7):40–49.

Rushton, C., S. Swoboda, N. Reller, K. Skrupski, M. Prizzi, P. Young, and G. Hanson. 2021. Mindful ethical practice and resilience academy: Equipping nurses to address ethical challenges. *American Journal of Critical Care* 30(1):e1–e11. doi: 10.4037/ajcc2021359.

Russell, K. 2020. Components of nurse substance use disorder monitoring programs. *Journal of Nursing Regulation* 11(2):20–27.

Rutherford, D. E., G. L. Gillespie, and C. R. Smith. 2019. Interventions against bullying of prelicensure students and nursing professionals: An integrative review. *Nursing Forum* 54(1):84–90.

Salyers, M. P., K. A. Bonfils, L. Luther, R. Firmin, D. White, E. Adams, and A. Rollins. 2017. The relationship between professional burnout and quality and safety in healthcare: A meta-analysis. *Journal of General Internal Medicine* 32(4):475–482. doi: 10.1007/s11606-016-3886-9.

SAMHSA (Substance Abuse and Mental Health Services Administration). 2000. Ethical issues. In *Substance abuse treatment for persons with HIV/AIDS*. Treatment Improvement Protocol (TIP) Series, No. 37. Rockville, MD: Center for Substance Abuse Treatment, Substance Abuse and Mental Health Services Administration. https://www.ncbi.nlm.nih.gov/books/NBK64933 (accessed April 9, 2021).

Sampson, M., B. M. Melnyk, and J. Hoying. 2019. Intervention effects of the MINDBODYSTRONG cognitive behavioral skills-building program on newly licensed registered nurses' mental health, healthy lifestyle behaviors and job satisfaction. *Journal of Nursing Administration* 49(10):487–495.

Sampson, M., B. M. Melnyk, and J. Hoying. 2020. The MINDBODYSTRONG intervention for new nurse residents: 6-month effects on mental health outcomes, healthy lifestyle behaviors, and job satisfaction. *Worldviews on Evidence Based Nursing* 17(1):16–23.

Sarna, L., S. A. Bialous, K. Nandy, A. L. M. Antonio, and Q. Yang. 2014. Changes in smoking prevalences among health care professionals from 2003 to 2010–2011. *Journal of the American Medical Association* 311(2):197–199. https://doi.org/10.1001/jama.2013.284871.

Sarna, L., P. J. Hollen, J. Heath, and S. A. Bialous. 2019. Increased adoption of smoke-free policies on campuses with schools of nursing. *Nursing Outlook* 67(6):760–764.

Sauerland, J., K. Marotta, M. A. Peinemann, A. Berndt, and C. Robichaux. 2014. Assessing and addressing moral distress and ethical climate, part 1. *Dimensions of Critical Care Nursing* 33(4):234–245.

Schulte, P. A., G. R. Wagner, A. Ostry, L. A. Blanciforti, R. G. Cutlip, K. M. Krajnak, M. Luster, A. E. Munson, J. P. O'Callaghan, C. G. Parks, P. P. Simeonova, and D. B. Miller. 2007. Work, obesity, and occupational safety and health. *American Journal of Public Health* 97(3):428–436.

Schuster, M., and P. A. Dwyer. 2020. Post-traumatic stress disorder in nurses: An integrative review. *Journal of Clinical Nursing* 29:2769–2787. doi: 10.1111/jocn.15288.

Shanafelt, T. D., and J. H. Noseworthy. 2017. Executive leadership and physician well-being: Nine organizational strategies to promote engagement and reduce burnout. *Mayo Clinic Proceedings* 92(1):129–146.

Shanafelt, T. D., L. N. Dyrbye, C. Sinsky, O. Hasan, D. Satele, J. Sloan, and C. P. West. 2016. Relationship between clerical burden and characteristics of the electronic environment with physician burnout and professional satisfaction. *Mayo Clinic Proceedings* 91(7):836–848.

Shanafelt, T. D., D. J. Lightner, C. R. Conley, S. P. Petrou, J. W. Richardson, P. J. Schroeder, and W. A. Brown. 2017. An organization model to assist individual physicians, scientists, and senior health care administrators with personal and professional needs. *Mayo Clinic Proceedings* 92(11):1688–1696.

Shapiro, M. 2020. *Johns Hopkins helps patients and families stay connected when COVID-19 prohibits visits*. https://www.hopkinsmedicine.org/coronavirus/articles/stay-connected.html (accessed December 13, 2020).

Shapiro, S., J. Astin, S. Bishop, and M. Cordova. 2005. Mindfulness-based stress reduction for health care professionals: Results from a randomized trial. *International Journal of Stress Management* 12:164–176.

Shay, J. 2014. Moral injury. *Psychoanalytic Psychology* 31(2):182–191.

Shechter, A., F. Diaz, N, Moise, D. E. Anstey, S. Ye, S. Agarwal, J. Birk, D. Brodie, D. Cannone, B. Chang, J. Claassen, T. Cornelius, L. Derby, M. Dong, R. Givens, B. Hochman, S. Homma, I. Kronish, S. Lee, W. Manzano, L. Mayer, C. McMurry, V. Moitra, P. Pham, L. Rabbani, R.

Rivera, A. Schwartz, P. Shapiro, K. Shaw, A. Sullivan, C. Vose, L. Wasson, D. Edmondson, and M. Abdalla. 2020. Psychological distress, coping behaviors, and preferences for support among New York healthcare workers during the COVID-19 pandemic. *General Hospital Psychiatry* 66:1–8. doi: 10.1016/j.genhosppsych.2020.06.007.

Singleton, O., B. K. Hölzel, M. Vangel, N. Brach, J. Carmody, and S. W. Lazar. 2014. Change in brainstem gray matter concentration following a mindfulness-based intervention is correlated with improvement in psychological well-being. *Frontiers in Human Neuroscience* 8:33.

Sinsky, C. L., and M. Linzer. 2020. Practice and policy reset post COVID-19: Reversion, transition, or transformation? *Health Affairs* 8:1405–1411.

Sinsky, C., L. Colligan, L. Li, M. Prgomet, S. Reynolds, L. Goeders, J. Westbrook, M. Tutty, and G. Blike. 2016. Allocation of physician time in ambulatory practice: A time and motion study in 4 specialties. *Annals of Internal Medicine* 165(11):753–760.

Slavin, S. J., D. Schindler, J. T. Chibnall, G. Fendell, and M. Shoss. 2012. PERMA: A model for institutional leadership and culture change. *Academic Medicine* 87(11):1481.

Smiley, R., and K. Reneau. 2020. Outcomes of substance use disorder monitoring programs for nurses. *Journal of Nursing Regulation* 11(2):28–35.

Song, Y., and R. Lindquist. 2015. Effects of mindfulness-based stress reduction on depression, anxiety, stress and mindfulness in Korean nursing students. *Nurse Education Today* 35(1):86–90.

Spence Laschinger, H. K., and R. Fida. 2014. New nurses burnout and workplace well-being: The influence of authentic leadership and psychological capital. *Burnout Research* 1(1):19–28.

Spence Laschinger, H. K., M. Leiter, A. Day, and D. Gilin. 2009. Workplace empowerment, incivility, and burnout: Impact on staff nurse recruitment and retention outcomes. *Journal of Nursing Management* 17(3):302–311.

Spence Laschinger, H. K., C. Wong, and A. Grau. 2012. The influence of authentic leadership on newly graduated nurses' experiences of workplace bullying, burnout and retention outcomes: A cross-sectional study. *International Journal of Nursing Studies* 49(10):1266–1276.

Speroni, K. G., T. Fitch, E. Dawson, L. Dugan, and M. Atherton. 2014. Incidence and cost of nurse workplace violence perpetrated by hospital patients or patient visitors. *Journal of Emergency Nursing* 40(3):218–228.

Squires, A., M. Clark-Cutaia, M. Henderson, G. Arneson, and P. Resnik. 2020. *Working paper: Working the frontlines of the COVID-19 pandemic: Perspectives of US nurses*. New York: Rory Meyers College of Nursing.

Stacey, G., G. Cook, A. Aubeeluck, B. Stranks, L. Long, M. Krepa, and K. Lucre. 2020. The implementation of resilience based clinical supervision to support transition to practice in newly qualified healthcare professionals. *Nurse Education Today* 94:104564.

Stanulewicz, N., E. Knox, M. Narayanasamy, N. Shivji, K. Khunti, and H. Blake. 2020. Effectiveness of lifestyle health promotion interventions for nurses: A systematic review. *International Journal of Environmental Research and Public Health* 17(1):17. doi: 10.3390/ijerph17010017.

Stephens, T. M. 2013. Nursing student resilience: A concept clarification. *Nursing Forum* 48(2): 125–133.

Stimpfel, A. W., D. Sloane, and L. Aiken. 2012. The longer the shifts for hospital nurses, the higher the levels of burnout and patient dissatisfaction. *Health Affairs (Millwood)* 31(11):2501–2509. doi: 10.1377/hlthaff.2011.1377.

Stimpfel, A. W., C. S. Brewer, and C. T. Kovner. 2015. Scheduling and shift work characteristics associated with risk for occupational injury in newly licensed registered nurses: An observational study. *International Journal of Nursing Studies* 52(11):1686–1693.

Stokes-Parish, J., R. Elliott, K. Rolls, and D. Massey. 2020. Angels and heroes: The unintended consequence of the hero narrative. *Journal of Nursing Scholarship* 52(5):462–466.

Strobbe, S., and M. Crowley. 2017. Substance use among nurses and nursing students: A joint position statement of the Emergency Nurses Association and the International Nurses Society on Addictions. *Journal of Addictions Nursing* 28(2):104–106.

Subhi, Y., S. H. Bube, S. Rolskov Bojsen, A. S. Skou Thomsen, and L. Konge. 2015. Expert involvement and adherence to medical evidence in medical mobile phone apps: A systematic review. *JMIR mHealth and uHealth* 3(3):e79.

Sue, D. W., C. M. Capodilupo, G. C. Torino, J. M. Bucceri, A. M. B. Holder, K. L. Nadal, and M. Esquilin. 2007. Racial microaggressions in everyday life: Implications for clinical practice. *American Psychologist* 62(4):271–286.

Szanton, S. L., L. K. Mihaly, J. Alhusen, and K. L. Becker. 2010. Taking charge of the challenge: Factors to consider in taking your first nurse practitioner job. *Journal of the American Academy of Nurse Practitioners* 22(7):356–360.

Tai-seale, M., C. Olson, J. Li, A. Chan, C. Morikawa, M. Durbin, W. Wang, and H. Luft. 2017. Electronic health record logs indicate that physicians split time evenly between seeing patients and desktop medicine. *Health Affairs* 36(4):655–662.

Tarcan, M., N. Hikmet, B. Schooley, M. Top, and G. Y. Tarcan. 2017. An analysis of the relationship between burnout, socio-demographic and workplace factors and job satisfaction among emergency department health professionals. *Applied Nursing Research* 34:40–47. doi: 10.1016/j.apnr.2017.02.011.

Taylor, R. A. 2019. Contemporary issues: Resilience training alone is an incomplete intervention. *Nurse Education Today* 78:10–13.

Terry, D., Q. Le, U. Nguyen, and H. Hoang. 2015. Workplace health and safety issues among community nurses: A study regarding the impact on providing care to rural consumers. *BMJ Open* 5(8):08306. PMID: PMC4538262.

Thomas, L. J., and S. H. Revell. 2016. Resilience in nursing students: An integrative review. *Nurse Education Today* 36:457–462.

Thompson, L. J. 2018. *Moral dimensions of wellbeing*. Paper presented at the Society for Business Ethics Annual Conference, Chicago IL, August 10–12, 2018.

Traudt, T., J. Liaschenko, and C. Peden-McAlpine. 2016. Moral agency, moral imagination, and moral community: Antidotes to moral distress. *Journal of Clinical Ethics* 27(3):201–213.

Trinkoff, A. M., J. M. Geiger-Brown, C. C. Caruso, J. A. Lipscomb, M. Johantgen, A. L. Nelson, B. A. Sattler, and V. L. Selby. 2008. Personal safety for nurses. In *Patient safety and quality: An evidence-based handbook for nurses*. Advances in Patient Safety. Rockville, MD: Agency for Healthcare Research and Quality.

Trotochaud, K., H. Fitzgerald, and A. D. Knackstedt. 2018. Ethics champion programs. *American Journal of Nursing* 118(7):46–54.

Ulrich, B., C. Barden, L. Cassidy, and N. Varn-Davis. 2019. Critical care nurse work environments 2018: Findings and implications. *Critical Care Nurse* 39(2):67–84.

Ulrich, C. M. 2020. The moral distress of patients and families. *American Journal of Bioethics* 20(6):68–70.

Ulrich, C. M., and C. Grady (eds.). 2018. *Moral distress in the health professions*. Cham, Switzerland: Springer Nature.

Ulrich, C. M., C. H. Rushton, and C. Grady. 2020. Nurses confronting the coronavirus: Challenges met and lessons learned to date. *Nursing Outlook* 68(6):838–844.

Ünal, A., and S. Seren. 2016. Medical error reporting attitudes of healthcare personnel, barriers and solutions: A literature review. *The Journal of Nursing Care* 5:1–8.

Vaismoradi, M., S. Tella, P. A. Logan, J. Khakurel, and F. Vizcaya-Moreno. 2020. Nurses' adherence to patient safety principles: A systematic review. *International Journal of Environmental Research and Public Health* 17(6).

Van Hoek, G., M. Portzky, and E. Franck. 2019. The influence of socio-demographic factors, resilience and stress reducing activities on academic outcomes of undergraduate nursing students: A cross-sectional research study. *Nurse Education Today* 72:90–96.

Waite, R., and D. Nardi. 2019. Nursing colonialism in America: Implications for nursing leadership. *Journal of Professional Nursing* 35(1):18–25.

Walsh, E. S., and D. Freshwater. 2009. The mental well-being of prison nurses in England and Wales. *Journal of Researching in Nursing* 14(6):553–564.

Wang, K., D. S. Varma, and M. Prosperi. 2018. A systematic review of the effectiveness of mobile apps for monitoring and management of mental health symptoms or disorders. *Journal of Psychiatric Research* 107:73–78.

Wasson, R. S., C. Barratt, and W. H. O'Brien. 2020. Effects of mindfulness-based interventions on self-compassion in health care professionals: A meta-analysis. *Mindfulness* 11(8):1914–1934.

Weaver, K. B. 2013. The effects of horizontal violence and bullying on new nurse retention. *Journal for Nurses in Professional Development* 29(3):138–142. PMID: 23703273.

Wech, B. A., J. Howard, and P. Autrey. 2020. Workplace bullying model: A qualitative study on bullying in hospitals. *Employee Responsibilities and Rights Journal* 32(73):73–96.

Wei, H., K. A. Sewell, G. Woody, and M. A. Rose. 2018. The state of the science of nurse work environments in the United States: A systematic review. *International Journal of Nursing Sciences* 5(3):287–300.

Welker-Hood, K. 2014. Underfunding and undervaluing the public health infrastructure: Reinforcing the haves and the have-nots in health. *Public Health Nursing* 31(6):481–483.

WHO (World Health Organization). 2004. *Promoting mental health—Concepts, emerging evidence, practice: Summary report*. World Health Organization, Department of Mental Health and Substance Abuse, in collaboration with the Victorian Health Promotion Foundation and the University of Melbourne. Geneva, Switzerland: World Health Organization.

WHO. 2011. mHealth: New horizons for health through mobile technologies. *Global Observatory for eHealth Series* 3. https://www.who.int/goe/publications/goe_mhealth_web.pdf (accessed April 9, 2021).

Williams, D. R., and L. Cooper. 2019. Reducing racial inequities in health: Using what we already know to take action. *International Journal of Environmental Research and Public Health* 16. doi: 10.3390/ijerph16040606.

Williams, D. R., J. A. Lawrence, and B. A. Davis. 2019. Racism and health: Evidence and needed research. *Annual Review of Public Health* 40:105–125.

Williams, R. D., J. A. Brundage, and E. B. Williams. 2020. Moral injury in times of COVID-19. *Journal of Health Service Psychology* 46:65–69. doi: 10.1007/s42843-020-00011-4.

Wocial, L. D., M. Hancock, P. D. Bledsoe, A. R. Chamness, and P. R. Helft. 2010. An evaluation of unit-based ethics conversations. *JONA's Healthcare Law, Ethics and Regulation* 12(2):48–54.

Wojciechowski, M. 2020 (July 2). Racism: Beginning the conversation. *Minority Nurse Blog, Nursing Diversity*. https://minoritynurse.com/racism-beginning-the-conversation (accessed April 9, 2021).

Wolf, L. A., C. Perhats, A. M. Delao, M. D. Moon, P. R. Clark, and K. E. Zavotsky. 2016. It's a burden you carry: Describing moral distress in emergency nursing. *Journal of Emergency Nursing* 42(1):37–46. doi: 10.1016/j.jen.2015.08.008.

Wolf, A. T., K. R. White, E. G. Epstein, and K. B. Enfield. 2019. Palliative care and moral distress: An institutional survey of critical care nurses. *Critical Care Nurse* 39(5):38–49.

Wood, A. E., P. Prins, N. E. Bush, J. F. Hsia, L. E. Bourn, M. D. Earley, R. D. Walser, and J. Ruzek. 2017. Reduction of burnout in mental health care providers using the provider resilience mobile application. *Community Mental Health Journal* 53(4):452–459. doi: 10.1007/s10597-016-0076-5.

Woodward, E. L., L. Northrop, and B. Edelstein. 2016. Stress, social support, and burnout among long-term care nursing staff. *Journal of Applied Gerontology* 35(1):84–105.

Worley, J. 2017. Nurses with substance use disorders: Where we are and what needs to be done. *Journal of Psychosocial Nursing and Mental Health Services* 55(12):11–14.

Yau, Y. H., and M. N. Potenza. 2013. Stress and eating behaviors. *Minerva Endocrinology* 38(3):255–267.

Yu, F., D. Raphael, L. Mackay, M. Smith, and A. King. 2019. Personal and work-related factors associated with nurse resilience: A systematic review. *International Journal of Nursing Studies* 93:129–140.

Yue, L., V. Plummer, and W. Cross. 2016. The effectiveness of nurse education and training for clinical alarm response and management: A systematic review. *Journal of Clinical Nursing* 26:2511–2526.

11

The Future of Nursing: Recommendations and Research Priorities

The next 10 years will test the nation's nearly 4 million nurses in new and complex ways. Nurses live and work at the intersection of health, education, and communities. In the decade since the prior *The Future of Nursing* report was published (IOM, 2011), the world has come to understand the critical importance of health to all aspects of life, particularly the relationship among social determinants of health (SDOH), health equity, and health outcomes. Consistent with this broader understanding, the National Advisory Council on Nurse Education and Practice (NACNEP) (2020) advanced an important set of recommendations that the committee endorses. The NACNEP report *Integration of Social Determinants of Health in Nursing Education, Practice, and Research* conveys the importance of investing in SDOH and research to strengthen the nursing workforce and help nurses provide more effective care, as well as design, implement, and assess new care models.

In a year that was designated to honor and uplift nursing (the International Year of the Nurse and the Midwife 2020[1]), nurses have been placed in unimaginable circumstances by the COVID-19 pandemic. The decade ahead will demand a stronger, more diversified workforce that is prepared to provide care; promote health and well-being among nurses, individuals, and communities; and address the systemic inequities that have fueled wide and persistent health disparities.

The COVID-19 pandemic has revealed in the starkest terms that illness and access to quality health care are unequally distributed across groups and commu-

[1] See https://www.who.int/campaigns/annual-theme/year-of-the-nurse-and-the-midwife-2020 (accessed April 12, 2021).

nities, and has spotlighted the reality that much of what affects health happens outside of medical care. The pandemic and continued calls for racial justice have illuminated the extent to which structural racism—from decades of neglect and disinvestment in neighborhoods, schools, communities, and health care to discrimination and bias—has placed communities of color at much higher risk for poor health and well-being.

The committee's recommendations call for change at both the individual and system levels, constituting a call for action to the nation's largest health care workforce, including nurses in all settings and at all levels, to listen, engage, deeply examine practices, collect evidence, and act to move the country toward greater health equity for all. The committee's recommendations also are targeted to the actions required of policy makers, educators, health care system leaders, and payers to enable these crucial changes, supported by the research agenda with which this chapter concludes. With implementation of this report's recommendations, the committee envisions 10 outcomes that position the nursing profession to contribute meaningfully to achieving health equity (see Box 11-1).

In this chapter, the committee provides its recommendations for charting a 10-year path forward to enable and support today's and the next generation of nurses to create fair and just opportunities for health and well-being for

BOX 11-1
Achieving Health Equity Through Nursing: Desired Outcomes

- Nurses are prepared to act individually, through teams, and across sectors to meet challenges associated with an aging population, access to primary care, mental and behavioral health problems, structural racism, high maternal mortality and morbidity, and elimination of the disproportionate disease burden carried by specific segments of the U.S. population.
- Nurses are fully engaged in addressing the underlying causes of poor health. Individually and in partnership with other disciplines and sectors, nurses act on a wide range of factors that influence how well and long people live, helping to create individual- and community-targeted solutions, including a health in all policies orientation.
- Nurses reflect the people and communities served throughout the nation, helping to ensure that individuals receive culturally competent, equitable health care services.
- Health care systems enable and support nurses to tailor care to meet the specific medical and social needs of diverse patients to optimize their health.
- Nurses' overarching contributions, especially those found to be beneficial during the COVID-19 pandemic, are quantified, extended, and strengthened, including the removal of institutional and regulatory barriers that have pre-

everyone. These recommendations are aimed at all nurses, including those working in hospitals, schools, and health departments; policy makers; educators; health care system leaders; and payers. The chapter concludes with a research agenda to fill current and critical gaps that would support this future-oriented path.

CREATING A SHARED AGENDA

In order for nurses to engage fully in efforts to achieve health equity, it will be necessary for nursing organizations to work together to identify priorities for education, practice, and policy, and to develop mechanisms for leveraging existing nursing expertise and resources. Creating a shared agenda will focus efforts and ensure that all nurses—no matter where they are educated or where they practice—are prepared, supported, and empowered to address SDOH and eliminate inequities in health and health care.

Recommendation 1: In 2021, all national nursing organizations should initiate work to develop a shared agenda for addressing social determinants of health and achieving health equity. This agenda should include explicit priorities across nursing practice, education, leadership, and health policy

vented nurses from working to the full extent of their education and training. Practice settings that were historically undercompensated, such as public health and school nursing, are reimbursed for nursing services in a manner comparable to that of other settings.

- Nurses and other leaders in health care and public health create organizational structures and processes that facilitate the profession's expedited acquisition of relevant content expertise to serve flexibly in areas of greatest need in times of public health emergencies and disasters.
- Nurses consistently incorporate a health equity lens learned through revamped academic and continuing education.
- Nurses collaborate across their affiliated organizations to develop and deploy a shared agenda to contribute to substantial, measurable improvement in health equity. National nursing organizations reflect an orientation of diversity, equity, and inclusion within and across their organizations.
- Nurses focus on preventive person-centered care and have an orientation toward innovation, always seeking new opportunities for growth and development. They expand their roles, work in new settings and in new ways, and markedly expand their partnerships connecting health and health care with all individuals and communities.
- Nurses attend to their own self-care and help to ensure that nurse well-being is addressed in educational and employment settings through the implementation of evidence-based strategies.

engagement. The Tri-Council for Nursing[2] and the Council of Public Health Nursing Organizations,[3] with their associated member organizations, should work collaboratively and leverage their respective expertise in leading this agenda-setting process. Relevant expertise should be identified and shared across national nursing organizations, including the Federal Nursing Service Council[4] and the National Coalition of Ethnic Minority Nurse Associations. With support from the government, payers, health and health care organizations, and foundations, the implementation of this agenda should include associated timelines and metrics for measuring impact.

Specific actions should include the following:

- Within nursing organizations:
  - Assess diversity, equity, and inclusion, and eliminate policies, regulations, and systems that perpetuate structural racism, cultural racism, and discrimination with respect to identity (e.g., sexual orientation, gender), place (e.g., rural, inner city), and circumstances (e.g., disabilities, depression).
- Across nursing organizations:
  - Develop mechanisms for leveraging the expertise of public health nursing (e.g., in population health, SDOH, community-level assessment) as a resource for the broader nursing community, health plans, and health systems, as well as public policy makers.
  - Develop mechanisms for leveraging the expertise of relevant nursing organizations in care coordination and care management. Care coordination and care management principles, approaches, and evidence should be used to create new cross-sector models for meeting social needs and addressing SDOH.
  - Develop mechanisms for prioritizing and sharing continuing education and skill-training resources focused on nurses' health, well-being, resilience, and self-care to ensure a healthy nursing workforce.

---

[2] The Tri-Council for Nursing includes the following organizations as members: the American Association of Colleges of Nursing, the American Nurses Association, the American Organization for Nursing Leadership, the National Council of State Boards of Nursing, and the National League for Nursing.

[3] The Council of Public Health Nursing Organizations includes the following organizations as members: the Alliance of Nurses for Healthy Environments, the American Nurses Association, the American Public Health Association—Public Health Nursing Section, the Association of Community Health Nursing Educators, the Association of Public Health Nurses, and the Rural Nurse Organization.

[4] The Federal Nursing Service Council is a united federal nursing leadership team representing the U.S. Army, Air Force, Navy, National Guard and Reserves, Public Health Service Commissioned Corps, American Red Cross, U.S. Department of Veteran Affairs, and the Uniformed Services University of the Health Sciences Graduate School of Nursing.

These resources should be used by nurses and others in leadership positions.

- External to nursing organizations:
    - Develop and use communication strategies, including social media, to amplify for the public, policy makers, and the media nursing research and expertise on health equity–related issues.
    - Increase the number and diversity of nurses, especially those with expertise in health equity, population health, and SDOH, on boards and in other leadership positions within and outside of health care (e.g., community boards, housing authorities, school boards, technology-related positions).
    - Establish a joint annual award or series of awards recognizing the measurable and scalable contributions of nurses and their partners to achieving health equity through policy, education, research, and practice. Priority should be given to interprofessional and multisector collaboration.

SUPPORTING NURSES TO ADVANCE HEALTH EQUITY

Promoting health and well-being for all should be a national priority, and a collective and sustained commitment is needed to achieve this priority. To chart this path, nurses should be fully supported with robust education, resources, and autonomy. Key stakeholders should commit to investing fully in strengthening and diversifying the nursing workforce so that it is sufficiently prepared to promote health and appropriately reflects the people and communities it serves. Nursing schools, health care institutions, and public health and community health organizations can do significantly more to empower nurses to raise their voices and use their considerable expertise to improve people's lives, health, and well-being.

Recommendation 2: By 2023, state and federal government agencies, health care and public health organizations, payers, and foundations should initiate substantive actions to enable the nursing workforce to address social determinants of health and health equity more comprehensively, regardless of practice setting.

This can be accomplished through the following actions:

- Rapidly increase both the number of nurses with expertise in health equity and the number of nurses in specialties with significant shortages, including public and community health, behavioral health, primary care, long-term care, geriatrics, school health, and maternal health. The Health Resources and Services Administration (HRSA), the Substance

Abuse and Mental Health Services Administration, the Centers for Disease Control and Prevention (CDC), and state governments should support this effort through workforce planning and funding.

- Provide major investments for nursing education and traineeships in public health, including through state-level workforce programs; foundations; and the U.S. Department of Health and Human Services' (HHS's) HRSA (including nursing workforce programs and Maternal and Child Health Bureau programs), CDC (including the National Center for Environmental Health), and the Office of Minority Health.
- State governments, foundations, employers, and HRSA should direct funds to nurses and nursing schools to sustain and increase the gender, geographic, and racial diversity of the licensed practical nurse (LPN), registered nurse (RN), and advanced practice registered nurse (APRN) workforce.
- HRSA and the Indian Health Service (IHS) should make substantial investments in nurse loan and scholarship programs to address nurse shortages, including in public health, in health professional shortage areas for HRSA, and in IHS designated sites; and invest in technical assistance that focuses on nurse retention.
- In all relevant Title 8 programs, HRSA should prioritize longitudinal community-based learning opportunities that address social needs, population health, SDOH, and health equity. These experiences should be established through academic–community-based partnerships.
- Foundations, state government workforce programs, and the federal government should support the academic progression of socioeconomically disadvantaged students by encouraging partnerships among baccalaureate and higher-degree nursing programs and community colleges; tribal colleges; historically Black colleges and universities; Hispanic-serving colleges and universities; and nursing programs that serve a high percentage of Asian, Native Hawaiian, and Pacific Islander students.
- HHS should establish a National Nursing Workforce Commission or alternatively, significantly invest in and enhance the current capacity of HRSA's National Advisory Council on Nurse Education and Practice. The membership of this body should comprise public and private health care payers, employers, government agencies, nurses, representatives of other health professions, and consumers, all from diverse backgrounds and sectors. This entity would:
    - Report on and propose actions to fill critical gaps in the current nursing workforce and prepare the future workforce to address health equity.

- Use findings, including those from workforce centers, on the diversity, capacity, supply, and distribution of nurses; associated competencies; and organizational support for the nursing workforce in addressing social needs, SDOH, and health equity. Recommend actions to ensure nurses' continued engagement in these areas.
- Further develop recommendations for nursing education and practice with respect to addressing social needs, SDOH, and health equity, and assess the implications of these changes for nurse credentialing and regulatory actions.
- Identify and address gaps in evidence-based nursing and interprofessional and multisectoral approaches for addressing social needs, SDOH, and health equity.
- Provide information to the secretary of HHS regarding activities of federal agencies that relate to the nursing workforce and its impact on health equity.

- Public health and health care systems should quantify nursing expenditures related to health equity and SDOH. This includes providing support for nurses in activities that explicitly target social needs, SDOH, and health equity through health care organization policies, governance and related advisory structures, and collective bargaining agreements.
- Representatives of social sectors, consumer organizations, and government entities should include nursing expertise when health-related multisector policy reform is being advanced.
- State and federal governments should provide sustainable funding to prepare sufficient numbers of baccalaureate, APRN, and PhD-level nurses to address SDOH, advance health equity, and increase access to primary care.
- Employers should support nurses at all levels in all settings with the financial, technical, educational, and staffing resources to help them play a leading role in achieving health equity.

PROMOTING NURSES' HEALTH AND WELL-BEING

During the course of their work, nurses encounter physical, mental, emotional, and ethical challenges, and burnout is an increasingly prevalent problem. The COVID-19 pandemic has only exacerbated these issues. In order for nurses to help others be healthy and well, they must be healthy and well themselves; a lack of nurse well-being has consequences for nurses, patients, employers, and communities. As nurses are asked to take a more prominent role in advancing health equity, it will become even more imperative that all stakeholders—including educators, employers, leaders, and nurses themselves—take steps to ensure nurse well-being.

Recommendation 3: By 2021, nursing education programs, employers, nursing leaders, licensing boards, and nursing organizations should initiate the implementation of structures, systems, and evidence-based interventions to promote nurses' health and well-being, especially as they take on new roles to advance health equity.

This can be accomplished by taking the following steps:

- Nursing education programs:
  - Integrate content on nurses' health and well-being into their programs to raise nursing students' awareness of the importance of these concerns and provide them with associated skill training and support that can be used as they transition to practice.
  - Create mechanisms, including organizational policy and regulations, to protect students most at risk for behavioral health challenges, including those students who may be experiencing economic hardships or feel that they are unsafe; isolated; or targets of bias, discrimination, and injustice.
- Employers, including nurse leaders:
  - Provide sufficient human and material resources (including personal protective equipment) to enable nurses to provide high-quality person-, family-, and community-centered care effectively and safely. This effort should include redesigning processes and increasing staff capacity to improve workflow, promote transdisciplinary collaboration, reduce modifiable burden, and distribute responsibilities to reflect nurses' expertise and scope of practice.
  - Establish a culture of physical and psychological safety and ethical practice in the workplace, including dismantling structural racism; addressing bullying and incivility; using evidence-informed approaches; investing in organizational infrastructure, such as resilience engineering;[5] and creating accountability for nurses' health and well-being outcomes.
  - Create mechanisms, including organizational policy and regulations, to protect nurses from retaliation when advocating on behalf of themselves and their patients and when reporting unsafe working conditions, biases, discrimination, and injustice.
  - Support diversity, equity, and inclusion across the nursing workforce, and identify and eliminate policies and systems that perpetuate structural racism, cultural racism, and discrimination in the nursing profession, recognizing that nurses are accountable for

[5] Resilience engineering is focused on "understanding the nature of adaptations, learning from success and increasing adaptive capacity" (Anderson et al., 2016, p. 1).

building an antiracist culture, and employers are responsible for establishing an antiracist, inclusive work environment.

- Prioritize and invest in evidence-based mental, physical, behavioral, social, and moral health interventions, including reward programs meaningful to nurses in diverse roles and specialties, to promote nurses' health, well-being, and resilience within work teams and organizations.
- Establish and standardize institutional processes that strengthen nurses' contributions to improving the design and delivery of care and decision making, including the setting of institutional policies and benchmarks in health care organizations and in educational, public health, and other settings.
- Evaluate and strengthen policies, programs, and structures within employing organizations and licensing boards to reduce stigma associated with mental and behavioral health treatment for nurses.
- Collect systematic data at the employer, state (including state workforce centers and state nursing associations), and national levels to better understand the health and well-being of the nursing workforce. This enhanced understanding should be used to inform the development of evidence-based interventions for mitigating burnout; fatigue; turnover; and the development of physical, behavioral, and mental health problems.

CAPITALIZING ON NURSES' POTENTIAL

Nurses often have untapped potential to help people live their healthiest lives because their education and experience are grounded in caring for the whole person and whole family in a community context. However, this potential is too often underutilized. Nurses, particularly RNs, need environments that facilitate their ability to fully leverage their skills and expertise across all practice settings—in hospitals, primary care settings, rural and underserved areas, homes, community organizations, long-term care facilities, and schools. To engage fully in advancing health equity, all nurses need the autonomy to practice to the full extent of their education and training, even as they work collaboratively with other health professionals. They are, however, frequently hindered in this regard by restrictive laws and institutional policies. Policy makers and health care systems need to lift permanently all barriers that stand in the way of nurses in their efforts to address the root causes of poor health, expand access to care, and create more equitable communities.

Recommendation 4: All organizations, including state and federal entities and employing organizations, should enable nurses to practice to the full extent of their education and training by removing barriers that prevent them from more fully addressing social needs and social determinants of

health and improving health care access, quality, and value. These barriers include regulatory and public and private payment limitations; restrictive policies and practices; and other legal, professional, and commercial[6] impediments.

To this end, the following specific actions should be prioritized:

- By 2022, all changes to institutional policies and state and federal laws adopted in response to the COVID-19 pandemic that expand scope of practice, telehealth eligibility, insurance coverage, and payment parity for services provided by APRNs and RNs should be made permanent.
- Federal authority (e.g., Veterans Health Administration regulations, Centers for Medicare & Medicaid Services [CMS]) should be used where available to supersede restrictive state laws, including those addressing scope of practice, telehealth, and insurance coverage and payment, that decrease access to care and burden nursing practice, and to encourage nationwide adoption of the Nurse Licensure Compact.[7]
- The Health Care Regulator Collaborative should work to advance interstate compacts and the adoption of model legislation to improve access, standardize care quality, and build interprofessional collaboration and interstate cooperation.

PAYING FOR NURSING CARE

Nurses are bridge builders, engaging and connecting with individuals, communities, public health and health care, and social services organizations to improve health for all. Without strong financial and institutional support, however, their reach and impact are limited. How care is paid for can determine one's access to and the quality of care. Thus, it is important to improve and strengthen the design of public and private payment models so nurses are supported, encouraged, and incentivized to bridge health and social needs for people, families, and communities. Nurses also can play a key role in helping to design those models. Also important is for local, state, and federal governments to place more value

[6] The term "commercial" refers to contractual agreements and customary practices that make antiquated or unjustifiable assumptions about nursing.

[7] Under the Nurse Licensure Compact (NLC), "nurses can practice in other NLC states without having to obtain additional licenses. The current NLC allows for RNs and LPNs/licensed vocational nurses (LVNs) to have one multistate license in any one of the 35 member states" (see https://www.ncsbn.org/nlcmemberstates.pdf). According to the National Council of State Boards of Nursing (NCSBN), "An APRN must hold an individual state license in each state of APRN practice" (see https://www.ncsbn.org/2018_eNLC_FAQs.pdf). There is a movement, organized by the National Council of State Boards of Nursing, to have an APRN Compact (see https://aprncompact.com/about.htm) (all accessed April 12, 2021).

on the vital role of school and public health nurses in advancing health equity by adequately funding and deploying these nurses where they are needed to promote health in communities.

Recommendation 5: Federal, tribal, state, local, and private payers and public health agencies should establish sustainable and flexible payment mechanisms to support nurses in both health care and public health, including school nurses, in addressing social needs, social determinants of health, and health equity.

Specific payment reforms should include the following:

- Reform fee-for-service payment models by
  - ensuring that the Current Procedure Terminology (CPT) code set includes appropriate codes to describe and reimburse for such nurse-led services as case management, care coordination, and team-based care to address behavioral health, addiction, SDOH, and health equity, and that the relative value units attached to the CPT codes result in adequate and direct reimbursement for this work;
  - reimbursing for school nursing; and
  - enabling nurses to bill for telehealth services.
- Reform value-based payment by
  - using clinical performance measures stratified by such risk factors as race, ethnicity, and socioeconomic status;
  - supporting nursing interventions through clinical performance measures that incentivize reductions in health disparities between more and less advantaged populations, improvements in measures for at-risk populations, and attainment of absolute target levels of high-quality performance for at-risk populations; and
  - incorporating disparities-sensitive measures that support and incentivize nursing interventions that advance health equity (e.g., process measures such as care management and team-based care for chronic conditions; outcomes such as prevention of hospitalizations for ambulatory care–sensitive conditions).
- Reform alternative payment models by
  - providing flexible funding (capitated payments, global budgets, shared savings, per member per month payments, accountable health communities models) for nursing and infrastructure that address SDOH; and
  - incorporating value-based payment metrics that enable nurses to address SDOH and advance health equity.
- Create a National Nurse Identifier to facilitate recognition and measurement of the value of services provided by RNs.

- Ensure adequate funding for school and public health nursing by
  - implementing state policies that allow school nurses to bill Medicaid and supporting schools, particularly rural schools, in meeting documentation requirements;
  - reimbursing school nursing services that include collaboration with clinical and community health care providers;
  - promoting new ways of financing public health to address SDOH in the community (e.g., having federal, state, and local leaders, along with public health departments and organizations, partner with payers, health systems, and accountable health communities, and blend or braid multiple funding sources);
  - creating funding mechanisms and joint accountability metrics for the efforts of the health, public health, and social sectors to address SDOH and advance health equity that align incentives and behavior across the various stakeholders, including school health;
  - leveraging nonprofit hospital community benefit requirements to create partnerships with and among school and public health nursing, primary care organizations, and other social sectors; and
  - using pay scales for public health nurses that are competitive with those for nursing positions in other health care organizations and sectors, and that provide equal pay when the services provided (e.g., immunizations) are the same.

USING TECHNOLOGY TO INTEGRATE DATA ON SOCIAL DETERMINANTS OF HEALTH INTO NURSING PRACTICE

The advent and adoption of new technologies have dramatically changed nursing practice over the past several decades, and will continue to do so into the future. Given the rapid acceleration of technical advances, nurses practicing in the coming decade will need to be adept at and comfortable with using emerging technology and have the skills to support others in doing the same. Nurses are well positioned to design, adopt, and adapt new technologies in practice and leverage data on SDOH to identify and address the needs of populations, individualize care, and reduce health disparities. With care expanding beyond the walls of traditional health care settings, including hospitals and clinics, the deployment of such advanced technologies as artificial intelligence and telehealth can assist nurses in connecting to health care networks, reaching individuals in their homes and other settings, and promoting health and well-being within communities. As key stakeholders in the design, adoption, and evaluation of new care tools, nurses also need to understand how to use new technologies to reduce rather than exacerbate inequities.

Recommendation 6: All public and private health care systems should incorporate nursing expertise in designing, generating, analyzing, and applying

data to support initiatives focused on social determinants of health and health equity using diverse digital platforms, artificial intelligence, and other innovative technologies.

This can be accomplished through the following actions:

- With leadership from CMS and The Office of the National Coordinator for Health Information Technology, accelerate interoperability projects that integrate data on SDOH from public health, social services organizations, and other community partners into electronic health records, and build a nationwide infrastructure to capture and share community-held knowledge, facilitate referrals for care (including by decreasing the "digital divide"), and facilitate coordination and connectivity among health care settings and the public and nonprofit sectors.
- Ensure that existing public/private health equity data collaboratives (e.g., the Gravity Project[8]) encompass nursing-specific care processes that improve visualization of data on SDOH and associated decision making by nurses.
- Employ nurses with requisite expertise in informatics to improve individual and population health through large-scale integration of data on SDOH into nursing practice, as well as expertise in the use of telehealth and advanced digital technologies.
- To personalize care based on person- and family-centered preferences and individual needs, give nurses in clinical settings responsibility and associated resources to innovate and use technology, including in the use of data on SDOH as context for planning and evaluating care; in the design of personal and mobile health tools; in coordination of community and public health portals across care settings; in methods for effective communication using technology; in evaluation of datasets and artificial intelligence algorithms (e.g., for racial bias); and in partnerships with corporate settings outside of health care delivery (e.g., large technology organizations, private insurers) that are addressing health equity in the nonclinical setting.
- Provide supportive resources to facilitate the provision of telehealth by nurses by
    - expanding the national strategy for a broadband/5G infrastructure to enable comprehensive community access to these services; and
    - increasing the availability of the necessary hardware, including smartphones, computers, and webcams, for high-risk populations.

[8] See https://sirenetwork.ucsf.edu/TheGravityProject (accessed April 12, 2021).

STRENGTHENING NURSING EDUCATION

Regardless of the setting in which they work or their level of education, nurses of the future will be expected to have a sophisticated understanding of social needs, SDOH, and health equity and to be capable of applying this knowledge in their practice. The World Health Organization has emphasized the importance of monitoring equitable service coverage across wealth and education gradients as part of achieving universal health coverage. Similarly, leading public health researchers have advocated for using markers of health equity to monitor health and health care as a first step in confronting inequities. Recognizing and meeting social needs could both lower health care spending and improve health outcomes.

Nursing schools need to prepare nurses to understand and identify the social, economic, and environmental factors that influence health by embedding content on SDOH throughout their curricula. Schools need to ensure that nurses have substantive, enduring, relevant community-based experiences and that they value diverse perspectives and cultures in order to help all people and families thrive. Nurses should have this content updated and reinforced throughout their careers through continuing education.

Recommendation 7: Nursing education programs, including continuing education, and accreditors and the National Council of State Boards of Nursing should ensure that nurses are prepared to address social determinants of health and achieve health equity.

To implement this recommendation, deans, administrative faculty leaders, faculty, course directors, and staff of nursing education programs should take the following steps:

- Integrate social needs, SDOH, population health, environmental health, trauma-informed care, and health equity as core concepts and competencies throughout coursework and clinical and experiential learning. These core concepts and competencies should be commensurate and seamless with academic level and included in continuing education.
- By the 2022–2023 school year, initiate an assessment of individual student access to technology, and ensure that all students can engage in virtual learning, including such opportunities as multisector simulation. Access to nursing education for geographically and socioeconomically disadvantaged students should be ensured through the development and expansion of the use of remote and virtual instructional capabilities. For rural areas, emphasis should be on baccalaureate preparation given the lower proportion of nurses educated at this level.
- To promote equity, inclusivity, and diversity grounded in social justice, identify and eliminate policies, procedures, curricular content, and clin-

ical experiences that perpetuate structural racism, cultural racism, and discrimination among faculty, staff, and students.

- Increase academic progression for geographically and socioeconomically disadvantaged students through academic partnerships that include community and tribal colleges located in rural and urban underserved areas.
- Recruit diverse faculty with expertise in SDOH, population health (including environmental health), and health equity and associated policy expertise, and, through evidence-based and other training, develop the skills of current faculty with the objective of ensuring that students have access across the curriculum to expertise in these areas. Faculty should also have the technical competencies for online teaching.
- Ensure that students have learning opportunities with care coordination experiences that include working with health care teams to address individual and family social needs, as well as learning opportunities with multisector stakeholders that include a focus on health in all policies and SDOH. Learning experiences should include working with underserved populations in such settings as federally qualified health centers, rural health clinics, and IHS designated sites.
- Incorporate in all nurse doctoral education content related to SDOH, population health, environmental health, trauma-informed care, health equity, and social justice. All graduates of doctoral programs should have competencies in the use of data on SDOH as context for planning, implementing, and evaluating care and for improving population health through the large-scale application of these data.
- Ensure that PhD nursing graduates are competent to design and implement research that addresses issues of social justice and equity in education and/or health and health care and informs relevant policies. Increase the capacity of these graduates to apply research and scale interventions to address and improve social needs, SDOH, population health, environmental health, trauma-informed care, health equity, the well-being of nurses, and disaster preparedness and to inform relevant policies.
- Prepare all nursing students to advocate for health equity through civic engagement, including engagement in health and health-related public policy and communication through traditional and nontraditional methods, including social media and multisector coalitions.

Accreditors should take the following actions:

- Incorporate standards and competencies for curriculum that reflect the application of knowledge and skills to improve social needs, SDOH, population health, environmental health, trauma-informed care, and health equity.

- Incorporate standards for increasing student and faculty diversity.
- Require nursing education programs to initiate curricular assessments in 2022–2023 and phase in curricular changes that integrate social needs, SDOH, population health, environmental health, trauma-informed care, and health equity throughout the curriculum and are assessed in subsequent midterm and accreditation reporting. These curricular changes and their impact should be subject to continuous accreditation review processes.
- Include standards for nurses' well-being and ethical practice in accreditation guidelines, and include such content on nurse licensing and certification exams.

The National Council of State Boards of Nursing and specialty certification organizations should take the following action:

- Incorporate test questions on meeting social needs through care coordination and on meeting population health needs, including addressing SDOH, through multisector coordination.

Continuing education providers should take the following action:

- Evaluate each offering for the inclusion of social needs, SDOH, population health, environmental health, trauma-informed care, and health equity and strategies for associated public- and private-sector policy engagement.

PREPARING NURSES TO RESPOND TO DISASTERS AND PUBLIC HEALTH EMERGENCIES

The COVID-19 pandemic has magnified the vital role of nurses on the front lines of crises—whether in the hospital intensive care unit, a community testing site, or an emergency shelter—in keeping communities safe and healthy and helping people and families cope. They are reliable, trusted, experienced, and proven responders during both public health emergencies and natural disasters, such as hurricanes and wildfires. But fundamental reforms and a stronger disaster preparedness infrastructure are needed to improve nursing education, practice, and policy so nurses are fully protected during such events and can better protect and care for recovering populations.

Recommendation 8: To enable nurses to address inequities within communities, federal agencies and other key stakeholders within and outside the nursing profession should strengthen and protect the nursing workforce during the response to such public health emergencies as the COVID-19 pandemic and natural disasters, including those related to climate change.

To this end, the following steps should be taken:

- CDC should fund a National Center for Disaster Nursing and Public Health Emergency Response, along with additional strategically placed regional centers, to serve as the "hub" for providing leadership in education, training, and career development that will ensure a national nursing workforce prepared to respond to such events.
- CDC, in collaboration with the proposed National Center for Disaster Nursing and Public Health Emergency Response, should rapidly articulate a national action plan for addressing gaps in nursing education, support, and protection that have contributed to the lack of nurse preparedness and disparities during such events.
- The Office of the Assistant Secretary for Preparedness and Response, CDC, HRSA, the Agency for Healthcare Research and Quality, CMS, the National Institute of Nursing Research (NINR), and other funders should develop and support the emergency preparedness and response knowledge base of the nursing workforce through regulations, programs, research, and sustainable funding targeted specifically to disaster and public health emergency nursing.
- The American Association of Colleges of Nursing, the National League for Nursing, and the Organization for Associate Degree Nursing should lead transformational change in nursing education to address workforce development in disaster nursing and public health preparedness. NCSBN should expand content in licensing examinations to cover actual responsibilities of nurses in disaster and public health emergency response.
- Employers should incorporate the expertise of nurses to proactively develop and implement an emergency response plan for natural disasters and public health emergencies in coordination with local, state, national, and federal partners. They should also provide additional services throughout a disaster or public health emergency, such as support for families and behavioral health, to support and protect nurses' health and well-being.

BUILDING THE EVIDENCE BASE

Strengthening and diversifying the nursing workforce of the future, fostering nurse well-being, and developing strong and impactful nurse leaders so that nurses can fully address the wide and persistent health disparities in the United States will require a robust and rigorous evidence base. Below, the committee prioritizes the research needs and identifies gaps in the knowledge base that, if filled, would substantially move the nursing profession forward in the future.

Recommendation 9: The National Institutes of Health, the Centers for Medicare & Medicaid Services, the Centers for Disease Control and Prevention, the Health Resources and Services Administration, the Agency for Healthcare Research and Quality, the Administration for Children and Families, the Administration for Community Living, and private associations and foundations should convene representatives from nursing, public health, and health care to develop and support a research agenda and evidence base describing the impact of nursing interventions, including multisector collaboration, on social determinants of health, environmental health, health equity, and nurses' health and well-being.

These efforts should be focused on the following actions:

- Develop mechanisms for proposing, evaluating, and scaling evidence-based practice models that leverage collaboration among public health, social sectors, and health systems to advance health equity, including codesigning innovations with individuals and community representatives and responding to community health needs assessments. This effort should emphasize rapidly translating evidence-based interventions into real-world clinical practice and community-based settings to improve health equity and population health outcomes, and applying implementation science strategies in the process of scaling these interventions and strategies.
- Identify effective multisector team approaches to improving health equity and addressing social needs and SDOH, including clearly defining roles and assessing the value of nurses in these models. Specifically, performance and outcome measures should be delineated, and evaluation strategies for community-based models and multisector team functioning should be developed and implemented.
- Review and adapt evidence-based approaches to increasing the number and diversity of students and faculty from disadvantaged and traditionally underrepresented groups to promote a diverse, inclusive learning environment and prepare a culturally competent workforce.
- Determine evidence-based education strategies for preparing nurses at all levels, including through continuing education, to eliminate structural racism and implicit bias and strengthen the delivery of culturally competent care.
- Augment the use of advanced information technology infrastructure, including virtual services and artificial intelligence, to identify and integrate health and social data, including data on SDOH, so as to improve

nurses' capacity to support individuals, families, and communities, including through care coordination.

Across all of these efforts, nurses should partner with key community stakeholders in research design; identification of the characteristics of new health models; and the development of related institutional and public policies at the health system, public health, and community levels. To expand the cohort of nurse researchers engaged in this research agenda, NINR should offer continuous summer intensive seminars to build expertise in population health, SDOH, and health equity. Table 11-1 summarizes gaps in the current research base that have been identified throughout this report.

TABLE 11-1 Research Topics for the Future of Nursing, 2020–2030

Topic	Relevant Areas in Which More Research Is Needed
Addressing Health Equity	Examine the roles of all nurses, particularly acute and long-term care, school, public health, and community-based nurses, in addressing health equity and reducing health disparities. This research would include nurses' roles in local contexts.
	Study interventions that target disadvantaged groups and whether and how they reduce disparities among groups.
	Conduct longitudinal studies to observe the sustained health impacts and effectiveness over time of nurse-involved/nurse-led interventions to advance health equity.
Disaster Preparedness and Public Health Emergency Response	Assess gaps in nurses' preparedness for their roles in disaster preparedness and public health emergency response to improve the profession's capacity and ability to advocate for population health and health equity in the context of such events.
	Establish a research agenda regarding nurses' roles in these areas based on a thorough needs assessment and documentation of gaps in the research literature, nursing knowledge and skills, and available resources. This research would include an emphasis on intervention studies using mixed-methods designs.
Paying for Health Care	Assess how nurses contribute to producing high-value care in value-based payment and alternative payment models. Value would be measured by examining both the outcomes obtained by nurses and the costs of the resources used to produce those outcomes.
	Examine the role and value of school nurses—the most accessible providers for school-age children—particularly with respect to how they affect students in underresourced rural and urban school districts. This would include current and post-COVID-19 research.
	Study the effects of the COVID-19 pandemic on the organization, financing, and care quality of the nation's health systems and associated changes in demand for nurses.

continued

TABLE 11-1 Continued

Topic	Relevant Areas in Which More Research Is Needed
Nursing Workforce	Assess the economic and noneconomic effects of COVID-19 on nurses currently in the workforce. Study and monitor entry into and exit from the workforce, and determine effects on the future supply of nurses. Examine efforts to increase nurses' ability to • improve access to mental and behavioral health care, and ensure the effectiveness of related interventions and services; • improve access to primary health care and ensure the effectiveness of primary care delivery systems; • improve maternal health outcomes and the delivery of maternal health care; • improve the care provided to the nation's aging population, particularly frail older adults; and • control health care spending, reduce costs, and increase the value of nurses' contributions to improving health and health care delivery. Examine approaches that can effectively prepare faculty to teach content related to SDOH, health equity, and structural racism. Evaluate characteristics of pipeline programs for licensed practical nurses/licensed vocational nurses that are effective with respect to program graduates matriculating to the bachelor's in nursing/registered nurse level, with a particular focus on minority and rural nurses. Examine how more effectively to recruit nurses into underenrolled specialties, including long-term care and geriatrics, school nursing, public health, and rural nursing. This research would include identification of barriers and successful approaches to scaling these strategies. Investigate and evaluate the efficacy of technology-based innovations in nursing education, such as virtual teaching and virtual reality simulations, and their impact on accessibility among rural and minority nursing students. Develop, implement, and evaluate interventions to eliminate implicit bias and structural racism in nursing education for students, faculty, staff, and administrators.

TABLE 11-1 Continued

Topic	Relevant Areas in Which More Research Is Needed
Nurse Well-Being	Include measures of physical, mental, social, and moral well-being in national surveys of the nursing workforce.
	Study the well-being of nurses outside of clinical care settings, including public health and school nursing.
	Develop, implement, and conduct rigorous evaluations of interventions to prevent compassion fatigue.
	Investigate the relevance of moral injury in nurses and its relationship to various measures of well-being and moral resilience.
	Implement and evaluate alternatives-to-discipline programs for addressing substance use disorders in nurses. This research would include an examination of the essential components of such programs.
	Consider differences among bullying, lateral violence, and incivility. Develop, implement, and conduct rigorous evaluations of interventions for addressing these phenomena, including simulations and other promising programs. Examine the relationship between bullying and workplace hierarchies, as well as factors within organizations that decrease bullying and incivility.
	Investigate how to ameliorate workplace violence among nurses and other health care workers, and such violence stemming from family members, visitors, and patients. Replication and rigorous randomized controlled trials are needed for promising interventions, including hybrid in-person and online interventions.
	Investigate the effects of mobile health technologies on nurses' well-being.
	Design, implement, and rigorously evaluate interventions that build psychological safety among health care teams.

FINAL THOUGHTS

The nursing profession is vital to the nation's creation of a culture of health, reduction of health disparities, and improvement in the health and well-being of the population. The committee's nine recommendations provide a comprehensive path forward for policy makers, practicing nurses, educators, health care system leaders, researchers, and payers to enable and support the nurses of today and the future in creating fair and just opportunities for health and well-being for everyone. The social, political, and health care trends discussed in this report, while replete with myriad challenges, also offer nurses new opportunities for practice and collaboration. Nurses will need to continue to adapt and respond to new and developing health problems at both the individual and community levels, and to deepen their understanding of how social, economic, and environmental issues and systemic barriers affect the health and well-being of the people and communities they serve. The rapidly deployed changes in community-based and clinical care, nursing education, nursing leadership, and nursing–community partnerships resulting from the COVID-19 pandemic have amplified those challenges. The deployment of all levels of nurses across the care continuum, including in collaborative practice models, will be necessary to address the challenges of building a more equitable and accessible health care system.

The United States is at an inflection point with respect to addressing disparities in health and well-being that have adversely impacted too many people for too long. The nation's health care system is also at an inflection point in terms of meeting consumers' health needs in ways and in places commensurate with their preferences. It is imperative that the nursing profession focus on the training and competency development needed to prepare nurses, including advanced practice nurses, to work competently in home and community-based as well as acute care settings and to lead efforts to build a culture of health and health equity. There is no time to waste. Over the next 10 years, nurses will assume even greater responsibility for helping to build an accessible, equitable, high-quality public health and health care system that works for everyone. The recommendations in this report are aimed at ensuring that nurses are inspired, supported, valued, and empowered in pursuing that goal so that by 2030, all individuals and communities will have the opportunities they need to live healthy lives.

REFERENCES

Anderson, J. E., A. J. Ross, J. Back, M. Duncan, P. Snell, K. Walsh, and P. Jaye. 2016. Implementing resilience engineering for healthcare quality improvement using the CARE model: A feasibility study protocol. *Pilot and Feasibility Studies* 2(61). doi: 10.1186/s40814-016-0103-x.

NACNEP (National Advisory Council on Nurse Education and Practice). 2020. *Integration of social determinants of health in nursing education, practice, and research*. 16th Report to the Secretary of the U.S. Department of Health and Human Services and the U.S. Congress. Washington, DC: Health Resources and Services Administration.

Appendix A

Biographical Sketches of Committee Members and Project Staff

COMMITTEE MEMBERS

Mary K. Wakefield (*Co-Chair*) is a visiting professor at The University of Texas at Austin. Previously, she served as the acting deputy secretary of the U.S. Department of Health and Human Services in the Obama administration, where she led strategic department-wide initiatives in key health policy areas, with a particular focus on health and human services programs for vulnerable populations. Her domestic policy work largely focused on improving the health status for underserved populations, including strengthening health programs for Native Americans and Alaska Natives and improving data analysis to better understand the health needs of rural populations. She also previously initiated and led program improvements as the administrator of the Health Resources and Services Administration to further strengthen the health care workforce, build healthier communities, increase health equity, and provide health care services to people who are geographically isolated or economically or medically vulnerable. Her public service career also includes work as a legislative assistant and later as the chief of staff to two North Dakota senators. Her extensive academic experience includes serving as the associate dean for rural health at the School of Medicine and Health Sciences and as a faculty member and area chair in the College of Nursing, both at the University of North Dakota, and as the director of the Center for Health Policy, Research and Ethics at George Mason University. She has also worked onsite as a consultant to the World Health Organization's Global Programme on AIDS in Geneva, Switzerland. She is a member of the National Academy of Medicine and a fellow of the American Academy of Nursing. She has served on a number of public and not-for-profit boards and committees, bringing expertise in nursing, health care quality, access to care, and the health workforce. She was a member of the committees that produced the landmark reports *To Err Is Human: Building a Safer Health System* and *Crossing the Quality Chasm: A New Health System for the 21st Century*. She co-chaired the committee that produced *Health Professions Education: A Bridge to Quality* and chaired the committee that produced *Quality Through Collaboration: Health Care in Rural America*. She has a B.S. in nursing from the University of Mary in Bismarck and an M.S. and a Ph.D. in nursing from The University of Texas at Austin. She also completed the Program for Senior Managers in Government at the Harvard Kennedy School.

David R. Williams (*Co-Chair*) is the Florence and Laura Norman Professor of Public Health and the chair of the Department of Social and Behavioral Sciences at the T.H. Chan School of Public Health at Harvard University, where he is also a professor of African and African American studies and sociology. His prior academic appointments were at Yale University and the University of Michigan. He is an internationally recognized authority on social influences on health and the author of more than 450 scientific papers focusing on the complex ways in which race, socioeconomic status, stress, racism, health behavior, and religious involvement can affect health. He has played a visible, national leadership role in raising awareness levels of the problem of health inequalities and identifying interventions to address them. This role includes his service as the staff director of the Robert Wood Johnson Foundation's Commission to Build a Healthier America and as a key scientific advisor to the award-winning PBS film series Unnatural Causes: Is Inequality Making Us Sick? The Everyday Discrimination Scale that he developed is one of the most widely used measures of discrimination in health studies. He is a member of the National Academy of Medicine and the American Academy of Arts & Sciences. He has received distinguished contributions awards from the American Sociological Association, the American Psychological Association, and The New York Academy of Medicine. He has been ranked as one of the top 10 most-cited social scientists in the world and as the most-cited Black scholar in the social sciences. Thomson Reuters, a media company, ranked him as one of the world's most influential scientific minds. His research has been featured by some of America's top print and television news organizations and in a recent TED talk. He holds an M.P.H. from Loma Linda University and a Ph.D. in sociology from the University of Michigan.

Maureen Bisognano is the president emerita and a senior fellow at the Institute for Healthcare Improvement (IHI), where she previously served as the president and the chief executive officer (CEO) for 5 years, and, before that, as the executive vice president and the chief operating officer (COO) for 15 years. She is also an instructor of medicine at Harvard Medical School and a research associate in the Brigham and Women's Hospital Division of Social Medicine and Health

Inequalities. Prior to joining IHI, she served as the CEO of the Massachusetts Respiratory Hospital and as the senior vice president of the Juran Institute. As a prominent authority on improving health care systems, she advises health care leaders around the world, is a frequent speaker at major health care conferences on quality improvement, and works as a tireless advocate for change. She chairs the advisory board of the Well Being Trust, co-chairs the Massachusetts Coalition for Serious Illness Care (with Dr. Atul Gawande), and serves on the boards of The Commonwealth Fund, Indiana University Health, and Nursing Now. She is a member of the National Academy of Medicine. She began her career in health care as a staff nurse at Quincy Hospital in Quincy, Massachusetts, and subsequently served there as the director of nursing, the director of patient services, and as the COO. She holds a B.S. from the University of the State of New York and an M.S. from Boston University.

Jeffrey Brenner is the co-founder and the chief medical officer for a new primary care start-up, JunaCare, located outside of Philadelphia, Pennsylvania. Previously, he served as the senior vice president at United Healthcare, where he developed a national model, used in more than 20 states, for providing housing and support services to Medicaid members experiencing homelessness. His career has been focused on improving care for vulnerable populations, beginning as a family physician in Camden, New Jersey, where he owned and operated a solo-practice, urban family medicine office providing full-spectrum family health services for a Medicaid-enrolled population. Recognizing the need for a new way for hospitals, providers, and community residents to collaborate, he founded what would become the Camden Coalition of Healthcare Providers and served as its executive director from its incorporation. Under his leadership, the Camden Coalition launched the National Center for Complex Health and Social Needs. His innovative use of data to identify high-need, high-cost patients in a fragmented system and improve their care was profiled in the 2011 *The New Yorker* article "The Hot-Spotters" (by writer and surgeon Dr. Atul Gawande) and on PBS's *Frontline*. He is a recipient of the MacArthur "genius" fellowship for his work, and he is a member of the National Academy of Medicine. He holds a bachelor's degree in biology from Vassar College and an M.D. from the Rutgers Robert Wood Johnson Medical School.

Peter I. Buerhaus is a professor in the College of Nursing and the director of the Center for Interdisciplinary Health Workforce Studies at Montana State University. As a nurse and a health care economist, he is well known for his studies and publications focused on the nursing and physician workforces in the United States. Previously, he was the Valere Potter Distinguished Professor of Nursing and a professor of health policy at Vanderbilt University and an assistant professor of health policy and management at the Harvard T.H. Chan School of Public Health. He maintains an active research program involving studies on the economics of the nursing workforce, forecasting nurse and physician supply, developing and testing measures of hospital quality of care, determining public and provider opinions on issues involving the delivery of health care, and assessing the quantity and quality of health care provided by nurse practitioners. Five of his more than 150 publications are designated as "classics" by the Patient Safety Network of the Agency for Healthcare Research and Quality, and he is the co-author of *The Future of the Nursing Workforce in the United States: Data, Trends, and Implications*. He has editorial responsibilities with many peer-reviewed health services research and nursing journals, and he has advised policy makers and legislators on nursing workforce policy. He is a member of the National Academy of Medicine and a fellow of the American Academy of Nursing. He has served on the Advisory Council of the National Institutes of Health's National Institute of Nursing Research, the National Quality Forum's Steering Committee on Nursing Quality Performance Measures, the board of directors of Sigma Theta Tau International, The Joint Commission's Nursing Advisory Committee, AcademyHealth, and the Bozeman Deaconess Health System. He was an advisor for the Bipartisan Policy Center's health care workforce initiative, and he served on the Institute of Medicine's Committee on Graduate Medical Education Governance and Transparency. He served as the chair of the National Health Workforce Commission that was established under the Patient Protection and Affordable Care Act, which is intended to provide advice to Congress and to the president on national health care workforce policy. He has a bachelor's in nursing from Mankato State University, a master's in nursing health services administration from the University of Michigan, and a master's in community health nursing and a Ph.D. from Wayne State University. He has also been awarded honorary doctorates from the University of Maryland and Loyola University Chicago.

Marshall H. Chin is the Richard Parrillo Family Professor of Healthcare Ethics in the Department of Medicine at the University of Chicago and a general internist with extensive experience improving the care of vulnerable patients with chronic disease. He is also the co-director of the Robert Wood Johnson Foundation (RWJF) Advancing Health Equity: Leading Care, Payment, and Systems Transformation Program Office; the director of the Chicago Center for Diabetes Translation Research; the co-director of the Merck Foundation's national program office of Bridging the Gap: Reducing Disparities in Diabetes Care; and the associate chief and the director of research in the Section of General Internal Medicine and the associate director of the MacLean Center for Clinical Medical Ethics at the University of Chicago. He co-chaired the committee that wrote *A Roadmap for Promoting Health Equity and Eliminating Disparities: The 4 I's for Health Equity*. He has served on the Centers for Disease Control and Prevention's Community Preventive Services Task Force and the National Advisory Council to the National Institute on Minority Health and Health Disparities. He is currently improving diabetes care and outcomes on the South Side of Chicago through health care system and community interventions. He is co-directing a project evaluating the value of the national federally qualified health center system. He is also leading a research project funded by the Agency for Healthcare Research and Quality to improve shared decision making among clinicians and LGBTQ racial and ethnic minority patients. His work over the past decade leading RWJF's Finding Answers program led to the widely cited *The Roadmap to Reduce Disparities*. He is a member of the National Academy of Medicine, a fellow of the American College of Physicians, and a former president of the Society of General Internal Medicine. He is a graduate of Harvard College and the University of California, San Francisco, School of Medicine.

Regina S. Cunningham is the chief executive officer at the Hospital of the University of Pennsylvania and an adjunct professor and the assistant dean for clinical practice at the School of Nursing at the University of Pennsylvania. She is an accomplished nurse executive, scientist, and educator who has made significant contributions to advancing nursing practice and clinical care. Her extensive experience in the organization and delivery of nursing service across the care continuum has focused particularly on the utilization of nursing resources in care delivery systems. In her former role as the chief nurse executive, she was responsible for a broad array of strategic and operational functions, including the development of professional practice standards, oversight of quality, and strengthening the integration of scholarship within the practice of nursing. Her research interests include the effect of nursing on outcomes, clinical trials, and innovative models of care delivery. She was a Robert Wood Johnson Foundation executive nurse fellow and is a fellow of the American Academy of Nursing. She holds an M.A. in the delivery of nursing service from New York University and a Ph.D. from the University of Pennsylvania. She also completed a postdoctoral fellowship at Yale University.

José J. Escarce is a distinguished professor of medicine in the David Geffen School of Medicine at the University of California, Los Angeles (UCLA), where he also serves as the vice chair for academic affairs in the Department of Medicine and as a distinguished professor of health policy and management in the Fielding School of Public Health. He has published extensively on a variety of topics, including physician behavior, medical technology adoption, racial and socioeconomic differences in health care, and the effects of market forces on access, costs, and quality of care. His research interests and expertise include health economics, managed care, physician behavior, racial and ethnic disparities in medical care, immigrant health, and technological change in medicine. He is a member of the National Academy of Medicine and has served on the Institute of Medicine committee that produced *Unequal Treatment: Confronting Racial and Ethnic Disparities in Health Care* and the National Academies of Sciences, Engineering, and Medicine committee that produced the three volumes of *Accounting* *for Social Risk Factors in Medicare Payment*. He has also served on numerous federal committees and advisory boards, including the National Advisory Council for Health Care Policy, Research, and Evaluation of the U.S. Department of Health and Human Services, and on the board of directors of AcademyHealth. He is the former co-editor-in-chief of *Health Services Research*, one of the leading journals in the field. He has a bachelor's degree from Princeton University, an M.S. in physics from Harvard University, and an M.D. and a Ph.D. in health economics from the University of Pennsylvania.

Greer Glazer is the Schmidlapp Professor of Nursing, the dean of the College of Nursing, and the vice president for health affairs at the University of Cincinnati, combining teaching, research, practice, community service, and policy work. Previously, she served as the dean and a professor at the University of Massachusetts Boston College of Nursing, the director of parent–child nursing and a professor at Kent State University, and an assistant professor at Case Western Reserve University. She has worked in large and small higher education institutions; research-intensive and not research-intensive environments; public and private universities; and colleges that are part of an academic health center. She has taught both undergraduate- and graduate-level students and has developed new programs and educational models in several institutions. Holding an established history of commitment to diversity, equity, and inclusion, she has created, implemented, and supported programs that promote inclusion and the success of diverse populations, whether as patients, students, faculty, or staff. She has served as the principal investigator of initiatives that advance nursing education and create opportunity for underrepresented individuals in health care professions, which is best illustrated by her co-leadership of the National Study on Holistic Review. She has authored more than 100 publications and made more than 220 presentations, in addition to abstracts and contributions to newspapers, radio, and television. She is the co-author of *Nursing Leadership from the Outside In* and is the co-founder and the legislative editor of the *Online Journal of Issues in Nursing*. She has been a Fulbright scholar, an executive nurse fellow of the Robert Wood Johnson Foundation, and the chair of the American Nurses Association Political Action Committee. She is a recipient of the Mary Adelaide Nutting Award for Outstanding Leadership in Nursing Education from the National League for Nursing and the award for diversity, inclusion, and sustainability in nursing education lectureship from the American Association of Colleges of Nursing. She holds a bachelor's in nursing from the University of Michigan and a master's and a Ph.D. in nursing from Case Western Reserve University.

Marcus Henderson is a lecturer and a clinical instructor at the University of Pennsylvania School of Nursing, where he teaches undergraduate psychiatric and community health nursing. In his teaching, he strives to help students understand the complexities of community health, engagement, and the impact of social determinants of health. He also maintains an active clinical practice as a psychiatric-mental health nurse for adolescent services at Fairmount Behavioral Health System in Philadelphia, Pennsylvania. In this role, he manages a 32-bed inpatient unit and works closely with the nursing staff and multidisciplinary teams to ensure safe, comprehensive patient care. Previously, he served as the co-founder and the executive director of Up and Running Healthcare Solutions, a Philadelphia-based organization that provides nurse-led case management by community health workers and other supportive services to homeless people in the city. His work on health for homeless people and community health workers was funded by the 2017 President's Engagement Prize from the University of Pennsylvania and has been presented at local, state, and national conferences. For his work in the Philadelphia community, he was recognized as a community champion for positive change by the Independence Blue Cross Foundation. He is a member of the board of directors of the American Nurses Association. He holds a B.S. in nursing and an M.S. in nursing health leadership from the University of Pennsylvania School of Nursing, and he also holds a certificate in health care innovation from its Perelman School of Medicine.

Angelica Millan was the director of children's medical services in the County of Los Angeles Department of Public Health, where she administered the nursing programs for California children's services, child, health and disability prevention, and health care for children in foster care, overseeing close to 350 nurses. She currently continues as a clinical nursing instructor at the Los Angeles Community College. She is a commissioner of the California Healthcare Workforce Policy Commission, a member of the board of trustees for the Chamberlain College of Nursing, a board member of the Case Management Society Association, and a board member of the National Association of Hispanic Nurses (NAHN). She served as the president of NAHN. She has been a recipient of NAHN's Nurse of the Year Award, its Janie Menchaca Wilson Leadership Award, its Outstanding Latina of the Year, and the Leadership Network Award of the National Hispanic Medical Association. She has also been recognized by a California Legislature Assembly Resolution and is the recipient of the 22nd District, Senate Woman of the Year award. She is a fellow of the American Nursing Academy. The first in her family to graduate college, she has been a dedicated nurse for more than 25 years in Los Angeles. She has a B.S. and an M.S. in nursing from California State University and a doctorate of nursing practice from Western University of Health Sciences. She is also a graduate of the Women's Health Nurse Practitioner Program of the University of California, Los Angeles.

John W. Rowe is the Julius B. Richmond Professor of Health Policy and Aging at the Columbia University Mailman School of Public Health. Previously, he served as the chairman and the chief executive officer (CEO) of Aetna Inc. He also previously served as the president and CEO of Mount Sinai New York

University Health, one of the nation's largest academic health care organizations, and as the president of the Mount Sinai Hospital and the Icahn School of Medicine at Mount Sinai in New York City. Before joining Mount Sinai, he was a professor of medicine and the founding director of the Division on Aging at Harvard Medical School, as well as the chief of gerontology at Boston's Beth Israel Hospital. He was the director of the MacArthur Foundation Research Network on Successful Aging and is the co-author of *Successful Aging*. He currently leads the foundation's Research Network on an Aging Society. He is a fellow of the American Academy of Arts & Sciences and a member of the National Academy of Medicine. He serves on the boards of trustees of The Rockefeller Foundation and the Urban Institute and is the past chairman of the board of overseers of the Columbia University Mailman School of Public Health, the board of fellows of Harvard Medical School, and the boards of trustees of the University of Connecticut and the Marine Biological Laboratory. He has a B.S. from Canisius College and an M.D. from the School of Medicine and Dentistry of the University of Rochester.

William M. Sage is the James R. Dougherty Chair for Faculty Excellence in the School of Law and a professor of surgery and perioperative care in the Dell Medical School at The University of Texas at Austin. He previously served as the university's first vice provost for health affairs. He was previously a tenured professor of law at Columbia Law School and has been a visiting law professor at Yale University, Harvard University, Duke University, and Emory University. Before entering law teaching, he practiced corporate and securities law in Los Angeles and headed four working groups for the White House Task Force on Health Care Reform in the Clinton administration. He is a member of the National Academy of Medicine and serves on the Board on Health Care Services of the National Academies of Sciences, Engineering, and Medicine. He is an elected fellow of the Hastings Center, a research institute on bioethics, and serves on the editorial board of the journal *Health Affairs*. He has written more than 200 articles and has edited 3 books, including the *Oxford Handbook of U.S. Health Law*. His research has been supported by the Agency for Healthcare Research and Quality, the Robert Wood Johnson Foundation, The Commonwealth Fund, and The Pew Charitable Trusts. He holds an A.B. from Harvard College, medical and law degrees from Stanford University, and an honorary doctorate from Universite Paris Descartes. He completed his internship at Mercy Hospital and Medical Center in San Diego and served as a resident in anesthesiology and critical care medicine at Johns Hopkins Hospital.

Victoria L. Tiase is the director of research science and informatics strategy at NewYork-Presbyterian (NYP) Hospital. She has more than 20 years of experience in giving clinical input to technology projects in all areas, especially regarding the implementation of the NYP Hospital electronic medical record. She is responsible for supporting a range of clinical information technology projects related to patient engagement, alarm management, and care coordination. She was the nursing lead for the design, implementation, and rollout of an institution-developed personal health record, myNYP.org. In national informatics roles, she serves on the board of directors for the American Medical Informatics Association, the executive board of NODE.Health (Network of Digital Evidence in Health), the steering committee for the Alliance for Nursing Informatics, and the chair of the North American Nursing Informatics Committee of the Healthcare Information and Management Systems Society. She is a lecturer in the Division of Health Informatics of the Weill Cornell Graduate School of Medical Sciences. She is a fellow of the American Academy of Nursing. She has a bachelor's in nursing from the University of Virginia, a master's in nursing informatics from Columbia University, and a Ph.D. from The University of Utah with a focus on the integration of patient-generated health data related to the social and behavioral determinants of health into clinical workflows.

Winston Wong is a scholar in residence at the Kaiser Permanente Center for Health Equity at the Fielding School of Public Health at the University of California, Los Angeles. His career has encompassed leadership roles at community health centers and in federal service, most recently at Kaiser Permanente, where he served as the medical director for community benefit. At Kaiser Permanente, he was responsible for its national philanthropic strategies to support clinical and population management initiatives with the safety net and for its quality initiatives to address disparities among its 12 million members. His commitment to addressing health equity is anchored by his experience as a bilingual primary care community health center physician for the Asian immigrant community in the Oakland, California, Chinatown neighborhood. That experience led him to leadership roles in the U.S. Public Health Service, serving in the Health Resources and Services Administration of the U.S. Department of Health and Human Services (HHS) as the chief clinical officer for a region that spanned the Pacific and western United States. He is the current chair of the HHS Advisory Committee on Minority Health, having previously served as a member. At the National Academies of Sciences, Engineering, and Medicine, he chairs the Roundtable on the Promotion of Health Equity, and has served on the Board of Population Health and Public Health Practice. As a leader in philanthropy, he has active board roles at The California Endowment and Grantmakers in Health. He also previously served as the board chair for the School-Based Health Alliance and is the current acting chief executive officer and the chair of the National Council of Asian Pacific Islander Physicians. He is a fellow of the American Academy of Family Practice. His work in developing programs and policies to address health equity has been recognized by awards from the California Primary Care Association, Latino Health Access, the Minority Health Foundation, Asian Health Services, and Congresswoman Barbara Lee. He has a B.A. and an M.A.

from the University of California, Berkeley, and an M.D. from the University of California, San Francisco. He is also the recipient of a doctor of humane letters from the A.T. Still University of Osteopathic Medicine.

PROJECT STAFF

Suzanne Le Menestrel (*Study Director*) is a senior program officer with the Board on Health Care Services at the National Academies of Sciences, Engineering, and Medicine, where her responsibilities have included directing four consensus studies focused on children and adolescents from birth to age 21. Prior to her tenure with the National Academies, she was the founding national program leader for youth development research at 4-H National Headquarters, U.S. Department of Agriculture; served as the research director at the Academy for Educational Development's Center for Youth Development and Policy Research; and was a research associate at Child Trends. She was a founder of the *Journal of Youth Development: Bridging Research and Practice* and chaired its publications committee. She has published in numerous refereed journals and is an invited member of several advisory groups, including a research advisory group for the American Camp Association and the National Leadership Steering Committee for the Cooperative Extension System–Robert Wood Johnson Foundation Culture of Health Initiative. She holds a B.S. in psychology from St. Lawrence University and an M.S. and a Ph.D. in human development and family studies from Pennsylvania State University. She also has a nonprofit management executive certificate from Georgetown University, and she is a certified association executive.

Susan B. Hassmiller (*Senior Scholar in Residence*) is the senior scholar in residence and the senior advisor on nursing to the president of the National Academy of Medicine. She is also the Robert Wood Johnson Foundation senior adviser for nursing and, in partnership with AARP, she directs the foundation's Future of Nursing: Campaign for Action. This 50-state and District of Columbia effort strives to implement the recommendations of *The Future of Nursing: Leading Change, Advancing Health*, for which she served as the report's study director. Her work has included service in public health settings at the local, state, and national levels, including at the Health Resources and Services Administration of the U.S. Department of Health and Human Services. She taught community health nursing at the University of Nebraska and George Mason University. She is a member of the National Academy of Medicine and a fellow of the American Academy of Nursing. She serves on several advisory committees and boards, including the Hackensack Meridian Health System, UnitedHealth, Carrier Clinic, and the American Red Cross. She is the recipient of many awards and three honorary doctorates, most notably the Florence Nightingale Medal, the highest international honor given to a nurse by the International Committee of the Red Cross. She has a bachelor's and a master's in nursing from Florida State University, a master's in community health nursing from the University of Nebraska Medical Center, and a Ph.D. in nursing administration and health policy from George Mason University.

Jennifer Lalitha Flaubert (*Program Officer*) is on the staff of the Board on Health Care Services at the National Academies of Sciences, Engineering, and Medicine. Prior to her work on this project, she carried out research and analysis for four consensus studies sponsored by the U.S. Social Security Administration (SSA). The SSA studies focused on disability benefits for children with mental disorders and speech and language disorders; assistive products and technologies in eliminating or reducing the effects of impairments for adults; and functional assessment for adults with disabilities. Prior to joining the National Academies, she worked at the U.S. Food and Drug Administration, managing the Adverse Event Reporting System at the Center for Food Safety and Applied Nutrition. She has a B.S. in biology from the University of Maryland, Baltimore County, and a master's in health administration from the University of Maryland.

Adrienne Formentos (*Research Associate*) is on the staff of the Board on Health Care Services at the National Academies of Sciences, Engineering, and Medicine. Previously, she worked as a research assistant with Knowledge Ecology International, focusing on advocacy for access to medication and clinical trials at the National Institutes of Health and the U.S. Food and Drug Administration. She served as a volunteer with the American Red Cross on the disaster action team (DAT) and case management and as the DAT administrator in San Francisco County. She also served as a volunteer with RotaCare Bay Area as a patient services navigator, assisting uninsured patients with follow-up care and applications for health care coverage. Early in her career, she served as a volunteer in Los Angeles, working at St. Vincent Medical Center as a patient advocate and community services coordinator, organizing health fairs and outreach to uninsured and underinsured populations. She has a B.A. in political science and English with a writing emphasis from Dominican University of California, where her thesis and research focused on sex trafficking and security governance, and an M.S. in global health from Georgetown University, where she co-led and authored a qualitative study on adolescents with mental and neurological disorders in Kintampo, Ghana.

Tochi Ogbu-Mbadiugha (*Senior Program Assistant*) is on the staff of the Board on Health Care Services at the National Academies of Sciences, Engineering, and Medicine. Prior to joining the National Academies, she assisted the legislative practice at Powers, Pyles, Sutter & Verville, PC, tracking legislation relevant to the firm's health care, disability, and rehabilitation clients. She holds a B.S. in kinesiology from the University of Maryland, College Park, where she completed research on the correlation between built environments and chronic disease rates among adults in urban settings.

Ashley Darcy-Mahoney (*Distinguished Nurse Scholar-in-Residence*) is a neonatal nurse practitioner and an associate professor at the George Washington University School of Nursing. She has worked throughout her career to advance nursing research, education, and practice, with a focus on neonatology, infant health, and developmental pediatrics. Her research has led to the creation of programs that improve infant health and developmental outcomes for at-risk and pre-term infants. As the director of infant research at the George Washington University Autism and Neurodevelopmental Institute, she advances the body of research in infant health and developmental outcomes in high-risk infants with a focus on understanding the early brain and development trajectories in this population. Her program of research leverages her background in neonatal nursing, behavioral and cognitive assessment, and training in neuroimaging to inform an understanding of multimodal social learning and social perception among high-risk infants and toddlers. Her work has been supported by the National Institutes of Health, the Office of Minority Health, and the Health Resources and Services Administration of the U.S. Department of Health and Human Services; the Robert Wood Johnson Foundation; United Way; and the Josiah Macy Jr. Foundation, among others. She has published in peer-reviewed interprofessional journals. She is a fellow of the American Academy of Nurses and a Robert Wood Johnson Foundation nurse faculty scholar alumna, and she has recently been named a modern health care rising star in nursing. She has a B.S. in nursing from Georgetown University and an M.S. in nursing in the field of neonatal nurse practitioner and a Ph.D. in nursing from the University of Pennsylvania.

Allison Squires (*Distinguished Nurse Scholar-in-Residence*) is an associate professor and the director of the Florence S. Downs Ph.D. Program in Nursing Research & Theory Development at the Rory Meyers College of Nursing at New York University (NYU). In addition to her primary appointment at the College of Nursing, she holds affiliated faculty appointments with the Grossman School of Medicine, the Center for Latin American Studies, and the Center for Drug Use and HIV Research, all at NYU. Her work on this study was part of her service as the distinguished nurse scholar-in-residence for the National Academy of Medicine. An internationally recognized health services researcher, she has led or participated in studies covering 38 countries, with current active projects in the European Union, Ghana, and Mexico. She is also leading the international arm of a COVID-19 study that examines how the global pandemic has affected clinical nursing practice on the front lines. Domestically, her research focuses on improving immigrant and refugee health outcomes with a special interest in breaking down language barriers during health care encounters. Most recently, she completed a study, funded by the Agency for Healthcare Research and Quality, that analyzed how language barriers influence the risk for hospital readmission from home health care. She has authored more than 150 publications, including more than 100 in peer-reviewed journals. She serves as an associate editor of the *International Journal of Nursing Studies* (the top-ranked nursing journal in the world), a research editor for the *Journal of Nursing Regulation*, and an associate editor for *BMC Health Services Research*. Prior to entering academia full time, she worked as a staff nurse in solid organ transplant and as a staff educator in the U.S. health care system. She has a B.S. in nursing from the University of Pennsylvania, an M.S. in nursing from Duquesne University, and a Ph.D. from Yale University. She also completed a postdoctoral fellowship in health outcomes research at the University of Pennsylvania.

Sharyl Nass (*Senior Board Director*) serves as the senior director of the Board on Health Care Services and the co-director of the National Cancer Policy Forum at the National Academies of Sciences, Engineering, and Medicine. To enable the best possible care for all patients, the board undertakes scholarly analysis of the organization, financing, effectiveness, workforce, and delivery of health care, with emphasis on quality, cost, and accessibility. For more than two decades, she has worked on a broad range of health and science policy topics that includes the quality, safety, and equity of health care and clinical trials; developing technologies for precision medicine; and strategies for large-scale biomedical science. She has been the recipient of the Cecil Medal for Excellence in Health Policy Research, a Distinguished Service Award from the National Academies, the mentor award from the Health and Medicine Division of the National Academies, and the Institute of Medicine staff team achievement award (as team leader). She holds a B.S. and an M.S. from the University of Wisconsin–Madison and a Ph.D. in cell biology from Georgetown University. She also undertook postdoctoral training at the Johns Hopkins University School of Medicine, as well as a research fellowship at the Max Planck Institute in Germany.

Appendix B

Data Collection and Information Sources

The Committee on the Future of Nursing 2020–2030 was asked to chart a path forward for nursing to help reduce health disparities and produce a report providing recommendations on how nurses can improve the health of individuals, families, and communities by addressing the social determinants of health. The broad scope of this 2-year study included an examination of nursing education, practice, research, and policy with the purpose of promoting health equity.

The committee was composed of 15 members with expertise and experience in diverse areas, including nursing education and training, nursing practice, health professions training and education, health policy, health economics, workforce policy, health care quality, health care delivery, hospital and health plan administration, public and community health, business administration, health informatics, health insurance systems, sociology, and health equity. The committee convened for four in-person meetings and participated in several conference calls throughout the study to deliberate on the content of this report and its recommendations. To provide a comprehensive response to the Statement of Task, the committee tapped the wide-ranging expertise of its members and reviewed data from a variety of sources, including recent literature, public and stakeholder input gathered through a series of town halls, site visits to a variety of health care settings where nurses work, and commissioned papers on selected topics. This appendix describes the inputs on which the committee relied to inform its deliberations and the approaches used to reach conclusions and craft recommendations.

INFORMATION COLLECTION AND PUBLIC INPUT

The committee received data and input from multiple sources throughout the course of the study. To support the committee's deliberations, a broad literature search for relevant published articles and reports, including grey literature, was conducted. For specific questions related to the charge that required specialized knowledge and expertise not available within its membership, the committee commissioned white papers, received support from AcademyHealth for data analyses, and heard presentations from other experts at town hall meetings.

Literature Search

A broad search for published literature was conducted using the Cochrane Database of Systemic Reviews, Embase, Medline, the National Bureau of Economic Research, the Organisation for Economic Co-operation and Development, PubMed, and Scopus. These databases cover all the sources of published literature indexed by CINHAL and more. Search terms targeted nursing workforce, leadership, clinical redesign, resilience, burnout, and technology and innovation broadly among the nursing field; the intersection of nursing and social determinants of health; programs and interventions to address health disparities, social needs, social determinants of health, and health equity broadly; and projections about the nursing field related to changing demographics and population needs and technological advancements. Publication dates were limited to 2009 to the present to reflect current policy, health care systems, and nursing education and workforce data since the prior *The Future of Nursing* report (IOM, 2011). Although the primary search was conducted in April 2019, staff conducted an updated search in February 2020, and additional publications and reports of relevance were added through June 2020.

Grey literature was searched for reports and data from multiple sources, including federal agencies, professional organizations, and scientific and health policy–focused organizations. Searches of federal agencies included the Agency for Healthcare Research and Quality, the Centers for Disease Control and Prevention, the Health Resources and Services Administration, the National Institute of Nursing Research, the U.S. Department of Defense (Military Health System and Tricare), the U.S. Department of Health and Human Services, the U.S. Department of Health and Human Services' Office of Disease Prevention and Health Promotion, the U.S. Department of Labor, and the U.S. Department of Veterans Affairs. Professional organizations included the American Association of Colleges of Nursing (AACN) and others. Institutions that regularly conduct scientific and health policy research, including AcademyHealth, the Patient-Centered Outcomes Research Institute, RAND, the Robert Wood Johnson Foundation (RWJF), The Commonwealth Fund, and others were also reviewed for relevant information.

The committee also relied on a collection of other National Academies reports in addition to the two prior nursing reports (IOM, 2011; NASEM, 2016). They are cited as appropriate throughout this report. They include

- *Crossing the Quality Chasm: A New Health System for the 21st Century* (IOM, 2001)
- *Unequal Treatment: Confronting Racial and Ethnic Disparities in Health Care* (IOM, 2003)
- *A Framework for Educating Health Professionals to Address the Social Determinants of Health* (NASEM, 2016a)
- *Communities in Action: Pathways to Health Equity* (NASEM, 2017)
- *Integrating Social Care into the Delivery of Health Care: Moving Upstream to Improve the Nation's Health* (NASEM, 2019a)
- *Taking Action Against Clinician Burnout: A Systems Approach to Professional Well-Being* (NASEM, 2019b)
- *Vibrant and Healthy Kids: Aligning Science, Practice, and Policy to Advance Health Equity* (NASEM, 2019c)
- *Social Isolation and Loneliness in Older Adults: Opportunities for the Health Care System* (NASEM, 2020a)
- *Birth Settings in America: Outcomes, Quality, Access, and Choice* (NASEM, 2020b)

AcademyHealth

To support the committee with timely data generation, analysis, synthesis, and dissemination, RWJF simultaneously contracted with AcademyHealth to support the committee with critical information not available in the current literature. AcademyHealth created a research network from its membership of health policy and workforce researchers to respond to requests from the committee and anticipate needs throughout the study process. Research products generated by the AcademyHealth research network informed the committee's deliberations and supported the committee's conclusions.

AcademyHealth selected five experts to serve as research managers to conduct research and analyses. Their efforts were managed by AcademyHealth staff. All products generated by AcademyHealth in support of the committee are available by request through the committee's Public Access File.

White Papers

The committee commissioned two white papers to further its understanding and incorporate input from experts in other areas:

- Barton, A. J., B. Brandt, C. J. Dieter, and S. D. Williams. 2020. *Social determinants of health: Nursing, health professions and interprofessional education at a crossroads*. https://www.nap.edu/resource/25982/Barton%20et%al%20Commissioned%20Paper.pdf (accessed June 7, 2021).
- Needleman, J. 2019. *Paying for nursing care in fee-for-service and value-based systems*. Paper commissioned by the Committee on the Future of Nursing 2020–2030.

TOWN HALLS

In conjunction with the site visits, the committee also participated in public town halls that included in-person expert and technical panels and testimony from organizations and individuals. These meetings[1] were open to the public and were webcast live.[2] The first town hall meeting, in Chicago, was held at Malcolm X Community College, and the theme was "Social Determinants of Health: Education, Research, and Practice." Experts, stakeholders, school administrators, community health nurses, and clinicians presented information on how nurse education is adapting to include new competencies, nurse engagement in research on health equity, and how nursing practice in the United States is currently incorporating social determinants of health screening and targeted programs. The town hall in Philadelphia was held at the University of Pennsylvania School of Nursing, and the theme was "Payment and Care for Complex Health and Social Needs," which featured speakers who discussed the role of nurses in rural health, maternal health, healthy aging, school nursing, and how payment systems can be reformed to support nurses' work. The final town hall, in Seattle, was held at the School of Nursing at the University of Washington, and the theme was "High Tech to High Touch," which focused on medical technology and its application in advancing health equity and well-being and preventing burnout of nurses.

The town hall meetings were important sources of information from other experts on selected topics relevant to the committee's task. They also served as important venues to solicit and receive public input.

SITE VISITS

Site visits were held in three cities in the United States between June and August 2019 and focused on current programs that involve nurses and address social determinants of health. The sites were chosen for their unique position in relationship to their communities and served as examples of successful models

[1] The agendas for all of the town halls are at the end of this appendix.

[2] Recordings of the town hall meetings are available online at https://www.nap.edu/catalog/25982 (accessed June 9, 2021).

in deploying nurses and nurse leaders, identifying community and social needs, and implementing these models with measurable outcomes. Committee members were able to learn about the programs and observe how nurses worked to address the social needs and social determinants of health facing their clients. The first site visits took place in Chicago in June 2019 and included several programs supported by Rush University. Some committee members were able to visit Threshold Community Mental Health Center, Sue Gin Health Center, and Simpson School Based Health Center. In July 2019, committee members met with leaders and staff at Stephen and Sandra Sheller 11th Street Family Health Services in Philadelphia and Camden Coalition and several of its community partners in Camden, New Jersey. The third set of site visits took place in and around Seattle and nearby cities and towns in August 2019. Subgroups of committee members visited Downtown Emergency Services Center, Kline Galland, International Community Health Services, Seattle and King County Public Health, Seattle Children's Hospital, Kitsap Connect at the Salvation Army in Kitsap, and the S'Klallum Reservation in Port Gamble.

The site visits gave the committee members valuable context for how nurses are working with clients with complex health conditions and social services needs, the challenges of this work, and the impact that these nurses and programs have on their clients and communities. Because the committee members bring a variety of life and professional experiences, it was imperative for them all to observe nurses in action and working in settings to address social needs and social determinants of health.

PUBLIC INPUT

Throughout the duration of the study, the committee received testimony and comments from the public through several channels. At each open session and town hall meeting, the committee heard testimony from organizations and comments from individuals about the study. Any comments made by online viewers during those meetings were also made available to the committee. The National Academy of Medicine conducted Twitter chats in coordination with the town hall meetings and shared ideas put forward with the committee. Throughout the study process, the committee invited the public to share comments and supporting materials with the committee by email. All public comments, in person and online, helped the committee understand the issues important to nurses, students, educators, leaders, and colleagues.

OPEN MEETING AND TOWN HALL AGENDAS

Below, the agendas for each of the committee's open meetings and town halls are listed chronologically. They include an introductory open meeting in Washington, DC; town hall meetings in Chicago, Philadelphia, and Seattle; and a second open meeting in Washington, DC.

OPEN MEETING 1

Open Session Agenda
March 20, 2019
2101 Constitution Avenue, NW, Washington, DC 20418

1:30 p.m. **Welcome Study Sponsor and Introductory Remarks**
Sharyl Nass, MS, PhD, Senior Board Director, Board on Health Care Services, National Academies of Sciences, Engineering, and Medicine
Mary Wakefield, PhD, RN, FAAN, and David Williams, MPH, PhD, Committee Co-Chairs

1:40 p.m. **Remarks from the National Academy of Medicine**
Victor Dzau, MD, President, National Academy of Medicine

1:50 p.m. **Introduction to *The Future of Nursing* (2011) and Its Impact**
Susan Hassmiller, RN, PhD, FAAN, Senior Scholar in Residence and Advisor to the President on Nursing, National Academy of Medicine

2:10 p.m. **Introduction to the Future of Nursing: Campaign for Action at the Center to Champion Nursing in America and Its Impact**
Susan Reinhard, RN, PhD, FAAN, Senior Vice President and Director, AARP Public Policy Institute, and Chief Strategist, Center to Champion Nursing in America

2:30 p.m. **Charge to the Committee**
Paul Kuehnert, DNP, RN, FAAN, Associate Vice-President for Programs, Robert Wood Johnson Foundation

Open Q&A with the Committee

2:50 p.m. **Invited comments** (limited to 5 minutes each)

- *Ann Cashion, PhD, RN, FAAN, Acting Director and Scientific Director, National Institute of Nursing Research, National Institutes of Health*
- *Ann Cary, PhD, MPH, RN, FAAN, FNAP, Chair, Board for American Association of Colleges of Nursing*
- *Donna Meyer, MSN, RN, ANEF, FAADN, Chief Executive Officer, Organization for Associate Degree Nursing*
- *Loressa Cole, DNP, MBA, RN, NEA-BC, FACHE, Chief Executive Officer, American Nurses Association*

- *Linda H. Yoder, PhD, MBA, RN, AOCN, FAAN, Immediate Past President, Academy of Medical-Surgical Nurses*
- *Susan V. Coleman, MPH, BSN, RN, Representing the Quad Council Coalition of Public Health Nursing Organizations*
- *G. Rumay Alexander, EdD, RN, FAAN, President, National League for Nursing*

3:25 p.m. **Public Comments**
Comments will be limited to 2 minutes per person; select comments submitted by online viewers will be read.

4:00 p.m. **Adjourn Open Session**

Chicago Town Hall: Integrating Social Determinants of Health into Nursing Education, Research, and Practice

June 7, 2019
8:30 a.m. to 12:30 p.m. at Malcom X Auditorium

8:30 a.m. **Welcome**

- *Sue Hassmiller, RN, PhD, FAAN, Senior Scholar in Residence and Senior Advisor to the President on Nursing, National Academy of Medicine*
- *Mary Wakefield, PhD, RN, FAAN, Visiting Distinguished Professor, Georgetown University and The University of Texas at Austin*

8:40 a.m. **Integrating Social Determinants of Health and Health Equity into Nursing Education**

- *Pam McCue, PhD, RN, Chief Executive Officer, Rhode Island Nurses Institute Middle College Charter High School*
- *Susan Swider, PhD, PHNA-BC, FAAN, Professor, Rush University*
- *Philip Dickison, PhD, Chief Officer of Operations and Examinations, National Council of State Boards of Nursing*
- *Moderated by Karen Cox, PhD, RN, FACHE, FAAN, President, Chamberlain University*

9:35 a.m. **Break**

9:45 a.m. **Integrating Social Determinants of Health and Health Equity into Nursing Research**

- *Ann Cashion, PhD, RN, FAAN, Acting Director and Scientific Director, National Institute of Nursing Research*
- *Janice Phillips, PhD, RN, CENP, FAAN, Director of Nursing Research and Health Equity, Nursing Administration, Rush University Medical Center*
- *Robyn Golden, LCSW, Associate Vice President of Population Health and Aging, Rush University Medical Center*
- *Moderated by Elizabeth Aquino, PhD, RN, Assistant Professor, DePaul University; President, National Association of Hispanic Nurses-Illinois Chapter*

10:40 a.m. **Integrating Social Determinants of Health and Health Equity into Nursing Practice**

- *Coletta C. Barrett, RN, FACHE, Vice President of Mission, Our Lady of the Lake Regional Medical Center*
- *Whitney Fear, RN, BSN, Case Manager/Outreach Nurse, Family HealthCare*
- *Teanya Norwood, MBA, MSN, RN, Social Determinants of Health Outcomes Manager, Promedica*
- *Moderated by Elizabeth Aquino, PhD, RN, Assistant Professor, DePaul University; President, National Association of Hispanic Nurses-Illinois Chapter*

11:35 a.m. **Invited Comments** (comments will be limited to 5 minutes)

- *Mary Beth Kingston, PhD, RN, NEA-BC, President, American Organization for Nursing Leadership*
- *Patricia Kunz Howard, PhD, RN, CEN, CPEN, TCRN, NE-BC, FAEN, FAAN, President, Emergency Nurses Association*
- *Mark Pelletier, RN, MS, Chief Operating Officer and Chief Nursing Officer, The Joint Commission*
- *Kaye Englebrecht, Executive Director, American Association of Occupational Health Nurses*

11:55 a.m. **Public Comments** (comments will be limited to 2 minutes)

12:25 p.m. **Closing Remarks and Adjourn**
Mary Wakefield, PhD, RN, FAAN, Visiting Distinguished Professor, Georgetown University and The University of Texas at Austin

---

Philadelphia Town Hall: Payment and Care for Complex Health and Social Needs

July 24, 2019
8:30 a.m. to 12:30 p.m. at the University of Pennsylvania School of Nursing

8:30 a.m. **Welcome**

- *Sue Hassmiller, RN, PhD, FAAN, Senior Scholar in Residence and Senior Advisor to the President on Nursing, National Academy of Medicine*
- *Mary Wakefield, PhD, RN, FAAN, Visiting Distinguished Professor, Georgetown University and The University of Texas at Austin*

8:40 a.m. **Serving Populations with, and at Risk for, Complex Health and Social Needs: Introduction and Overview**

Moderator: Antonia M. Villarruel, PhD, RN, FAAN, Professor and Margaret Bond Simon Dean, University of Pennsylvania School of Nursing

- **Maternal Child Health, Nurse Family Partnership**
  Erin Graham, BSN, RN, IBCLC, Nurse Supervisor, National Nurse-Led Care Consortium
- **School Health**
  Robin Cogan, MEd, RN, NCSN, School Nurse, Camden City School District (Yorkship Family School)
- **Rural Health**
  Cheri Rinehart, RN, BSN, NHA, President and Chief Executive Officer, Pennsylvania Association of Community Health Centers
- **Aging**
  C. Alicia Georges, EdD, RN, FAAN, Chair, Department of Nursing, Lehman College; National Volunteer President, AARP

10:10 a.m. **Break**

10:20 a.m. **Paying for Care for Those with Complex Health and Social Needs: Introduction and Overview**

Moderator: Margaret Flinter, APRN, PhD, FAAN, c-FNP, Senior Vice President and Clinical Director, Community Health Center, Inc.

- **Federal Perspective on Payment**
  Ellen-Marie Whelan, PhD, NP, RN, FAAN, Chief Population Health Officer, Center for Medicaid and CHIP Services

- **State Perspective on Payment**
  Carole Johnson, Commissioner, New Jersey Department of Human Services
- **Local/Regional Perspective on Payment**
  Terrie P. Sterling, MSN, MBA, Executive Vice President, Strategic Initiatives, Our Lady of the Lake Regional Medical Center

11:35 a.m. **Invited Comments** (limited to 5 minutes each)

- *Kristene Grayem, MSN, CNS, PPCNP-BC, RN-BC, President, American Academy of Ambulatory Care Nursing*
- *Elise Krikorian, Nursing Student, Pennsylvania State University; Chair, Population and Global Health, and Board Member, National Student Nurses' Association*
- *Linda MacIntyre, PhD, RN, American Red Cross*
- *Johnathan Holifield, JD, MEd, Executive Director, White House Initiative on Historically Black Colleges and Universities*

11:55 a.m. **Public Comments** (limited to 2 minutes each)

12:25 p.m. **Closing Remarks and Adjourn**
Sue Hassmiller, RN, PhD, FAAN

Seattle Town Hall: High Tech to High Touch

August 7, 2019
8:30 a.m. to 12:30 p.m. at the University of Washington, Kane Hall, Room 210

8:30 a.m. **Welcome**

- *Sue Hassmiller, RN, PhD, FAAN, Senior Scholar in Residence and Senior Advisor to the President on Nursing, National Academy of Medicine*
- *Mary Wakefield, PhD, RN, FAAN, Visiting Distinguished Professor, Georgetown University and The University of Texas at Austin*

8:40 a.m. **Advancing Health Care Equity in the Digital Age**
Moderator: Sue E. Birch, MBA, BSN, RN, Director, Washington State Health Care Authority

- *Molly Coye, MD, Executive-in-Residence, AVIA*

- *Kenya Beard, EdD, AGACNP-BC, NP-C, CNE ANEF, FAAN, Dean of Nursing and Health Sciences, Nassau Community College*
- *Molly McCarthy, MBA, BSN, RN-BC, Chief Nursing Officer, Microsoft*

9:35 a.m. **Break**

9:45 a.m. **Technology to Inform Practice and Advance Equity**
Moderator: Sofia Aragon, JD, BSN, Executive Director, Washington Center for Nursing

- *Sheila K. Shapiro, MBA, Senior Vice President-National Strategic Partnerships, UnitedHealthcare Clinical Services*
- *Eli Kern, MPH, BSN, Epidemiologist, Public Health Seattle and King County*
- *Stefan J. Torres, BSN, RN, CEN, Registered Nurse, Swedish Medical Center*

10:40 a.m. **Nurse Well-Being and Impact on Patients and Caregivers**
Moderator: Kristen Swanson, RN, PhD, FAAN, Dean and Professor, Seattle University College of Nursing

- *Tim Cunningham, DrPH, MSN, RN, Corporate Director of Patient and Family Centered Care, Emory Healthcare*
- *Bernadette M. Melnyk, PhD, RN, FAANP, FNAP, FAAN, Vice President for Health Promotion, University Chief Wellness Officer, Dean and Professor, College of Nursing, The Ohio State University*
- *Jason Wolf, PhD, CPXP, President and Chief Executive Officer, The Beryl Institute*

11:35 a.m. **Invited Comments** (limited to 5 minutes each)

- *Susan Reinhard, RN, PhD, FAAN, Senior Vice President and Director, AARP Public Policy Institute; Chief Strategist, Center to Champion Nursing in America*
- *Karen Cox, PhD, RN, FACHE, FAAN, President, American Academy of Nursing*
- *Joyce Sensmeier, MS, RN-BC, CPHIMS, FHIMSS, FAAN, Vice President of Informatics, HIMSS*
- *Christina Dempsey, DNP, MSN, CNOR, CENP, FAAN, Chief Nursing Officer, Press Ganey*

11:55 a.m. **Public Comments** (limited to 2 minutes each)

12:25 p.m. **Closing Remarks and Adjourn**
Sue Hassmiller, RN, PhD, FAAN, Senior Scholar in Residence and Senior Advisor to the President on Nursing, National Academy of Medicine

---

OPEN MEETING 2

Open Session Agenda
November 20, 2019
500 Fifth Street, NW, Washington, DC 20001

Open Session

9:00 a.m. **Welcome and Introductory Remarks**
Mary Wakefield, Committee Co-Chair
Moderated by Maureen Bisognano, Committee Member

Technical Panel

9:05 a.m. **Center for Health Care Strategies**
Tricia McGinnis, Executive Vice President and Chief Program Officer

9:20 a.m. **CVS Health**
Angela Patterson, Chief Nurse Practitioner Officer, CVS MinuteClinic and Vice President, CVS Health

9:35 a.m. **Pacific Business Group on Health**
Elizabeth Mitchell, President and Chief Executive Officer (presentation by Zoom)

9:50 a.m. **American Hospital Association**
- *Priya Bathija, Vice President, The Value Initiative, American Hospital Association*
- *Robyn Begley, American Hospital Association Senior Vice President and Chief Nursing Officer, American Organization for Nursing Leadership*

10:05 a.m. **Q&A with the Committee**
Moderated by Maureen Bisognano, Committee Member

10:45 a.m. **Closing Remarks**

Technical Panel Adjourns

10:50 a.m. **Break**

11:00 a.m. **Future Trends**
Lori Melichar, Senior Director, Program, Robert Wood Johnson Foundation

11:55 a.m. **Closing Remarks and Adjourn**
David Williams, Committee Co-Chair

REFERENCES

IOM (Institute of Medicine). 2001. *Crossing the quality chasm: A new health system for the 21st century*. Washington, DC: National Academy Press.

IOM. 2003. *Unequal treatment: Confronting racial and ethnic disparities in health care*. Washington, DC: The National Academies Press.

IOM. 2011. *The future of nursing: Leading change, advancing health*. Washington, DC: The National Academies Press.

NASEM (National Academies of Sciences, Engineering, and Medicine). 2016a. *A framework for educating health professionals to address the social determinants of health*. Washington, DC: The National Academies Press.

NASEM. 2016b. *Assessing progress on the Institute of Medicine report* The Future of Nursing. Washington, DC: The National Academies Press.

NASEM. 2017. *Communities in action: Pathways to health equity*. Washington, DC: The National Academies Press.

NASEM. 2019a. *Integrating social care into the delivery of health care: Moving upstream to improve the nation's health*. Washington, DC: The National Academies Press.

NASEM. 2019b. *Taking action against clinician burnout: A systems approach to professional well-being*. Washington, DC: The National Academies Press.

NASEM. 2019c. *Vibrant and healthy kids: Aligning science, practice, and policy to advance health equity*. Washington, DC: The National Academies Press.

NASEM. 2020a. *Social isolation and loneliness in older adults: Opportunities for the health care system*. Washington, DC: The National Academies Press.

NASEM. 2020b. *Birth settings in America: Outcomes, quality, access, and choice*. Washington, DC: The National Academies Press.

Appendix C

Data Sources, Definitions, and Methods

This appendix describes the two main sources of data used to produce the tables and figures for Chapter 3 on the nursing workforce and provides definitions of key variables. To assist researchers interested in replicating the descriptive results presented in the chapter, step-by-step procedures are provided that identify how variables were defined and data analyzed.

U.S. CENSUS BUREAU, AMERICAN COMMUNITY SURVEY (ACS)

The ACS, an annual nationwide survey designed to supplement the decennial census, began reporting data in 2001. The survey is based on the decennial census long form and produces population and housing information every year instead of every 10 years. Annual estimates of demographic, social, economic, and housing characteristics are available for geographic areas with a population of 65,000 or more. This includes all states, the District of Columbia, all congressional districts, approximately 800 counties, and 500 metropolitan and micropolitan statistical areas. Multiyear estimates are available for smaller geographic areas. During the demonstration stage (2000 to 2004), the U.S. Census Bureau carried out large-scale, nationwide surveys and produced reports for the nation, the states, and large geographic areas. The full implementation stage began in January 2005, with an annual housing unit (HU) sample of approximately 3 million addresses throughout the United States and 36,000 addresses in Puerto Rico. And in 2006, approximately 20,000 group quarters were added to the ACS so that the data fully describe the characteristics of the population residing in geographic areas.

The ACS Public Use Microdata Sample (PUMS) files show the full range of population and housing unit responses collected on individual ACS questionnaires for a subsample of ACS housing units and group quarters persons. PUMS files covering a 5-year period, such as 2011–2015, contain data on approximately 5 percent of the U.S. population.

The survey is fielded annually and achieves a response rate exceeding 90 percent. The race/ethnicity questions are asked nearly identically in the National Sample Survey of Registered Nurses (NSSRN), with respondents first asked about Hispanic origin and then about race. Data were weighted using sampling weights provided by the Census Bureau. Registered nurses (RNs) and nurse practitioners (NPs) are reported as working on a full-time equivalent (FTE) basis, which was estimated by counting a 40-hour workweek as 1.0 FTE.

The ACS surveyed approximately 12,000 RNs in each year from 2001 to 2004, and more than 30,000 RNs in each year starting in 2005 (when the sample was enlarged).

Population data used to adjust estimates of advanced practice registered nurses (APRNs) were obtained from the ACS.

Projections of the NP workforce come from Auerbach, D., P. Buerhaus, and D. Staiger. 2020. Implications of the rapid growth of the nurse practitioner workforce. *Health Affairs* 39(2):273–279. doi: 10.1377/hlthaff.2019.00686. These projections used data from the ACS.

The ACS can be accessed from the Census Bureau: *About PUMs*. https://www.census.gov/programs-surveys/acs/technical-documentation/pums/about.html (accessed April 13, 2021).

Definition of an FTE Employed RN or APRN: Using the ACS, a 1.0 FTE = 40 hours, reported as usual weekly hours.

Replicating Results: So that others can replicate the results shown in tables and figures in Chapter 3, the following provides the procedures used to analyze data and, in this illustrative example, develop the information shown in Table C-1.

TABLE C-1 Demographic Characteristics of Full-Time Equivalent (FTE) Registered Nurses (RNs), 2001–2018

		Year			
Characteristics		2000	2004	2008	2018
Total FTE RNs		1,985,944	2,142,353	2,542,703	3,352,461
FTE RN/population		7.04	7.32	8.36	10.26
Gender	Men	157,285 (7.9%)	211,891 (9.9%)	244,363 (9.6%)	424,342 (12.7%)
	Women	1,828,709 (92.1%)	1,930,462 (90.1%)	2,298,340 (90.4%)	2,928,119 (87.3%)

TABLE C-1 Continued

Characteristics		Year			
		2000	2004	2008	2018
Race	White	1,571,136 (79.1%)	1,673,073 (78.1%)	1,906,756 (75.0%)	2,313,002 (69.0%)
	Black/African American	175,669 (8.8%)	191,102 (8.9%)	269,271 (10.6%)	401,755 (12.0%)
	Asian	128,064 (6.4%)	161,598 (7.5%)	211,751 (8.3%)	305,740 (9.1%)
	Other	37,266 (1.9%)	28,027 (1.3%)	37,370 (1.5%)	84,454 (2.5%)
	Hispanic	73,859 (3.7%)	88,553 (4.1%)	117,556 (4.6%)	247,511 (7.4%)
Education	Associate	703,959 (37.7%)	839,506 (37.4%)	997,671 (38.1%)	910,629 (29.3%)
	Baccalaureate	610,735 (32.7%)	778,513 (34.7%)	957,422 (36.6%)	1,411,525 (45.4%)
	Graduate	202,018 (10.8%)	296,245 (13.2%)	361,559 (13.8%)	644,764 (20.7%)
Employment	Hospital	1,307,476 (63%)	1,352,356 (63.1%)	1,606,924 (63.2%)	2,071,034 (61.8%)
	Nonhospital	778,461 (37%)	789,997 (36.9%)	935,779 (36.8%)	1,281,424 (38.2%)
Age	<35	895,759 (23.0%)	486,098 (22.7%)	584,982 (23.0%)	980,779 (29.3%)
	35–49	2,017,925 (51.8%)	968,308 (45.2%)	1,017,328 (40.0%)	1,202,345 (35.9%)
	50+	980,651 (25.2%)	687,947 (32.1%)	940,394 (37.0%)	1,169,337 (34.9%)
	Overall average	42.68	43.87	44.37	43.69

Step-by-step procedures for generating the data shown in Table C-1. (Note: Names of variables as they appear in the ACS are depicted in *italic*.)

1. Download ACS data for 2018 (https://usa.ipums.org/usa-action/samples) (accessed July 24, 2021).
2. Select RNs only, *occ* = 3255 to 3258. See https://usa.ipums.org/usa/volii/occ2018.shtml (accessed July 24, 2021).
3. Construct FTEs
   a. Keep RNs who are working (empstat = 1).
   b. Construct FTEs as the ratio of usual hours worked (*uhrswork*, top-coded at 60 hours) to 40.

4. Use survey weights: variable is *perwt*.
5. U.S. population taken from the U.S. Census Bureau.
6. Gender: variable "*sex*" coded male = 1, female = 2.
7. Define race/ethnicity
    a. The ACS variable "*race*" is coded in the following categories:
        i. White
        ii. Black/African American
        iii. American Indian or Alaska Native
        iv. Chinese
        v. Japanese
        vi. Other Asian or Pacific Islander
        vii. Other race, not elsewhere classified
        viii. Two major races
        ix. Three or more major races
    b. The ACS variable "*hispan*" denotes various categories of Hispanic ethnicity.
    c. Coding is as follows:
        i. Any nonzero value of "*hispan*" → **Hispanic**
        ii. *Hispan* = 0 AND Black/African American → **Black/African American**
        iii. *Hispan* = 0 AND (Chinese, Japanese, or OtherAsian or Pacific Islander) → **Asian**
        iv. *Hispan* = 0 AND White → **White**
        v. All others = **Other**
8. Define educational attainment
    a. Use variable *educd*.
        i. Associate's degree: (*educd* ≥0 & *educd* <101)
        ii. Bachelor's degree (*educd* = 101)
        iii. Graduate (*educd* >101)
9. Define employment setting
    a. Prior to 2003, hospital employed if = *ind1990* = 831.
    b. 2003 and later, hospital employed if *ind* >8189 and *ind* <8193.
    c. All other are considered non-hospital employed.
10. The variable indicating age is *age*.

2008 AND 2018 NATIONAL SAMPLE SURVEY OF REGISTERED NURSES (NSSRN)

The second major source of data for constructing the tables and figures describing the RN and APRN workforce was the 2008 and 2018 NSSRNs. According to excerpts from the Health Resources and Services Administration, the NSSRN is the longest-running survey of RNs in the United States. Since its inaugural assessment in 1977, the NSSRN has provided educators, health workforce leaders, and policy makers with key details and developments of the nursing workforce supply. The survey assesses the number of RNs in the United States and contains questions regarding RNs' educational background, employment setting, job position, salary, geographic distribution, social and demographic characteristics, job satisfaction, and other information. The NSSRN was fielded every 4 years from 1977 to 2008 and again in 2018, with most questions pertaining to the RNs' status as of December 31, 2017.

Considered the cornerstone of nursing workforce data, this comprehensive exploration provides a dynamic status of the RN population by revealing their demographics, educational attainment, licenses and certifications, and employment characteristics. These continued data collections have supported evaluations of government RN workforce programs, assisting in critical decision making affecting the U.S. health care system. Highlighting the intricacies of the current status of the RN workforce is essential for developing strategies that address present-day health care challenges and evolving nursing workforce needs. Following the 2008 survey, the NSSRN questionnaire underwent a complete content review, and large improvements were made based on changes in the U.S. health care landscape and best practices in survey methodology. The latest survey also aims to reduce redundancy in the collection of data and lower the response burden on participants.

The 2018 NSSRN comprises questions derived from both the National Sample Survey of Nurse Practitioners (NSSNP) and the NSSRN for one concise survey capturing a broader RN workforce and is the first production implementation that provides data for both RNs and NPs at the state and national levels. In collaboration with the U.S. Census Bureau, the National Center for Health Workforce Analysis administered the 10th NSSRN data collection in 2018. From April 2018 to October 2018, a total of 50,273 RNs completed the survey via a web instrument or paper questionnaire with an unweighted response rate of 50.1 percent (49.1 percent weighted). This instrument gathered data from participants with active RN licenses from all U.S. states, providing a comprehensive look at the RN workforce. The 2018 NSSRN heavily oversampled NPs and obtained a roughly 50 percent response rate for RNs and NPs, with a final sample of 28,489 RNs excluding NPs and 21,784 NPs.

Data from the 2008 and 2018 NSSRNs were used to produce tables and figures describing characteristics of both RNs and the APRN workforce, particularly NPs.

Definition of Employed APRNs Using the 2008 and 2018 NSSRNs: The following procedures were used to define employed APRNs:

1. The respondent to the NSSRN was identified as being educationally prepared as either a nurse practitioner (NP), clinical nurse specialist (CNS), certified nurse midwife (CNM), or certified nurse anesthetist (CNA);

2. The respondent was identified as employed in nursing and active in providing patient care in his/her primary nursing position.

For cases in which a respondent reported being active in providing patient care but who was identified as being educationally prepared in more than one APRN role (e.g., as both an NP and a CNS), the following methods were used to assign the type of APRN employment (i.e., employed as an NP versus employed as a CNS):

For the 2008 NSSRN, if the respondent reported an APRN job title, the observation was coded to match that job title. For example, if the respondent was identified as having been prepared as both an NP and a CNS, employed in nursing, and active in providing patient care in his/her primary nursing position but reported a job title of NP, the observation was coded "employed as NP."

The 2018 NSSRN did not ask individuals to report a job title; however, the survey did ask explicitly whether the individual was employed as an NP. As a result, individuals who were identified as being educationally prepared in more than one APRN role but reported employment as an NP were coded "employed as NP."

If the reported job title could not be used to assign APRN employment type (2008 NSSRN) or the respondent did not report being employed as an NP (2018 NSSRN), variables describing the patient population most often cared for and the reported clinical specialty area were examined. For example, if the respondent was identified as being prepared as both a CNM and an NP, employed in nursing, and active in providing patient care in his/her primary nursing position but reported caring primarily for a geriatric patient population, the respondent was coded "employed as NP." Similarly, if the respondent was identified as being prepared as both a CNM and a CNS, employed in nursing, and active in providing patient care in his/her primary nursing position but reported a clinical specialty of labor and delivery, the individual was coded "employed as CNM."

If the reported primary patient population or clinical specialty could not be used to determine the type of APRN employment, data were examined to determine whether the respondent was required by an employer to be state-licensed (2008) or nationally certified (2018) in one role but not the other. In such cases APRN employment was assigned to the role in which the respondent reported employer-required licensure or certification.

In the 2018 NSSRN, all sample cases were assigned to an APRN employment type using this approach. In the 2008 NSSRN, a total of 30 sample observations (out of 2,381) were excluded from the analysis of APRN employment because an individual's APRN employment type could not be determined. These 30 cases represented an estimated 2,727 employed nurses active in providing patient care in their primary nursing position.

Replicating Results: To assist individuals interested in replicating results shown in tables and figures in Chapter 3, the following provides the procedures used to generate the data included in Table C-2, which are representative of the descriptive analyses conducted of RNs and APRNs.

TABLE C-2 Number of Registered Nurses by Employment Settings, Average Annual Earnings, and Age, 2018

Employment Settings	All RNs	Percent of Total	Average Annual Earnings	RNs Older Than 50	Percent Over Age 50
Hospital (not mental health)					
Critical access hospital	309,822	11.2%	$77,122	120,353	38.8%
Inpatient unit, not critical access hospital	755,639	27.2%	72,668	210,958	27.9%
Emergency department not critical access hospital	161,603	5.8%	76,577	32,708	20.2%
Hospital-sponsored ambulatory care	253,347	9.1%	77,826	128,015	50.5%
Hospital ancillary unit	54,181	2.0%	82,063	23,514	43.4%
Hospital nursing home unit	13,288	0.5%	72,442	7,564	56.9%
Hospital administration	95,543	3.4%	110,396	54,103	56.6%
Other hospital setting	20,133	0.7%	88,454	8,054	40.0%
Other hospital setting (consultative)	49,717	1.8%	85,924	34,436	69.3%
Other Inpatient Setting					
Nursing home unit not in hospital	60,615	2.2%	69,479	30,557	50.4%
Rehabilitation facility/long-term care	110,554	4.0%	74,832	50,160	45.4%
Inpatient mental health	55,089	2.0%	68,044	24,091	43.7%
Correctional facility	13,775	0.5%	75,769	5,028	36.5%
Other inpatient setting	11,938	0.4%	70,729	4,414	37.0%
Clinic/ambulatory					
Nurse-managed health center	9,183	0.3%	91,244	2,594	28.2%
Private medical practice (clinic, physician	138,291	5.0%	72,787	58,379	42.2%
Public clinic (rural health center, federally qualified health center, Indian Health Service, tribal clinic, etc.)	33,484	1.2%	69,983	14,210	42.4%
School health service (K–12 or college)	65,015	2.3%	57,506	36,718	56.5%

continued

TABLE C-2 Continued

Employment Settings	All RNs	Percent of Total	Average Annual Earnings	RNs Older Than 50	Percent Over Age 50
Outpatient mental health/substance	14,995	0.5%	68,288	7,124	47.5%
Ambulatory surgery center (freestanding)	8,807	0.3%	63,668	3,062	34.8%
Other clinical setting	67,182	2.4%	71,599	28,773	42.8%
Other Types of Settings					
Home health agency/service	175,212	6.3%	71,277	96,400	55.0%
Occupational health or employee health	11,360	0.4%	77,556	8,346	73.5%
Public health or community health	41,176	1.5%	71,712	16,952	41.2%
Government agency other than public/community health or correctional facility	41,229	1.5%	81,423	23,777	57.7%
Outpatient dialysis center	27,704	1.0%	81,032	11,231	40.5%
University or college academic	34,698	1.2%	70,857	19,178	55.3%
Case management/disease management	78,637	2.8%	81,324	38,202	48.6%
Call center/telenursing center	15,935	0.6%	79,754	9,613	60.3%
Other type of setting	12,197	0.4%	89,431	7,298	59.8%
Other type of setting (consultative)	38,130	1.4%	92,522	21,366	56.0%
All	2,778,476	100.0%	76,180	1,137,176	

SOURCE: Calculations based on the 2018 National Sample Survey of Registered Nurses.

Step-by-step procedures to replicate the results for Table C-2 are shown below. Note that the variable names are the original variable names given in the 2018 NSSRN public use file.

1. Download the 2018 NSSRN public use data.
2. Define RNs as non-APRNs using the variable APN_COMBOS_PUF and respondents with value = 0.
3. Define an FTE as the ratio of hours worked (variable = HRS_YR) to 2000. FTEs = HRS_YR/2000.
4. Use the variable RKRNWGTA as the survey weight for all respondents.
5. Define RNs over age 50 using the variable AGE_PUF.
6. Tabulate employment settings using the variable PN_EMPSET_COMB_PUF, only for respondents who are an RN (step 2) and working at least 0.75 FTE (step 3), for both those under and over age 50 (step 5), employing survey weights (step 4), and for each value of PN_EMPSET_COMB_PUF, summarizing earnings using the variable PN_EARN_PUF.

In the case of Table C-3, which focuses on NP employment, the data shown in the table also were obtained from the 2018 NSSRN. Step-by-step procedures to replicate the results are shown below. Note that the variable names are the original variable names given in the 2018 NSSRN public use file.

TABLE C-3 Nurse Practitioner Employment Settings, 2018

Employment Setting	Number	Percent	Median FTE Annual Earnings
Clinic or Ambulatory Care Settings			
Nurse-managed health center	1,736	0.9%	$99,000
Private medical practice (clinic, physician office, etc.)	63,155	32.6%	100,000
Public clinic (rural health center, federally qualified health center, Indian Health Service, etc.)	16,309	8.4%	97,000
School health service (K–12 or college)	4,060	2.1%	90,000
Outpatient mental health/substance abuse	5,528	2.9%	110,000
Other clinic/outpatient/ambulatory setting	9,742	5.0%	106,000
Total	100,529	51.9%	
Other Settings			
Home health agency/service	4,118	2.1%	105,000
Occupational health/employee health service	1,459	0.8%	106,000
Public health/community health agency	995	0.5%	100,000
Government agency, other	3,558	1.8%	110,000
University or college academic department	2,021	1.0%	91,000
Case management/disease management insurance company	970	0.5%	114,000
Other setting (outpatient dialysis centers, call centers)	1,064	0.5%	100,000
Total	14,185	7.3%	105,000
Hospitals			
Critical access hospital	7,971	4.1%	112,000
Inpatient unit, not critical access hospital	28,855	14.9%	110,000
Hospital-sponsored ambulatory care	21,464	11.1%	109,000
Emergency department, not critical access hospital	6,077	3.1%	120,000
Other hospital-based setting	3,758	1.9%	105,000
Total	68,125	35.2%	112,000

continued

TABLE C-3 Continued

Employment Setting	Number	Percent	Median FTE Annual Earnings
Other Inpatient Settings			
Nursing home, nonhospital	2,687	1.4%	105,000
Rehabilitation facility/long-term care	3,705	1.9%	105,000
Inpatient mental health/substance abuse	2,502	1.3%	111,000
Correctional facility	1,567	0.8%	108,000
Other inpatient setting	288	0.1%	103,000
Total	10,749	5.6%	

SOURCE: Calculations from data in the 2018 National Sample Survey of Registered Nurses.

Employed NPs active in providing patient care were identified using the variables "NP_EMPL_17" and "PN_PATCARE"; for both variables, sample cases with a recorded value of "1." In Table C-3, the values of "PN_HOSPSET," "PN_INPSET_PUF," "PN_CLINSET_PUF," and "PN_OTHSET" were used to calculate estimated employment by work setting; within each broad group, specified settings with small sample sizes were recoded and combined with cases originally reported as "other setting." For example, in the broad group of "other setting," the small number of cases reported for "outpatient dialysis centers" and "call center/telenursing center" were recoded and combined with cases originally reported as "other setting." The variables "PN_EARN_PUF" and "EMP_STAT" were used to calculate median full-time annual earnings from the principal nursing position, by employment setting.

Appendix D

Glossary

Accountable care organizations: Groups of health care providers who work together to coordinate care for their patients who are covered by Medicare.

Advanced practice registered nurses (APRNs): Hold at least a master's degree in addition to the initial nursing education and licensing required for all RNs, and may continue in clinical practice or prepare for administrative and leadership positions.

Community resilience: "Community capabilities that buffer it from or support effective responses to disasters," and is of growing importance in disaster preparedness, particularly in underresourced areas (Wells et al., 2013, p. 1172).

Compassion fatigue: "A health care practitioner's diminished capacity to care as a consequence of repeated exposure to the suffering of patients, and from the knowledge of their patients' traumatic experiences" (Cavanagh et al., 2020, p. 640).

COVID-19: The official name for the disease identified as the cause of the novel coronavirus outbreak first identified in Wuhan, China, in 2019; CO stands for corona(virus), VI for virus, and D for disease. COVID-19 is a variant of a group of coronaviruses that can infect humans and animals and cause respiratory illnesses (CDC, 2020).

Cultural competency: "A set of congruent behaviors, attitudes, and policies that come together in a system, agency, or among professionals that enables effective work in cross-cultural situations. Competence implies the capacity to function effectively as an individual and an organization within the context of the cultural beliefs, behaviors, and needs presented by consumers and their communities" (Cross et al., 1989, p. 17).

Cultural humility: In health care, cultural humility is a goal in training and education that informs providers' relationships to patients and people and involves "developing mutually beneficial and non-paternalistic partnerships with communities on behalf of individuals and defined population" (Tervalon and Murray-Garcia, 1998, p. 118).

Cultural racism: "The ideology of inferiority in the values, language, imagery, symbols, and unstated assumptions of the larger society" (Williams et al., 2019, p. 110).

Cultural taxation: Refers to the phenomenon whereby faculty who are individuals of color are asked routinely to take on extra, uncompensated work to address a lack of diversity in their institutions.

Culture of health: The Robert Wood Johnson Foundation (RWJF, n.d.) defines a culture of health as "one in which good health and well-being flourish across geographic, demographic, and social sectors; fostering healthy equitable communities guides public and private decision making; and everyone has the opportunity to make choices that lead to healthy lifestyles."

Disaster: Defined as a serious disruption of the functioning of a community or a society at any scale due to hazardous events interacting with conditions of exposure, vulnerability, and capacity, leading to one or more of the following: human, material, economic, and environmental losses and impacts (UNDRR, 2017).

Discrimination: Occurs when people or institutions treat racial groups differently, with or without intent, and this difference results in inequitable access to opportunities and resources (Williams et al., 2019).

Downstream intervention: "Interventions and strategies that aim to provide equitable access to care and services to individuals, groups and communities, in order to mitigate the negative impacts of adverse health effects" (NCCDH, 2020). These interventions occur at the individual and family level.

Grey literature: Literature, writing, and research that is produced at all levels of government, academia, and private industry in both print and electronic formats but is not controlled by or associated with commercial publishers (Farace et al., 2005; Schöpfel and Farace, 2010).

Health care equity: Ensuring that access to health care and high-quality care are available to all individuals and communities.

Health disparities: Health differences that "adversely affect groups of people who have systematically experienced greater social or economic obstacles to health based on their racial or ethnic group, religion, socioeconomic status, gender, mental health, cognitive, sensory, or physical disability, sexual orientation, geographic location, or other characteristics historically linked to discrimination or exclusion" (Carter-Pokras and Baquet, 2002; HHS, 2016).

Health equity: "The state in which everyone has the opportunity to attain full health potential and no one is disadvantaged from achieving this potential because of social position or any other socially defined circumstance" (NASEM, 2017).

Health inequities: "Systematic differences in the opportunities that groups have to achieve optimal health, leading to unfair and avoidable differences in health outcomes" (NASEM, 2017).

Implicit bias: "Refers to the attitudes or stereotypes that affect our understanding, actions, and decisions in an unconscious manner" (Staats, 2013, p. 6).

Intersectionality: Recognizing the complex factors that contribute to health inequities by stressing the importance of the intersection of multiple interdependent social determinants that shape the health and well-being of individuals and communities. More specifically, the theoretical framework considers the intersection of these social determinants at the "micro level of individual experience to reflect multiple interlocking systems of privilege and oppression at the macro, social-structural level" (Bowleg, 2012, p. 1267).

Licensed practical nurses (LPNs)/licensed vocational nurses (LVNs): Support the health care team and work primarily under the supervision of a registered nurse (RN), advanced practice registered nurse, or physician. They perform basic tasks, such as taking vital signs; administering medications; changing wound dressings; and ensuring that patients are comfortable and receive nutrition and hydration. LPNs/LVNs complete a 12- to 18-month education program at a vocational/technical school or community college, and are required to take a nationally standardized licensing exam in the state where they begin practice (IOM, 2011). In nursing homes, where they predominate, they supervise nurse aides to oversee care. LPNs/LVNs can become RNs through associate's degree or baccalaureate in nursing bridge programs.

Microaggressions: "Brief and commonplace daily verbal, behavioral, or environmental indignities, whether intentional or unintentional, that communicate hostile, derogatory, or negative racial slights and insults toward people of color" (Sue et al., 2007, p. 273).

Midstream interventions: "Seek to reduce exposure to hazards by improving material working and living conditions, or to reduce risk by promoting healthy behaviors" (NCCDH, 2020). These interventions occur at a level between upstream factors (e.g., policy) and downstream factors (e.g., chronic illness), and often include a mixture of population- and individual-level factors, such as access to quality health care.

Moral well-being: "The highest attainable development of innate capacities that enable humans to flourish as embodied, individuated but necessarily interdependent social organisms by managing the adaptive challenges of vulnerability, constraint, connection, and cooperation in an uncertain, risky environment" (Thompson, 2018, p. 4).

Nursing informatics: "The specialty that integrates nursing science with multiple information and analytical sciences to identify, define, manage and communicate data, information, knowledge and wisdom in nursing practice" (ANA, 2015).

Population health: "The health outcomes of a group of individuals, including the distribution of such outcomes within the group" (Kindig and Stoddart, 2003, p. 381).

Posttraumatic stress disorder (PTSD): A "psychiatric disorder that may occur in people who have experienced or witnessed a traumatic event such as a natural disaster, a serious accident, a terrorist act, war/combat, or rape or who have been threatened with death, sexual violence or serious injury" (APA, 2020).

Public health: "The art and science of preventing disease, prolonging life and promoting health through the organized efforts of society" (Acheson, 1988).

Racism: "An organized social system in which the dominant racial group, based on an ideology of inferiority, categorizes and ranks people into social groups called 'races' and uses its power to devalue, disempower, and differentially allocate valued societal resources and opportunities to groups defined as inferior" (Williams et al., 2019, p. 106).

Registered nurses (RNs): Provide preventive, primary, and acute care in collaboration with other health professionals. Their roles vary enormously by setting but can include such activities as conducting health assessments and taking health histories, looking for signs that health is deteriorating or improving, providing counseling and education to promote health and manage chronic disease, administering medications and other personalized interventions and treatments, and coordinating care. RNs are required to take a nationally standardized licensing exam after completing a program at a community college, diploma school, or 4-year college or university.

Relational ethics: Defined in health care as actions that take place within relationships and consider the existence of the other (i.e., patient, nurse) (Bergum and Dossetor, 2005). Core tenets include mutual respect, engagement, embodied knowledge, environment, and uncertainty; the most important tenet is mutual respect (Pollard, 2015).

Resilience: Refers to "the capacity of dynamic systems to withstand or recover from significant disturbances" (Masten, 2007, p. 923).

Resilience engineering: Focused on "understanding the nature of adaptations, learning from success and increasing adaptive capacity" (Anderson et al., 2016, p. 1).

Social determinants of health (SDOH): The conditions of the environments in which "people live, learn, work, play, worship, and age that affect a wide range of health, functioning, and quality-of-life outcomes and risks." These conditions include education, employment, health systems and services, housing, income and wealth, the physical environment, public safety, the social environment (including structures, institutions, and policies), and transportation at the population level. SDOH are sometimes called social influences or social factors (HHS, 2020).

Social justice: The concept that everyone deserves equal rights and opportunities. In health care, it refers to the delivery of high-quality care to all individuals.

Social needs: A person-centered concept that incorporates a person's perception of her or his own health-related needs. Nonmedical social needs that may affect health can include housing instability, food insecurity, and exposure to violence that drives health care utilization and may impact health outcomes (NASEM, 2019).

Structural inequities: The personal, interpersonal, institutional, and systemic drivers—such as racism, sexism, classism, ableism, xenophobia, and homophobia—that make those identities salient to the fair distribution of health opportunities and outcomes (NASEM, 2017, p. 99).

Structural racism: "The processes of racism that are embedded in laws, policies, and practices of society and its institutions that provide advantages to racial groups deemed as superior, while differentially oppressing, disadvantaging, or otherwise neglecting racial groups viewed as inferior" (Williams et al., 2019, p. 107).

Systemic racism: According to The Aspen Institute, "In many ways 'systemic racism' and 'structural racism' are synonymous. If there is a difference between the terms, it can be said to exist in the fact that a structural racism analysis pays more attention to the historical, cultural and social psychological aspects of our currently racialized society" (The Aspen Institute, 2016).

Telehealth: "The use of electronic information and telecommunications technologies to support and promote long-distance clinical health care, patient and professional health-related education, and public health and health administration" (HHS, 2020).

Trauma-informed: "A program, organization, or system that is trauma-informed realizes the widespread impact of trauma and understands potential paths for recovery; recognizes the signs and symptoms of trauma in clients, families, staff, and others involved with the system; and responds by fully integrating knowledge about trauma into policies, procedures, and practices, and seeks to actively resist re-traumatization" (SAMHSA, 2014, p. 13).

Upstream interventions: These "interventions and strategies focus on improving fundamental social and economic structures in order to decrease barriers and improve supports that allow people to achieve their full health potential" (NCCDH, 2020). These interventions occur at the community and population levels.

Well-being: An inherently complex concept, encompassing an individual's appraisal of physical, social, and psychological resources needed to meet a particular psychological, physical, or social challenge (Dodge at al., 2012).

White privilege: Defined by The Aspen Institute (2016) as "whites' historical and contemporary advantages in access to quality education, decent jobs and liveable wages, homeownership, retirement benefits, wealth, and so on."

REFERENCES

Acheson, E. D. 1988. On the state of the public health [the fourth Duncan lecture]. *Public Health* 102(5):431–437.

ANA (American Nurses Association). 2015. *Nursing: Scope and standards of practice*, 3rd ed. Silver Springs, MD: Nursesbooks.org.

Anderson, J. E., A. J. Ross, J. Back, M. Duncan, P. Snell, K. Walsh, and P. Jaye. 2016. Implementing resilience engineering for healthcare quality improvement using the CARE model: A feasibility study protocol. *Pilot and Feasibility Studies* 2:61. doi: 10.1186/s40814-016-0103-x.

APA (American Psychiatric Association). 2020. *What is posttraumatic stress disorder?* https://www.psychiatry.org/patients-families/ptsd/what-is-ptsd (accessed April 10, 2021).

Bergum, V., and J. B. Dossetor. 2005. *Relational ethics: The full meaning of respect*. Hagerstown, MD: University Publishing Group.

Bowleg, L. 2012. The problem with the phrase women and minorities: Intersectionality—an important theoretical framework for public health. *American Journal of Public Health* 102(7):1267–1273.

Carter-Pokras, O., and C. Baquet. 2002. What is a "health disparity"? *Public Health Reports* 117(5): 426–434.

Cavanagh, N., G. Cockett, C. Heinrich, L. Doig, K. Fiest, J. Guichon, S. Page, I. Mitchell, and C. Doig. 2020. Compassion fatigue in healthcare providers: A systematic review and meta-analysis. *Nursing Ethics* 27(3):639–665.

CDC (Centers for Disease Control and Prevention). 2020. *About COVID-19*. https://www.cdc.gov/coronavirus/2019-ncov/cdcresponse/about-COVID-19.html (accessed April 10, 2021).

Cross, T. L., M. P. Benjamin, and M. R. Isaacs. 1989. *Towards a culturally competent system of care*. Washington, DC: CASSP Technical Assistance Center, Georgetown University Child Development Center.

Dodge, R., A. Daly, J. Huyton, and L. Sanders. 2012. The challenge of defining wellbeing. *International Journal of Wellbeing* 2(3):222–235. doi: 10.5502/ijw.v2i3.4.

Farace, D. J., J. Frantzen, Greynet, and Grey Literature Network Service. 2005. *Work on grey in progress*. Sixth international conference on grey literature, NYAM conference center, New York, December 2004. Amsterdam: TextRelease.

HHS (U.S. Department of Health and Human Services). 2016. *Disparities*. http://www.healthypeople.gov/2020/about/foundation-health-measures/Disparities (accessed January 28, 2016).

HHS. 2020. *Social determinants of health*. https://www.healthypeople.gov/2020/topics-objectives/topic/social-determinants-of-health (accessed April 10, 2021).

IOM (Institute of Medicine). 2011. *The future of nursing: Leading change, advancing health*. Washington, DC: The National Academies Press.

Kindig, D., and G. Stoddart. 2003. What is population health? *American Journal of Public Health* 93(3):380–383.

Masten, A. 2007. Resilience in developing systems: Progress and promise as the fourth wave rises. *Development and Psychopathology* 19:921–930.

NASEM (National Academies of Sciences, Engineering, and Medicine). 2017. *Communities in action: Pathways to health equity*. Washington, DC: The National Academies Press.

NASEM. 2019. *Integrating social care into the delivery of health care: Moving upstream to improve the nation's health*. Washington, DC: The National Academies Press.

NCCDH (National Collaborating Centre for Determinants of Health). 2020. *Glossary: Upstream/downstream*. https://nccdh.ca/glossary/entry/upstream-downstream (accessed April 10, 2021).

Pollard, C. 2015. What is the right thing to do: Use of a relational ethic framework to guide clinical decision-making. *International Journal of Caring Sciences* 8(2):362–368.

RWJF (Robert Wood Johnson Foundation). n.d. *What is a culture of health?* https://www.evidenceforaction.org/what-culture-health (accessed April 10, 2021).

SAMHSA (Substance Abuse and Mental Health Services Administration). 2014. *SAMHSA's concept of trauma and guidance for a trauma-informed approach*. HHS Publication No. (SMA) 14-4884. Rockville, MD: Substance Abuse and Mental Health Services Administration.

Schöpfel, J., and D. J. Farace. 2010. Grey literature. In *Encyclopedia of Library and Information Sciences*, 3rd ed., edited by M. J. Bates and M. N. Maack. Boca Raton, FL: CRC Press.

Staats, C. 2013. *State of the science: Implicit bias review*. Columbus, OH: Kirwan Institute for the Study of Race and Ethnicity. http://kirwaninstitute.osu.edu/docs/SOTS-Implicit_Bias.pdf (accessed April 10, 2021).

Sue, D. W., C. Capodilupo, G. Torino, J. Bucceri, A. Holder, K. Nadal, and M. Equilin. 2007. Racial microaggressions in everyday life: Implication for clinical practice. *American Psychologist* 64(4):271–286. doi: 10.1037/0003-066X.62.4.271.

Tervalon, M., and J. Murray-Garcia. 1998. Cultural humility versus cultural competence: A critical distinction in defining physician training outcomes in multicultural education. *Journal of Health Care for the Poor and Underserved* 9(2):117–125.

The Aspen Institute. 2016. *11 terms you should know to better understand structural racism*. https://www.aspeninstitute.org/blog-posts/structural-racism-definition (accessed March 3, 2021).

Thompson, L. J. 2018. *Moral dimensions of wellbeing*. Paper presented at the Society for Business Ethics Annual Conference, Chicago IL, August 10–12, 2018.

UNDRR (United Nations Office for Disaster Risk Reduction). 2017. *Terminology*. https://www.undrr.org/terminology/disaster (accessed June 9, 2021).

Wells, K. B., J. Tang, E. Lizaola, F. Jones, A. Brown, A. Stayton, A. Plough. 2013. Applying community engagement to disaster planning: Developing the vision and design for the Los Angeles County Community Disaster Resilience Initiative. *American Journal of Public Health* 103(7):1172–1180. doi: 10.2105/ajph.2013.301407.

Williams, D., J. Lawrence, and B. Davis. 2019. Racism and health: Evidence and needed research. *Annual Review of Public Health* 40:105–125. doi: 10.1146/annurev-publhealth-040218-043750.

Appendix E

The Future of Nursing 2020–2030: Meeting America Where We Are

Supplemental Statement of William M. Sage, M.D., J.D.

In 2019, the National Academies of Sciences, Engineering, and Medicine launched its second major consensus study (and third study in 15 years) of the future of the nursing profession in the United States, with an intended focus on community nursing and health equity. In 2020, the COVID-19 global pandemic changed how the United States understands its health and its health care system.

Such times cry out for policies with ambition and courage, especially from organizations such as the National Academies that serve as stewards and guardians of biomedical science and public health. I write separately today because, in my view, the conclusions and recommendations in this report are not sufficiently bold to fully meet the moment.

The committee's charge was amended in mid-2020, and the project's timetable extended, to consider COVID-19. Among other changes, the final report includes a COVID-focused chapter on "disaster preparedness." Given the systematic issues of injustice and avoidable harm that the COVID-19 pandemic has revealed, it is my view that the *least* important lessons for the future of nursing may be about disaster preparedness. The U.S. pandemic experience has made plain that illness is unequally distributed across groups and communities, that the burdens of illness track long-standing racial and socioeconomic injustices, that public engagement and education are critical components of health improvement, and that nurses are essential to an effective public health system now and in the future.

As this report was being drafted, heartbreaking headlines proclaimed growing numbers of sick and dying across the country and throughout the world. Most severely—and unfairly—affected were individuals and communities of color, who suffer from the compound disadvantages of racism, poverty, workplace hazards, compromised health care access, and preexisting health conditions resulting from the foregoing factors. Seniors in long-term care and other congregate settings were also profoundly endangered.

Nurses in COVID-19 hot spots went to work every day, often for extended shifts, caring for patients despite the hazard to themselves and their family members. Some nurses served on the front lines in hospital emergency departments and intensive care units, or in skilled nursing facilities. Many left loved ones to help strangers who were sick and dying, sometimes rendering care without adequate protective equipment. Other nurses have educated the public about COVID-related risks and protective measures, including overcoming vaccine hesitancy, while working to test communities and trace contacts of those infected. The rewards for such dedicated service are great, but so are the dangers of psychic trauma and moral injury to nurses and other health care workers. It seems likely that the scope and scale of post-pandemic stress on the health care workforce will be unprecedented in American history.

COVID-19 has also revealed profound problems with the financing and delivery of American health care, presenting both challenges and opportunities for nursing, and has reopened old wounds about lack of voice and subordination in professional hierarchies. Even as the pandemic raged, nurses with outstanding professional skills suffered economic hardship as reduced demand for nonemergency, specialized medical care and surgical procedures resulted in furloughs and layoffs. The value of nursing has often been obscured by hospital accounting practices that treat nurses as undifferentiated though dominant contributors to organizational "labor costs"—relegating them to the expense side of the ledger. This short-sightedness explains why nurses were among the first casualties of COVID-related financial pressures on many provider organizations.

Nurses cannot engage the social determinants of health as charity or in their spare time, but must be paid for the value they deliver, especially as hospitals and other major employers of nurses become accountable for population health. Considered as an engine of value creation, nursing is economically significant at the national level and in every community across the country. Nurses' cumulative national earnings total approximately $250 billion annually, as much as the entire economies of Connecticut, Oregon, and South Carolina. Registered nurses earn more in the aggregate than any occupational classification in the United States except "manager" and "chief executive"—more even than physicians. Secure employment at fair wages contributes to economic stability for nurses and their families. Because the United States spends health care dollars in every region, nurses' earnings also build health equity by helping to offset socioeconomic disadvantage, including in communities of color.

This supplemental statement focuses on missed opportunities—potential conclusions and recommendations within the project's Statement of Task, illuminated by the COVID-19 experience, that were not included in the report. I regard these as critical omissions because I do not think the goal of a National

Academies report should be to publish a tome, or to compile a long list of approved areas for possible funding and future policy development. In my view, its goal should be to make a compelling case for action and advocacy through clear, unmistakable statements combining data, insight, and purpose.

A futurist project on the nursing profession at this moment in our country's health care history demands the formulation of strong hypotheses for the post-COVID era, which ongoing research, some of it COVID-related, will continue to test. In my experience, moreover, major National Academies reports on health policy are most effective when they are self-critical. Some progress has been made since this report's 2011 predecessor (FON-1), but other recommendations in FON-1 have languished or stalled. Whatever has been accomplished since 2011, the COVID-19 pandemic shows that it was not enough. Nursing has far more to do, and nursing must be inspired and empowered to do it.

As a physician, I might seem an unlikely messenger to suggest that a report on the future of nursing lacks sufficient ambition. But physicians still hold the greatest public authority in U.S. health care, and they still wield the most power. If radical change in our health care system is required to promote both health and justice, physicians must open their tent and welcome nurses and others inside, an urgent set of tasks that the National Academies can help move forward. I therefore feel a special responsibility for the reach and quality of this critically important work.

The recommendations in this report are well-intentioned and well-expressed, and I wholeheartedly endorse their goals and most of their details. But, in my view, they dwell excessively on generalities regarding health equity and the social determinants of health. Using the right vocabulary is not enough—COVID-19 proves that talking the talk without walking the walk does not shorten the journey, much less reach the destination.

I believe that substantial evidence, including ongoing research in connection with COVID-19, supports the following additional conclusions and associated recommendations to improve the future of nursing and promote health equity as called for in the Statement of Task:

1. *Despite lavish expenditures, America's "medical-industrial complex" is failing to preserve and improve the nation's health*. COVID-19 has shown that core public and community health functions are inadequately supported and poorly coordinated. At the same time, major segments of our massive yet often elective clinical enterprise—which employs the majority of nurses—now demand even greater taxpayer subsidy as they struggle to continue their accustomed activities. The report recommends workforce expansion, but would finance it indirectly through existing clinical revenue streams that would serve mainly to further medicalize social problems. Instead, it should call for substantially greater direct

public funding of community and public health nursing as part of an overall redirection of investment from medical care to health. Enhanced support for public employment should be accompanied by an expansion of scope of practice that empowers bachelor's degree–trained RNs to serve their communities more effectively, amplifying the benefits of full practice authority for nurse practitioners and other advanced practice nurses.

2. *The nursing profession is an economic force for health improvement and should be treated as such by hospital systems, other clinical settings, and payers.* When a physician performs a clinical task, the presumption is that the physician will be paid for that task; when a nurse (leaving aside advanced practice) performs a clinical task, the presumption is that her or his work is subsumed in aggregate fees paid to the facility where she or he practices—even if both the physician and the nurse are employees of the same organization. Treating physician services as attracting revenue while nurse services impose costs disempowers nursing and favors procedural over community-oriented care. The report should devote greater attention to identifying, measuring, and rewarding the patient and public benefits of all nursing care, not just advanced practice—including facilitating revenue generation by nurses who improve quality, safety, and population health.
3. *Nursing is too siloed and too rivalrous, both within itself and with respect to other professions.* Significant gains in nurses' authority and performance with respect to community health and health equity are more likely to result from partnering than from climbing ladders and pulling them up afterwards. Yet, the nursing profession remains dominated by the largely White, nearly exclusively female groups that have been most successful in hospital-based settings with physician-led hierarchies. The report should be more self-aware and self-critical of nursing's professional blinders, including an acknowledgment and promise that the National Academies' repeated, well-funded attention to the future of nursing is intended to be inclusive of rather than competitive with other health professions. The report should also be more attentive to recommendations affecting the basic RN nursing workforce, which was relatively neglected in FON-1 compared with advanced practice; to the various aspects of professional diversity that follow from generational change; and to the important roles played by nursing aides, community health workers, and others who may not be fully qualified nurses but who are key contributors to health equity and community health.
4. *Fulfilling the promise of nursing means speaking truth to the medical establishment and making it acknowledge an ethical obligation to reform professional hierarchies.* The laws and norms that constrain nurses' ability to practice to the full extent of their skills and training were put

in place by physicians to protect their privileges, independence, and income. As the COVID-19 pandemic recedes, retrogressive lobbying campaigns by organized medicine have already resurfaced, aimed at rolling back improvements in nursing practice authority that were long overdue and that the report, admirably, speaks out to defend. Such outdated, unwarranted restrictions often apply not only to advanced practice nurses but also to other nurses and health professionals, and they include the payment policies that continue to fill health industry coffers primarily from orders, prescriptions, and referrals that originate with the physician's pen. The report should be more demanding and explicit about examining these pathways and providing nursing with a meaningful voice and greater parity with physicians in performing professional self-regulatory functions, whether adding a nursing organization to corporate membership in The Joint Commission or revisiting the American Medical Association's monopoly on clinical coding and its Medicare payment advisory structure (the "RUC"), which favors specialized physician services and retards progress on community health and health equity.

5. *Racism and discrimination affecting health are ubiquitous, often not vestigial, and not always unintentional.* The COVID-19 pandemic and the protests over racism in law enforcement synergized to raise public awareness of pervasive discrimination in today's America. Inequities associated with race have been evident in the heightened vulnerability to disease within communities of color, in the comorbidities originating in social determinants that increased COVID-19 mortality among those infected, and in the tiering of hospitals by wealth and demographics with respect to accessing personal protective equipment and other critical resources. Although health disparities based on race are well documented in the report, the purposefulness of discrimination is often obscured by the detached tone in which scientific research is presented. In my view, the report also underplays racism in formulating its recommendations, especially concerning nursing practice.
6. *Because disease tracks injustice, social advocacy is an essential element of nursing ethics.* With few exceptions, ethical advocacy by the health professions has observed a line between the medical and the social, focusing mainly on issues of health insurance, treatment relationships, and biomedical technology. A major lesson of the social determinants literature, further validated by the COVID-19 experience, is that the most meaningful health laws are those that increase and equalize wealth and power and education and opportunity, not those limited to medical care. Nurses (and physicians) therefore must change lanes in their ethical causes and advocacy strategies, which they seldom have the knowledge, training, or independence to do effectively. The report is not sufficiently

explicit about nurses' affirmative commitments to advocacy or about how to protect nurses who advocate from retaliation or discipline, nor does the report acknowledge that in a profession as large and diverse as nursing, a range of views and positions will be sincerely held and entitled to respect and discussion.

7. *Hospitals have special obligations to accelerate improvement in health equity through nursing.* America's hospital sector remains the greatest beneficiary of health care spending and the largest employer of nurses. Although the report invokes health equity as the primary objective for nursing over the coming decade, hospitals are barely acknowledged and almost never directly advised. Hospitals possess the capital, organization, and position within communities to play a leadership role in advancing health equity. Whether hospitals embrace that responsibility, or instead sit on the sidelines or even oppose necessary change, is far from certain. Some hospitals consider themselves primarily community institutions, while others function more as giant revenue-generating businesses, research powerhouses, or workshops for private physicians. A fundamental shift is required in how hospital management perceives nurses, and in how those perceptions are translated into strategic planning, budgeting, and operations. The report should be much clearer about incorporating health equity into hospitals' core clinical functions; about expanding leadership roles for nurses in forward-looking domains, such as informatics and community engagement; and about committing hospitals to respect and empower their nursing workforce while ensuring nurses' well-being and building their resilience.

Although I value my participation on this committee and have learned much from my colleagues, I feel personally obliged to offer these frank observations and the priorities for action that they convey. The massive health-related and social and economic upheavals consequent to COVID-19, the trepidation associated with nascent and impending climate crises, and the rapidity of technologic and generational change make this a teachable moment for the nursing profession and for the nation. The top-line message of this report should be more than that the National Academies agrees on the importance of health equity to nursing policy; it should be that the National Academies calls for action. The late Supreme Court Justice Ruth Bader Ginsburg, whose former faculty office at Columbia Law School I once had the privilege to call my own, wrote that "real change, enduring change, happens one step at a time." In my view, this report should do more to illuminate the path. It should see clearly, think deeply, lead, and inspire. It should help bend the arc of nursing, of health care, and of health toward justice.

Appendix F

Committee Response to Supplemental Statement

The committee has carefully considered Dr. Sage's supplemental statement (see Appendix E) and believes the report's findings and conclusions that form the basis for its recommendations are consistent with the evidence at hand. The Statement of Task for this consensus study on The Future of Nursing 2020–2030 directed the committee to chart a path for the nursing profession to help the nation create a culture of health, reduce health disparities, and improve the health and well-being of the U.S. population in the 21st century. The committee believes that an ambitious call for action associated with each component of the Statement of Task for this study is robustly addressed within the report and its recommendations even as the report content is guided by the standards for evidence-based recommendations of the National Academies of Sciences, Engineering, and Medicine. This report adheres to those requirements to present recommendations that are supported by evidence. The committee is not permitted to advance an advocacy agenda.

The committee members all agree that the report should illuminate a path for nursing that, if executed, would substantively address the serious issues of inequities in the nation that are clearly shown to adversely impact health status. Through its extensive exploration of issues and formulation of a set of recommendations that invites broad and deep engagement across multiple stakeholders, the committee believes it has developed a report that substantively addresses issues of inequities associated with health disparities. Committed to the National Academies' requirements to ground all conclusions and recommendations in sound science, the committee has directed nine action-oriented recommendations to specific actors with a specific timeline. Dr. Sage's recommendation that the committee formulate strong hypotheses for the post-COVID era is beyond the scope of the committee's Statement of Task and while interesting, would be inappropriate for this report. The remainder of this response by the committee addresses some of the specific points Dr. Sage makes in his supplemental statement.

NURSING'S ROLE IN DISASTER PREPAREDNESS

Dr. Sage states that the report does not focus sufficiently on nursing in the post-COVID period. We disagree strongly with this view. The committee has offered two recommendations related specifically to COVID-19 and future emergencies (see Recommendations 3 and 8 in Chapter 11) and devoted two chapters to the topic of disaster preparedness/public health emergencies and the well-being of the nursing workforce (see Chapters 8 and 10, respectively). Specifically, the committee has called out moral distress, stating: "Nurses in all roles and settings are confronted with ethical challenges that have the potential to cause moral suffering (ANA Code of Ethics, 2015), including moral distress or moral injury (Rushton, 2018). When nurses are unable to convert their moral choices into action because of internal or external constraints, moral distress ensues and threatens their integrity (Ulrich and Grady, 2018)." Conclusion 10-1 in Chapter 10 states: "All environments in which nurses work affect the health and well-being of the nursing workforce. Ultimately, the health and well-being of nurses influence the quality, safety, and cost of the care they provide, as well as organizations and systems of care. The COVID-19 crisis has highlighted the shortcomings of historical efforts to address nurses' health and well-being." Inclusion of further material regarding nursing in the post-COVID era would clearly be beyond the scope of this study and run the risk of creating an imbalance that would diminish the importance of the many other issues at the core of the committee's charge.

PROGRESS SINCE THE 2011 *THE FUTURE OF NURSING* REPORT

Dr. Sage states that the report's response to the lack of progress in some areas over the past decade is inadequate. We reject this view; the report emphasizes the need for additional progress throughout. The report addresses the important but insufficient progress in nurses achieving greater parity with physicians through an expanded scope of practice for advanced practice nurses that was recommended in the 2011 report, and includes a recommendation reiterating the need to continue this work. Recommendation 4 states: "All organizations, including state and federal entities and employing organizations, that prevent nurses from practicing to the full extent of their education and training by imposing regulatory barriers; public and private payment limitations; restrictive policies and practices within health care, public health, and other community-based organizations; and other legal, professional, and commercial impediments should remove those barriers so that nurses can fully address social needs and social determinants of health and improve health care access, quality, and value."

Most important, this report expands on the work identified in the 2011 report as needed to increase the diversity of the nursing workforce. (See, for instance, Conclusion 3-3 in Chapter 3: "As the nation's population becomes more diverse, sustaining efforts to diversify the racial, ethnic, and gender composition of the nursing workforce will be important.") The committee explicitly addresses racism, social determinants of health, and health equity throughout the report. Building on the need to expand diversity, this report describes the racism that is embedded in nursing education and practice and calls for nurses to address their own biases and address structural racism. The report also identifies opportunities to deploy more fully the expertise of baccalaureate and other nurses in a wide array of settings. And the report advances a set of recommendations that, if implemented, will align resources and attention to address contemporary and emerging challenges facing both the profession and the U.S. population—fully commensurate with the scope of this study.

ALIGNMENT ACROSS NURSING

We also emphatically disagree with Dr. Sage's remarks regarding the committee's treatment of opportunities for increased alignment across nursing organizations. The report's first recommendation focuses explicitly on the alignment of expertise and other resources within nursing profession associations and organizations, and this and other recommendations reflect the opportunity for partnerships with other professions and groups. Regarding the lack of sufficient recognition of the value of nursing, the report states that there must be direct public funding for both school nursing and public health. The two chapters that address this need are Chapter 4, "The Role of Nurses in Improving Health Care Access and Quality," and Chapter 5, "The Role of Nurses in Improving Health Equity." The committee also calls for workforce expansion (see Chapter 3) and adequate financing of the nursing workforce (see Chapter 6). In particular, the committee notes a number of ways in which public health nursing and school nursing can be bolstered in an effort to lead health equity efforts.

Taken together, the committee believes that this report and its recommendations, if implemented, will have far-reaching and meaningful impact on the education and practice of nurses at every level and specialty. Dr. Sage said that the goal of the report should be to make a compelling case for action and advocacy. The committee believes that a careful reading of the report will reveal that this has in fact been accomplished within the evidence-based tradition of the National Academies.

Appendix G

Profiles of Nursing Programs and Organizations

Appendix G is only available online at https://www.nap.edu/catalog/25982.